Esther Urdang, PhD

Human Behavior in the Social Environment
Interweaving the Inner and Outer Worlds

Pre-publication REVIEWS, COMMENTARIES, EVALUATIONS . . .

"This book will serve as a superb introduction to human behavior, normal and pathologic, not only for graduate social work students, but also for anyone who is curious about the vicissitudes of the human condition. The students who use this book will be lucky, indeed.

Dr. Urdang has produced a splendid book that encompasses an enormous body of knowledge about the human condition in a most readable manner. The integration of clinical material and theory is particularly outstanding, as are the chapters on development throughout the life cycle."

Calvin A. Colarusso, MD
*Clinical Professor of Psychiatry,
University of California at San Diego;
Training and Supervising Analyst,
Adult and Child Psychoanalysis,
San Diego Psychoanalytic Institute*

"Urdang has provided us with a text that is usable with first-year master's students and that draws heavily on psychodynamic theory—something that has been sorely needed for many years.

Using a constructivist framework for integrating a variety of theoretical perspectives, including ego psychology, self psychology, object relations, systems theory, and cognitive-behavioral theory, Urdang's book uses language that is accessible for the beginner without becoming simplistic. Numerous case illustrations help the reader understand the relevance of the theories presented.

Perhaps most important, Urdang's book integrates perspectives on culture, diversity, poverty, and oppression into her psychodynamic approach, thereby avoiding a split between inner and outer worlds."

Carolyn Saari, PhD
*Professor,
School of Social Work,
Loyola University, Chicago*

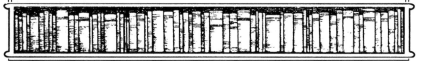

More pre-publication
REVIEWS, COMMENTARIES, EVALUATIONS . . .

"**B**uilding on her extensive experiences as a practitioner, consultant, and teacher, Esther Urdang offers an exciting and comprehensive text on human behavior and the social environment. Particularly noteworthy are her emphasis on a psychodynamic approach within a biopsychosocial perspective; clear presentation of ideas and theories; imaginative use of practice examples; and inclusion of illustrative materials from philosophers, historians, and poets.

The text is most appropriate for graduate social work students in the required initial course in the human behavior and social environment sequence. It will also interest beginning and advanced practitioners in the field of human services. Readers will be inspired to help their clients in confronting life challenges in a dynamic and growth-producing manner."

Anthony N. Maluccio, DSW
Professor, Boston College
Graduate School of Social Work

The Haworth Social Work Practice Press
An Imprint of The Haworth Press, Inc.
New York • London • Oxford

Human Behavior
in the Social Environment
Interweaving the Inner and Outer Worlds

Human Behavior in the Social Environment
Interweaving the Inner and Outer Worlds

Esther Urdang, PhD

The Haworth Social Work Practice Press
An Imprint of The Haworth Press, Inc.
New York • London • Oxford

Published by

The Haworth Social Work Practice Press, an imprint of The Haworth Press, Inc., 10 Alice Street, Binghamton, NY 13904-1580.

All particulars relating to case material that are in any way distinctive of those involved have been sufficiently altered to render such persons unidentifiable.

Cover design by Marylouise E. Doyle.

Library of Congress Cataloging-in-Publication Data

Urdang, Esther.
    Human behavior in the social environment : interweaving the inner and outer worlds / Esther Urdang.
        p.   cm.
    Includes bibliographical references and index.
    ISBN 0-7890-0716-9 (alk. paper)—ISBN 0-7890-1522-6 (alk. paper)
    1. Social psychology. 2. Developmental psychology. 3. Human behavior. I. Title.

HM1033 .U73 2002
302—dc21

2001024391

To my parents

Rose Klepper
1909-1999

and

Mendel Klepper, MD

ABOUT THE AUTHOR

Dr. Urdang brings to the writing of this book a strong background as a clinician, supervisor, and social work educator. She received her master's degree in social work at Adelphi University and her PhD in social work from Simmons College School of Social Work. She has practiced in a variety of settings including mental health clinics, family agencies, and hospitals. Dr. Urdang was on the faculty of the Boston College Graduate School of Social Work for 27 years, where she taught human behavior—the required clinical courses and psychopathology—as Adjunct Associate Professor. She was actively involved in the Field Education Department, serving as Assistant Director of Field Education, did extensive faculty advising, and developed and taught the Seminar for Field Instructors.

Dr. Urdang's published articles have centered on social work education, chiefly focusing on the processes of student learning and the development of the professional self, and have been published in journals including *The Clinical Supervisor, Smith College Studies in Social Work, Clinical Social Work Journal, Journal of Teaching in Social Work,* and *Social Casework.* One journal article, discussing the use of a video lab, received the Simmons Alumni Special Recognition Award in 1999.

Currently, Dr. Urdang is involved in writing, in a private clinical practice, and in providing supervision and consultation. She was a research advisor to the Smith College School of Social Work from 1998 to 2001.

CONTENTS

Preface

This book is intended for graduate social work students, although all readers, beginning and advanced in the field of human services, may find this a helpful review or source of new knowledge.

This text is intended to accompany the one-semester course of the Human Behavior Sequence, focusing on maturation through the life cycle, psychological development, and family life. Physical illness and disability are also addressed, as our biological makeup and infirmities affect our well-being and social functioning. Many people today live long lives with major disabilities and illnesses; we must be sensitive to their needs and aspirations. Loss, which permeates the life cycle, is often a key dynamic in psychosocial problems and is stressed here, as this painful subject is frequently avoided by clients, students, and clinicians.

Many mental states, such as anxiety, depression, dissociative experiences, and psychosomatic involvement, are part of the human condition. When sufficiently intense they may impair functioning, in which case we regard them as pathological. Because we think of these states along a continuum, psychopathology is included here—rather than excluded as it often is from human behavior courses—because it is viewed as a content area separate from "normal" behavior. Furthermore, people with severe mental illness are encountered in social work practice in many different contexts; they face the same life-cycle dilemmas as those judged to be "mentally healthy." Excluding them from a human behavior text would mirror the exclusion they often experience in society.

Although diversity, race, culture, and systemic issues, such as housing, social discrimination, violence, social policies, politics, and organizations, are included and integrated into the text, they are not extensively addressed; it is assumed these subjects will receive major attention in a second-semester course.

Although this is not a text on clinical practice, special attention is given to problems students often encounter in practice, and many case illustrations are presented with relevant theory discussed. This is based on the conviction that a firm foundation in human behavior provides the underpinning for a sound perspective when contending with human problems.

In writing this text, I have drawn upon my vivid experiences as a social work educator for twenty-seven years, teaching human behavior and clinical social work, advising students, and serving as Assistant Director of Field

Education at Boston College Graduate School of Social Work. I have also drawn upon my ongoing involvement in clinical practice.

These experiences have involved me in an active way with the puzzles, conundrums, and rewards of clinical work and have sensitized me to students' struggles in mastering the intellectual and emotional demands of social work training. In sharing my insights, I have highlighted problems that are particularly troublesome for students in the field, such as the feelings of incompetence often aroused by clients who have a history of rejecting and distorted relationships.

Of course, some social work students do not plan to enter direct clinical practice but rather to become involved in administration, research, or social planning. Nevertheless, the emphasis on clinical work in this text is intended to provide *all* future social workers with the core understanding of individual and family functioning, which is indispensable in both clinical and policy work.

For example, whether working with foster children directly, administering child-welfare agencies, or developing related policy at the governmental level, social workers who lack an in-depth understanding of the intense emotional impact of attachment, separation, loss, and maltreatment will be unable either to offer adequate clinical help or to design adequate social services and policies for this vulnerable population.

A biopsychosocial perspective is emphasized throughout this book. Although this has been the traditional foundation of social work, its psychodynamically based psychological component has gradually been depreciated. It has been displaced by an emphasis on cognitive-behavioral approaches, quantitative research-based outcome measures, and brief solution-focused treatments currently designed to meet the requirements of managed care.

In addition, the field has moved toward emphasizing the amelioration of social problems, with reliance on educational approaches for vulnerable populations and the promotion of social policy at the expense of the development of clinical social work. This book, while recognizing the importance of the outer social world, highlights the significance of the *inner world* of people, which shapes their sense of self-worth as well as their relationships and behaviors. Emphasis is therefore given to a psychodynamic perspective incorporating psychoanalytic, ego psychology, object relations, and self psychology theories within a developmental framework.

As the title of this book suggests, when viewed comprehensively life is characterized by a constant interweaving of inner and outer worlds; this is the perspective I wish to present. Accepting psychodynamic theory does not mean turning our backs on the "real" world with its troubling problems and inequities. Homelessness is a serious social problem requiring economic solutions and new housing policies. But we also need to understand and help homeless individuals, many of whom have deep underlying emotional problems, such as depression (leading to unemployment) and major mental illness (often untreated in today's climate of deinstitutionalization). We need to understand the homeless teenager, the "throwaway" child who has run away from abuse and neglect often as a result of and resulting in psychological traumatization and conflict that must be addressed.

Human behavior in the social environment is more than a subject for a textbook. It is the interwoven fabric of the world around us and the world within us. Although it is the subject matter of psychology and sociology, it has also been of profound concern to philosophers, historians, writers, and poets throughout the ages. To reflect this, I have incorporated materials from biographies, literature, and newspapers to enrich your understanding. As we begin this journey of learning together, I hope it will be with open eyes, inquisitive minds, and compassionate hearts that can see beneath surface explanations and superficial solutions.

Acknowledgments

This book is written for social work students and is based on my work with many students over the years who have been a constant source of stimulation and learning. I thank them for contributing to my own development and for the inspiration working with them has provided me in writing this book. My special thanks are also extended to those unnamed students who have given me their papers discussing their work with clients, adding greatly to the depth of this presentation.

Warmest thanks are extended to my husband, Elliott B. Urdang, MD, who has been a constant source of support and encouragement as well as an active participant in this project in terms of vital editorial and technical assistance.

Carolyn Thomas, PhD, Professor Emeritus at Boston College Graduate School of Social Work, has provided editorial advice as well as great ongoing support.

The unending moral support of my children, Erik and Gwen, their respective spouses, Nan and Jerry, and my dear grandchildren is deeply appreciated.

During the writing of this book, I have supervised four outstanding social workers from the Groden Center, a facility that specializes in work with autistic and other developmentally disabled children and has a specialized foster home unit. Bill Carey, Susan Garland, Maria Mishkind, and Michael Pendergast have shared their work with me, and our discussions were continually a source of stimulation. They have also contributed thoughts and editorial comments about the book, which are highly appreciated.

SECTION I:
THE BIOPSYCHOSOCIAL PERSPECTIVE

Chapter 1

Overview

For every complex problem, there is a solution that is simple, neat, and wrong.

H. L. Mencken

INTRODUCTION

Human behavior is extraordinarily varied and complex. The unexpected behaviors of others often astound us, and, on occasion, we find ourselves bewildered by our own actions. We like to think of ourselves as logical and entirely in control of our lives. However, the directions we sometimes take, the people we marry (and perhaps divorce), and the dreams we follow may be dictated by strong emotional forces that do not necessarily flow from logic and may not even be entirely in our conscious awareness. As we pursue our dreams and desires, we do so within the social context of our lives, the constitutional makeup of our physical being, and the physical environment surrounding us, which also may decisively influence our destinies.

This book examines such complex questions as: Why do foster children placed in "good" homes run away and return to abusive parents? Why do people "who should know better" repeatedly reenter self-destructive relationships? Why does an intelligent, well-functioning person in a stable family situation plunge the family into serious debt through persistent and chronic gambling?

As we observe people in the former Yugoslavia who once lived peacefully as neighbors now ruthlessly massacre one another, we wonder about the intensity of the ethnic and political forces which have swept away reason. As we look at our own country, how did we become the "most violent country in the industrialized world, with violence having reached epidemic proportions as we approach[ed] the end of the 20th century" (Osofsky, 1997, p. 3)? How do we explain the paradox of being a child-centered society while, at the same time, "the social record of America is clouded by steep declines in the quality of life for children in the 1980s and 1990s" (Fraser, 1997, p. 1)?

3

The biological world also affects and can determine our destinies. Throughout history, epidemics—such as the bubonic plague during the Middle Ages, the influenza epidemic after World War I, and now AIDS (acquired immunodeficiency syndrome)—have taken countless lives and wreaked havoc among the survivors. We watch helplessly as powerful manifestations of the physical environment, such as hurricanes, tornadoes, and volcanic eruptions, assert destructive power over individual lives as well as the fabric of whole communities and sometimes entire countries.

For centuries, comets, a celestial manifestation of the physical environment, have had a disturbing influence on people. "Whenever the predictable clockwork of the heavens has been jarred by a comet hurtling unexpectedly through the sky, people throughout the ages have feared that unthinkable horrors would inevitably follow" (Johnson, 1997, p. A9). This country reacted with disbelief and puzzlement when thirty-nine members of the Heaven's Gate cult in Southern California took their own lives as the Hale-Bopp comet crossed the sky. How did the convergence of the comet's flight, the members' life courses, adherence to a rigid cult culture, and the faith that an extraterrestrial spaceship awaited them lead to this organized and communal suicide?

When observing people over the trajectory of their lives, other paradoxes and puzzles emerge. Why do some people, with average expectable environments as children, seem unable to function as adults? On the other hand, how do some, wounded in childhood, evolve into creative and productive individuals? Let us consider the development of three young girls, who, having lost their mother at an early age, were raised by a rigid maiden aunt and an often-aloof father. As children they lost two older sisters and later saw their only brother become addicted to drugs and alcohol. They grew up socially alienated from others in their small village. It would not surprise us to learn that they struggled with depressive feelings during their lives. But how can we explain their creative genius and fame as the Brontë sisters?

How did a slave, who never knew who his father was and who was separated at an early age from his mother, somehow martial his strengths and become a famous abolitionist and orator known to the world as Frederick Douglass?

Why do "ghosts" from the past haunt some parents, inhibiting them in their ability to love, whereas other parents are free from these "ghosts" (Fraiberg et al., 1975)? Ordinarily, we consider babies a source of great joy. Relatives and friends can have an evening's entertainment watching a baby begin to crawl or start to babble. The cooing baby with its foot in its mouth demonstrates a love of life and a pleasure of being in the world. This love of being is infectious; emotionally tuned-in adults can also feel happiness radiating from a child. It is perhaps one of the greatest tragedies in life that some adults cannot feel this happiness and are frozen in their response to their babies.

The actions and attitudes of human beings in their world are replete with conundrums and enigmas. Well-known female writer Jan Morris was born biologically a male and lived as a male for many years, marrying and having children. But since the age of four she felt that she was a female, rather than a male; this secret tormented her for many years. She concluded that the only way to achieve inner peace was to realize her true identity: to transform "himself" into "herself," to physically change identity, which was accomplished through medical and surgical treatment. In her beautifully written book *Conundrum* (1997), she describes both her conflict and transformation. This book, which paints a poignant picture of Jan Morris and her life, ends on a note of uncertainty.

> My loves remain the same loves. . . . Have I discovered . . . the real purpose of my pilgrimage, the last solution to my Conundrum . . .? Sometimes down by the river I almost think I have: but then the light changes, the wind shifts . . . and the meaning of it all once again escapes me. (p. 160)

Such uncertainties often lead students to despair of ever grasping the complexities involved in case situations and to flee toward certainty, simplicity, and solutions. After many years as both a practitioner and teacher of clinical social work, I remain a student of human behavior, still puzzling over the conundrums and enigmas of life. I invite you to share this search for understanding with me, as we contemplate the human condition, the social environments in which people live, and the dynamic interplay of psychological, physical, and social forces in life.

This book is written in the spirit of Winnicott, who values "ambiguity, openness and creativity" in his search for understanding (Grolnick, 1990, p. 188).

GOALS OF THIS BOOK

This book is intended for only *one semester* of the basic Human Behavior in the Social Environment course, which focuses on individual development and the life cycle. It is my assumption that a second course will focus on systems, organizations, and culture and will use a different text, covering these issues more deeply. It is written for the master's-level social work student, although undergraduate students may find it helpful. It may also prove useful for practitioners wishing to review and resynthesize their knowledge about human behavior. Those practitioners who have not been exposed to psychodynamic thinking in their training may find these ideas serve as an orientation to further study.

Although this book utilizes a clinical perspective, it is not intended only for clinical students. Those specializing in policy, administration, or community organization also need a firm foundation in human behavior to be able to design policies and programs that meet human needs and analyze the consequences of policy decisions more fully. If one understands, for example, the depth of attachment and loss issues, one is in a better position to understand not only the need for family preservation programs and sound adoptive programs, but also the complexities in getting them to work. Understanding human motivations and biopsychosocial features in human existence requires considerable knowledge, sensitivity, and skill.

Clinical students must acquire a systemic perspective so that they can appreciate how sound programs and policies can affect the quality of their clients' lives and help them adapt to difficult situations. They should understand the significance of and need for special projects that can dramatically impact social and emotional problems, such as those facing grandparents who have custodial responsibility for their grandchildren. One such program is the GrandFamilies House, which was recently established in Boston. This is the "first housing development in the nation to cater to one of the fastest growing family groups, older adults raising their children's children" (Dowdy, 1998, p. B1).

It is indeed a daunting task to write a book about human nature and the social world, because no boundaries exist to this assignment. Where does one begin, and what does one include? Endless theories and perspectives exist. Each person has his or her own story, each culture has its own intricacies, and the interactions of people can take infinite forms. In attempting to resolve this conundrum, I have drawn from my many years of experience as both a clinical social work practitioner and a social work educator. Doing so has helped me form the book's goal: to impart to social work practitioners the basic knowledge to provide a firm beginning foundation for practice and for developing a professional self.

I have elected to emphasize a *psychodynamic* approach within a *biopsychosocial* perspective because I believe this provides the deepest understanding of people and their relationships to the world around them. It is not possible within the scope of this book to give equal time to all theories or even to give total coverage to those theories I am discussing. Two basic considerations have determined my choices: (1) presentation of ideas and theories that students can directly relate to practice issues, and (2) the need to present sufficient theoretical background so that students will be able to understand their conceptual context.

To bring human behavior theories to life, case vignettes taken from clinical practice are included. Occasionally constructed case examples will be presented, representing a composite mosaic of clients and problems. Excerpts from novels, biographies, and autobiographies have also been included. Readers may gain insights from the reflectiveness and sensitivities of writers to their own inner worlds as well as to their social and political worlds. Goldstein (1990) values the humanities, through which "we discover that our own and our clients' triumphs and struggles have been played out in a multitude of ways in an effort to make sense of living and find meaning within it" (p. 41). Resonating with the spirit of this book, the humanities, he adds, "do not profess to offer answers; rather, they encourage the kind of disciplined questioning and reflection that are fundamental to what effective practice may be" (Goldstein, 1990, p. 41).

References to newspaper and magazine articles are also included in this book. They have much to say about human nature, social and political issues, systemic processes, and competing values and conflicts. Knowledge about human behavior and the social environment exists only in a limited form in textbooks. New knowledge, along with companion conundrums, come into being every day. Even old knowledge, looked at with fresh eyes, can offer new insights. Our clients, educated and uneducated, young and old, well or disabled, have much to tell us about the riddle we call life. A psychodynamic perspective instructs us how to ask them to become our teachers, to share with us their own discoveries as well as their perplexities about the meanings of their lives. Psychodynamic exploration also provides us with the opportunity to look beneath surface adaptations to life and to understand subjective inner worlds.

This text aims to suggest ways of looking at the world around us, the world within us, and the world between us and to suggest ways of listening, observing, understanding, and inquiring that will lead to an ongoing search for and discovery of meanings and answers.

STRUCTURE OF THE BOOK

This book is divided into four major sections. The first section discusses the major theoretical orientations; the second, human development and behavior over the life span; and the third, special issues. The final section integrates the major points in the book.

Each chapter includes suggested readings so that readers can expand their understanding of the materials presented and explore relevant new areas. Chapters also incorporate suggested learning exercises, which are intended as vehicles for students to become involved with the materials and to do their own research concerning people and the world around them.

Section I. The Biopsychosocial Perspective

This section includes seven chapters, six of which discuss the main perspectives as outlined in the Overview.

1. Overview
2. Psychoanalytic and Ego Psychology Theories
3. Object Relations, Self Psychology, and Cognitive-Behavioral Theories
4. Social Systems and the Community
5. Culture and Diversity
6. The Family: Forms and Organization
7. The Family: Internal Structures and Special Family Problems

Section II. The Life Cycle

The second section of the book presents a picture of the life cycle from conception through old age. Biological, social, cultural, and familial factors are interwoven into this discussion. Emphasis is given to issues of attachment and loss, separation/individuation, violence, resilience, and creativity as they pertain to people at different life stages. This section includes the following three chapters:

8. Reproductive Issues, Infancy, and Early Childhood Development
9. Middle Childhood and Adolescence
10. Adult Development

Section III. Special Issues

In this section, special issues discussed in this overview chapter are presented. The three chapters under this section include:

11. Life Transitions, Crises, and Loss
12. Illness and Disability
13. Mental Health Problems

Section IV. Integration

In this final section, the perspectives discussed in this book are summarized and integrated.

14. Conclusion

THEORETICAL PERSPECTIVES

Psychodynamic Theory

A psychodynamic stance within a systemic and ecological framework has been chosen for this book, as this approach will provide readers with a sound and comprehensive *foundation* for exploring the human condition. A psychodynamic approach, in this case, will provide the best *tools* for exploration, listening, and understanding.

Critics of psychodynamic thinking seem oblivious to the rich tapestry of thought this paradigm encompasses, often criticizing this theoretical framework as though it were limited to early Freudian thinking centered on drive theory. Today, it in fact encompasses divergent and rich schools of thought, including ego psychology, object relations, and self psychology. Constructivism argues that all theories (including the ones discussed here) are created by people, who impart their own meanings and values to the theories they construct. A constructivist perspective compels us to look at our theoretical perspectives in a relativistic manner and to examine both the client's and our own belief systems within a cultural and social context.

To emphasize psychodynamic understanding does not imply an exclusive reliance on psychodynamic treatment modalities nor on long-term treatment models, nor does it mean that other theoretical orientations, such as learning theory, family dynamics, or group approaches, should be ignored. These frameworks as well as systemic and ecological theories are incorporated into this book. Biological factors, such as genetics, physical growth and maturation, sexuality, and psychosomatic issues, are also discussed. As it is not possible to understand people fully without knowing their cultural context, this perspective will be interwoven throughout. This approach parallels that of Woods and Hollis (1990): *"In our psychosocial approach, ecological systems and psychodynamic perspectives have become inseparable"* (p. 9).

We would agree with the statement by Berzoff and colleagues (1996) that insights afforded by a psychodynamic approach are not only valuable in diagnostic assessments and long-term psychotherapy but also when "one is making a hospital discharge plan or completing a housing application. Clinical knowledge grounded in psychodynamic theory is one of the most powerful ways we have to look inside someone's heart and mind. Without it, we are almost blind, limited to the surface" (pp. 5-6).

Psychoanalytic Theory

We reexamine aspects of Freudian theory and glean from it insights that continue to have relevance. Many social workers and others in the mental health field are intensely antagonistic to Freudian thinking, based on political, philosophical, and empirical research issues and possibly because we all seem to prefer to view ourselves as entirely free of inexplicable motivations. Freud's views on women and homosexuality are seen by some as prejudicial; his emphasis on drive theory is considered outmoded; his lack of quantitative research has led others to dismiss his work as unsubstantiated. However, we are discarding an invaluable legacy if we ignore contributions that shed light on the buried mysteries of the mind.

In his review of Jonathan Lear's book *Open Minded: Working Out the Logic of the Soul,* Edmundson (1998) asserts that Lear holds that "democracy needs Freud," because "without him . . . people will go around thinking they are acting rationally . . . all men and women should comprehend their proclivities for destructiveness and self-idealization in order to make the best-informed choices" (p. 10). Freud also taught clinicians the importance of listening to themselves, in the service of awareness of their own attitudes which may distort their perceptions of and responses to clients. This self-awareness can often be a difficult and disturbing process. More recently it has been discovered that "listening to ourselves" can be a useful guide for picking up clues regarding clients.

Learning how to listen to clients, to understand the world as they perceive and experience it, rather than assuming we know just what they mean is one of the contributions to our profession coming from psychoanalysis. Freud learned to listen intently to each patient. A lasting legacy has been the manner in which Freud "listened, heard, and understood his patients" (Edward, 1996, p. 23). His "respectful attitude . . . expressed through his communicative approach continue to influence analytically and many non-analytically oriented therapists today, irrespective of . . . their theoretical outlooks" (Edward, 1996, p. 23).

A psychodynamic approach can also help us to understand internalized psychological conflict, in which a person is "at war" with himself or herself. A struggle might ensue between the person's wishes and instinctual life (such as sexual feelings), as opposed to his or her conscience (or superego) with its self-prohibitions (e.g., against sexual activity). Even in our relatively sexually permissive society people often struggle with these conflicts, as we demonstrate in our case illustration at the end of the chapter. *Superego guilt,* a concept introduced by Freud, was much earlier described by Shakespeare, who created Hamlet, a character brooding with guilt.

Lewis Carroll, author of *Alice in Wonderland,* a man of imagination and wit, has puzzled his biographers as aspects of his psychological self remain hidden. Cohen (1996) discusses the continual *internal conflicts* (and superego guilt) he believed Carroll experienced in relation to his attraction to prepubescent girls.

Beneath the bubbles and the froth lived yet another force, however, a brooding guilt. . . . He was a good practicing Christian, but he nevertheless saw himself as a repeated sinner. Stern Victorian that he was, he could never give voice or employ pen and ink to record the nature of his sins, but the painful appeals to God for forgiveness that he confided to his diary reveal a man in spiritual pain for transgressions that surely go beyond ordinary failings like idleness or indolence. Lewis Carroll's strong and virile imagination must also have bred sexual fantasies. His dreams probably reached out beyond what he considered accepted terrain and ventured into dangerous precincts. A severe disciplinarian, he never transgressed propriety or violated innocence. He was . . . superhuman, in today's terms, in controlling his impulses during waking hours. But the nights brought troubled thoughts for which he saw himself a miscreant. (p. xxi)

The development of *affect* and the transmission of affect to others are also of special interest to the psychodynamic social worker. Psychodynamic theorists recognize the power and significance of feelings in people: the *motivating* force of affects; the importance of recognizing and expressing feelings; the ability to modulate and keep feelings under control. "It is the nature and intensity of the affect generated by or in connection with a particular event that determines one's behavioral reaction: *affect is the gateway to action*" (italics added) (Basch, 1988, p. 65).

A psychodynamic frame of reference also enables us to understand how the past can still live in the present, providing another tool for further understanding. Some social workers, as well as other mental health professionals, consider a person's past irrelevant and prefer to deal only with the here and now. Moultrup (1981) questions this stance, for inasmuch as "each moment passes into the past instantly, it would seem to be logically impossible to deal strictly with the 'present' " (p. 120). He adds that although the objective past is significant, so also is "that which might have been, i.e., fantasy, hopes, etc., . . . they are a part of an individual's or family's experience" (p. 120). Some cultures place emphasis on the past. Believers in Confucianism, Buddhism, and Taoism have "reverence for the family's past and its ancestors . . . [which] provides a strong sense of continuity and obligation" (Germain, 1991, p. 111).

People experiencing trauma in their *adult past* may find it affects the rest of their lives. In fact, trauma in the life of parents can be *transmitted* to their children, who are growing up in an otherwise trauma-free environment. Anxiety experienced by Holocaust survivors, for example, can be experienced by their children who never experienced the Holocaust and who may not even understand the source of this feeling. There are "intergenerational patterns . . . *common everyday patterns* through which anxiety and silence are transmitted"; although the parents may be silent, this does not impede the transmission of anxiety. "Unexplained silences further intensify the affective, fearful power of children's fantasies" (Brown, 1998, p. 270).

Attention has been focused in recent years on the issue of violence in the United States. Glodich describes the situation as an epidemic, directly or indirectly threatening the youth population in particular (Glodich, 1998). One of the behaviors observed in children who have experienced trauma is the reenactment, in various forms, of the traumatic experience. Glodich (1998) finds Freud's concept of the *repetition compulsion* to be an important concept to utilize in working with this population. Glodich notes that Freud observed patients exhibiting compulsive repetition of threatening or alarming actions to achieve mastery. Such mastery often implies a reversal of the passive role of the victim in the traumatizing situation to an active role of victimizer or provoker of further victimization in scenarios reminiscent of the original trauma.

Glodich (1998) cites Freud's statement that a person " 'reproduces it [the trauma] not as a memory but as an action; he repeats it, without knowing, of course, that he is repeating, and in the end, we understand that this is his way of remembering' " (p. 336). Glodich finds this concept to be an extremely useful one in understanding reenactments by children and adolescents.

Freud's important legacies have naturally been both further developed and criticized by later theorists. Many reject his emphasis on the primacy of the drives, or instinctual life, without giving due weight to issues of attachment, relationship, and the impact of the external world on human development. Others partially or fully accept Freud's emphasis but at the same time redress it by giving much greater theoretical weight to issues on which he did not focus. In the following section, advances and additions that were made to psychodynamic theory are discussed.

Ego Psychology

An important component of personality is the ego, that portion of personality structure which, in Freud's basic conceptualization, mediates between the id (the unconscious contents of the mind, especially those linked with instinctual forces or drives) and the superego (the conscience). (These terms are used in full recognition that they are not concrete actualities but useful constructs.)

Heinz Hartmann (1958), the "father of ego psychology," developed and expanded the Freudian concept of the ego to focus on its interaction with and adaptation to the external world. He spoke of autonomous ego functions (such as the development of language and memory) that develop in the conflict-free sphere of the ego (that part of the ego that is not involved with "settling conflicts" between the id and the superego). "As a result, ego psychology encourages practitioners to think about developmental processes across the life cycle, about the unfolding of human capacities in response to the interaction between environmental influences and inborn developmental potentials" (Schamess, 1996, p. 68).

Ego psychology also offers a window of insight into psychological defenses and ego functions. The clinician's assessment of the ego functions can contribute greatly to understanding people and their adaptation to life. Does a person have good reality testing? What can be seen about the individual's ability to function on a daily basis? Is he or she capable of good judgment? Is there cohesiveness of personality, or is there a tendency to slip into psychosis under stress? Ego functions are discussed at greater length in Chapter 2.

The major ego defenses are examined so that we can understand what they mean and how they may be used. The defenses are chiefly unconscious mental mechanisms that help an individual ward off anxiety, protecting him or her from unwanted thoughts and feelings. Defenses can be both adaptive and maladaptive, depending on the context and how they relate to a person's functioning and accurate perception of the world. People with problems of alcoholism, for example, frequently use the defense of denial (and often their family members do the same) to avoid confronting the problem and the consequences of the drinking behavior. In this context, the defense is maladaptive, as denial facilitates continued drinking, which can have serious detrimental effects on the person's health, job functioning, and social relationships. The utilization of this defense, however, does enable the drinker to continue to fulfill whatever emotional needs are met (or felt to be met) by the drinking.

Ego defenses were first discussed by Freud, elaborated on by Anna Freud, and expanded by object relations theorists. Freud introduced the defense of repression, which is receiving a great deal of attention recently in regard to the major controversy related to recovering repressed memories of childhood abuse.

Developmental Theory

Developmental theory, within a biopsychosocial model, considers individuals and their biopsychosocial development over the trajectory of life. Knowing where people are in the life cycle can be an important aid when undertaking comprehensive assessments. For example, in working with an adolescent boy who is depressed, understanding his *age-specific needs,* which would include his developing sexuality and the impact of peer group influences on him, would help to clarify his problems contextually. In helping children faced with specific trauma, such as the death of a family member, understanding their developmental level is significant in understanding the impact on the child. Children may react differently to violence according to their ages and "emotional, cognitive, and physical capacities" (Marans and Adelman, 1997, p. 202), which must be considered in a developmental framework.

Adult development, from early adulthood through aging, has been a neglected subject until recent years, as an earlier belief existed, influenced by psychoanalytic thinking, that major developmental and maturational landmarks were achieved by the end of adolescence. It is recognized today that many developmental and psychological changes continue in the adult personality (Levinson et al., 1978; Levinson and Levinson, 1996; Nemiroff and Colarusso, 1990). Emphasis, for example, has been placed on reciprocity (between parents and child) in the parenting relationship and on the fact that the child influences the parent as much as the parent affects the child. The experience of parenthood can have a major impact on the further psychological development of parents (Benedek, 1970; Fischer, 1994).

Development is also examined in a cultural context. For example, standard U.S. culture stresses independence and encourages the young adult to move away from the parental home, while "a young Chinese man's failure to leave home is often seen as a sign of pathology in this [the standard U.S.] culture" (Tang, 1997, p. 337). From the Chinese point of view, on the other hand, "a great deal of the oldest son's self-esteem lies in the proper fulfillment of his duties [necessitating] living with the parents and seeing to their needs" (Tang, 1997, p. 337).

Object Relations Theory

Object relations theory contributes to a deeper understanding of the complex relationships people develop, which are colored by their *internalized* images of themselves as well as of other important people in their lives. In the following example, we can see the client, Meg, struggling with her feelings of discomfort in a social situation, which can be best understood from an object relations perspective.

> Meg discussed her experience when she was invited to a dinner party. She was introduced to a man who was friendly and who expressed an interest in her work. She was relaxed and animated as she talked to him. Later in the conversation, when she learned that he was a judge, she immediately felt anxious and frozen. She felt intimidated by his "authority," although, she admitted, he was not "acting like an authority." She could feel herself starting to respond in an inhibited manner.

Meg was not reacting to this man's genuine acceptance and warmth objectively. She perceived him internally as a critical judge of her; she *pro-*

jected her internalized negative feelings about herself onto him and reacted to him as though he were indeed critical.

In object relations theory, *objects* refer to people. (The rather unusual meaning of the term in this context is derived from early Freudian usage, when the mother was seen as the object of the infant's needs and drives.) Object relations is concerned not only with the real-world relationships people have with one another, but also their internal reactions to and conceptions of other people as well as their inner feelings about themselves.

> In addition to our loves, friendships, and rivalries, we have intricate relationships within us. They are not static images, but rather, powerful influences on how we feel about ourselves and relate to others. The people around us also affect us within ourselves. The exploration of these internal and external relationships has led to a growing body of knowledge called object relations theory. (Hamilton, 1990, p. 3)

Object relations theory has also contributed to a deeper understanding of the *"use of self"* of the clinician. Clinicians can obtain a valuable understanding of clients and their inner worlds by tuning in to their own feelings *evoked* by clients' attitudes and behaviors toward them. "Feelings in the therapist can provide important information about the patient's deepest and most disturbing affects" (Hamilton, 1990, p. 91).This use of self is one important aspect of *intersubjectivity,* a concept receiving increasing recognition in clinical work. Intersubjectivity is concerned with the reciprocal subjective reactions and interactions of the client and clinician (Stolorow et al., 1994). The "use of self" in the service of others is a key to professional development (Urdang, 1999).

Winnicott, an object relations theorist, has been gaining increasing recognition in the social work literature. Many of his ideas "lend depth and precision to social work's person-in-environment perspective" (Applegate and Bonovitz, 1995, p. 8). Winnicott's concepts include: the good-enough mother, transitional objects, play, the false self, the capacity to be alone, and the development of creativity.

Winnicott has applied his concept of *holding environment*—which means that parents provide nurturing and a sense of security to their children—to case management with disturbed children and adults. The "impersonal" case-management service is potentially ego supportive when accompanied by caring and empathy. Elements analogous to parental nurturing and growth-promoting actions can be reproduced by the social worker's support and the provision of supportive services and environments appropriately matched to the needs of the client (Kanter, 1990). (Although Winnicott includes the father as an important figure, he stresses the relationship to the mother as the primary caregiver, which, in the context of his times, was usually the case. Today we recognize the significance of the father, even during the very early days of the child's life, and generally refer to "parenting" rather than "mothering.")

The *bonding* and *attachment* behaviors of parents and children in the common everyday patterns of life are of great interest to the psychodynamic theorist. Interest has focused on how good bonding leads to good ego development, whereas poor bonding can have an adverse effect on all areas of physical, social, and emotional development (Bowlby, 1988; Goldberg, 1995; Holmes, 1995; Talbot, 1998). Attachment theories are relevant to many child welfare issues: to family reunification programs, which aim to maintain a degree of connection of children to their families, from whom they have been separated by some type of out-of-home care (Maluccio et al., 1996); to child maltreatment (Morton and Browne, 1998); and to early intervention programs (Shapiro and Gisynski, 1989). Attachment theory also can shed light on issues of intimacy and commitment with which adults struggle.

Mahler and colleagues (1975) explore the separation/individuation process in detail. They focus on the processes by which infants move away from the close maternal orbit, explore the world, develop a sense of individuality apart from mother, and, finally, negotiate the right "space" between themselves and mother to maintain closeness without losing autonomy. Although Mahler and colleagues (1975) assert that these developments occur primarily within the first three years of life, they do note that separation/individuation issues reverberate throughout the life cycle. Adolescents go through a "second step in individuation" (Blos, 1962, p. 12). Adolescents' normal storms and rebellions can be viewed as part of their struggle to separate and to continue to develop their own identities.

Kramer and colleagues (1997) argue that people grapple with separation/individuation issues throughout their lives. "In her presidential address to the American Psychological Association, Janet Spence (1985) . . . asserted that the conflict between individuation and fusion is one of the central issues of all human development" (Stevens-Long, 1990, p. 157). Issues of *loss* are also present throughout the life cycle, not only through death, the ultimate separation, but through the many vicissitudes of traversing the life cycle.

Psychodynamic theory also helps us to understand the formation of *identity,* our sense not only of "who we are, but that we are" (Mahler et al., 1975, p. 8). While ecological theory stresses the importance of self-esteem and self-efficacy, object relations theory and self psychology stress the deeper-lying structure of self-identity, the vicissitudes of its development, and the attainment of *self-cohesion.*

Self Psychology

An important concept relating to self-cohesion is that of *selfobjects,* as seen in *Vivienne: The Life and Suicide of an Adolescent Girl* (Mack and

Hickler, 1981). The book reports that Vivienne took her own life at the age of fourteen years and four months by hanging herself (after several previous suicide attempts). She had struggled for a long time with feelings of low self-esteem and depression but felt uplifted when a new teacher entered her school and provided her with a warm and supportive relationship. The loss she felt when he left the school and moved across the country appears to have been devastating. "Well over a year before he left, Vivienne anticipated that she would feel deeply bereaved, and wrote that her 'joy will be gone in a year'" (p. 101). The departure of the teacher had "a greater significance than his loss as a person. It struck at the core of Vivienne's psychological vulnerability" (Mack and Hickler, 1981, p. 101).

Here we see in operation the notion of the selfobject. This concept suggests that individuals from infancy onward derive subjectively determined, need-fulfilling assessments of their own worth from actual relationships with others. The attitude toward such subjectively derived assessments may range from profound dependency on them, with needs for continuing and immediate reaffirmation by the external source, to relative freedom from such dependency. Selfobject experiences are important throughout the life cycle. "Indeed, the need for selfobject responses is always present, waxing and waning with the ups and downs of the strength and vulnerability of the self" (Wolf, 1994, p. 81).

> Kohut postulates that if there had been a significant disturbance in the parent-child relationship . . . the child will be left especially vulnerable to later injuries to self-esteem . . . [and] will then seek idealized parent figures in adolescence or adult life . . . to replace something missing in the self . . . losses of these objects at critical times will bring about not merely a loss of self-esteem but terrible emotional pain, a sense of nothingness, and, potentially, a dissolution in the structure of the self. (Mack and Hickler, 1981, p. 107)

Self psychology contributes other important ideas to our understanding of people, including the importance of self structure and empathy, which are discussed further in Chapter 3.

Constructivism

A constructivist perspective compels us to look at our theoretical perspectives in a relativistic manner and to examine both the client's and our own belief systems within a cultural and social context. In the treatment situation, the therapist is not the detached authority but is a participant in the therapeutic dialogue. Finally, this perspective emphasizes the importance of looking at people's values and meanings in life, which are often motivating factors in themselves. People can have strong religious, political, or social beliefs which can take dominant roles in their lives. The constructivist perspective sheds light on how competing values between groups of people can be major forces in producing conflict; for example, religious wars, the pro-choice/pro-life battles, and the often intense wars between disciples of differing (and sometimes the same) psychological theories.

Constructivism as a theory asserts that "there is no ultimate objective truth, that each person interprets experience in terms of his/her background, cultural and personal" (Turrini, 1996, p. 447). Some writers see this theory as a movement away from the "positivistic assertions of the scientific basis of psychoanalysis of Freud and others to increasingly subjective and relativistic theoretical developments" (Coleman, 1996, p. 47). Mitchell (1988) emphasizes that we are actively involved in the creation of our world, noting that "the analysand is not just the fly caught in the web, but is the spider, the designer of the web as well" (p. 257).

Cultural perspectives take an important place in social constructivist theory, as we can see in the following excerpt from an article describing the treatment from a generative social constructivist perspective of Leon, a fifteen-year-old Ojibwa youth who made a failed suicide attempt (Angell et al., 1998). The authors note that by reframing suicide in accordance with this view, it was possible to generate an approach to the problem of integrating the client's cultural outlook. In this way, "the burden for change became a shared responsibility rather than an 'Indian problem'," and a "conscientious effort was made [to] integrate the use of Ojibwa culture into the helping process" (p. 19). Through using this framework, "the client's Native worldview became the foundation for . . . treating his suicidality" (Angell et al., 1998, p. 19).

THE EMBATTLED PLACE
OF PSYCHODYNAMIC THEORY

Psychodynamic theory is currently losing ground, for many reasons, in social work education (Sanville, 1994; Mishne, 1982). "Many schools of social work, counseling programs, and psychiatric residencies have cut back or dropped their psychodynamic curricula" (Berzoff et al., 1996, p. 3). In the future, treatment plans "will frequently be guided by established 'critical path models,' where the most effective service plans are determined in advance for a given difficulty and psychosocial profile" (Strom-Gottfried, 1997, p. 12). The use of computers has evolved from use in case record keeping to proposed applications for direct clinical work.

Computer therapies are already being developed, and Kreuger (1997) presents a somewhat exaggerated, but nevertheless chilling scenario for the future. "Already emerging are myriad on-line and computer-based software therapies that minimize the need for live, face-to-face, clinical intervention. Social work clinicians . . . will thus be replaced by on-line cyberstewards, who, acting as librarians armed with an assortment of consciousness-altering solutions, find the proper electronic solvents to be applied" (p. 20). Students won't need to establish caring professional relationships in such a world! (Urdang, 1999, p. 8)

One factor militating against the use of psychodynamic understanding is the long-standing schism in social work between advocates of work with the individual and advocates of social policy and social change. This conflict is reflected today in social work education (Urdang, 1999).

Psychodynamic clinical social work is dismissed by some faculty as irrelevant, as a means to "blame the victim" rather than change the injustices in society. This schism is not new, and has been with social work throughout its history. Austin (1997) notes that "in the widely read *Unfaithful Angels: How Social Work Has Abandoned Its Mission,* Specht and Courtney (1994) cited Jane Addams as the prophet of social work's true vision and called on the profession to reject an individual psychotherapy model in favor of a practice model based on the community as the unit of intervention and on group work and adult education as the primary interventive approach" (p. 608). (Urdang, 1999, p. 12)

Examining the diminishing role of psychodynamic theory in social work education from a *systemic perspective,* it becomes apparent that a powerful controlling force today in the present mental health field is *managed care.* The force behind this is primarily economic; keeping costs down is the primary goal. Brief treatment and supposedly efficient case management are given emphasis: "The spectre of managed care was propelling clinical social workers, responsible for the majority of therapy in the nation, to find short and simple solutions to long and complex problems" (Rose, 1996, p. xix). Coupled with this emphasis on short-term models has been the preference accorded to cognitive-behavioral constructs. (In this theoretical approach, emphasis is placed on models teaching people to "think differently" as well as to change their behaviors into more constructive actions.) Quantitative outcome measures are given priority, as empiricism is king, and statistical verification, rather than psychodynamic understanding, becomes the "royal road" to insight into the human condition.

It is regrettable that divisiveness exists within the profession on the subject of community and the individual. The uniqueness of social work has been the melding of the two. The *psychosocial* perspective, which deals concurrently with the individual (psyche) and the social, now augmented by a biological perspective (the biopsychosocial), has been the unshakable focus of the field in modern times. Every person has an inner world; every person has a social context. In fact, constant interaction and often conflict occurs between the two worlds.

Furthermore, social action and advocacy are important tools of the clinical social worker who works with individuals. If people are starving, food is a priority. If children live in crime-ridden neighborhoods where they see their friends murdered, safety is a priority. If gays and lesbians are harassed and beaten, protection is a priority. If adolescents are becoming infected with HIV and develop AIDS, treatment and prevention are priorities.

However, the community is not a corporate mass; it is composed of individuals, each unique. Historically, one of the highest values of the social work profession has been to recognize and respect the uniqueness of the individual—to appreciate the humanity, the suffering, the human dignity, and the spirit of every person (Chenot, 1998). Chenot cites Pray (1991), who has said that " 'honoring the uniqueness of the individual is central to social work practice, " and is " 'the core social work value' " (p. 80) (Chenot, 1998, p. 302).

It is indeed paradoxical that the time-honored social work values of caring for and individualizing the person are placed in opposition to the equally time-honored values of social policy and change, often to the disadvantage of the former in social work education. Yet nothing in principle dictates that one cannot be oppressed and suffer from inner emotional conflict at the same time. If children see their friends murdered, they often suffer emotionally, have nightmares, and experience other trauma-related symptoms. Gays and lesbians need protection from harassment, but they also may need help with the same myriad life issues that heterosexual people do. If adolescents are becoming infected with HIV and develop AIDS, they need individualized support as they face this life-threatening illness. Poor people are no less entitled to skilled professional help simply because they are poor; they also struggle with the purportedly "middle-class" problems of depression, marital conflict, and substance abuse.

It is also ironic that as we learn more about the human condition, about attachment theory (through infant research), object relations theory, intersubjectivity, constructivism, and self psychology, many in the social work profession have moved away from these approaches and emphasize systems theory and cognitive-behavioral and task-oriented models. We are not arguing for an exclusive emphasis on psychodynamic thinking: our argument is that this approach is a cornerstone, a sound foundation for exploring the human condition. Without it, complexities that are relevant and determining in all spheres of life, and at all levels—and therefore of interest in all types of social work practice—are glossed over.

Students today are responsible for dealing directly with increasingly complex problems within complex fieldwork systems. "Multiproblem clients, over-burdened supervisors, fewer agency resources, and increases in home-based services result in some students handling more difficult cases with reduced or inadequate supervision, and working in riskier environments" (Jarmon-Rohde, 1997, p. 33). It becomes more critical than ever before that students enter the field with a strong foundation in human behavior, based in a sound knowledge of psychodynamic concepts to help them maintain a firm footing as they are buffeted by multiple pressures. At the same time, this psychodynamic understanding must be embedded in a systems perspective.

Systems Theory

As the poet Donne reminds us: "No man is an island, entire of itself." We are all part of multiple systems. In talking directly to you, if you are a student, I note that you are currently part of a social work school system where the rules, expectations, actual work demands, peer relationships, involvement with faculty, and tuition you pay all have an impact on you. Socially, outside of school, you have friends, family, perhaps belong to organizations, have a religious affiliation, or a political orientation. Your current student status (with its accompanying time constraints) may affect all of your social involvements. You may be a long-standing member of your community; you may be a newcomer, perhaps just moving here to go to school. You live in housing that may be comfortable, or you may be sharing an apartment with six people, which may be stressful (or stimulating) for you. You may or may not have a system of social supports.

You have ethnic, racial, cultural, religious (or nonreligious) backgrounds and a sexual orientation, all of which affect your identity, your values, and your current perspectives on life and social work training. You come from a family with whom you may or may not be currently involved in complex ways. You may be in good health, or you may be having health problems (or concerned about someone else's health). It would not be unusual if you were feeling some degree of anxiety and self-doubt as you begin your new career. You know you will probably change in relation to your graduate training, but you do not know how this will happen, nor the nature of that eventual change.

Thinking in these terms exemplifies a systemic approach, a perspective to be applied to all client work and agency activity. *Macrolevel* systems include society, community, and organizations; *microlevel* systems include individuals, families, and groups. As a student, your school, placement agency, and organizations would be examples of *macrosystems*. Your friends, colleagues, and family are part of your *microsystem.* Micro- and macrolevel systems often interconnect and interact.

Macrosystem issues, such as managed care, may affect the funding of your agency, which means you may not have enough cases assigned to you (because you won't be covered by insurance payments), which means you may not be able to write the necessary papers for school, which may cause you worry about passing. This anxiety may be transmitted to your family, which may increase the stress they feel about your education in the first place.

Ecological theory, as defined by Germain, "studies the relations between organisms and their environments . . . [which are] characterized by continuous reciprocal exchanges or transactions, in which people and environments influence, shape, and sometimes change each other" (1991, pp. 15-16). Ecological theory leans heavily on the concepts of *adaptation* and *coping* (Fraser, 1997; Germain, 1991).

Systemic thinking will be addressed from two perspectives: the first involves the *processes* of systemic interactions (as we noted above when we discussed the chain of events that could affect you as students in relation to managed care). The second aspect of a systems perspective involves looking at major systemic *issues* and how they affect people. For example, while we study children from a developmental and psychodynamic perspective, it is also important to understand some of the general macrosystems issues many children in America face today (Fraser, 1997).

> Beginning in the last quarter of the century, both the relative and official rates of childhood poverty climbed. . . . Between 1985 and 1993, the percentage of babies born weighing less than 5.5 pounds . . . rose 6 percent. . . . The violent death rate for teenagers increased 10 percent, the birthrate for teenagers increased 23 percent. . . . Children of color . . . disproportionately bear the burden of poverty. (Fraser, 1997, p. 1)

We look at many systemic issues, including poverty, homelessness, divorce, violence, sexual abuse, and addictions. Special attention is paid to the subject of *violence* and *sexual abuse* because of their prevalence both in larger society and the family. "The major setting for violence in America is the home. Intrafamilial abuse, neglect, and domestic battery account for the majority of physical and emotional violence suffered by children in this country" (Perry, 1997, p. 126). Although it has been difficult to obtain precise statistics on the prevalence of child sexual abuse, it is nevertheless "clear that the sexual abuse of children is a significant and relatively common problem of childhood" (Conte, 1995). Women are often victims of domestic abuse (Longres, 1995b). Recent attention has been paid to the presence of physical abuse in gay and lesbian couple relationships (Carlson and

Maciol, 1997). Physical and sexual abuse can have a significant psychological impact on individual adults and dramatically affect a child's development (Glodich, 1998; Kilgore, 1988; Osofsky, 1997).

We also address discrimination against various groups in our society, including racial minorities, women, homosexuals, the elderly, and the disabled, and examine both women's rights and the men's movement. Currently, many advances are taking place in civil rights, progress is being made by racial and ethnic minorities, and greater acceptance of gays and lesbians is occurring; we also see serious regressions and backlashes. Matthew Shepard, a gay man, was brutally murdered and his body stretched along a Wyoming fence one day after National Coming Out Day. There followed a large gathering protesting this crime.

> Three days after Shepard died, a crowd of around 5,000 gathered in the night on the steps of the Capitol in Washington, in a candlelight vigil that struggled to make another argument and extract another message from his death. Ellen DeGeneres, Ted Kennedy and Barney Frank, the openly gay Massachusetts Congressman—all the expected speakers took the microphone. What was less expected was the sheer turnout of lawmakers at a moment when Congress was embroiled in the crazy closing hours of the budget deal. So many members showed up to voice their grief that House minority leader Richard Gephardt had time only to read their names. "It speaks volumes about how much progress we've made," says Winnie Stachelberg, lobbyist for the Human Rights Campaign, the nation's biggest gay-rights group. "Yet Matthew's death shows how much farther we have to go." (Lacayo, 1998, pp. 33-34)

Ecological theory contributes many important ideas to social work practice, such as exploration of the *nature of communities* and the utilization of *social networks* and *social supports* to enable people to lead more productive lives (Germain, 1991). The ecological concept of *goodness-of-fit* describes the matching of a person with specific needs (such as an employment problem), with someone or some place (such as an employment service) in the environment where the best chance for meeting these needs can occur. For example, a man with creative abilities was placed in a job requiring rote mechanical skills and did poorly. When alternatively transferred to a position where his creative abilities were used, he flourished. In support of the goodness-of-fit approach, Woods and Hollis (1990) note: "An individual's temperament, needs, and preferences and the available opportunities can be evaluated and, whenever possible, matched to better suit both sides. This perspective contributes to a 'no-fault' approach to reducing person-situation disequilibrium" (p. 29).

Culture

There can be cultures based on race, ethnicity, sexual orientation, or disability, such as deafness. Some people have combined cultural backgrounds; for example, they may have a multiethnic heritage, or they may be part of two cultures such as being black and gay. Cultures are not static; there may be changing cultural values and varying degrees of adherence to cultural patterns. Conflict often occurs within cultures as well as between cultures. This book's aim is to enable the reader to become more culturally sensitive, to learn how to take the cultural aspects of a client's life into account, and to see the subtleties and nuances involved in cultural values, identities, and conflicts. Notable differences exist, for example, between Chinese and U.S. cultures in the ways mothers handle the developmental vicissitudes of their children, such as the separation-individuation crisis (Tang, 1997).

Many Americans today are immigrants living the immigrant experience with varying degrees of comfort and distress. We will examine aspects of immigration, including issues of acculturation and marginality, and its effect on the evolving self-identity of the immigrant.

> Immigration from one country to another is a complex and multifaceted psychosocial process with significant and lasting effects on an individual's identity. Leaving one's country involves profound losses ... [and] a renewed opportunity for psychic growth and alteration. (Akhtar, 1995, p. 1052)

A cultural perspective is included in the discussion of adolescent suicide, a very serious problem today. The suicide rate for Native Americans is "1.5 times greater than any other group in America. . . . However, it is particularly high among young males 15-34 years of age for whom it is the second leading cause of death" (Angell et al., 1998, p. 2). Recently, a sharp increase has been reported in the rate of suicide for black teenagers, which "might reflect the strain some black families feel in making the transition to middle-class life" (Belluck, 1998a, p. A1). It is not clear to what extent homicide, the leading cause of death of black youths, might mask underlying suicidal behaviors as a path perceived as more acceptable to some cultural groups. Suicidal behavior in black and Hispanic adolescents, for example, is found to be influenced by cultural attitudes regarding self-destructive behavior (Wyche and Rotheram-Borus, 1990). These authors believe that suicide tends to be seen in these groups as "a passive response to frustration" and "dying is . . . more honorable if it occurs in rage and aggression rather than in passive solitude. Provoking a fight and being killed as a result may be culturally more appropriate as an expression of suicidal intent" (p. 327).

Families

It is generally acknowledged that families are vital for the child's basic nurturance and socialization into society. Family members are involved (or not involved) with each other in varying degrees and patterns over the course of the life cycle and can be critically involved (or absent) as parents age and look for (or cannot obtain) nurturance from their adult offspring. The family can be a source of emotional refueling, support, and love; it can also be a source of tension and violence, and may itself ultimately dissolve. Going home to family makes Thanksgiving the most heavily traveled day in this country; having no family to go home to can produce sadness or despair. A foster child who says "I don't belong anywhere" yearns for a family he or she may never have.

Family life takes many forms today, at the dawn of the twenty-first century in America. This includes single-parent, blended, gay, foster, kinship caring, and adoptive families as well as "grandfamilies" (where grandparents are custodial parents) (Dowdy, 1998). Traditionally, the nuclear family consisted of a husband and wife, and several children (and maybe a dog and some goldfish). Today, we are aware of the changing nature of families and family structure. In a discussion of adoption as one of the "many ways that men and women create families," Fein (1998) wrote that "the panorama of the American family now includes children born through advanced reproductive technology, some conceived with donated sperm and eggs; families broken apart by divorce then blended through remarriage; families created by single parents and by gay men who have hired a surrogate to bear a child" (p. 30).

Cultural and systemic issues affecting families today (such as both parents in the workplace) are addressed. The following are among the aspects of family structure and process discussed: The *internal structure* of families (for example, boundaries and subsystems); enmeshed and disengaged families (Minuchin, 1974); *communications patterns* in family life, which can be functional or dysfunctional (Satir, 1967); *intergenerational* aspects of family life (Bowen, 1985); and an *object relations* perspective in marital and family life (Scharff and Scharff, 1987).

ADDITIONAL PERSPECTIVES

Biological Orientation

The biological is a critical aspect of human behavior and human development, starting with the commencement of our physical existence and culminating in its ending. Biological factors include: reproductive technologies and physical aspects of maturation, development, and aging over the life cycle. People's inborn constitutions, including attributes, limitations, and temperaments, will be addressed from both a biological and interactional perspective. When a mother's alcoholism affects her baby's physical development in utero, causing the baby to be born with fetal alcohol syndrome, manifesting excessive crying or withdrawal, the mother's response to this "difficult" infant will be affected; the interaction between them may spiral into dysfunction.

Sexuality—a biological drive that has psychological, social, and cultural ramifications—is presented, including the dramatic hormonal surges at puberty, sexual issues in adult relationships, and the often-ignored topics of sexual feelings in elder adults and in people with developmental disabilities. Homosexuality is addressed from a life-span perspective and also from a systemic perspective, including issues such as homophobia.

Physical illness and disability are discussed later in this chapter.

Cognitive Development

Cognition is given emphasis in a broad perspective, including: cognitive-behavioral theoretical approaches and the development of cognitive schema; the development of thought, following Piaget's theories as well as impairments in brain functioning related to developmental disabilities, alcoholism, and Alzheimer's disease; the cognitive unconscious; the form and content of schizophrenic thought; and the effect of traumatic experiences on children's neurodevelopment.

The close relationship between cognition and psychodynamic understanding is highlighted, as cognitive functioning and the intellect are central to making sense of one's experience and dynamics, inter- and intrapersonal. It is impossible to imagine insight-oriented therapy without the capacity to conceptualize and abstract.

Resilience

The observation that some children who live under adverse conditions and/or who have lived through multiple stresses do not experience symptoms of psychopathology but "remain invulnerable or resilient, able to cope with the effects of misfortune and adversity" (Cohler, 1987, p. 363) is one of the conundrums of human behavior. Studies of such children have shown that positive forces and protective factors are important variables. Protective factors have been defined "as both the internal and external forces that help children resist or ameliorate risk" (Kirby and Fraser, 1997, p. 16). Kegan (1982) suggests that there may be qualities within the child that may serve to "recruit" others in providing external supports. "Our survival and development depends on our capacity to recruit the invested attention of others to us. Nature is nowhere more graceful than in the way she endows each new-born infant with seductive abilities" (Kegan, 1982, p. 17). Do some children have greater recruitment capacities than others? Resilience is examined from multiple perspectives as we look at biopsychosocial development over the life course.

Creativity

Creativity, highly prized in our society, is a complex phenomenon requiring high-level ego development including the capacity for abstract thinking. In addition to aesthetic satisfaction, creativity may offer adaptive strategies. The capacity to play and to be creative bear a relationship. "The child at play and the creative writer are alike in that both create a new world or rearrange aspects of their own experience in new ways" (Colarusso, 1993, p. 235).

While Maslow (Longres, 1995b) suggests that self-actualization (Maslow's "highest level of need") is achieved only after other lower-order needs, such as self-esteem needs, have been met (p. 27), further examination reveals a more complex picture. Creativity, perhaps one of the highest forms of self-actualization, can itself be used in the service of adaptation to satisfy lower-level needs. Storr (1988) argues that artistic endeavors are not merely adaptive or compensatory mechanisms but have a special life in and of themselves—they have a special meaning, providing a sense of self-fulfillment.

Can childhood losses serve to promote special abilities and strengths, including an appreciation of solitude and an enriched inner life? It is known that many writers have experienced "rather solitary childhoods" (Storr, 1988, p. 106). But, Storr adds, "unless those circumstances are so inimically severe that they cause mental disintegration, absence of, or partial deprivation of, interpersonal relationships encourages imagination to flourish" (p. 106).

The importance of imagination, creativity, and play and their development in the life cycle are discussed.

SPECIAL ISSUES

Three issues of special significance merit separate chapters. Chapter 11 focuses on life changes, transitions, crises, loss, and death. Chapter 12 focuses on illness and disability, and Chapter 13 discusses mental health problems.

Life Transitions, Crises, and Loss

Life is full of changes, and we face many transitions and continually make new adaptations. Sometimes we are faced with life crises which can be overwhelming but often can serve as an opportunity for growth. These subjects are addressed in Chapter 11, which also incorporates the subjects of death and loss.

Loss accompanies us through the life cycle sometimes in lesser ways, such as the feelings evoked by graduation from high school (although it may not feel very "small" at the time), or in major ways, such as through divorce, loss of physical abilities, or the death of loved ones. "Despite the centrality of grief as a universal response to loss, and its prevalence in the social work domain, little empirical attention has been given to the impact of grief instruction in social work courses" (Kramer, 1998, p. 211). Grieving or the lack of grieving can have important emotional consequences for us. *Unresolved grief* can result in psychosomatic disorders, depression, or disturbed relationships.

William Styron (1990), the well-known novelist, experienced a bout of serious depression and wrote an autobiographical account of his illness describing his despair and preoccupation with suicide. Suddenly, he had a dramatic breakthrough, and became aware of unresolved grief as the root of his depression.

> I'm persuaded that an even more significant factor was the death of my mother when I was thirteen . . . the death or disappearance of a parent, especially a mother, before or during puberty—appears repeatedly in the literature on depression as a trauma sometimes likely to create nearly irreparable emotional havoc . . . especially . . . if the young person is affected by . . . "incomplete mourning" has . . . been unable to achieve the catharsis of grief, and so carries within himself through later years an insufferable burden of which rage and guilt, and not only dammed-up sorrow . . . become the potential seeds of self-destruction. (pp. 79-80)

Issues of death, loss, and grief will also be discussed from a cultural perspective. Native Americans, for instance, have traditional patterns of experiencing their grief. The Lakota grief experience (Brave Heart, 1998) includes the display of "visible signs of grief," such as "cutting one's hair and at times one's body, symbolizing the psychic pain of the bereaved" (p. 290). In addition, "the bereaved give away possessions" and the "Spirit keeping ceremonies allow the bereaved to mourn . . . while keeping the soul of the deceased. A 'releasing of the spirit ceremony' is held at the end of the mourning period" (p. 290).

Illness and Disability

Illness and disability (Chapter 12) affect patients and their families profoundly and are integral to understanding human behavior. Illness and disability have profound and widespread biopsychosocial effects on patients, their families, and social networks. *Psychological* sequelae can include: feelings of loss, changes in self-image and self-esteem, shame, depression, and sometimes suicidality. Barbara Ceconi, an MSW in social work, lost her eyesight suddenly while in college due to juvenile diabetes.

Her initial feelings and experiences in relation to her blindness were "akin to those of grieving the loss of a significant friend or family member. I was mourning the loss of my eyesight" (Ceconi and Urdang, 1994, p. 181). She experienced rapid mood changes, feeling "anger, depression, fear, and isolation. . . . Being helpless, not able to function independently, not having a career were the thoughts running through my head" (p. 181). Barbara's statement resonates with one made by Reverend Thomas Carroll who said, " 'It is superficial, if not naive, to think of blindness as a blow to the eyes only, to sight only. It is a destructive blow to the self-image which man has carefully, though unconsciously constructed throughout his lifetime, a blow almost to his being itself' " (Ceconi and Urdang, 1994, p. 181).

Family members may experience feelings of loss, anger, and depression and may also assume caretaking functions (which can prove stressful). They may need to make adjustments (which they may be unable to make) in their family structure. Systemic issues, such as societal attitudes toward the disabled, the limited availability of medical and support services, and the impact of managed care on patient treatment are also important variables. The mind-body interaction has been receiving increasing attention. These subjects are included in the discussion in Chapter 12.

Psychopathology

Psychopathology (disturbances of thinking and feeling) is not exclusively the province of the so-called "mentally ill" but is experienced by all human beings to varying degrees. Feelings of depression and anxiety, for instance, fade in and out of our state of mind and are included in our consideration of human behavior. Mental health problems, such as schizophrenia, substance abuse, and post-traumatic stress disorder (related to issues of violence and child abuse) are included in Chapter 13.

Many people in this country are affected directly (as patients) or indirectly (as families or friends of patients) by various types of mental illness, including *schizophrenia, mood disorders, anxiety disorders,* and *characterological or personality problems.* Children of depressed mothers, for example, are at serious developmental risk (Brody, 1998). Material related to psychopathology is often isolated in a separate course, as the human behavior course supposedly stresses "normal" functioning only. However, the line between normal emotional states and pathological conditions is not always easy to draw. An intimate relationship exists between serious psychological problems, and many social problems such as violence, sexual abuse, suicide, the breakdown of the family, and homelessness.

A brief overview of the four major types of mental disorders referred to above will be given. Special emphasis, however, is given to depression, the addictions (including gambling), borderline pathology, and anxiety, including panic disorders and post-traumatic stress disorder, which is often a consequence of abuse and violence. Developmental disabilities, including retardation and autism, are also discussed in this section.

The strengths perspective is emphasized in current social work literature (Saleebey, 1992); the use of psychopathological diagnoses or concepts is often criticized, as it is felt to impose the "medical model" on treating people, to ignore the "social processes," and to "blame the victim" instead of "changing society."

Yet "pathology" (or disorder, disturbance, dysfunction) is part of the human psychological condition, just as physical pathologies such as cancer and heart disease can be part of the human physical condition. It is important not to pathologize the person with cancer or with manic-depressive illness, but we need to recognize that pathological functioning exists in both conditions and that it may be tenacious.

It is incontestable that we must support a patient's strengths; this support is the basis of providing hope and enhancing functioning. But if we fail to comprehend or respect the intensity of certain mental states, we cannot free the strengths from what enslaves them. What may disempower people in a profound way is not always an unjust society (although society's provisions of care for the mentally ill are often unjust; and some societal factors may precipitate breakdowns in people). Strong biological forces, which may coexist with psychosocial factors, are often at work in the etiology of mental problems. Patients themselves can resist getting better; they sometimes prefer aspects of remaining ill to regaining strengths.

Kay Redfield Jamison, a professor of psychiatry at Johns Hopkins School of Medicine and a prolific author on manic-depressive illness, is herself afflicted (or blessed, as she sometimes feels) with manic-depressive illness. In her impressive autobiography, *An Unquiet Mind* (1996), she shares her struggles with her illness with us. Although she is a person of unquestionable strengths, the tenacity and chronicity of this illness remain with her. She also describes her resistance to fighting this illness.

> Even though I was a clinician and a scientist, and even though I could read the research literature and see the inevitable, bleak consequences of not taking lithium, I for many years after my initial diagnosis was reluctant to take my medication as prescribed. . . . Why did it take having to go through more episodes of mania, followed by long suicidal depressions, before I would take lithium in a medically sensible way?

Some of my reluctance, no doubt, stemmed from a fundamental denial that what I had was a real disease. . . . Moods are such an essential part of the substance of life, of one's notions of oneself, that even psychotic extremes in mood and behavior somehow can be seen as temporary, even understandable, reactions to what life has dealt. In my case, I had a horrible sense of loss for who I had been and where I had been. *It was difficult to give up the high flights of mind and mood, even though the depressions that inevitably followed nearly cost me my life.* [italics added] (Jamison, 1996, p. 91)

ILLUSTRATION OF THE BIOPSYCHOSOCIAL APPROACH TO A CASE

In concluding this overview, the case of Mrs. Billings is presented to illustrate how the biopsychosocial approach can be applied in a clinical social work situation.

Mrs. Billings, a thirty-two-year-old Caucasian woman, was admitted to an inpatient psychiatric facility for treatment of depression. She was tired, felt tearful, and stated that her symptoms were increasing. She had one previous psychiatric hospitalization for a suicide attempt and depression. She has very low self-esteem, strong feelings of guilt, and is very self consciousness. "It is hard for me to make friends . . . I am uncomfortable with people." She is married, to Mr. Billings, thirty-six, who runs a store in their small rural town; they have two children, Susan, ten, and Todd, eight. The family lives on a 100-acre farm with cows and horses.

As we think about Mrs. Billings, several questions suggest themselves for further exploration. First, let us consider her relationship with her husband. Is he a potential source of support? Might conflict in their relationship be contributing to her depressive feelings? Mr. Billings drove some distance to the hospital to visit with his wife, and he readily accepted the recommendation for a social work interview. Both Mr. and Mrs. Billings were seen individually for one session and then had a joint interview.

Mr. B., thirty-six, relates well and seemed insecure, passive, and eager to please. He is concerned about his wife but feels helpless in terms of knowing what to do for her. He tries to help her at home . . . "maybe she feels guilty about that . . . I wash dishes for her . . . she fusses at me for this . . . tells me to do my farm work." Both Mr. and Mrs. B. feel that something is missing in their relationship; they each see their own involvement in their marital problems. Mr. B. stated: "We don't sit down and talk to each other . . . that is one of our problems . . . I can't stand to have her mad at me." He added that his wife "just holds her feelings inside . . . things keep building up in her." Mrs. B. commented that she likes her husband. "I feel as comfortable with him as I ever did . . . can be myself with him."

Mrs. B. talked openly about her sexual problems. There is a "coolness between my husband and myself. . . . I won't let him kiss me or hold my hand. . . . I don't want him to touch me . . . can't tolerate the idea of sex." When first married, "I enjoyed sex," but since the birth of her two children she has had a fear of getting pregnant. "Why I'm that way, I don't know." Concerning their present sexual life, Mr. B. stated: "We don't talk about it."

The communication patterns of this couple seem impaired; they know this but seem unable to move ahead on their own to correct the problem. They both express caring feelings for each other, relate well to the interviewer, and have a basic capacity to relate, but at present this seemed *inhibited*. Sexual problems seem serious, although the baseline of their sexual functioning was at a higher level in the past. Mrs. B. reports sexual fears and relates this to a horror of becoming pregnant. Her general sense of superego guilt is pervasive (she may have an excessively punitive, critical superego); problems and conflicts about "mothering" also seem key issues in her fear of becoming pregnant. The transactional nature of the marital problems become obvious; the inner conflicts of Mrs. B. affect her response to Mr. B., which in turn affect his response to her, so the spiral escalates. As we examine the interaction of this couple, Mrs. B's inner state, conflicts, and anxieties come into focus. We can observe that her self-esteem is low, and her self-image is poor.

Mrs. B. has fears of pregnancy, which we hypothesized are related to her anxieties about mothering. What is her relationship to her two children like? To what extent are they a source of pleasure to her; to what degree a source of conflict?

Mr. B. states that the children are doing well and get along in school. He feels that they (especially his daughter) "get on his wife's nerves." Mrs. B. expressed concern that her behavior affects both children. Her son is "bordering on an ulcer." She finds that she "fusses at them for small things . . . I'm afraid I'm making them high strung." Recently her daughter came home from school with school pictures of herself and started crying while showing them to her mother. Mrs. B. said that she used to be the same way: ". . . I was ashamed of my looks . . . did not want to show my pictures."

We can observe the effects of the mother's temperament and depression on the children. The interactional nature of the family system becomes apparent. We see the expression of ambivalence, as she shows some concern and empathy as well as irritation toward her children. We see the possible beginnings of a psychosomatic condition, as the son may be developing an ulcer. The object relations perspective helps us to understand how her daughter has internalized some of her mother's attitudes and feelings.

It will be instructive to look at the family in the larger system of work, extended family, friends, and community. As we proceed with this exploration, we can see that the family, especially Mrs. B., while having some social contacts, has relatively closed boundaries with the outside world; socially they are relatively isolated.

> Mr. Billings works in a store, which he now owns after making a financial arrangement with Mrs. B's father who had owned it previously. Mr. B. works his farm by himself "every spare minute I have." He enjoys living in this small town, has friends, and meets many people in the store. But he finds that it is a "relief to get out on the farm . . . you can fed up with the public . . . they are hard to please." Mrs. B. works as a salaried bookkeeper for her father. Although she likes office work because "it is methodical," she is under some pressure working for her father "who leaves too much to her."
>
> The Billings have no outside interests, except camping, which they do once a year. Mr. B. reports that his wife "doesn't enjoy this, does it mostly for the kids . . . would really rather go to a motel." He feels he should take his wife out more. "It's a help for her to eat out . . . but I would just as soon eat home." Mr. B. would like to go to church (which Mrs. B. refuses to attend because of her weight) and to lodge meetings, "but I don't want to leave her and the kids alone." Mrs. B. has no "real close friends." They don't visit or have others come to the house. "She worries because the house is not polished." Mrs. B.'s mother comes over once a week to help her clean the house. Mrs. B. has complained to her husband about her mother "being a problem to her . . . mother cries on her shoulder."

We find an *enmeshed family system* in which the Billings' economic and employment situations are intertwined with those of Mrs. B.'s parents. There is not a goodness-of-fit between Mrs. B. and her social environment. For Mrs. B., working for her father and having her mother help at home weekly adds to her distress, rather than her pleasure. Her resentment is internalized, adding to her depressed feelings. Her poor self-image makes having friends a difficult chore for her. She states that it is "hard for me to make friends . . . I am uncomfortable with people." A complex interaction exists:

she would probably benefit from having friends but seems unable to do so at the present time, and her isolated life style adds to her depressed feelings. Also, we can see her depressed moods controlling the family's activities to some extent. Mrs. B. has little pleasure in her life. *Anhedonia,* the inability to experience pleasure, is one of the symptoms of depression; for Mrs. B., it also seems characterological, i.e., part of her personality, in that it has been an entrenched feature since her early life. In terms of the ego function of management of needs and feelings, there is great inhibition of both aggressive and pleasurable feelings, and an abundance of superego guilt.

Turning to biological factors, we see that Mrs. B. complains of fatigue, which is a symptom of depression; but this could be related to other illnesses, such as anemia. She complains of dizziness and shortness of breath. She had gained forty pounds in the last three years, adding greatly to her self-consciousness. Mr. B. noted: "When she is nervous, she tends to eat more." Her physical problems were evaluated; nothing significant was found. She was then referred to the psychiatric service.

Researchers have found evidence for a biological basis for depression; Mrs. B. may be constitutionally prone to this disorder. However, to see her depression exclusively in biological terms would blind us to the complex psychosocial factors in her life. Medication was helpful to her, but individual and marital therapy might help her live a more satisfying life. We saw earlier that her son might be developing an ulcer, a condition with psychosomatic implications. When Mrs. B. came to the hospital to be evaluated, her mother also came for an evaluation for stomach problems.

In an effort to understand how her past might live in the present, Mrs. Billings was asked about her early family life. She described a number of family problems and she, on her own, related them to her present sense of self. From a self-psychological perspective, we can see that she experienced serious empathic failures on the part of her parents and did not receive adequate mirroring, or admiration, from them. She did not receive sufficient acceptance from her family to build healthy self-esteem.

> Mrs. B. was the second of three children and "got along well her parents," but "blamed them for many of my problems . . . never felt I could talk to them." With some guilt she added, "They never had a chance themselves." Mrs. Billings' mother was six months old when her own mother died. Mrs. Billings' mother was then raised by an aunt in a large family, not receiving much attention herself. Mrs. Billings' parents were "never free in their praise of me . . . maybe they did praise me when I got good grades . . . but never for anything else." If something "bothered me, I would bottle it up and brood over it . . . I imagine that's what I've been doing now."

Sex was never discussed at home; she never saw her parents kiss or hold hands. Her own femininity was never encouraged. "I never learned to wear make-up . . . still can't fix my hair . . . was never told I was pretty." In growing up, she usually had a few "fairly close friends . . . was never very comfortable with people at large." Mrs. B. graduated from high school, then went to business school, worked successfully, and had ambitions to be a doctor, which she never pursued.

Looking at Mrs. B.'s background from an object relations perspective, we see that the early loss of her mother's mother was a significant factor, probably affecting her mother's ability to mother, and then, subsequently, Mrs. B.'s capacity to mother. Also some role reversal is occurring, at least presently, as Mrs. B. complains that her mother tends to lean on her emotionally. We can also see how she has internalized many of the interactions with her family, and that this has played a large role in her psychological development, including her self-image as well as present relationships with others.

CONCLUSION

This chapter has presented an overview of the philosophy and format of this book. I incorporate a biopsychosocial perspective with an emphasis on psychodynamic understanding. Because this perspective leans so heavily on psychodynamic thinking, these concepts are presented first, in the next section of the book.

LEARNING EXERCISES

1. *Small Group Exercise.* In small groups, discuss the systemic issues affecting your life now as social work students; each group can then share its thoughts with the class.
2. *Newspaper Assignment.* Select a newspaper article that illustrates an interesting aspect of peoples' behaviors, social problems, or systemic processes. Analyze this article from a biopsychosocial perspective.
3. *Biographical Analysis.* Select a well-written biography or autobiography and begin to read this. At the end of the course, compose a biopsychosocial assessment of the person who is the book's subject and analyze the combination of strengths and vulnerabilities that exist. What are the main factors you see as contributing to the person's successes and difficulties?

SUGGESTED READINGS

Articles

Ceconi, B. and Urdang, E. (1994). Sight or insight? Child therapy with a blind clinician. *Clinical Social Work Journal, 22,* 179-192.

Glodich, A. (1998). Traumatic exposure to violence: A comprehensive review of
the child and adolescent literature. *Smith College Studies in Social Work, 68,*
321-345.

Books

Frank, M. G. (1996). A clinical view of the use of psychoanalytic theory in front-
line practice. In J. Edward and J. Sanville (Eds.), *Fostering healing and growth:
A psychoanalytic social work approach* (pp. 59-76). Northvale: Jason Aronson
Inc.

Germain, C. (1991). The ecological perspective. In *Human behavior in the social
environment* (pp. 9-37). New York: Columbia University Press.

Kirby, L. D. and Fraser, M. W. (1997). Risk and resilience in childhood. In
M. W. Fraser, (Ed.), *Risk and resilience in childhood: An ecological perspective*
(pp. 10-33). Washington: NASW Press.

McFeely, W. S. (1991). *Frederick Douglass.* New York: W. W. Norton and Co.

McGoldrick, M. (1982). Ethnicity and family therapy: An overview. In M. McGoldrick, J. K. Pearce, and J. Giordano (Eds.), *Ethnicity and family therapy* (pp. 3-30).
New York: The Guilford Press.

Chapter 2

Psychoanalytic and Ego Psychology Theories

Tell me where is fancy bred,
Or in the heart or in the head?
How begot, how nourished?

William Shakespeare
Merchant of Venice

INTRODUCTION

This chapter encompasses psychoanalytic and ego psychology theories, particularly the ego functions and defense mechanisms. Psychodynamic understanding is relevant to clinical interventions in any social work setting; although they may not be asking for help in altering it, all clients do have a psychological life. People dealing with medical problems, aging parents, or child welfare issues are coping with critical life issues to which they bring their unique personalities, vulnerabilities, and ways of relating. The deeper our understanding and sensitivity to their underlying needs, feelings, ego functioning, and defensive operations, the better able we are to help them and to anticipate and deal with the complexities of working with them, their relationship demands on others and ourselves, and the resulting dilemmas in which we can become entangled. This chapter aims to enable students to begin to appreciate the complexities of human behavior and to approach their participation in the joint clinical endeavor with greater objectivity.

PSYCHOANALYTIC THEORY

Freud felt that it was his fate to "'agitate the sleep of mankind'" (Gay, 1988, p. xvii). The agitation he produced was pronounced in his day and persists to the present. Now, as in the late nineteenth century, Freud has staunch adherents and strong opponents. "Freud has been called genius, founder, master, a giant among the makers of the modern mind, and no less emphatically, autocrat, plagiarist, fabulist, the most consummate of charlatans" (Gay, 1988, p. xvi). The goal of psychoanalysis, he asserted, was to "struggle with the 'demon'—the demon of irrationality—in a 'sober way' " (Gay, 1988, p. xvii). Freud noted that "this very sobriety, which reduces that demon to a 'comprehensible object of science,' only made his ideas about the nature of human nature seem all the more dismaying, all the more unacceptable. No wonder that mankind has for the most part defended itself against Freud's message with angry denials" (Gay, 1988, p. xvii).

Freud was born in 1856, eventually began his medical practice in Vienna as a neurologist, and, in 1885, studied with Charcot, who was treating patients with hysterical symptoms, such as paralysis or blindness, for which no physical basis existed. From Charcot, Freud learned how to remove these symptoms through hypnotic suggestion and utilized this method "with varying degrees of success" (Brenner, 1974, p. 6). Freud became frustrated with hypnosis, finding that it was often difficult to induce, that the cures were often transitory, and that during the course of this treatment some women patients became "sexually attracted to him . . . something which was most unwelcome to him" (Brenner, 1974, p. 7).

Freud's early collaborator, Breuer, told him about an earlier case he had treated; Freud wrote about this as the famous case of Anna O. Breuer's work, and Freud's understanding of the implications of this work, led to a major breakthrough for the development of psychoanalysis. For Breuer, however, this case led to flight from the fledgling psychoanalysis. Anna O. was later identified as Bertha Pappenheim, who became famous as a feminist reformer and social worker (Swenson, 1994).

Joseph Breuer, a general physician, was asked to treat Bertha for a number of medical problems, including a cough, which her mother was concerned could be tuberculosis. Bertha's father was at the time terminally ill with this disease, and Bertha and her mother were caring for him at home (Rosenbaum and Muroff, 1984).

> When Breuer came to attend Bertha Pappenheim, he found more than the cough. She had paralysis of the right arm, both legs were paralyzed, and she could move only the fingers of her left hand. She was unable to feed herself, and she was barely able to turn her head because of what appeared to be a paralyzed neck muscle. She complained of visual difficulty, so that she could neither write nor read. Other specialists had been consulted before Joseph Breuer, and they could find no physical basis for Bertha's complaints. Breuer recognized at once the mental and emotional problems that were involved. (Rosenbaum and Muroff, 1984, p. 2)

During the course of therapy, when she was under hypnosis (or put herself into a hypnotic trance), Bertha was able to talk about her symptoms, adding information related to her background. As she did so, her symptoms began disappearing. Bertha referred to this talking as " 'chimney sweeping' " (Rosenbaum and Muroff, 1984, p. 4) and to the treatment as " 'the talking cure' " (p. 5). Talking included the recollection of a significant dream involving a snake about to attack her father; when she tried to prevent this, her arm became paralyzed. Apparently, after recounting this dream and her anxiety surrounding it, "her right arm was no longer paralyzed" (Rosenbaum and Muroff, 1984, p. 5). Breuer, satisfied with the results, then terminated treatment, not anticipating what followed.

> That very evening Breuer was called to the Pappenheim home, and there he found Bertha in a hysterical state imagining that she was giving birth to a child, which she told Breuer was his. Although he was in a state of shock, he managed to hypnotize her and calm her. He left the Pappenheim apartment in what he later described as a "cold sweat." He never returned to the Pappenheim family. . . . (Rosenbaum and Muroff, 1984, p. 5)

The case of Anna O. led Freud to the exploration of the vital role of unconscious processes and to an understanding of how "neurotic symptoms will disappear when the unconscious cause or causes are permitted to come to awareness" (Rosenbaum and Muroff, 1984, p. 11). Anna O.'s discovery of the "talking cure" led to Freud's development of the use of free association in treatment. Freud did not "discover" the unconscious; earlier philosophers and writers, including Descartes, Goethe, Schiller, Coleridge, Words- worth, Leibnitz, and Schopenhauer had described aspects of the unconscious (Rosenbaum and Muroff, 1984). Shakespeare also wrote of deep inner forces and understood that dreams had power and meaning. However, Breuer and Freud "originated . . . the first systematic study of the unconscious. Freud applied his scientific training so that he could study the irrational and unconscious and make it rational and conscious" (Rosenbaum and Muroff, 1984, p. 11).

The Anna O. case highlights some of the enduring contributions of psychoanalysis, including the power of the unconscious, the appearance of repressed conflicts in neurotic symptom formation, and the therapeutic utilization of dreams. It also highlights the importance of *transference* and *countertransference* issues, although, at that time, these were not well understood. Breuer did not see Anna O. in his office; he came to her home for treatment, at times twice daily. Bertha indicated that he was the "only one who could feed, understand, console, or help her. There was a considerable amount of touching—she recognized him at times by touching him; he gave her massages" (Swenson, 1994, p. 157). Breuer "abandoned" Anna O. abruptly, as her father had abandoned her by dying. Both Anna O. and Breuer were young, attractive people. The feelings that were stirred toward each other (and by each other) were never addressed, and the fact that Anna O. had transferred some of her love and sexualized feelings for her father onto Breuer were not understood by him, although later, when hearing about the case, Freud did understand this.

Drive Theory

Anna O. affords us a glimpse into the "subterranean" world of feelings so deep and so powerful that they can overpower the intellect and the body as well as alter behavior. Freud stressed the importance of instinctual forces in the development of the personality, emphasizing the role of the drives of sexuality (libido) and aggression. "The psychological theories which Freud developed were always physiologically oriented as far as it was possible for them to be so" (Brenner, 1974, p. 15). Although some psychodynamic theorists today dismiss Freud's emphasis on the primacy of sexuality and/or aggression in psychological development, the concept of the intensity of drives and feelings has been expanded and transposed to other areas of development, such as the innate drive for attachment. If looked at in this broader perspective, we can observe intense feelings become driving forces which fuel (with psychic energy) human motivation and behavior. Basch (1988) has referred to affect as *"the gateway to action"* (p. 65).

If a drive or need, such as sexuality or attachment, is not met by an external agency, for example, nurturance, love, or by the executor actions of the individual independently, the energies of drives or needs and their associated affects (feelings) seek gratification or satisfaction through substitute means.

> A social work student was assigned the case of Joan, a young, unmarried, overwhelmed, and neglectful mother who took little interest in her child. The student built a positive relationship with Joan, connected her with appropriate community resources, enabled her to return to school, and helped her feel more competent. Joan continued to show no interest in her child and could not bond with her. She cognitively reexamined her life goals and felt it was in the baby's best interest as well as her own to give this child up for adoption. Shortly after the adoption was finalized, the woman became pregnant again.

We can hypothesize that Joan, deprived of adequate maternal nurturing herself, had a deep unmet need to be nurtured, to feel "full" and "not empty," and was seeking a special connectedness that she never experienced and did not know how to re-create. Her strong affective, or drive-directed need to become pregnant again was stronger than her cognitive understanding of the present inappropriateness of motherhood for her. Joan's behaviors are familiar to child welfare workers who see mothers with similar attachment conflicts.

Freud analyzed childhood development in terms of age-related drives and the means of their gratification as playing a dominant role in the psychological development of the child. Every child, for example, passes through the *oral stage,* where the needs for eating and sucking predominate; if these needs are not met, problems, such as thumb sucking or overeating, needing immediate gratification, and becoming chronically dependent may develop and continue throughout life. Freud's "psychosexual drive theory synthesized the concept of children's erogenous zones as being associated with the kinds of relationships, attachments, symptoms, character traits, and psychological preoccupations they face at each stage of development" (Berzoff, 1996b, p. 29). The five developmental stages Freud discussed are: the *oral phase* of infancy, the *anal phase* of toddlers, the *oedipal phase* of the preschool child, the *latency phase* of the school-age child, and the *genital phase* of adolescence. These stages are discussed in Chapters 8 and 9 on childhood development.

The *id,* the repository of instinctual feelings, drives, and needs, is a dynamic force that presses to be discharged. The id does not concern itself with reality; a timelessness, a rulelessness, and a peremptory quality exists in the id. The id, however, does not exist in isolation but is part of a larger psychological system including the *ego* and the *superego,* postulated by the *structural theory,* which will now be addressed.

Structural Theory

Structural theory explains how drives are expressed and mediated and how conflict between drives and expectations of the external world are resolved. Examining the Latin meanings of the three key mental structures we find: the id means "it," suggesting the primal, given engine of behavior; the ego means "I," suggesting the notion of the executor self; and the superego means "the higher ego." The id "comprises the psychic representatives of the drives, the ego consists of those functions which have to do with the individual's relation to his environment, and the superego comprises the moral precepts of our minds as well as our ideal aspirations" (Brenner, 1974, p. 35).

The ego and the id can have a cooperative relationship, as the ego deals with the environment "for the purpose of achieving a maximum of gratification or discharge for the id . . . the ego is the *executant* for the drives" (Brenner, 1974, p. 37). However, the id, ego, and superego may come into conflict both as a normal, manageable phenomenon or as a disruptive one.

If we reexamine the Anna O. case from this perspective, we can see that her deep feelings related to her attachment to her father as well as conflict about nursing him might not have been acceptable to her superego (or conscience). The "war" between these segments of her psychic apparatus was too strong for the ego to mediate; the result was symptom formation, in which the conflict (and the underlying wishes) are expressed in a substitute (albeit uncomfortable and dysfunctional) manner. When some of her conflict is resolved through the "talking cure," the symptoms abate. In everyday life, we continually deal with conflicts between our wishes, our reality, and the "rules" we must live by; we usually handle these conflicts with the help of our *defense mechanisms,* which operate predominantly on an unconscious level. We shall return to the defense mechanisms in the next section.

Distinctive types of thought processes are associated with the id and the ego. *Primary process* thinking is associated with the id; *secondary process* thinking refers to the ego. In reading this book, you are engaging in structured secondary process thinking as you attempt to comprehend the ideas and to integrate your understanding with other learning and life experiences. Secondary process thinking is "ordinary, conscious thinking as we know it from introspection, that is, primarily verbal and following the usual laws of syntax and logic" (Brenner, 1974, p. 48). Primary process thinking relates to the id, and its representations are those of the instinctual life. Logic, the constraints of time, and the need for consistency are not relevant in primary process thought. Artists may gain inspiration for their painting through primary process mechanisms, but in order to execute the painting they must purposefully and coherently apply secondary thought processes to obtain the needed materials, decide on colors, brushes, composition, subject matter, etc.

Primary thought processes are often manifested in serious mental illness in which break down in formal thought processes and content, and a serious break with reality takes place. However, primary process thinking is not per se pathological. Developmentally it tends to color the thinking of young children. In waking thought, it gradually comes more and more under the influence of secondary process (verbal, logical thought). A schizophrenic patient may have no sense of time in a realistic sense, but this is also true of the young child. "It is several years before a child develops a sense of time, before there is anything comprehensible to him but the 'here and now' " (Brenner, 1974, p. 49). The presence of primary process thinking does not in itself indicate mental illness; "it is the dominance or exclusive operation of the primary process that constitutes an abnormality when it occurs in adult life" (Brenner, 1974, p. 49). An excellent example of the pairing of both types of thinking is found in dreams, with daydreams as an intermediate form.

Dreams

The interpretation of dreams was and remains an essential part of the psychoanalytic process. Freud (1959) wrote that "psychoanalysis is founded upon the analysis of dreams; the interpretation of dreams is the most complete piece of work the young science has done up to the present" (p. 28). Dreams allow the repressed thoughts and affects (in disguised form) into consciousness while in the dream state, as sleep tends to "produce a relative weakening of the defenses" (Brenner, 1974, p. 166), as well as a paralysis of action. Freud (1959) has described the state of sleep.

> We are not accustomed to expend much thought on the fact that every night human beings lay aside the garments they pull over their skin, and even also other objects which they use to supplement their bodily organs . . . for instance their spectacles, false hair or teeth, and so on. In addition to this, when they go to sleep they perform a perfectly analogous dismantling of their minds—they lay aside most of their mental acquisitions. . . . The feature characterizing the mind of a sleeping person is an almost complete withdrawal from the surrounding world and the cessation of all interest in it. (Freud, 1959, p. 28)

Dreams have both *latent* and *manifest* content. The manifest content is the story of the dream, those aspects that the dreamer may be able to recall. The latent content is the "unconscious thoughts and wishes which threaten to waken the dreamer" (Brenner, 1972, p. 150). The unconscious mental processes "by which the latent dream content is transformed into the manifest dream we call the *dreamwork*" (Brenner, 1974, p. 150).

The following dream was related to me in a personal communication.

> A young woman reported a dream in which she was putting her bicycle inside her coat (the manifest content). Upon awakening, she was quite puzzled by her actions in the dream. "But why my bicycle?" Suddenly, in a flash memory, she recalled that she used to refer to her bicycle as her "baby" (latent content). She realized that a meaning of the dream was that she was wishing for a baby *(dream work),* which she could acknowledge as a true desire.

In the following case, utilizing play therapy with an eight-year-old boy, *fantasy* and *dreams* were significantly pertinent to the treatment (Barton and Marshall, 1986). The case, recorded by two social workers, emphasizes the impact of termination on a child. The termination phase led to him revealing new material about past trauma, which he shared before "it was too late."

Brian's parents divorced when he was three; he remained with his mother under very chaotic and neglectful circumstances. His father, now remarried, was seeking legal custody of Brian. Brian was initially seen with "disturbances in sleeping, eating and toileting, excessive clinging, and distractibility at school" (Barton and Marshall, 1986, p. 141). Play therapy with Brian and family work with his father and stepmother were undertaken. A number of themes appeared in the early phase of Brian's treatment. These "involved fears of annihilation, abandonment, and the fusion of generational boundaries" (Barton and Marshall, 1986, p. 142). They suggest that Brian "was also concerned with issues of self esteem, his worth and integrity as an autonomous individual, and his believability" (p. 142).

> One extended fantasy involved Brian being pursued by a faceless man who pushed him off the Washington Monument into a pond of hungry sharks. When the President and a policeman appeared, they were more concerned with locating the culprit than with rescuing Brian. Brian was disinclined to draw their attention to him since "their backs are turned, they can't see me and they don't care anyway." (Barton and Marshall, 1986, p. 142)

Brian made very good progress during his eight months of treatment, and two months were used in preparation for termination. During the termination phase, Brian reported a bad dream that involved "a glove reaching up from the bed and pulling him into a black, bottomless hole. . . . Brian associated to times in his biological mother's household when he had experienced the same nightmare" (Barton and Marshall, 1986, p. 144). Brian's play enactments and discussion of more fantasy material led to the revelation of his sexual abuse by his mother, her boyfriend, and "all former household members" (p. 145). In the following passage, veiled hints of abuse are symbolically represented in the fantasy material.

> Utilizing anatomically correct dolls . . . the boyfriend was described [by Brian] as "gay" and was manipulated to make seductive-assaultive gestures in attempts to quiet the frightened boy doll. . . . The adult male doll, dressed in women's underwear, chased the boy doll out the window into a tree, from which the adult fell into a pond of hungry dolphins, and was jailed. . . . With a pair of scissors [Brian] made stabbing motions at the genitalia of the adult male doll, then at his own genitals. Finally, he cut a lock of his own hair, then the corners of a calendar on which [his therapist] had marked the date of their last session.
>
> Th[is] fantasy . . . was a symbolic reformulation of Brian's fantasy with the Washington monument and the sharks. This time, however, anger was directed not towards the self, but more appropriately toward

the object of his anxiety: the boyfriend was victimized and punished. . . . In addition, Brian's subliminal manipulation of the scissors was interpreted . . . as the signs and symptoms of the type of unresolved intrapsychic conflict which is typical of sexual abuse. (Barton and Marshall, 1986, pp. 144-145)

The clinician's knowledge of Freud's contributions led to the understanding of the anxiety, unconscious fantasy, symbolic content of dreams, and internalization of guilt (blaming the self), which are all present here. The utilization of these fantasies within the context of Brian's life led the clinician to help Brian disclose the abuse and helped him and his father to cope with the trauma.

Today, some clinicians work actively with dreams; others dismiss them as irrelevant and/or unscientific (they are not "observable" behaviors). Some practitioners with a strong biological orientation assert that dreams are only a manifestation of REM brain activity found in sleep and have no other meaning. Some psychodynamically trained clinicians use the method of *free association* to understand the unconscious meaning of dreams; other clinicians may use dream interpretation in a modified form.

Sackheim (1974), a social worker, advocates the use of dreams in casework treatment, noting that "like any other life experience, they admit of interpretation on varying levels" (Sackheim, 1974, p. 29). Catalano (1990) uses children's dreams in his clinical social work practice. Research has provided "insight into the dreams of children and adolescents with emotional disturbances and how they differ from those without such disturbances. . . . Dreams provide a wealth of useful material about the issues, feelings, and memories most important to the child" (Catalano, 1990, p. 139).

Discussion

Looking at dreams and other unconscious mental processes beneath the surface of human behavior can be overwhelming and frightening to some; it is more comfortable to explore surface issues exclusively.

This agitation of the "sleep of mankind" (Gay, 1988, p. xvii) is one of the most insurmountable sources of resistance to Freudian thought. Further complicating this picture of resistance to Freud was the resistance *by* Freud and his inner circle to deviations from orthodox theory, a kind of fortress mentality. Although Freud revised his theory as he deemed necessary based on *his* new insights, he did not welcome serious disagreement from his followers. Many bitter and acrimonious intellectual and personal disputes followed and led to the establishment of divergent schools of thought by such disciples as Jung, Adler, and Rank. Tensions have existed among theoreticians of human behavior since the time of Freud, including both external battles between those of competing theories, such as between behaviorists and psychodynamic practitioners, as well as internal battles among adherents of the same school.

The intensity of the theoretical wars tended to keep adherents of the various psychoanalytic approaches from seeing the commonalities of their ideas (Mitchell, 1988). These conflicts also kept disciples of competing approaches from seeing how their differences might complement each other.

Psychoanalysis seems to have lost much of its influence today. Goode (1999d) notes that analysts are currently on the sidelines of an arena in which pharmacotherapy and "short-term talking therapies predominate" (p. D1).

However, the profession has responded with a renewed vitality and a willingness to deal with change. One now finds "only an occasional . . . nostalgia . . . [and] the threat of extinction has inspired . . . self-examination and the urge to . . . connect with the world at large" (Goode, 1999d, p. D1). Additionally, "a retrofitted psychoanalysis . . . [has become] more tolerant . . . [and] orthodoxy . . . has gradually given way to a gentler theoretical pluralism" (Goode, 1999d, p. D1). Social workers are among the nonmedical applicants "flocking" to analytic institutes (Sanville, 1994, p. 131).

We will now turn our attention to a very important outgrowth of psychoanalytic theory: Heinz Hartmann's ego psychology.

EGO PSYCHOLOGY

The ego is that portion of personality structure that, in Freud's basic conceptualization, mediates between the id (the unconscious contents of the mind and drives), and the superego (the conscience). Heinz Hartmann (1958), the "father of ego psychology," developed and expanded the Freudian concept of the ego to focus on its nonpathological interaction with and adaptation to the external world as well as the internal realm. He defined adaptation as "primarily a reciprocal relationship between the organism and its environment" (Hartmann, 1958, p. 24).

Hartmann (1958) did not dispute the notion of the ego as a mediator of conflicts; however, his interest in development was broader than the study of intrapsychic conflict. He asserted that "not every adaptation to the environment, or every learning and maturation process, is a conflict" (p. 8). It was his proposal that "we adopt the provisional term *conflict-free ego sphere* for that ensemble of functions which at any given time exert their effects outside the region of mental conflicts" (Hartmann, 1958, pp. 8-9). Hartmann describes these maturational processes:

I refer to the development *outside of conflict* of perception, intention, object comprehension, thinking, language, recall-phenomena, productivity, to the well-known phases of motor development, grasping, crawling, walking, and to the maturation and learning processes implicit in all these and many others. (Hartmann, 1958, p. 8)

These [autonomous] ego functions develop as they meet the "average expectable environmental conditions" (Hartmann, 1958, p. 46) and require such an environment to thrive. This is analogous to the development of a flower. Assuming that the seeds are "good" and not "damaged," a plant will grow, develop roots, buds, a flower, etc., but only if the environmental conditions of soil, sunshine, and water are propitious. On the other hand, as we shall discover, when "the average expectable environment" is not present, as when an infant raised in an orphanage does not receive adequate nurturing, the ego apparatuses will not mature; developmental landmarks of walking, language, logical thought, etc., might be extremely delayed and distorted.

The notion of the ego embodies the capacity to integrate and synthesize external and internal reality, "past and present," and ideas and feelings (Vaillant, 1993, p. 7). The ego encompasses adaptation, mental synthesis, defensive operations, and "adult development and creativity" (Vaillant, 1993, p. 8). The primary ego functions will be discussed in detail now, followed by a section on ego defenses.

Ego Functions

Classifications of ego functions vary from author to author; Upham's (1973) classification of seven ego functions is utilized in this discussion:

1. Perception
2. The cognitive function
3. The management of drives, needs, and feelings
4. The management of object relationships
5. The executive function
6. The integrative function
7. Ego identity

In practice, it is important to assess the baseline of a given ego function, which means looking at the person's past attainment of a specific function prior to the present evaluation.

The ego is more than the summation of these seven functions. "Contemporary ego psychologists assume that the ego has successfully accomplished its organizing and synthesizing functions when individuals experience themselves as coherent, functional human beings with an enduring sense of personal identity" (Schamess, 1996, p. 70). Individuals can have uneven patterns of ego functioning, in which one ego function—for instance, perception—may be well developed, whereas identity formation might be shaky. "A working understanding of ego functions is enormously helpful both in evaluating client's strengths and weaknesses, and in predicting how they are likely to respond to different therapeutic interventions" (Schamess, 1996, p. 71).

Perception

Outer perception is concerned with the ability to perceive the world in a realistic manner; *inner perception* refers to the capacity to turn attention inward and to observe one's feelings and motivations (Upham, 1973).

Outer perception. People have attained good outer perception when they are able to orient themselves to "reality," to the "social world" surrounding them, especially to "human relationships," and can view their concerns, circumstances, and the people they relate to "in a reasonably realistic way without significant distortion" (Upham, 1973, p. 123). *Reality testing* "differentiates cues coming from within from those which come from external reality. It prevents assigning [one's] own ideas and feelings to sources outside of [one's] self" (Upham, 1973, p. 122). If a man will not enter a store because he is convinced everyone inside is spying on him, we might speculate that he has a serious problem with reality testing (unless he is indeed under surveillance).

An example from practice: Ms. O'Toole had difficulty distinguishing between her internal feelings and wishes, on one hand, and reality, on the other.

> Ms. O'Toole told her therapist that she had killed her neighbor. She hated this man who was very mean and wished he would die. Shortly afterward, he died; she was convinced she had murdered him because of her strong wishes. Her therapist, Mrs. Wendorer said, "Suppose I did not feel like coming to work today and wished it would snow. If it started to snow, did I do that?" Ms. O'Toole looked at her therapist, smiled, and said: "Oh, you are funny, Mrs. Wendover." The therapist was explicitly using the function of reality testing to help Ms. O'Toole realize that she was not omnipotent enough to cause her neighbor's death through her thoughts.

It is not uncommon for people to feel guilty about bad wishes toward others that later become actual in some independent way, but it is less common for individuals to be convinced that they were perpetrators of this reality.

This is an example of *magical thinking,* which Piaget (Elkind, 1981) finds universally present in early childhood but which is largely modified in essentially normal individuals by continual retesting of reality. Persistence of fixed magical thinking along especially absurd lines is characteristic of abnormal mental states.

Although perhaps not manifesting serious difficulties with reality testing, people can have problems with outer perception, sometimes *chronic,* sometimes *situational.* People witnessing a car accident might report differing perceptions of what happened, distorted by their anxiety. Family members involved in conflict might not accurately perceive each other's intentions or messages.

> Sarah was expressing anger with her husband because of his inattentiveness. She thought that he was being particularly unfair because he would not let her buy a new pair of shoes. Her therapist asked if she had told him she wanted new shoes. Oh, no, she replied, he should have known—he should have asked!

Sarah expected her husband to be able to read her mind—another form of primitive or magical thinking.

Connoisseurs of detective literature realize the importance of gathering the "facts," the relevant descriptive details of interactions and time sequences—rather than suppositions that are then regarded as facts.

Clinicians must distinguish their own perceptions, prejudices, and biases, which may color their assessment of the client's perceptions, from ascertainable facts. Cultural contexts should likewise be considered, as clients may be perceiving certain events and relationships in ways shaped by their culture—which may not be readily understood by a clinician who is an outsider to that culture.

Inner perception. Inner perception enables people to observe and reflect on themselves and their feelings, as well as on "the related awareness of the effect of their own urges, feelings, and activities on other persons" (Upham, 1973, p. 122).

In training social work students, the attainment of self-awareness is a highly valued goal. For example, Jane, an MSW student, realized through supervisory discussion that she tended to "push" her client away because she felt threatened by the hostile feelings the client expressed toward her. In this realization, Jane reveals a good capacity for inner perception (and, correspondingly, to utilize social work training).

Clients too may develop increased self-awareness or inner perception through the therapeutic process.

Jessica reported the following incident to her therapist: A friend who had moved to Europe visited Jessica after many years of absence. After several happy days together, the friend returned to Europe, and Jessica felt sad and cried, not knowing when she would see her friend again. At the same time, Jessica was joyful as she told of her sadness. She was happy that she had experienced her sadness; in the past, she would not have known she was sad—a black wave of depression would have descended upon her instead.

The Cognitive Functions

Cognitive functions encompass capacities such as thinking, remembering, using language, planning, problem solving, and making judgments.

A person may have had a baseline of good cognitive functioning that has become temporarily diminished due to extreme stress, serious physical illness, or emotional turmoil. "Clinicians base their assessment of cognitive capacity: 1) on the client's ability to present a clear and coherent picture of his difficulty and to respond appropriately to the practitioner's verbal communication, and 2) on evidences of previous levels of development" (Upham, 1973, p. 128).

Alzheimer's disease, affecting older adults, seriously impairs memory and leads to a general decline of cognitive functions. Strokes can have a major impact on cognitive functioning, destroying centers of the brain involved with thinking, information processing, and communicating. Severe alcoholism can permanently damage brain tissue.

People with mental retardation may have cognitive deficits, but, on the other hand, severely "limited understanding and ability to communicate" may be aggravated "by the widespread under-estimation by others of their capacity to learn and to make choices and participate in decision making" (Mittler, 1992, p. 163).

People with various problems, including attention deficit disorder, learning disabilities, or chronic dependent characterological issues may have difficulty thinking through situations and understanding both causes and effects of behavior and may not have acquired successful problem-solving techniques. They may need help thinking through problems and solutions to them.

Some people persistently use poor judgment in situations, as we can observe in the following account of Mr. Morgan.

Mr. Morgan had not been employed for a year and was eager to obtain a job offered to him. He arrived half an hour late for his interview because he stopped to buy some lottery tickets and, although there was a line, he thought that if he could win the lottery, a lot of his problems would be solved. When he was questioned about being late, he insulted the interviewer because he felt the man had no right to question him about his use of time. He launched into a tirade about the importance of lottery tickets and how winning one was a much better way of living than sweating over a bum forty-hour-a-week job with lousy pay. Mr. Morgan did not receive this position and complained to his friends about the injustices of the world. Mr. Morgan has an impaired capacity to assess cause and effect and to use sound judgment. He has limited capacity for inner perception in terms of self-reflection and seeing his effect on others.

Cognitive functions are typically impaired and distorted in psychotic states. A major diagnostic sign of schizophrenia is a thought disorder, a gross impairment in thinking capacity. Patients may exhibit problems in their content of thought (what they are thinking about) and in their thought process (or forms and coherence of thought). A man with a delusion that he is Napoleon is having a problem in his content of thought; if challenged he may also demonstrate illogic in arguing the basis for this belief. If he has racing thoughts or thought blocking, he would be having difficulty with the process of thought (Kaplan et al., 1994).

Basic logic is regularly impaired by the schizophrenic process; the individual suffering from schizophrenia tends to regress to a lower level of logicality. "Schizophrenic cognition in some aspects corresponds to the primary process of the Freudian school" (Arieti, 1974, p. 571). The logic often used is "paleologic, based on a principle enunciated by von Domarus" (Arieti, 1974, p. 574). For instance, a patient might argue: "All deer are swift. All marathon runners are swift. Therefore, all deer are marathon runners." This is termed identification through the predicate (which refers to finding similarities in the characteristics of the subject). *"Whereas the normal person accepts identity only upon the basis of identical subjects, the paleologician accepts identity based upon identical predicates"* (Arieti, 1974, p. 574). By applying von Domarus's principle, "even bizarre and complex schizophrenic delusions can be interpreted" (Arieti, 1974, p. 575). In other words, meaning and "logic" exist beneath thought processes that, on the surface, appear totally meaningless and illogical.

People may have a basic capacity for cognitive functioning but show faulty reasoning, such as having a self-defeating way of thinking of themselves or reasoning about certain emotionally charged situations in nonproductive ways. Cognitive therapy (discussed in the following chapter) was developed as a method for correcting the faulty thinking that may be the basis for dysfunctional attitudes, feeling states, and behavior (Beck, 1976).

In summation, assessment of cognitive functioning can guide a therapist in deciding what level of treatment might be appropriate and which limitations in thinking, appraising, and judging must be taken into account in selecting a treatment approach or which can possibly be strengthened. Clinicians should consider differences in education, culture, and language in appraising a person's cognitive functioning.

Management of Needs and Feelings

Managing one's needs and feelings involves the capacity to recognize what one is feeling and to recognize and accept one's emotional needs while meeting these needs in a realistic and socially appropriate way. It "include[s] the capacity to tolerate frustration, to postpone gratification, to find substitute gratifications, to find detour routes to satisfaction when a given route is blocked, to reconcile and synthesize conflicting needs, feelings, or aims, and to handle related feelings" (Upham, 1973, p. 131). In discussing Mrs. Billings in the last chapter, we noted that anhedonia, the inability to experience pleasure, was one of her depressive symptoms, as well as an entrenched personality feature. Mrs. Billings had a severe inhibition of both aggressive and pleasurable feelings and an abundance of superego guilt. This suggests major disturbances in the management of needs and feelings.

In discussing the related concept of *autonomous gratification,* Arieti and Bemporad (1978) refer to people's ability to obtain "self-esteem or pleasure through their own efforts" (p. 166). For example, when a client spoke of her delight in drinking a cup of coffee each morning at the window while she watched the boats glide past on the water, she demonstrated her love of life and her capacity for *autonomous gratification.* Arieti and Bemporad assert that the inability to experience this gratification as well as the driven need to gain self-esteem through the approval of others (the dominant other) is related to the development of the depressive state, as seen in their case illustration below.

Nancy, a highly successful executive who began psychotherapy after years of visiting internists with vague pains and insomnia, exemplified this fear of autonomous gratification. Although she . . . made an attractive salary, she could not bring herself to furnish her apartment comfortably or live in a manner commensurate with her income. She considered anything spent on herself to be a shameful extravagance, but would buy inordinately expensive gifts for her parents. Nancy was equally self-sacrificing with her free time and canceled social engagements if her boss asked her to work late or if her father asked to see her. In actuality Nancy was unable to enjoy a social evening unless she could somehow relate it to her work. . . . She found it difficult to date and dreaded sexual confrontation. . . . Eventually Nancy confessed that even her work, which seemed to be her major concern in life, brought her no pleasure in itself but only served as a means of pleasing her boss. Whenever she gained recognition from him or when she was praised by her father, Nancy become ecstatic with a great sense of well-being and felt vibrant and alive. (Arieti and Bemporad, 1978, p. 166)

Related to autonomous gratification is the capacity to *self-soothe:* to be able to console or comfort oneself not only when life is comfortable but during times of stress as well. This behavior is described as being good to oneself or permitting oneself to feel better. Listening to music, painting, gardening, and taking a warm bath are examples of what some people do to soothe themselves when under stress.

Some choose methods of self-soothing that may be maladaptive, such as excessive drinking. Others, including borderline personalities who do not have the capacity to self-soothe, need selfobjects (dependence on others to meet unmet emotional needs) to provide this relief (Adler, 1985). When this is not available, they are "faced with the ultimate threat of disintegrative annihilation of the self" (Adler, 1985, p. 34).

Borderline personalities also lack inhibition of feelings and may express anger explosively; they have difficulty with impulse control. Many people other than borderline personalities may also have difficulty controlling and directing their feelings in adaptive ways. Freud commented that " 'the postponement of gratification is the hallmark of maturity' " (Vaillant, 1993, p. 70).

In assessing the baseline of impulse control, we explore whether chronic problems have been present (such as a pattern of violence or perpetrating sexual abuse) or a new behavior, perhaps reactive to situational stress, has appeared. People may lose control when intoxicated; sometimes loss of control may be related to a neurological disorder. Kaplan and colleagues (1994) refer to assessment of impulse control as part of the mental status exam to determine the patient's sense of social appropriateness and possible dangerousness. Cognitive disturbances, psychoses, and chronic characterological defects may impair impulse control, which may be assessed in the interview from current history and observed behavior.

People can become flooded with feelings of anxiety that they are unable to control—sometimes in response to a crisis, sometimes as part of an ongoing anxiety state. Many people suffer from problems with anxiety, including panic disorders, in which they can temporarily be so overcome with anxiety that they may feel "out of control" and unable to function.

Management of needs and feelings is a critical area to assess and covers the wide range of issues previously alluded to.

The Management of Object Relationships

The individual's capacity to relate to others and the quality and patterns of these relationships are important aspects of ego functioning. "It is the single most important function of the ego because it enables the child to become human" (Upham, 1973, p. 139). Noam and Fischer (1996) comment that "people are fundamentally social, and relationships . . . especially close ones, form an essential foundation for the development of human beings, molding each person's mind and behavior" (p. ix). The importance of early relationships for attachment and trust has been widely recognized (Bowlby, 1988; Kohut, 1971; Mahler et al., 1975; Mitchell, 1988; Winnicott, 1965), although some disagreement exists about how permanent the effects of these early interactions are, and how later events and relationships may modify early patterns. Mitchell (1988) argues for the importance of understanding past experiences not because "the past lies concealed within or beneath the present, but because understanding *the past provides clues to deciphering how and why the present is being approached and shaped the way it is*" [italics added](p. 149).

Many writers, particularly those with a psychodynamic orientation, stress the importance of parental nurturance, warmth, acceptance, the development of secure attachment, and the provision of a "holding environment" (Winnicott, 1965) for the development of good adaptation and mental health. The ego functions will flourish in the "average expectable environment" (Hartmann, 1958). However, growth and development are not without conflict even under optimal conditions. Normal conflict is inherent in separation and individuation (Mahler et al., 1975), since as Mitchell (1988) asserts, "Being a self with others entails a constant dialectic between attachment and self-definition, between connection and differentiation, a continual negotiation between one's wishes and will and the wishes and will of others" (Mitchell, 1988, p. 149).

Close relationships within the family and with others can also be a source of great distress (Noam and Fischer, 1996). "The most extreme example . . . is maltreatment, including the injuries of physical abuse and the boundary transgressions of sexual abuse. . . . Developmental consequences can be devastating" (Noam and Fischer, 1996, p. xii). Daily events much less conspicuously severe than these can also produce serious consequences. "It is the day-to-day conflicts and small abandonments, the chronic sense of not being listened to that often create long-lasting effects" (Noam and Fischer, 1996, p. xii).

Object relations theory, to which we shall return in the next chapter, offers many insights into the development and complexity of human relationships. Cultural factors can also affect patterns of relationships.

Executive Functioning

The executive function of the ego involves the ability to carry out everyday goal-directed activities. "This function makes it possible to decide and to act effectively and in ways which demonstrate social competence" (Upham, 1973, p. 142). Social workers may assess the executive functioning of clients to determine if they can care for themselves or their families. For example, an elderly woman, living alone, may at times appear confused but upon assessment is found to be capable of shopping, cooking, and caring for herself and her apartment. Her executive functioning appears adequate to warrant her living independently without the need for protective services, although at a later date she may consider assisted living arrangements.

A person with a baseline of excellent executive functioning may be temporarily incapacitated due to illness or extreme stress. "Anxiety caused by stress, trauma, or hopelessness and discouragement may interfere with the client's use of previously adequate patterning of executant ability. He may seem immobilized" (Upham, 1973, p. 144). On the other hand, some clients may have a history of poor executive functioning, such as the schizophrenic patient who may need long-term external supports, including a day program and job training, to support executive functioning. A person with temporarily impaired executive functioning due to anxiety or stress may also need some type of external supports, although probably only on a short-term basis.

Overwhelmed parents, unable to cope adequately with the needs of their children, may be responsive to supportive services offered (which may be thought of acting as auxiliary executive ego functions).

> Mrs. Kramer, an African-American woman, lived on the fifteenth floor of a housing project with her husband and ten children. She was overwhelmed by life and her large family. She rarely went outside as she had no carriage for the baby, and taking her family downstairs in the elevator was too stressful. Children ran pell-mell over the small apartment; little goal-directed activity or play material existed. The children were all well fed, adequately clothed, and attended school, and no evidence existed of either physical abuse or serious neglect.
>
> Mrs. Kramer was very responsive to the supportive services offered by a social worker and a homemaker. The homemaker did not "take over" and do things for her but involved her in working out a realistic schedule and engaging in household activities together. The older children were enrolled in after-school activities, the younger ones in preschool programs. Mrs. Kramer began to go outside. When Mrs. Kramer gave birth to her eleventh child, she decided to have a tubal ligation. When the case was terminated, Mrs. Kramer and her family had achieved an overall higher level of executive functioning.

The Integrative Function

The active but often unnoticed process of integration occurs when social work students apply classroom learning by recalling a concept from class when working with clients. Integration is the "act of bringing together the parts into an integral whole. . . . The singleness of individual parts remains a characteristic of the mind during the greater part of the infantile period. . . . Gradually . . . the individual parts begin to act in cooperation with one another. It is the harmonizing of separate parts that is called integration" (Campbell, 1989, p. 377). The ability to "learn and to integrate new patterns into ego functioning exemplifies the integrative or synthetic function" (Upham, 1973, p. 146). The capacity to *integrate* implies that a person can "flexibly learn and adaptively change his behavior patterns to fit reality. He can then integrate these patterns into his total functioning" (Upham, 1973, p. 147).

Each social work student usually finds that his or her ways of intervening with people are modified gradually, and a professional self evolves, without the individual necessarily realizing that his or her integrative capacity has been developing. A student, for example, may initially react to a client's acting-out behavior with anger but gradually, while being aware of feeling angered by a client's behavior, will not retaliate with anger; instead, the student develops a deeper understanding of the sources of the client's anger as well as a greater responsiveness to the client's feelings.

The capacity for integration underlies a person's ability to utilize therapy for gaining insight and learning new coping skills. Some clients may show good intellectual understanding of their issues but lack the integrative capacity to translate their understanding into change. Others may appear to be making no changes but, through a slow process, often imperceptible, suddenly feel "everything is coming together." Integration is an elusive process.

Ann, a first year MSW student, was the volunteer subject of a study in which her learning and professional development were examined over the course of her first year of graduate social work school. One of the goals of the study was to gain a deeper understanding of the factors that contributed to her learning.

> One day in February, Ann came into my office with a good deal of animation and buoyancy. All seemed to be gong well: "Things are looking up . . . I received my grades and I have three A's . . . I feel better about myself . . . about school . . . about my placement. . . . Education can be fun!" Leaning forward expectantly, I asked: "What is making it work? What is happening?" And Ann answered: "I don't know!" . . . And yet, perhaps this very lack of clarity was indeed quite profound! Because what Ann was reporting was the experience of *integration*,

and indeed, true integration is often so profound that it leaves the person with a sense of the "inexplicable." (Urdang, 1974, p. 94)

Ego Identity

Ego identity encompasses the development of a sense of self, self-esteem, sexual identity, and physical identity (including such attributes as "beauty" or "disability") and may also contain elements of religious, cultural, racial, professional, and social group identities. The development of identity gives us our sense of not only "who we are, but *that* [italics added] we are" (Mahler et al., 1975, p. 8).

Object relations theory and self psychology stress the deeper-lying structure of self-identity, the vicissitudes of its development, and the attainment of self-cohesion. Upham (1973) asserts that "through the sense of identity, the individual integrates all of his ego functioning and achieves a feeling of wholeness and relatedness, both within himself and in respect to his place in society" (p. 148).

By examining the baseline of a person's sense of identity, we can begin to determine if we are looking at a person with a long-standing stable pattern of self-identity who has currently regressed, or if a chronically unstable pattern is the case. Many types of traumatic experiences "may disturb a previously well-formed identity" (Upham, 1973, p. 150). Certain losses, such as going through an unwanted divorce or living in a dysfunctional relationship, can affect one's sense of identity. "Loss of a sexual organ or bodily part changes body and self-image from intact and reliable to damaged and unreliable" (Upham, 1973, p. 150).

Members of minorities may continually experience discrimination and rejection to the degree that "their sense of self worth is more or less constantly assaulted . . . there is . . . cumulative impact of chronic narcissistic injury caused by poverty, emotional neglect, environmental violence, and inferior status in society" (Pérez Foster et al., 1996, p. xv).

A strong relationship exists between ego identity and the development of object relationships, as the sense of self develops in relation to the nurturing received and "messages" conveyed about self that come from the family and other significant others. Children must separate from but concurrently remain attached to the family and distinguish themselves as separate from others. Some may never fully develop a sense of an autonomous self but remain perpetually dependent on another (sometimes termed the dominant other or selfobject) for self-esteem needs.

People with a strong sense of ego identity can differentiate themselves from others, and therefore are said to have good ego boundaries. They can feel they are separate from another in the sense of being a distinct personality as opposed to merging with another—in effect, being lost as a separate individual or, to use earlier terminology, be "swallowed up" by the other. People with distinct and stable ego boundaries can tell the difference between what is "inside" and what is "outside" themselves and can differentiate what they feel from what others are feeling.

Mark Vonnegut (1975) experienced a severe schizophrenic episode after his graduation from Swarthmore College and his move to a commune in British Columbia. After his recovery, he wrote a very sensitive and insightful autobiography describing his experiences with this illness. Slipping into a psychotic world was a very frightening experience; his sense of reality as well as his sense of self became very confused, diffuse, and unreliable. He wondered if a part of him was attempting to hypnotize himself day and night by repeating the idiosyncratic phrase: "Is the tea in the tongue or in the leaves?" The boundaries between his self and others were so porous that he feared that others would go down into his psychosis with him. Speaking to his friend Simon, he said: "Sometimes I think I'm being hypnotized by compost. . . . I guess I'm afraid of losing control somehow and running amuck and so *if you could hypnotize me then you could control me and everything would be all right* [italics added]" (Vonnegut, 1975, p. 80).

Fluidity of identity boundaries can be a normal developmental phenomenon and challenge as well. Social work students may themselves face many professional boundary issues in their work with clients. Foster children may wish the clinician to become a replacement for their parents; but clinicians cannot simply adopt them or take them home. The professional-client boundary must be clear.

In an assessment of ego boundaries, a cultural perspective must be taken, as the processes and parameters of the delineation of appropriate boundaries and parental management of separation-individuation issues may vary among cultural groups.

Before leaving the subject of ego functioning, I will add two related concepts to the discussion: (1) strengths and competence, and (2) the superego and moral development.

Competence

Competence and mastery refer to a person's capacity to deal effectively with life and to experience a sense of accomplishment. White and Allport (Maluccio, 1980) stress the motivational importance of competence which " 'is an important force in human behavior' " (p. 285). In White's formulation, the major ingredients of competence are: " 'self-confidence, ability to make decisions, and trusting one's judgment. The ego is strengthened through the cumulative experience of producing desired effects upon one's surroundings' " (Maluccio, 1980, p. 284). Saleebey's (1992) strengths perspective is popular in current social work literature. Recognizing and supporting clients' strengths can promote their feelings of competence.

A child gains satisfaction from building a structure of blocks; a student is pleased with himself for passing a difficult examination; a woman is proud that she now has mastered the skills of driving—all are examples of the achievement of competence.

Clinical social workers aim to help clients gain greater competence in social functioning as well as to help them enjoy their achievements with enhanced perceptions of themselves as competent, adequate, and effective. A variety of therapeutic interventions, including environmental modifications, are used to achieve this; adjusting the environment can help people gain a sense of competence. For instance, providing wheelchair access enables some to master mobility in the world; special education, providing children with education appropriate to their needs, can help them achieve a sense of mastery, rather than failure. The ecological perspective stresses competence and goodness-of-fit between the person and the environment.

Linda Valli attended weekly psychotherapy sessions for anxiety and low self-esteem. In this encounter, her determination, recognized by the clinician, led Linda to discuss her strengths further.

> Linda commented that she was feeling better and making an effort to face herself more. She drove to the clinic (driving was initially anxiety provoking), deciding that "the dependency would make it worse." She also went to a large party Saturday and stayed after experiencing some initial anxiety, which disappeared in half an hour. When the therapist commented that Linda's actions seemed to demonstrate a lot of determination, she agreed and said that she had been determined to put herself through culinary school and had accomplished this. She worked nights to support herself through school.

In addition to supporting her existing strengths, examining her pain (such as grief over the loss of her mother), her negative feelings about herself, and her difficulty acknowledging aggressive feelings also helped her to develop feelings of competence and self-worth. Linda had a tendency to internalize her negative and painful feelings; if she were angry, it would be manifested in feelings of guilt as well as in her phobic symptoms. She felt her mother was angry with her before she died, and Linda regarded herself as bad and at fault. She never fully grieved for her mother; feelings of loss were not expressed but instead she experienced anxiety and inner constriction. If we fail to comprehend or respect the intensity of certain mental states as these, we cannot free the strengths from what enslaves them.

Developing ego strengths is one aspect of a general process that includes moral development as a component task (Vaillant, 1993, p. 116), which is discussed in the next section.

Moral Development

Superego and moral development refer to the development of a conscience, that is, the inner voice that reflects a sense of what is right and wrong and the development of values. Upham notes that the "core of moral character lies in the capacity to identify with another human being . . . to become able to empathize with other persons, and to feel remorse for transgressions against others" (Upham, 1973, p. 152). Freud introduced the concept of the ego ideal, which represents "those standards of behavior toward which we aspire" (Nemiah, 1961, p. 37). The ego ideal reflects positive, approving aspects of the superego, while the conscience reflects more the prohibitions of the superego, its negative or critical aspects.

An important distinction exists between guilt and shame. Guilt is concerned with internal matters that present conflict (within the internal mental system of) the individual and is thus an attitude of the self toward the self. Lewis Carroll was evidently tormented with brooding guilt as he struggled with his sexual attraction to prepubescent girls (Cohen, 1996).

Shame, on the other hand, is concerned more with how we feel others are perceiving us—whether we will lose face because of our actions. "Shame implies the failure of the ego to live up to an ego ideal and can result in the loss of self-esteem and depression . . . [it] contrasts with guilt, which is a transgression of the ego that conflicts with the superego" (Tang, 1997, p. 335). In Western or American culture, people might feel shame when being fired (or even "downsized") from a job, not graduating on time, having a physically handicapped or mentally ill relative, or when a mother has a child taken away because of a drinking problem. In China, which "values relationships above all else, it is not surprising that shame plays a more important role in shaping a child than guilt" (Tang, 1997, p. 335). People often try to defend themselves from the painful feelings of guilt and shame.

Vaillant (1993) has noted that the ego's "wisdom also encompasses defense" (p. 8), which is presented next.

Ego Defenses

Defenses are normal, healthy, and necessary for everyday functioning, protecting the self (ego) from experiencing anxiety and other forms of inner tension. The "defenses—like . . . immune mechanisms—protect us by providing a variety of illusions to filter pain and to allow self-soothing" (Vaillant, 1993, p. 1).

Ego defenses were first discussed by Freud, then elaborated by Anna Freud, and later expanded by object relations theorists. Freud's model of defenses stressed internal drives and feelings, seeking outlets in action, which the ego had to regulate and control. However, this model has subsequently been expanded to include the impact of outside forces and relationships that a person may need to defend against. The external as well as the internal may be perceived as threatening. "Thus the ego must control . . . desire, conscience, people, and reality" (Vaillant, 1993, p. 7).

Any individual may utilize any of the defenses over the course of a lifetime. A close relationship exists between the utilization of defenses and their effects on the ego functions. A key issue in assessment is the extent to which the defenses control or dominate a person's ego functioning, producing serious distortions in reality testing and judgment, problematic relationships, and destructive or self-destructive behaviors.

Vaillant (1993) has classified the defenses into four categories: (1) psychotic defenses; (2) immature defenses; (3) neurotic (intermediate) defenses; and (4) mature defenses. Schamess (1996), while adapting Vaillant's classification, nevertheless has reservations about this classification, since well-functioning individuals "actually employ a wide range of defenses, including some that are categorized as developmentally early or immature. It seems likely that the ability to call on, as needed, a wide range of different defenses is an indication of mental health" (p. 85). Kaplan and colleagues (1994) refer to the psychotic defenses as "narcissistic defenses" (p. 250). Following is a list of fifteen defenses (another defense, *splitting,* is added in the next chapter) that are generally accepted by social workers. I will amalgamate the classifications of Vaillant (1993) and Kaplan and colleagues (1994).

Developmentally Early/Psychotic Defenses

Denial. This defense fends off awareness of some aspect of external reality that is painful or threatening; people with substance abuse problems and their families tend to deny that a problem exists. A mother might deny signs that her boyfriend is making sexual overtures to her daughter. A man with a tumor growing on his neck may deny its existence to avoid facing anxiety at the prospect of cancer. A close friend may plan to move far away, but we may remain "oblivious" to this event, denying the situation by not facing or talking about it.

In psychotic denial, external reality may be severely distorted. Vaillant (1993) notes that it is normal to employ "denial in fantasy; our deceased loved ones come alive in our daydreams . . . psychotic denial leads us to set a place for them at the . . . table" (p. 43). Denial can serve adaptive uses in everyday life. We all know that we will die someday; but we usually deny this fact as we go about our daily business.

Projection. Projection is related to blame. A man might be described as projecting the blame for a divorce onto his wife. However, technically, when used as a defense, projection refers to the attribution of a wish or impulse (which is disavowed) onto some other person or some nonpersonal object in the outside world. In other words, I don't feel angry at you—you are angry at me. "It is the act of giving objective or seeming reality to what is subjective. The expression implies that what is cast upon another is considered undesirable to the one who projects" (Campbell, 1989, p. 563).

As with the other defenses, projection has a spectrum of use: from the "normal," in which reality testing is still reasonably intact (for example, Susan believes that Jim is attracted to her, when the reverse—that is, she is attracted to him—is the case) to its manifestation in mental illness, in which the capacity to test reality has been lost. William, who is mentally ill, first disavowed his angry feelings and then projected them onto the FBI and the communists; he felt he was in danger from both groups and led his life so as to prevent detection. Projection is one of the major defenses in *paranoid schizophrenia* and other paranoid conditions.

An extension of this defense is *projective identification,* a concept attributed to Melanie Klein, one of the early object relations theorists. Projective identification is a complex defense and has been "defined differently by almost every chronicler of defenses . . ." (Vaillant, 1993, p. 58). This is a defensive process in which an individual avoids recognizing and taking responsibility for or ownership of traits that are threatening to him or her, and in a complex way, ascribing these attitudes to (or projecting them onto) another person. This is done in such a way that the other person reacts with the same kind of behavior or attitudes being disavowed by the person utilizing this defensive maneuver.

If Bill, the client, feels disorganized and is afraid to own these feelings, he projects them onto or ascribes them to Sally, the therapist, interacting with her in such a manner that she may actually conform to these projected feelings and act as though she feels disorganized. In this scenario, Bill might behave in such a confused manner (attempting, for example, to subtly demand that Sally understand and comment on his incoherent story) that Sally (making an earnest attempt to follow this illogical account) may likewise become confused and disorganized. Bill might take this one step further and criticize Sally for being too incompetent to follow a simple story.

This entire process may be further reflected subsequently in supervision, where the therapist (who is unaware of this at the time) continues to respond to the client's feeling state and reenacts these feelings while in session with her supervisor (Kahn, 1979). This behavior has been referred to as *parallel process.* In the following excerpt, we can see how the supervisee has absorbed the helplessness and disorganization of her client (Kahn, 1979). By contrast with her prior well-defined presentations, the worker came across as disorganized and diffuse: "The supervisor . . . suggested that there might be a similarity between her feelings and those of the client. The worker . . . said that this client had aroused so much disorganized feeling . . . that she felt almost helpless and in despair" (Kahn, 1979, p. 525).

Bowen (1985) discusses the *family projection process,* a specific variation of projective identification that takes place within a family. A mother may feel helpless but, rather than owning the feeling, projects it onto the child, so that not only does she perceive this child to be helpless but may be so overprotective and infantilizing that the child may feel helpless, and act helpless; therefore, the mother can be the strong one, caring for the needy, weak child. "With her adequate self she mothers her weak self which is perceived to be in the child" (Bowen, 1985, p. 8). In this process, "the mother's attention was determined from inside herself rather than the reality of the situation" (Bowen, 1985, p. 8). This process occurs in all families to some degree; however, it becomes a more serious problem when it is a chronic pattern of interaction, and the child becomes "fused" (i.e., does not develop adequate ego boundaries and does not feel a sense of autonomy and differentiation in relation to the mother).

Projective identification is a major defense in *borderline personality disorder.* The clinician is often the unwitting actor in the scenario created by the patient's projecting disavowed feelings onto the therapist.

> Ms. Schmidt, a child welfare worker, was asked by her client, Mrs. Bosworth, to place her son, whose oppositional behavior she could not handle. When Ms. Schmidt attempted to carry out the plan, the mother became very angry, verbally attacking the social worker. She concluded her tirade by stating: "There are plenty of children out there that you can help. Why don't you go and help them?" Mrs. Bosworth subsequently called up Ms. Schmidt's supervisor to complain about Ms. Schmidt's incompetence. In these instances, Mrs. Bosworth was disavowing her own angry feelings toward her son and her wish to "be rid of him." She involved Ms. Schmidt in acting out this wish for her, then attacked her for this "hostile" act, while she could remain the innocent victim of this "outrage." The extreme disowning of and distancing of oneself from one's own feelings and attitudes here verges on the delusional.

Projective identification, when understood and processed by the clinician, can be used to encourage the psychological growth of the patient. If therapists can feel the clients' projected feelings arising within themselves, such as suddenly feeling incompetent or helpless when with the clients, they can utilize this insight therapeutically rather than act out the feeling by becoming helpless (or defend against it by proving the opposite, that they are not incompetent or helpless). "It may be that the essence of what is therapeutic" resides in a "therapist's ability to receive the patient's projections, utilize facets of his own mature personality system to process the projection, and then make the digested projection available . . . [to the patient] through the therapeutic interaction" (Ogden, 1982, p. 20). Understanding projective identification is a critical factor in the work of utilizing intersubjectivity, the reciprocal subjective reactions and interactions of the client and clinician (Stolorow et al., 1994).

Immature Defenses

Vaillant (1993) states that he does not use the term "immature defenses" in a judgmental manner, but to stress that the "ego develops into adult life" (p. 45).

Acting out. Acting out is defined as "the direct expression of an unconscious wish or impulse . . . to avoid being conscious of the affect" and the associated ideation (Vaillant, 1993, pp. 52-53). In acting out, the person, through action, experiences relief from psychological tensions and conflicts. In utilizing this defense, some individuals engage in many "impulsive delinquent acts and temper tantrums" that explode so violently "as to allow the user to be unaware of their passion" (Vaillant, 1993, p. 53). The risk-taking behaviors of some teenagers may be a form of acting out. As a rule, "adolescent streetwalkers are running from the risk of incestuous molestations or other abuse at home" (Vaillant, 1993, p. 52).

Passive aggression. In passive aggression, the individual defends against the awareness of the aggressive nature of his or her behavior by concealing the aggression in the disguise of apparent passivity. For example, rebelliousness and resistance are cloaked in procrastination. We have all encountered the adolescent who seems outwardly to comply ("Oh yes, I will definitely get my paper in on time") but then procrastinates or makes excuses ("I finished typing it, but the wind blew it away").

Vaillant (1993) views the so-called defense mechanisms referred to as "turning against the self" as a form of passive aggression. In serious situations of turning against the self, adolescents might burn themselves, deliberately cut themselves, or attempt suicide. This mechanism may represent aggression expressed in an extremely disguised form, turning it as far away as possible from its real object and putting oneself in its place; ordinary passive aggression, however, in which little harm is inflicted on the individual except in the sense that the behavior may be socially self-defeating, should not be conceived of as turning against the self.

The unconscious object of suicidal behavior may also be the internal image of another person (such as a rejecting spouse) who is the target of the suicidal individual's rage. This rage is in profound conflict with the same individual's love for that object.

Identification with the aggressor. When utilizing the defense of identification with the aggressor, first described by Anna Freud (1946), an individual identifies with certain characteristics of a person by whom he or she is threatened rather than reject the aggressor outright, when the aggressor is more powerful and at some level needed by the less powerful individual. In a famous kidnapping case, the victim appeared to have taken on similar characteristics as her captors, participating with them in a bank robbery. "Introjection of a feared object serves to avoid anxiety when the aggressive characteristics of the object are internalized, thus placing the aggression under one's own control" (Kaplan et al., 1994, p. 250). It also avoids a feared loss of the relationship.

Anna Freud (1946) cites the example of a girl who was afraid of ghosts but soon found a solution.

> She would run across the hall, making all sorts of peculiar gestures as she went. Before long, she triumphantly told her little brother the secret of how she had got over her anxiety. "There's no need to be afraid in the hall . . . you just have to pretend that you're the ghost who might meet you." This shows that her magic gestures represented the movements which she imagined that ghosts would make. (Freud, 1946, p. 119)

This mechanism is often present in childhood games in which children's anxiety is "converted into pleasurable security" (Freud, 1946, p. 119) by pretending to become the very things they dread. A boy who underwent a difficult medical procedure might imitate this procedure in his play, where he (as doctor) performs the procedure on a teddy bear.

Anna Freud (1946) cites a case of a boy in an elementary school involving identification with the aggressor, in which the psychologist, August Aichorn, consulted.

> The boy was brought to him because of a habit of making faces. The master complained that the boy's behavior, when he was blamed or reproved, was quite abnormal. On such occasions he made faces which caused the whole class to burst out laughing. . . . When master, pupil and psychologist were together, the situation was explained. Observing the two attentively, Aichorn saw that the boy's grimaces were simply a caricature of the angry expression of the teacher and that, when he had to face a scolding by the latter, he tried to master his anxi-

ety by involuntarily imitating him. The boy identified himself with the teacher's anger and copied his expression as he spoke, though the imitation was not recognized. Through his grimaces he was assimilating himself to or identifying himself with the dreaded external object. (Freud, 1946, p. 118)

It is important to be aware of identification with the aggresssor because of its common usage in psychological life and because of its special prominence in cases involving physical and sexual abuse. It is not uncommon, for example, to see an abused child attack another child, attempting to overcome the trauma by acting out the role of the aggressor.

Somatization. In somatization, a conversion of psychological tensions and conflict into somatic (physical) problems and complaints occurs. A person might experience headaches, for example, when in conflict, but the nature of the conflict causing the tension might not be apparent; people often present in a general practitioner's office with physical complaints that may be masking and at the same time reflecting depression (apart from the common somatic manifestations of depression, such as loss of appetite, constipation). In such instances "psychic derivatives are converted into bodily symptoms, and the person tends to react with somatic manifestations, rather than psychic manifestations" (Kaplan et al., 1994, p. 251). Somatization can be found in a number of emotional disorders including somatization disorder, conversion disorder, and post-traumatic stress disorder; it is a common defense in victims of child abuse (Kilgore, 1988).

Some cultural groups may present more readily with somatic rather than psychological problems. In China, for example, "because individual feelings are considered unimportant but close attention is paid to physical needs," many patients with underlying depressive symptoms "often presented with somatic complaints. In a world view that makes no distinction between the mind and the body, it is the body that carries the 'illness' in a socially acceptable way and without the shame that goes along with mental weakness" (Tang, 1997, pp. 335-336).

Regression. Regression behaviorally and/or attitudinally to a more immature, earlier level of development operates as a defense by allowing the individual to play out the role of the more dependent, less socially accountable child as well as permitting more direct forms of instinctual gratification and aggression. This may occur at any age.

One of the most universally known manifestations of regression is seen in young children experiencing the arrival of a new sibling. Children who have attained good language skills, some self-care skills (such as feeding themselves), and good toilet training may suddenly regress in language skills (to baby language), in self-care skills (to demanding to be fed), and in toilet training (to wetting or soiling themselves). "Through regression, the person attempts to return to an earlier libidinal phase of functioning to avoid the tension and conflict evoked at the present level of development. It reflects the basic tendency to gain instinctual gratification at a less-developed period" (Kaplan et al., 1994, p. 251).

To determine whether (and to what extent) regression has taken place, it is important to obtain a baseline of previous functioning. Was the child previously described ever proficient in self-care skills, language, and toilet training? The same principle applies in the assessment of older individuals.

At the same time, regression is essential to healthy development, as the ability to regress permits people to play, relax, enjoy vacations, gain pleasure from sexual activity, and, periodically, withdraw strategically from the demands of the world in general. Regression is also considered to be "an essential concomitant of the creative process" (Kaplan et al., 1994, p. 251).

Regression in the service of the ego is also an important phenomenon. A child may regress before a new developmental landmark is achieved; a patient in therapy may regress prior to an advance in growth; in both instances, the ego is in the process of synthesizing and consolidating old patterns to prepare for the integration of new development. Regression in the service of the ego can also be observed during times of illness: a man having a heart attack who allows himself to be treated in a dependent or more regressed manner will do better medically than one who denies his illness and resists "being taken care of."

Regression as a permanent state can present serious problems in functioning, depending on how chronic and pervasive it is. In schizophrenia, a marked regression occurs in various areas of functioning and cognitive processes. However, *schizophrenic regression* is different from other forms of regression (if thought of in psychological terms) "because it usually fails in its purpose and still further regression is necessary until, finally, the process may lead to complete dilapidation" (Campbell, 1989, p. 626).

Neurotic Defenses

According to Vaillant (1993), neurotic defenses are "closer to reality [than psychotic and immature defenses]. . . . The user feels responsible for his or her conflicts, and neurotic defenses often reflect compromise" (p. 60).

Displacement. A boss yells at his employee, who yells at his wife, who yells at her son, who kicks the dog; this is displacement. The affect, anger, is experienced and owned (not disavowed as in projection), but displaced onto what is perceived to be a safer object than the one toward whom it is really directed. Safer, in this sense, refers to psychological rather than physical safety. To feel and express anger directly can be threatening to the psychological integrity of the person, as anger may produce anxiety related to superego guilt, fear of rejection or abandonment by the object of the anger, psychological retaliation, etc. Thus, the employee felt safer being angry at his wife than the boss. Although a reality element may have been present, i.e., the possibility of loss of job, we can hypothesize that a psychological prohibition against expressing anger toward a person in authority may also have been at work.

Displacement "permits the symbolic representation of the original idea or object in a way that . . . evokes less distress than the original" (Kaplan et al., 1994, p. 251). During displacement, "the source and aim of the instinct remain constant; it is only the object that varies" (Hall and Lindzey, 1979, p. 50).

Displacement is the primary defense in *phobias* (Kaplan et al., 1994). On the surface the patient is fearful of something in the external world (such as elevators or dogs), which is seen (by psychodynamic therapists) as a displacement from a feeling (or a person) causing anxiety. The anxieties underlying phobias can result from many sources. In agoraphobia (the fear of open spaces and traveling away from home) "separation anxiety clearly plays a leading role" (Kaplan et al., 1994, p. 593). Therefore, one is not likely to get to the bottom of "phobics' anxiety by questioning . . . [them] about the exact object of their fears. . . . We must look everywhere else for the source of their distress" (Vaillant, 1993, p. 24).

Displacement is seen in play therapy. "Parent dolls are murdered and put in garbage cans. The result is relief, not guilt" (Vaillant, 1993, p. 60). The child is relieved because not only has he preserved his real parents, but he has gained emotional release by expressing or displacing his anger onto a safe object: the dolls. A foster child who correctly sensed that he was about to be removed from his foster home was playing a telephone game with his therapist. He said to her: "Tell Harold [his foster-home caseworker] that the bank is on the phone—he owes them a lot of money, and they are going to take away his house!" (The caseworker becomes "dispossessed" rather than the child.)

Displacement is also observed in transference, when the patient displaces feelings from a past significant person (often the parents) onto the therapist.

> A client said to her therapist: "I feel you are sitting there judging me." The therapist asked if she were doing or saying anything to give her client this impression. "No," the patient replied. "I guess I feel that way about everyone." "It is not surprising," the therapist replied. "You have told me how judgmental your mother has always been toward you."

As the therapist was not in fact being judgmental, we can say that displacement was occurring.

Isolation. Isolation or isolation of affect, as it is sometimes called, refers to the disowning of feelings associated with a given idea or event even though the idea or event might be recalled. Citing Freud, Campbell (1989) noted that when using this defense "what remains in consciousness is nothing but an ideational content which is perfectly colorless and is judged to be unimportant" (p. 386).

Why do "ghosts" from the past haunt some parents, inhibiting them in their ability to love their children, whereas other parents are free from these "ghosts" (Fraiberg et al., 1975)? The authors focus on parents who have been abused and make a distinction between those who subsequently abuse their own children and those who do not. Those formerly abused parents who do *not* become abusers can remember not only the event, but their feelings associated with this event. "These are the parents who say: I remember what it was like. . . . I would never let my child go through what I went through" (Fraiberg et al., 1975, p. 419). According to this formulation, when parents become abusers, two defenses have been at work. In the first, identification with the aggressor, the parents have formed a pathological identification with their own abusing parents. In the second, although they could vividly recall the abuse, they could not recall the associated feelings; isolation of affect was at work. The dissociated/isolated affect, presumably rage and the associated tension, cannot remain totally hemmed in but must be discharged at least in part through reenactment of the abuse.

Although the concept of social isolation, in which a person remains removed from other people, is an important object relations concept, it should not be confused with isolation of affect, which is a unique defense mechanism.

Dissociation. Dissociation is a complex mental process, one of the first major pathological phenomena to receive scientific attention in the last century ("Dissociation: Part I," 1992). Subsequently, psychiatric interest in dissociation greatly diminished until about twenty years ago, when the mental health field again became interested in it along with a parallel interest in trauma. The relationship between this defense and abuse is an important one to note, as dissociation is often referred to as a defense against external trauma. People, however, can also experience mild, everyday forms of dissociative reactions ("Dissociation: Part I," 1992) but without obvious antecedent trauma. Dissociation has also been noted to occur in hypnosis, in the religious experience of spirit possession, in temporal lobe epilepsy, in amnesia (of psychological origin), and in multiple personalities (where there is also a strong connection to past abuse) ("Dissociation: Part I," 1992; Kaplan et al., 1994).

Dissociation can be a common phenomenon of everyday life ("Dissociation: Part I," 1992).

According to one survey, almost a third of people say they occasionally feel as though they are watching themselves in a movie.... Fourteen percent say they sometimes look into a mirror and momentarily cannot recognize themselves. Up to 70 percent of young adults may have brief episodes in which they momentarily feel as though the world is dreamlike or they are not themselves. ("Dissociation: Part I," 1992, p. 1)

In dissociation a disruption occurs in the person's sense of identity or consciousness.

Dissociation can be described as a process or experience in which the unity of consciousness is disrupted, [and] normal integrated awareness is disturbed. . . . Connections, continuity, and consistency are lost; the sense of identity changes; groups of memories, feelings, and perceptions are relegated to separate compartments or buried in oblivion from which they may suddenly emerge ("Dissociation: Part I," 1992, p. 1).

One form of dissociative experience that often occurs is *depersonalization*—"an elusive sensation of being not human, not alive, or disconnected from parts of one's body" ("Dissociation: Part I," 1992, p. 3). In more extreme cases the world may not appear real and "other people may appear to be dead or automatons" ("Dissociation: Part I," 1992, p. 2).

Hypnosis is an example of a "dissociative state in normal people" (Kaplan et al., 1994, p. 638). When acting under a hypnotic command, a person may carry out an order that he or she does not "own" (i.e., relinquishes self-awareness and thus ownership of his or her will to the hypnotist).

Traumatic events, such as childhood physical and sexual abuse, can lead to the development of dissociative symptoms and disorders (Kaplan et al., 1994; Kilgore, 1988). Dissociated states have been reported in victims of state-sanctioned terror (Bloche and Eisenberg, 1993). Social work students will probably encounter this defensive state in children who are victims of physical and/or sexual abuse, in adults who are survivors of past abuse, and in people who have lived through other traumas. Many immigrants, such as refugees from war-torn or terror-torn Cambodia or Vietnam, suffer from post-traumatic stress disorder, and dissociation is often one of their prominent symptoms.

People suffering from post-traumatic stress disorder no longer know themselves, so their actions and emotions may feel inauthentic, unreal. They usually do not want to talk or think about the trauma, and may eventually find that more and more things will not bear examination. Alienated memories and feelings return involuntarily in a dissociated form. ("Dissociation: Part II," 1992, p. 3)

The presence of dissociation in the adult incest survivor presents therapeutic complexities to both the patient and the therapist, as "dissociative defenses play havoc with analysis by complicating the patient's identity and ego functions" (Hegeman, 1995, p. 187). Furthermore, as these experiences have not been processed by the ego, when this "dissociated material . . . reemerges into awareness it is as terrifying and overwhelming as when it first occurred" (Hegeman, 1995, p. 187).

Although dissociation is often seriously dysfunctional for the patient, it nevertheless serves a protective function. Traumatic experiences are usually so catastrophic that they are often described as "an event that is outside the range of ordinary human experience" ("Dissociation: Part II," 1992, p. 2). What is involved supersedes resolution of psychological conflicts; "survival is at stake" ("Dissociation: Part II," 1992, p. 2). Rather than repressing a wish struggling to emerge from the unconscious, the "dissociative barrier . . . separates two sets of equally complex experiences and memories" ("Dissociation: Part II," 1992, p. 2).

Multiple personality or dissociative identity disorder is an extreme dissociative phenomenon (Kaplan et al., 1994). This disorder is characterized by a plurality of separate personalities within the same individual; some or all of the personalities may have no awareness of the others (Kaplan et al., 1994). There has been some criticism of the use of the term *multiple personality,* as some feel it is "misleading; they prefer 'self-integration disorder,' which implies that these people are suffering from the loss of a unified control system rather than a proliferation of selves. In a sense they have less than one complete personality instead of more than one" ("Dissociation: Part I," 1992, p. 3).

In most cases of multiple personality disorder, conflicting self-representations are kept in isolated compartments (Kaplan et al., 1994). The unitary self, the product of the integration of elements of the individual's singular persona, is lost in the dissociative disorders, with resulting fragmentation of identity (Kaplan et al., 1994).

Trauma, including violence, sexual abuse, and incest, are discussed in later chapters. Post-traumatic stress disorder will be addressed at length in Chapter 13.

Reaction formation. Reaction formation involves the presence of two similar but opposing attitudes, such as anger and love. One of these attitudes (anger) becomes unconscious, and the other (love) emerges into consciousness in an exaggerated form. A person utilizing this defense might talk of a love for someone (or an idea) in such a way that it does not quite ring true.

An overemphasis on cleanliness might mask a wish to be dirty. Reaction formation "keeps both idea *and* affect in mind; only the value is reversed. . . . Reaction formation . . . turns a wish into its opposite" (Vaillant, 1993, p. 65). An example of the "development of an attitude diametrically opposed to the id desires" would be that of a person "with strong homosexual impulses [who] may crusade against homosexuality" (Wolman, 1973, p. 313).

Sometimes the suppressed impulse breaks through and the person acts out the feelings and wishes that had been under control. Vaillant (1993) discusses a well-publicized situation of a crusading religious leader who had regularly denounced the " 'decline of morals and decency in our country,' " yet who subsequently was discovered to have had sexual relations with both a male and female student where he taught and then went on to officiate at their wedding (p. 78).

In discussing the Chinese culture, Tang (1997) points out that because a strong prohibition against anger exists within this population, reaction formation is a major defense. This is often "manifested in an oscillation between a ready compliance to authority and murderous, antiauthority rampages such as occurred during the Cultural Revolution from 1966-1976" (Tang, 1997, p. 336). The occurrence of the "rampages" would be another example of the acting out of the suppressed side of angry feelings held in control by the reaction formation.

Repression. When utilizing the defense of repression, thoughts and feelings perceived to be dangerous by the ego are rendered unconscious; a person may have no recollection of an emotionally painful experience. It is "the active process of keeping out and ejecting, banishing from consciousness, ideas or impulses that are unacceptable to it" (Campbell, 1989, p. 631). Kaplan and colleagues (1994) make a distinction between primary and secondary repression. When individuals use primary repression, they are not admitting mental/affective activity into consciousness in the first place. It is "the curbing of ideas and feelings before they have attained consciousness; secondary repression excludes from awareness what was once experienced at a conscious level" (Kaplan et al., 1994, p. 251).

Freud's (Brenner, 1974) discussion of the mechanisms of dreaming is based on the concept of repression, which banishes from waking thought forbidden ideas and impulses, which then may return in disguised form at night in dreams. From this viewpoint, it is understandable that Freud referred to the analysis of dreams as the "royal road to the unconscious" (Brenner, 1974, p. 150).

Repression plays an important role in psychological functioning. We repress aspects of our instinctual life (and primary process thinking) to some extent and develop secondary process thinking to adapt to external reality.

It might be helpful to view repression on a continuum; a sufficient amount of repression is needed to enable us to function and not be continually diverted by pressing internal preoccupations, while permitting us to be attuned to our feelings and wishes. Insufficient repression, appearing in psychotic states, may result in such primitive and inappropriate ways of thinking, relating, integrating, and adapting that the individual may not be able to function adequately in the real world to the point of severe impairment. Severe repression, on the other hand, can require the expenditure of so much psychic energy that the ego may become constricted, resulting in, among other problems, a rigidity of personality, lack of spontaneity and imagination, and an inability to play. People with severe repression can experience somatic symptoms, such as migraine headaches and conversion phenomena, depression, anxiety states, etc.

Although on the surface dissociation and repression may seem to be similar, the psychological processes involved in each are different. Repression appears to achieve its defensive aim by impeding the access of troubling mental contents as a whole to consciousness, whereas dissociation appears to achieve its defensive aim by breaking connections between components of troubling mental contents, thus submerging the essential significance of the underlying whole.

A current controversy exists over the issue of the accuracy of repressed memories of sexual abuse. Alpert (1995) summarizes this conflict.

> The controversy over the validity and impact of adult memories of childhood abuse has been oversimplified by the media and has resulted in a division. One side of the controversy acknowledges that memories for childhood abuse may be delayed and recalled decades after the abuse. The other side believes that recovered memories of childhood trauma are more likely the result of suggestion from misinformed therapists, self-help books, or other forms of influence. This dialogue . . . has been harmful to the mental health professions, practitioners, and the people served by them. (p. xix)

There is probably truth in both arguments; many people have been abused and may not recover memories until later in life. There are also indications that some people may be suggestible and "fantasize" about events that may not have occurred. Furthermore, evidence of manipulative behaviors exists in this arena; it is not unknown for parents in custody disputes to prompt their children to accuse a parent of abuse which may never have occurred; strong suspicion exists that similar manipulations may occur in some instances on the part of police, prosecutors, and mental health professionals. In this emotional sphere, the importance of maintenance of objectivity is a critical factor, as this uncharted realm continues to be explored.

Mature Defenses

The mature defenses enable people to integrate conflicts, to "balance and attenuate the four lodestars of reality, people, conscience, and desire" (Vaillant, 1993, p. 67).

Sublimation. Sublimation is the conversion of feelings and impulses into socially acceptable and constructive behavior. In this formulation, the child, rebelling against toilet training, sublimates the wish to control his or her feces into playing with mud or with clay. Many adult activities, including various forms of artistic expression, are examples of successful sublimation. "Sublimation allows instincts to be channeled, rather than blocked or diverted" (Kaplan et al., 1994, p. 252).

Humor. Humor, as a defense, can help people handle stress or conflict by draining the seriousness from situations. "Freud suggested [humor] 'can be regarded as the highest of these defensive processes'" (Vaillant, 1993, p. 72). We can all think of many examples of how people have related a distressing event, but which they have mastered to a sufficient degree so that it becomes a funny story in the telling, which can serve the goal of further mastery.

Characterological Mechanisms of Defense

Another dimension of defensive operations is that which can become incorporated into character, and that which can be designated as adaptational behavior. Heinz Hartmann (Vaillant, 1993) stated that "'defensive processes may simultaneously serve both control of the instinctual drive and adaptation to the external world'" (p. 116). The development of creativity, for example, is a "striking example of adaptation to instinctual conflict evolving into sustained behavior" (Vaillant, 1993, p. 116). These defensive operations can be adaptive or maladaptive or both, in the sense that what may be adaptive in one sphere of life (a high degree of organization at work) might be maladaptive in another sphere (a spouse might complain of a partner's "overorganization" and "control" at home).

Characterological mechanisms of defense can develop in relation to traumatic experiences. In one study, adults were interviewed twenty years after they had survived the disastrous Buffalo Creek flood as children (Honig et al., 1993). The researchers were struck by the fact that while few symptoms of post-traumatic stress disorder remained in these former survivors, they had developed "'patterns of adaptation' which may have originated as coping responses to the trauma" (Honig et al., 1993, p. 334). They added that these patterns, which could develop into "characterological mechanisms of defense, appeared to be more or less adaptational from the perspective of the individual's subsequent emotional development and from the perspective of the individual's capacity to confront other stressful events" (Honig et al., 1993, p. 334). In one case study, Henry, who assumed a great deal of responsibility for others during the flood crisis, was found twenty years later to have incorporated "this strong sense of responsibility" (Honig et al., 1993, p. 340) as a fixed, predominant aspect of his personality and functioning.

Discussion. Finally, we all need and utilize defenses; they protect the ego from perceived internal and external dangers. Key considerations in examining defenses include assessing the strength, flexibility, or rigidity of the defenses; their utilization for adaptation and coping; whether they help the person deal with reality or provide a false sense of the world; and the extent to which defenses constrict or promote a person's emotional and cognitive life.

A clinician may immediately wish to confront a client's unhealthy defenses and replace them with healthy ones; however, one should interpret defenses cautiously and supportively, exploring underlying conflicts and offering "an alternative mode of coping" (Vaillant, 1993, p. 111). It can be reassuring to students who are afraid of harming clients through their interventions to learn of Vaillant's observation that the "ego is wily, resilient, and wise." People will not "give up defenses they need just because we point them out" (Vaillant, 1993, p. 111).

CONCLUSION

A discussion has been presented of psychoanalytic and ego psychology theories, including ego functions and the defense mechanisms, as it is my conviction that this will enable the reader to gain a deeper understanding of the complexities of human behavior. Students generally have a strong wish to help clients and tend to feel responsible for their successes and failures as well as to personalize therapeutic relationship demands and difficulties. It is important to realize that clients come with a life history, with established patterns of relating to people, varying levels of trust, and an ego organization that may be solid or unstable. We can get caught up in a whirlwind of relationship tangles and "crunches" (emotionally charged impasses) with clients; we may feel overidentified or repulsed, or confused and helpless. Learning how to analyze ego functions, defense mechanisms, and other psychological processes enables us to reach more deeply the pain and suffering of the client without losing ourselves in the process. Although some social workers will argue that we are medicalizing and pathologizing the client, we would argue that we are aiming for as much objectivity as it is possible to muster in intense clinical situations. We would agree with the social work emphasis of developing a caring relationship and developing a client's strengths, but, to do so, we must know our clients in the full dimensionality of their psychological lives.

If we learn how to listen and what to listen for, we will be able to go beneath the surface communications of people to ascertain what underlying thoughts and feelings are present. Scuba-diving instructors might suggest to students, about to go beneath the surface of the water, what types of undersea life to look for and where they can be found. Then the learners are ready to observe the wonders of the undersea world for themselves and continue their own explorations. These students, however, first must accept that there could be a world under the sea; if they believe that all that exists are the waves, seaweed, and shells and crustaceans that are washed ashore, that is all they will ever know. So I ask the reader to look at what is not visible—the unconscious, internal representations, defenses, and internal conflict—rather than remain with superficial knowledge. I hope that the awesomeness of your explorations will enrich your understanding of people and enable you to be a more sensitive clinician.

Discussion of psychodynamic theories continues in Chapter 3, looking at object relations theory and self psychology, and adding the perspectives offered by cognitive and behavioral theories. The puzzling question of how some children and adults who have had difficult life experiences but appear to adapt well is discussed in the chapter's final section on resilience.

LEARNING EXERCISES

1. Review one of your cases (or a printed case, if you do not have one of your own). Assess the client in terms of the ego functions and defenses that you see operating. Look for both strengths and areas of vulnerability.
2. In a group exercise, each group should be assigned several ego functions and defenses and prepare to explain these with examples to the class.

SUGGESTED READINGS

Articles

Swenson, C. J. (1994). Freud's "Anna O.": Social work's Bertha Pappenheim. *Clinical Social Work Journal, 22,* 149-163.

Books

Berzoff, J., Flanagan, L. M., and Hertz, P. (Eds.) (1996). *Inside out and outside in: Psychodynamic clinical theory and practice in contemporary multicultural contexts.* Northvale: Jason Aronson Inc.

Mackey, R. A. (1985). *Ego psychology and clinical practice*. New York: Gardner Press, Inc.

Putnam, F. W. (1997). *Dissociation in children and adolescents: A developmental perspective*. New York: The Guilford Press.

Vonnegut, M. (1975). *The Eden Express: A personal account of schizophrenia*. New York: Praeger Publishers.

Chapter 3

Object Relations, Self Psychology, and Cognitive-Behavioral Theories

We are at times as different from our real selves as from other people.

La Rochefoucauld
Maximes, No. 135, 1665

INTRODUCTION

In Chapter 2, I traced the development of psychoanalysis and the influence of ego psychology on psychodynamic thought. We now turn our attention to further psychodynamic developments, including object relations theory, with its emphasis on issues of attachment, internalization of representations of self and other, and separation-individuation. This is followed by a discussion of self psychology, with its assertion of the central roles in psychological development played by identity and self-cohesion. Some of the major ideas of cognitive and behavioral theories are then presented, discussing ways these theories diverge from psychodynamic theory and suggesting how contributions from this viewpoint can be used in complementary ways with psychodynamic thinking. The chapter concludes with a discussion of resilience, examining the puzzle of how some children and adults who have been through extreme stress and trauma appear to have adapted well.

OBJECT RELATIONS THEORY

In the context of this theory, objects refer to people toward whom the self (the subject) is drawn; presumably it refers back to the general notion of the "love object" in Freud's works. Object relations theory emphasizes internal reactions to and conceptions of others, as well as inner feelings about oneself.

The projection of feelings onto others, activated by internalized objects, is seen in the following example.

> A client, who was very engaging and appeared positively involved in her clinical treatment, commented that she was always very anxious before she came to the office. She was afraid that the therapist would be judgmental and critical. When the clinician asked if she had done or said anything to give this impression, the client remarked: "Not yet!" The discussion turned to the client's mother, who could be supportive and sympathetic at times but who overall tended to be critical of the client; her surprise "attacks" could not be anticipated by the client. It became clear that the client was expecting and attempting to "defend" herself against similar behavior from the clinician.

In this example, the client's internalized view of her mother (an internal object) was coloring her feelings about her present relationship with the clinician and, correspondingly, her behavior in this relationship. This root of her anxious, self-critical attitude was also adversely affecting her self-image (her self-representation). Mother's estimation of her must be the correct one!

Melanie Klein was the first psychoanalyst to revise Freud's theory (while retaining the concepts of the instinctual drives) by adding the perspective of interpersonal relationships (St. Clair, 1986). Fairbairn (St. Clair, 1986), utilizing Klein's theory, departed completely from Freudian drive theory by proposing a " 'pure' object relations position, which asserts that the main drive that a person has is *a drive for a relationship* [italics added], not the satisfaction of biological instinct" (St. Clair, 1986, p. 13). Fairbairn asserted that "the seeking out and maintaining of an intense emotional bond with another person" is the fundamental motivation in life (Mitchell, 1988, p. 27).

The emotional connection to parents is a matter of utmost importance to the child, to be maintained at all costs. Understanding this, Fairbairn gained an insight into the paradoxical situation of the "loyalty of abused children to their abusing parents" (Mitchell, 1988, p. 26). Foster children often need to blame someone for being removed from their homes; often they blame themselves, enabling them to retain the belief that their parents will come back for them and to deny that the parents are to blame. "No matter how weak or abusive are the parents, the child needs to believe that they are the best of all possible parents" (Levine, 1990, p. 58).

Foster children may have difficulty attaching to their foster families because of a pattern of insecure attachments; they may also feel that loving their foster parents is a betrayal of their biological parents. The often "punishing" rejection of the foster parents by the child and overt aggression directed toward them can be a difficult burden for the foster parents to accept (Levine, 1990).

People who have had secure attachments to a nurturing figure generally have a solid sense of self and tend to have positive and pleasurable interpersonal relationships. Those who have received inadequate nurturance and support, developing a "shaky" sense of self, may avoid intimate relationships with others out of fear of closeness, or they may constantly seek deeply involving relationships, in which they demand total attention and nurturing. Sometimes this works; the person finds another with a need to nurture, so a complementary relationship may develop. However, people in need of nurturing often are attracted to those with similar needs, which can lead to disappointment and conflict, as neither person can meet the deep needs of the other.

Some emotionally needy people become engaged in enmeshed relationships in which the individuality of each is lost, as they fuse into a unit, always together (but frequently not "tuned in" to each other). Some enmeshed couples follow this pattern into the divorce process, finding they cannot get along with each other but are not able to let go (Kressel, 1997). Enmeshed families are discussed further in Chapter 7.

Social workers encounter many people who have entered into self-destructive relationships, which serve "as vehicles for *the perpetuation of early ties to significant others* [italics added]. The child learns a mode of connection . . . and these learned modes are desperately maintained throughout life" (Mitchell, 1988, p. 27). Looked at from this vantage point, the perplexing picture of a woman growing up with an abusive father and then marrying a man who is abusive to her becomes more understandable. It is not uncommon to see children born to teenage unmarried mothers becoming teenage unmarried parents themselves.

The intergenerational transmission of child maltreatment has been observed when an object relations perspective is applied to the study of child abuse (Hughes, 1998; Morton and Browne, 1998; Zeanah and Scheeringa, 1997). If children receive "insensitive parenting" (Morton and Browne, 1998, p. 1098), they will introject an image of themselves as unlovable and deficient; subsequently, they are unable to develop caring, consistent relationships with their own children. "This may be the primary process by which child maltreatment continues from one generation to the next. Thus, it is the caregiving relationship that is transmitted across the generations rather than violence per se" (Morton and Browne, 1998, p. 1098). Mitigating circumstances (or protective factors enhancing resilience) can prevent this transmission; these include supportive substitute care when growing up, current involved and supportive spouses, and the development of self-awareness about their abusive experiences (often with the assistance of therapy) (Morton and Browne, 1998).

Object relations theory has also contributed to a deeper understanding of the use of self by the clinician; its concepts promote the clinician's attunement to feelings evoked in them by their clients; these feelings are then explored in a therapeutic manner.

> Dan, who had a history of disturbed attachments, engaged in therapy, presenting with many anxieties and deep insecurities about himself. On several occasions, when the clinician made a sensitive and attuned comment to Dan, he would laugh in what felt to the clinician to be a disparaging manner. Instinctively, the clinician felt defensive, wondering if she was off the mark, and changed the subject. During one session, when Dan again laughed "at her," she realized that she was feeling put down. This time, she brought this behavior to his attention. She asked him if he realized that when she said something of a sensitive nature, he would laugh at it. He was able to discuss his discomfort with the feelings she evoked in him, which led to a meaningful interchange. The clinician speculated that perhaps his put-down of her was the way he was made to feel when he had tried to express painful feelings to others in his past.

In this illustration, the clinician, although initially thrown off balance by the client's disparagement of her insights, was able to use her defensive emotional reaction by processing it within her self, and then sharing this with her client. She was utilizing the concept of *intersubjectivity,* which refers to the reciprocal subjective reactions and interactions of the client and clinician. This concept has been receiving increasing attention (Schamess, 1999; Mattei, 1999; Stolorow et al., 1994).

In Chapter 2 we discussed the projective identification defense whereby clients can project their own disavowed feelings, such as guilt, onto their therapists. This process may evoke irrational guilt in clinicians, the source of which may be quite unclear initially, and thus they may unwittingly react to those feelings. Ogden (1982) recommended that therapists become aware of these projections from the client within themselves, "utilize facets of [their] own mature personality system to process the projection, and then make the digested projection available . . . [to the patient] through the therapeutic interaction" (p. 20). This therapeutic utilization of projective identification by the clinician is an important component of intersubjectivity. Object relations family therapists actively utilize projective identification in their treatment of families (Scharff and Scharff, 1987). The following is an example from the practice of a clinician making therapeutic use of projective identification.

A family therapist, in talking with a couple, found that the wife was often sarcastic to both her husband and to himself. He found himself getting angry at the wife and was inclined to make "hostile" interpretations to her, under the guise of increasing her insight. He subsequently realized that her interactional style must also be affecting her husband, who had a need to deny the force of his wife's anger, and that the wife's hostility had origins in her embattled childhood family. The therapist's intervention involved dealing with the wife's hostility in a direct but empathic manner and relating this both to her present interactions and past history.

Object relations family therapy is discussed further in Chapter 7. *Attachment theory,* a major component of object relations theory, discussed next, sheds light on the meaning and importance of relationships throughout the life cycle.

Attachment Theory

"Human development begins with people in relationships" (Noam and Fischer, 1996, p. xvii). Although some debate exists as to whether (and to what extent) later reparations can make up for early deprivations in nurturing relationships, it is generally accepted that babies need to be held, hugged, smiled at, and talked to. "Attachment behaviors have as their objective the promotion of proximity and contact. The loss of the mother, whether she is absent or unable to provide adequate nurturing, has major consequences that lead to a specific sequence of reactions which Bowlby called protest, despair, and detachment" (Frankel, 1994, pp. 87-88).

Bowlby and Spitz observed, many years ago, the effects of institutionalization on children, such as failure to thrive (sometimes culminating in death), anaclitic depression, and failures in attachment (Karen, 1990). Worldwide attention recently focused on the serious physical and psychological damage to children who were exposed to severe deprivation of basic caretaking and nurturing. Talbot (1998) describes the horrendous experiences (and subsequent developmental impairments) of infants in Romanian and Soviet orphanages who were confined "to cribs in . . . gloomy, ill-heated orphanage[s] with a small, rotating staff of caretakers who might spend an average of 10 minutes a day talking to them or holding them" (p. 26); many of these children have been adopted by Europeans and Americans. There "are more than 18,000 of these adoptees in the United States now, and the most traumatized among them—roughly 20 to 30 percent, according to researchers—are becoming one of the most scrutinized and therapeutically manipulated populations in the annals of psychology" (Talbot, 1998, pp. 26-27).

Although many of these neglected children developed severe attachment disorders, attachment disorders have also been observed in a number of children in this country whose caretakers are unable to nurture them adequately; many of these children are served by child welfare agencies. *Reactive attachment disorders* have been diagnosed in children under five years of age; one early manifestation is a failure to thrive syndrome, in which the infant may appear seriously malnourished, apathetic, and display a sad affect (Kaplan et al., 1994). This particular syndrome does not result from physical illness (such as a gastrointestinal malabsorption disorder) but is related to inadequate nurturing.

With time, others symptoms of a reactive attachment disorder may develop. According to the American Psychiatric Association's *Diagnostic and Statistical Manual of Mental Disorders,* Fourth Edition (DSM-IV) (1994), an attachment disorder is marked by "disturbed and developmentally inappropriate social relatedness in most contexts . . . and is associated with grossly pathological care" (p. 116). This disorder is distinguished from *pervasive developmental disorders* (such as *autism,* an extreme lack of social relatedness, with a presumed biological basis), whereas attachment disorders are reactive to poor caretaking.

> In the *Inhibited Type* [italics added], the child persistently fails to initiate and to respond to most social interactions in a developmentally appropriate way. The child shows a pattern of excessively inhibited, hypervigilant, or highly ambivalent responses. In the *Disinhibited Type* [italics added], there is a pattern of diffuse attachments. The child exhibits indiscriminate sociability or a lack of selectivity in the choice of attachment figures. (DSM-IV, 1994, p. 116)

Hughes (1998) discusses the case of Katie who was subjected to "physical abuse, verbal and emotional abuse, and long periods of emotional neglect" during her first five years (p. 19). Emotional neglect has its own toxic effects.

> The endless acts of emotional violation to Katie's heart and soul through [maternal] looks of disgust, screams of rejection, and the deadly silence of indifference were what led to her losing her desire to form an attachment with her parents. The trauma of sexual and physical violence is well documented. The "trauma of absence," which characterizes neglect, is less obvious to many. The cycle of abuse that leads inexorably from one generation to the next is powered most forcefully by the inability to enter and maintain meaningful attachments. (Hughes, 1998, pp. 19-20)

Sometimes children have specific characteristics that may contribute to the parent's difficulties in nurturing, such as disabilities in the child or temperamental incompatibilities. Children may also have attachment problems due to circumstances such as loss of parents and/or multiple placements out of the home (Kaplan et al., 1994).

Bowlby (1988) postulates deep instinctual needs for attachment and asserts that "emotionally significant bonds between individuals have basic survival functions," i.e., humans require each other for basic biological survival. Bowlby's findings have been supported by Main (1995), along with Ainsworth, who have done extensive research into the formation of childhood attachments, observing the importance of children bonding with their caretakers, leading to the development of a "secure base." Main (1995) discusses classification of attachment behaviors into four categories: the *secure* attachment, *insecure-avoidant* attachment, *insecure-resistant/ambivalent* attachment, and *disorganized/disoriented* attachment. These patterns are discussed at length in Chapter 8.

Bowlby asserts that a biological basis exists for attachment behaviors in humans, as in many animals, as the "cybernetic systems situated within the CNS [central nervous system] of each partner . . . have the effect of maintaining proximity to each other" (1988, p. 29). In keeping with Bowlby's use of *ethology* (the study of the behavior of animals and human beings, especially in their natural environments) to describe attachment theory, the following narrative account of an American on vacation in Britain conveys the intensity of attachment behavior in sheep.

> Ingrid loved sheep, and she loved the Yorkshire Dales. Wandering the footpaths, she passed mother ewes with their lambs, noticing their continual awareness of each other; if the distance between them became too great, they would search until they found each other.
>
> Ingrid and her husband enjoyed listening to the evening song of the sheep, in a wide range of melodies and pitches, answered by equally varied calls in other tones. A farmer's wife told them that the music of the sheep was their calling to one another; lamb and mother recognize each other's unique calls. These calls became intense at shearing time, as mothers are temporarily separated from their lambs. High pitched and intense bleating would occur as they sought reunion. Ingrid could not forget the image or sound of this frantic, intense searching. This is akin, she thought, to what human babies and mothers experience at the preverbal level.

Bowlby refers to the importance of internalizations and object representations during the attachment process. "Each partner builds in his or her mind working models of self and of other and of the patterns of interaction that have developed between them" (Bowlby, 1988, p. 29). This means that each person develops internalized pictures or images (representations) of the self and other people in his or her mind, as well as a picture of mutual patterns of attachment and expectations, along with the associated feeling states. Bowlby hypothesizes that the way in which attachment bonds "develop and become organized during . . . infancy and childhood . . . are major determinants of whether a person grows up to be mentally healthy" (1988, p. 29). Bretheron (1996) asserts that relationships between parents and children that are "characterized by emotionally open and sensitive communications are the royal road to the development of adequate and flexible internal working models of self and other" (p. 16).

One of the criticisms leveled against attachment theory is its emphasis on the bonding of the child and mother, especially during the first three years of life, which raises three major objections: (1) children usually form multiple attachments; (2) insufficient credit is given to the child's capacity for adaptation; and (3) positive changes in later stages of a child's life (such as good parenting through adoption) can help repair earlier deprivations, while negative effects, such as the death or mental illness of a parent of a secure child, can "increase the child's vulnerability" (Frankel, 1994, p. 86). Schaffer (1994) claims that "a child's future is not shaped by events in the early, so-called formative years; development is rather a matter of a slow process of genetic and environmental interactions that continue throughout the time of psychological growth" (p. 39). The child's adaptation to early deprivations and the development of resilience is discussed in the final section of this chapter.

Research points to the multiple attachments children develop in addition to mother-child bonds, which include bonds to their fathers, their extended family, and their siblings (Frankel, 1994; Lieberman, 1984). Relationships to siblings can "ease adjustment to conflicts and stresses by providing a positive source of reference and sense of support through sibling bonds" (Thomlison, 1997, p. 58). The dramatic increase in utilization of day care today, for infants as well as older children, has demonstrated the child's capacity to adapt to multiple caretakers and has also raised questions about whether subtle negative effects may show up later in development; this is discussed further in Chapters 6 and 8.

While attachment and bonding are vital to children's physical and emotional well-being, each child also needs to move away from the intensity of the maternal orbit, to walk, to develop autonomy, and to tolerate solitude, while still maintaining an emotional connection to mother and others. Margaret Mahler and her associates (1975) have done extensive research on this very complex process of separation-individuation in the human infant.

Mahler: Separation and Individuation

Mahler's work "has been of central importance to virtually all American object relations theories" (Hamilton, 1990, p. 56) and provides many concepts useful in the understanding of diverse situations encountered in social work practice in a wide range of settings (for example, adoption work, placement of the aged, parent-child relationships).

Mahler and colleagues (1975) carried out a longitudinal study of normal children using observations in a nursery school setting and in the home. They explored "the psychological birth of the human infant," the establishment of a sense of identity, and psychological separation from as well as the maintenance of connection with the mother. In this context, separation refers to the feeling of being a separate individual—"the intrapsychic achievement of a sense of separateness from mother" (Mahler et al., 1975, p. 8).

Four major subphases have been identified in the separation-individuation process: (1) differentiation; (2) practicing; (3) rapprochement; and (4) the beginnings of emotional object constancy.

Forerunners of Separation-Individuation

There are two phases the child must pass through before reaching the four major subphases of the separation-individuation process. These are the normal *autistic* (nonpathological) and *symbiotic* phases.

Autistic phase. According to Mahler and colleagues (1975), during the first few weeks of life the child is in an autistic (auto: by one's own agency) stage of total absorption, has an "inborn unresponsiveness to outside stimuli" (p. 41), and lacks awareness of a mothering person. Current early infant research indicating that children have greater perceptual awareness and more interaction with the mother and the environment than previously recognized has led to criticism of Mahler's characterization of this phase. Disagreement has also arisen because the term autistic has been applied to the pathological states of *infantile autism* and the autistic thinking characteristic of schizophrenia; nevertheless, Mahler obviously did not apply the term here in any pathological sense but rather in its general meaning of inwardly focused self-absorption.

Acknowledging the new infant research, Mahler sought a more normalizing and less pathological term for this stage (Edward et al., 1992). However, she remained committed to the idea that there is an "early period in human existence when the infant's focus is directed inward and during which awareness of the outside is relatively minimal" (Edward et al., 1992, p. 13).

Symbiotic phase. From the second month on, the child enters the symbiotic phase, becoming aware of its mother, and forming a "dual unity" with her, an "omnipotent system" (Mahler et al., 1975, p. 44). There is a sense of "oneness," of sharing a common boundary. This dual unity "forms the primal soil from which all subsequent human relations form" (Mahler et al., 1975, p. 48). The mother's holding, cuddling, having eye contact, and talking to the child are important in this stage. Modifying this concept later, Mahler (Edward et al., 1992) "described symbiosis as referring to two organisms, intimately tied to each other, developing along in parallel" (p. 14). This interaction *"shapes not only the personality of the child, but also that of the mother"* [italics added] (Edward et al., 1992, p. 14). Parents may also develop psychologically as they enter the developmental stage of parenting.

The concept of symbiosis enables us to understand a number of both normal and pathological phenomena in life. "The wish to merge and the fantasy of merging with another are commonplace in the language of love and in love itself" (Edward et al., 1992, p. 31). The research of Silverman, Lachmann, and Milich (Edward et al., 1992) suggests that symbiotic wishes are part of "everyday experiences and activities such as love, religion, meditation, and even jogging" (Edward et al., 1992, p. 31).

The concept of symbiosis offers insight into "what it means for the psychotic individual to lose the distinction between self and object" (Edward et al., 1992, p. 31). These concepts illuminate the "profound feelings of panic or dissolution of the self under the impact of separation or loss" (Edward et al., 1992, p. 31). Ms. O'Toole (discussed in Chapter 2), who believed she had murdered her neighbor because she had wished him dead, later suffered a psychotic break. Her clinician, Mrs. Wendover, visited her in the hospital.

> When Mrs. Wendover entered the visiting room, Ms. O'Toole greeted her, saying: *"I am Mrs. Wendover."* Mrs. Wendover replied: "No, I am Mrs. Wendover." Ms. O'Toole found chairs for them and brought over two glasses of water. When it was time to leave, Mrs. Wendover said good-bye and walked toward the elevator. When she looked back, she noticed that Ms. O'Toole had picked up Mrs. Wendover's glass and was holding it in a secretive manner, trying to hide her action as she drank from it.

Ms. O'Toole is suffering from a major disruption in her ego boundaries. She is not indicating that she wants to be like Mrs. Wendover, which would be an identification. She thinks she *is* Mrs. Wendover, which illustrates a psychotic merger. Drinking from her therapist's glass is probably indicative of her wish to incorporate her therapist as part of herself. If this bizarre behavior is examined in the light of Mahler's theory of the symbiotic phase, we can view it as a regression to the symbiotic state; from that perspective, it is not outside of the normal human condition.

Ego functioning will thrive in the close human attachment of the symbiotic stage (Mahler et al., 1975) if this stage is progressive and nurturing.

This conceptualization is similar to Hartmann's (1958) observation that the "autonomous ego functions" will grow in the "average expectable environment." If the child does not receive adequate nurturing, not only will relationship capacities become potentially impaired, but the other ego functions will not adequately develop. "In the context of the symbiotic exchange . . . ego functions such as anticipation, frustration tolerance, delay of drive discharge are developed and the ego as a whole becomes increasingly organized and structured" (Edward et al., 1992, p. 32).

The First Subphase: Differentiation and the Development of the Body Image

At about four to five months old, children move out of the symbiotic orbit, beginning the process of *differentiation* from mother. Mahler and colleagues (1975) describe the very beginnings of this event as hatching. The child's facial expressions begin to change, and a "certain new look of alertness, persistence, and goal-directedness [emerges]. . . . An infant with this look has "hatched" (Mahler et al., 1975, p. 54). Infants at about six months of age reach to touch mother and pull at her nose, her hair, or her necklace. The child begins "straining his body away from mother in order to have a better look at her . . . in contrast to simple molding when held" (Mahler et al., 1975, p. 54). This arching away from mother has a serious developmental purpose, as the child begins to move toward individuation.

The child develops an interest in transitional objects during this phase, a concept Mahler and colleagues (1975) attribute to Winnicott. The child is beginning to self-soothe, with an object that is like mother but is not mother, and one which he or she can control. Linus's blanket is a well-recognized transitional object. Citing Greenacre, Mahler and colleagues (1975) note that the child's needs for physical contact with the mother are "touchingly expressed in the infant's insistent preference for an object which is lasting, soft, pliable . . . and remain[s] saturated with body odors" (p. 54). Mahler and colleagues (1975) add that "the mother's preferred soothing or stimulating pattern is taken over . . . and so becomes a *transitional pattern*" [italics added] (p. 55).

The concept of transitional objects is relevant to clinical practice and can add subtle dimensions to the client-worker relationship.

> Gloria told her therapist that she was dreading her daughter's wedding, an event which would have normally filled her with pride, but, due to her recent divorce, complicated family relationships were interfering with her anticipating pleasure in the event. After discussion, Gloria felt empowered to deal with the wedding in a more positive way, but the clinician, concerned that Gloria might feel somewhat iso-

lated and unsupported at the wedding, asked her to bring in a picture of this event. Gloria smiled with pleasure and said that she would. The clinician did not want Gloria to feel "alone" at this wedding but to feel the clinician's presence and support, even if she was not to be there. The request for a picture would hopefully evoke for the client the memory of this discussion and reinforce the idea that she would be returning with an evocative object from the celebration. The picture and the evoked memory of the therapist (and their discussion) were considered transitional objects.

The Second Subphase: Practicing

The practicing subphase (occurring between age ten to twelve months to sixteen to eighteen months) is accompanied by an increase in physical mobility; crawling and walking enable infants to greatly increase their exploratory forays into the world. This (in the "average expectable environment") fills children with joy; at times they appear more interested in their explorations than in their mothers. Borrowing Greenacre's term, Mahler and colleagues (1975) speak of the child's " 'love affair with the world' " (p. 70), adding that the child "seems intoxicated with its own faculties and with the greatness of his own world" (p. 71).

During the practicing subphase, as children becomes more autonomous and delighted with new discoveries—including discoveries of their own new-found abilities—they seem to lose interest in mother. Perhaps, these feelings are also related to "the elated escape from fusion with, from engulfment by mother" (Mahler et al., 1975, p. 71). However, the child still needs its mother and will periodically return to her for comfort. This *emotional refueling* "perks him up and restores his previous momentum to practice and explore" (Mahler et al., 1975, p. 290). The child can also maintain a connection to mother through seeing and hearing her.

The Third Subphase: Rapprochement

While exciting, the practicing stage has its psychological dangers. When they become aware of their separateness from their mothers, children often develop *separation anxiety*. Yet children do not want to regress to the symbiotic orbit; they are having too much fun! But how to create the right distance between closeness and independence, between autonomy and connection? This is the dilemma of *rapprochement* (occurring between eighteen and twenty-four months) as described by Mahler and colleagues (1975).

Around 18 months our toddlers seemed quite eager to exercise their rapidly growing autonomy to the hilt. Increasingly, they chose not to be reminded that at times they could not manage on their own. Conflicts ensued that seemed to hinge upon the desire to be separate, grand, and omnipotent, on the one hand, and to have mother magically fulfill their wishes. . . . The prevalent mood changed to that of general dissatisfaction, insatiability, a proneness to rapid swings of mood and to temper tantrums. The period was thus characterized by the rapidly alternating desire to push mother away and to cling to her—a behavioral sequence that the word "ambitendency" describes most accurately. (Mahler et al., 1975, p. 95)

Intense rapprochement struggles are also very typical of adolescence; however rapprochement issues present a dilemma throughout the life cycle, as we negotiate distance-closeness issues in relationships with others. The philosopher Arthur Schopenhauer was reported to have observed that porcupines struggle to find the right distance between each other. They move closer together for warmth on a cold night; finding that their quills hurt each other, they move apart, only to be too cold again. Finding the right distance is not only a problem for porcupines but for people as well. It is a crucial problem for the borderline personality, as those with this disorder continually struggle to maintain the right distance in all their relationships. One client stated: "I don't want to be submerged and yet I'm scared of being too much of an individual."

In the Japanese culture, the emphasis is on integration into one's family and social networks rather than on differentiation and autonomy, as stressed on the whole in contemporary American culture (Tamura and Lau, 1992). Yet a newly married Japanese couple also needs to work out closeness and separation issues in their relationships with each other as well as finding a way to incorporate the extended family into this new unit.

Major tasks of a marriage in any culture are the formation of a secure marital relationship and the realignment of relationships with the members of the extended families of both spouses. It is complicated and difficult for Japanese couples to achieve both because relationship with the extended family is more emphasized. In Japan there is a popular phrase: *A distance where soup does not get cold;* that is, the ideal distance between the parents' and children's households would be a few blocks away where they can easily deliver foods without the soup getting cold. The soup would be too hot if the two generations live together, but too cold if they live far apart. (Tamura and Lau, p. 327)

The Beginnings of Emotional Object Constancy

In this final phase (occurring between twenty and twenty-two months until thirty and thirty-six months), some very important and complex developmental phenomena occur. First, children internalize an image of their mother, which can comfort them in her absence (termed *object constancy*). Then, after internalizing an image of mother as a good, comforting presence, children will internalize a positive image of themselves.

The child's internalization of the mother's image is a very important psychological event, denoting the beginning of the development of the constancy of the object. The child's negative and positive images of the mother become fused into one consistent image (representation) of her. This enables children to modify their angry feelings toward mother and to experience anger while still having loving feelings toward her. If all goes well, children will normally develop feelings of ambivalence, wherein both good and bad feelings toward a loved person can coexist. A mother, for example, might resent her child's demands at times, but her overwhelmingly positive feelings for the child predominate and thus help her temper or modulate her angry feelings. It is, therefore, conversely important for the child to develop object constancy as this "fosters the fusion of the aggressive and libidinal drives and tempers the hatred for the object [mother] when aggression is intense" (Mahler et al., 1975, p. 110).

When object constancy does not develop, and the child experiences a conflictual relationship with its mother, if the mother goes away, however temporarily, it "stirs up considerable expressed or unexpressed anger and longing; under such conditions, the positive image of the mother cannot be sustained" (Mahler, 1975, p. 114).

The defense that develops in response to inadequate development of object constancy is *splitting*. In splitting, the good and bad feelings (about the self or another or a situation) are handled by assigning them in a relationship in an all-or-none fashion at any given time. Ambivalence per se is unstable and not sustainable, and the psychological dilemma is "solved" allowing either the positive or the negative, but not both simultaneously, into consciousness, with dissociation of the other (Shapiro, 1978). "In splitting, the positive and negative fantasized relationships remain alternatively in consciousness with the complementary side dissociated" (Shapiro, 1978, p. 1307). Splitting occurs in everyone to some degree; however, many object relations theorists see splitting in the borderline personality as a predominating and immature defense (Shapiro, 1978).

Kernberg suggested that borderline patients' core difficulty lies in their inability to bring together and integrate loving and hating aspects of both their self-image and their image of another person. [They] cannot sustain a sense that they care for the person who frustrates them. Kernberg saw this characteristic failure in the achievement and tolerance of ambivalence . . . as diagnostic. He suggested that loving fantasized relationships and hating ones are internally 'split' for the borderline patient to prevent the anxiety that would result if they were experienced simultaneously. (Shapiro, 1978, p. 1307)

The splitting of staff by borderline patients is often observed on inpatient psychiatric units. Patients will, often successfully, manage to pit the "good" staff (those who appear to favor them) against the "bad" staff (those who appear to disfavor them) (Tashjian, 1979). Tashjian provides the following example, illustrating such splitting by K, a young adult man in a psychiatric hospital.

Indeed, he devalued the whole hospital experience as he mythologized his high school years, endowing them with success and freedom from conflict. He attempted to split the staff by identifying the "good" and the "bad" and, in doing so, alienated most of them. For instance, he had a special fixation about a black psychiatric technician on the basis of his color. He saw himself as better than blacks, yet feared them because of a projected retaliatory rage. He repeatedly called this man a "jungle bunny," yet could not see why the man would be sensitive to such an epithet. K tried to get me to fire the technician (who was remarkably patient with K's abuse) and, when I would not entertain such thoughts, saw us as aligned against him. He was relentless in his attack as, at the same time, he pleaded for help. He wore the staff out, driving them beyond their capacity to understand him or to listen to my explanations of his patterns of maladaptive object relations; by the end, the staff's countertransference reactions were negative and apparent. Thus the milieu, which ideally should have aided him in working through his conflicts and strengthening his ego, became an arena for continued destructive behavior and sterile repetition compulsion. (Tashjian, 1979, pp. 44-45)

Internalization is "the key concept in modern psychoanalytic developmentalism" (Grolnick, 1990, p. 28). The development of object constancy and its reliance on the process of internalization, as described in Mahler's work, sheds light on the process of identity formation. Identity formation (successful or failed) and struggles in its formation are universal. Although many cultural variations in identity formation exist, nevertheless the process of identity formation is universal, "resulting in different external expressions of similar internal occurrences" (Lieberman, 1984, p. 158).

Winnicott has also contributed to our understanding of the development of identity, developing through the "holding environment" of good nurturing (Grolnick, 1990).

Winnicott

> The writings of any one of us must be to some extent plagiaristic. Nevertheless I think we do not copy; we work and observe and think and discover, even if it can be shown that what we discover has been discovered before. (Winnicott, 1965, p. 11)

The process of discovery is one of Winnicott's major themes; how the child discovers himself, his environment, the capacity to be alone. Winnicott's playful approach, including playing with ideas (Grolnick, 1990), is a cornerstone of his therapeutic approach. "For Winnicott, treatment was more of a dialogue of mutual discovery than the exercise of interpretive finesse by a clinician-expert" (Applegate and Bonovitz, 1995, p. 83). Winnicott tended to develop "individualized" theories, related to each case, as he "entered the 'swampy lowlands' of messy, confusing difficulties that elude objectively derived solutions, challenge existing theory, and are characterized by uncertainty, ambiguity, and unpredictability" (Applegate and Bonovitz, 1995, p. 18). Rather then seeing uncertainty as an obstacle, he felt this was "an opportunity for exploration, for becoming fruitfully confused" (Applegate and Bonovitz, 1995, p. 19).

Yet Winnicott's work is not devoid of valuable generalizations and formulations; indeed, he developed many important theoretical ideas. "He has helped us all to use theory and not allow it to use us" (Grolnick, 1990, p. xiii).

Winnicott's important concepts include: the *holding environment,* the *good enough mother, transitional objects,* the *capacity to be alone,* the *importance of play,* and the development of the *false self.* Applegate and Bonovitz (1995) assert that Winnicott's theories have direct relevance to clinical social work practice. "The developmental and clinical theories of . . . Winnicott offer a uniquely useful set of concepts for articulating the 'silent,' supportive and sustaining, relationship-focused interventions that constitute the core praxis of social work *across service settings*" [italics added] (p. 7).

The Holding Environment and the Good Enough Mother

Winnicott's holding environment and Mahler's symbiotic phase emphasize providing closeness, nurturing, and security to the infant. The holding environment refers to the mother's capacity "to create the world in such a way [that] the baby . . . feels held, safe, and protected from dangers without and protected as well from the danger of emotions within" (Flanagan, 1996, p. 137). The good enough mother providing this holding environment need not be perfect or ever present. In addition to support, "optimal frustration . . . is necessary for ego building. . . . The good enough mother implies that she settles for a good enough child" (Grolnick, 1990, p. 31). The underlying contrast to "good enough" is "ideal" or "perfect." The parallel in the therapeutic situation would appear to be a "*good enough therapist* treating a *good enough patient*" (Grolnick, 1990, p. 31).

This concept is critical for students struggling to be *perfect* therapists (Brightman, 1984-1985). A good enough patient eludes precise definition, and each therapist probably has evolved different criteria for this category. However, in this context, what appears to be implied is a patient (by contrast with the imaginary "perfect" patient) who is not immediately "cured," is not necessarily compliant with the therapist's suggestions and interpretations, and who may exhibit vicissitudes in forming the therapeutic relationship. It also assumes the possibility of struggles, ambivalence, attempts to negotiate mutual understandings, and the acceptance of uncertainty and not knowing on the part of both partners in the therapeutic dyad.

Winnicott's holding environment can be applied to case management with clients (Kanter, 1990). Winnicott stressed providing emotional support and appropriate environmental modifications to disturbed clients. Patients being released from a psychiatric hospital or discharged from a medical facility with a diagnosis of cancer often respond very positively to the provision of needed services, such as a day treatment program for the psychiatric patient and a home health aide for the cancer patient. Both will be aided by the emotional support of others. "Winnicott viewed this work as the 'professionalized aspect of the normal (holding) function of parents and (communities),' a 'holding of persons and situations, while growth tendencies are given a chance'" (Kanter, 1990, p. 35).

The False Self

Children in the care of good enough mothers develop a sense of security, "feel real," and subsequently "the true self becomes the source of personal authenticity and creativity" (Applegate and Bonovitz, 1995, p. 72). However, when the child's needs are not met and/or recognized and instead the child merely gratifies the needs of the caretaker, "in time, the infant subsumes his own needs to those of the caregiver, and becomes overly attentive to the caregiver's needs. Such children become expert at picking up cues that others need attention and supplying it in ways that squelch their own strivings. . . . The false self 'lacks . . . the essential element of creative originality'" (Applegate and Bonovitz, 1995, p. 72).

Seneca, a young woman in Toni Morrison's (1999) novel *Paradise,* reflects on her past experience as a foster child; although not uncared for or even unloved, she clearly doubted that she was approved of for herself. She evidently sensed that she had gained approval though conformity, through the fact that "she took reprimand quietly, ate what was given, shared what she had and never ever cried" (Morrison, 1999, p. 135). As Seneca adapted to her foster homes by external compliance to her perceptions of expected behaviors, her false self evolved.

"Parentified" children of alcoholic parents often sacrifice their true selves while assuming caretaking functions and effecting parental wishes. The depressive person's reliance on the dominant other (Arieti and Bemporad, 1978) bears a resemblance to the false self. Winnicott (Giovacchini, 1993) discusses a "continuum of the false self 'ranging from the healthy, polite aspect of the self to the truly split-off, compliant, false self that is mistaken for the whole person'" (p. 254).

The Capacity to Be Alone

The capacity to be alone "is one of the most important signs of maturity in emotional development" (Winnicott, 1965, p. 29). The experience of a close nurturing relationship fosters tolerance for and even pleasure in aloneness. "The basis of the capacity to be alone is the experience of being alone in the presence of someone" (Winnicott, 1965, p. 36). With good enough mothering, the child is not alone when alone, as the image of the mother has become internalized and is available through a "self-evocative function" (Grolnick, 1990). This self-evocative function is similar to the development of object constancy (Mahler et al., 1975). The capacity to be alone can encourage the "imagination to flourish" (Storr, 1988, p. 106).

Self psychology was developed by Kohut in the 1970s and 1980s and has similarities to object relations theory, as both study the development of the self; but each theory has a different perspective, and each offers unique insights.

SELF PSYCHOLOGY

Kohut's theory of self psychology discusses the development of the self, emphasizing the development of cohesion of the self; when the self does not cohere, "fragmentation and emptiness of the self" occur (Wolf, 1988, p. 11). Understanding the subjective world of the individual is a cornerstone of Kohut's theory; empathic responsiveness of the therapist becomes the key to effective treatment. Kohut has broken with Freud's drive and conflict theories, as have other object relations theorists, such as Fairbairn and Winnicott. Through the utilization of a healing therapeutic relationship, which becomes the focus of treatment, the patient is enabled to achieve a firmer, more stable sense of self and self-esteem. The examination of the therapeutic relationship (or selfobject transference) becomes the major goal of treatment; when interpretations are made, they encompass *"reactivated selfobject needs"* [italics added] of the patient, which have been evoked by the treatment (Donner, 1991, p. 57).

Selfobjects

Selfobjects essentially refer to people who meet a person's needs for developing and sustaining a sense of self and self-esteem. The presence of positive selfobjects (nurturing parents or parent-substitutes) during childhood is critical for the development of a cohesive sense of self; however, selfobject experiences are needed throughout adulthood (both through close relationships with others and through evoked memories of past selfobjects). "Along with food and oxygen, every human being requires age-appropriate selfobject experiences from infancy to the end of life" (Wolf, 1988, p. 11).

In Chapter 1, we discussed Vivienne, who committed suicide when she was fourteen. Her depression and shaky self-esteem had improved during the period when she received a great deal of support from a teacher who was warm and empathic with her. However, when he left the school to move across the country, she could not replace this loss and was overcome with depressed feelings. The teacher was not merely an idealized older person to her; he was needed to "replace something missing in the self" (Mack and Hickler, 1981, p. 107). Therefore, his leaving was more than a sad loss; it produced a "terrible emotional pain, a sense of nothingness, and, potentially, a dissolution in the structure of the self" (Mack and Hickler, 1985, p. 107). From the self psychology perspective, Vivienne appears to have related to the teacher as a selfobject.

If Vivienne had received therapy with a self psychology orientation, the emotions and wishes for need fulfillment that she had directed toward this teacher might have been transferred to her therapist, and this selfobject transference might have been brought out into the open in an empathic manner and worked through; Vivienne might then have developed a firmer sense of self, without needing others so desperately to give her permission to feel good about herself.

In her novel, *Villette,* Charlotte Brontë (Bell/Brontë, 1853) describes Paulina, six, who comes to live with Mrs. Bretton for several months. Paulina's mother has recently died, and her father, brooding and overcome by guilt, is prescribed travel as a remedy by his doctors. So he temporarily leaves Paulina with Mrs. Bretton, an old family friend. Paulina is grief stricken when he leaves, but "repressed it. That day she would accept solace from none; nor the next day: she grew more passive afterwards" (Bell/ Brontë, 1853, p. 18). She then develops a relationship with Graham, Mrs. Bretton's sixteen-year-old son. Her world centers around Graham, who becomes her selfobject (although, of course, this was Brontë's artistic and human insight in 1853, more than a century before Kohut developed his concept). In the mornings, Paulina would persuade Mrs. Bretton to include a sweet cake for Graham to take to school, insisting that "he would like it" (Bell/Brontë, 1853, p. 21).

> Graham did like it very well, and almost always got it. To do him jus-tice, he would have shared his prize with her [Paulina] to whom he owed it; but that was never allowed: to insist, was to ruffle her for the evening. To stand by his knee, and monopolize his talk and notice, was the reward she wanted—not a share of the cake.
>
> With curious readiness did she adapt herself to such themes as in-terested him. One would have thought the child had no mind or life of her own, but must necessarily live, move, and have her being in an-other: now that her father was taken from her, she nestled to Graham, and seemed to feel by his feelings: to exist in his existence. (Bell/Brontë, 1853, pp. 21-22)

An interesting note is that Charlotte Brontë wrote this (and her earlier novels) under the name Currer Bell. She and her two sisters (Anne and Em-ily), also important writers, wrote under pseudonyms, and each chose a man's first name. This was done to help ensure publication, as there was a good deal of discrimination against women writers at that time.

Empathy

A major tenet of self psychology is the understanding and use of empa-thy. Empathy is the ability to "participate in another's feelings and experi-ences and to understand them" (Sutherland, 1989, p. 137). The appropriate application of empathy is the affective cornerstone of self psychology ther-apy. When the client feels understood, "new 'compensatory structures' are built" and a "stronger, more cohesive self structure" can gradually emerge (Lynch, 1991, p. 16). Empathy is vital in any form of clinical work; it allows the client "to feel understood in a way that connects the person to others" (Donner, 1991, p. 54).

> Empathy is a message . . . coming from a selfobject, that one is a hu-man among humans. The most disavowed thoughts and affects . . . held by a client to be out of the realm of "normal" . . . human experi-ence can, in the context of empathy, be brought into the thinkable

sphere of self experience. . . . Immersion in a therapeutic relationship characterized by sustained empathy can increase ownership of self. . . . This . . . inevitably expands one's ability to view others through a more empathetic lens. (Donner, 1991, pp. 54-55)

The development of empathy is one of the major skills for clinical social work students to acquire in developing a professional self (Urdang, 1999). However, the therapeutic use of empathy can create complexities; receiving an empathic response from the therapist can create anxiety in some patients (Kohut, 1971). The "immediate pleasure" of feeling understood can be followed by the fear of "a regressive merger experience" with the therapist in certain kinds of clients (Kohut, 1971, p. 306). Patients can also be afraid of giving up the security of their "narcissistic isolation" as they face the risks of getting close to others. Kohut (1971) describes a patient whose fears of "empathic contact with another person and of participation in the world, were movingly portrayed . . . in [the following] dream" (p. 306).

This man had lost his mother in very early childhood and had lost a number of other mother figures subsequent to the first loss. He dreamed that he was alone in his house, his fishing equipment by his side, looking out the window. Through the window he saw numbers of fishes swimming by, big and little, and attractive, and he was yearning to go fishing. He realized, however, that his house was at the bottom of the lake and that as soon as he opened the window to fish the whole lake would flood the house and drown him. (Kohut, 1971, pp. 306-307)

Case Illustration

Kohut (1971) developed self psychology through his work with patients with narcissistic personality disorders, a group of self-centered and self-absorbed patients who had been difficult to treat with standard psychoanalytic techniques. Self psychology has subsequently been extended to the treatment of many "disorders of the self" (Wolf, 1988, p. 24), including: treatment of alcoholism and other addictions, in which alcoholism is considered "a disorder of the self" (Levin, 1991, p. 3); treatment of eating disorders, which involve many " 'self' issues" ("self-esteem and self-cohesion") (Barth, 1991, p. 223); and in the treatment of depression, where the therapist's "empathic attunement to the emergence of the selfobject transferences . . . [can lead to] the restoration of the patient's . . . sense of cohesion" (Deitz, 1991, p. 201).

Wagner (1991) applies self psychology concepts to treating abusing parents who were often abused themselves as children. "Bereft of empathic

selfobjects [that is, nurturing caretakers] . . . [and] subject to multiple traumatic empathic failures, they were unable to develop a cohesive sense of
self" (p. 249). Unable to meet their children's needs, the parents turned to
their children (as selfobjects) to meet *their* needs; when the children are unable to nurture their parents and appear "unresponsive, the parent feels injured and may respond with infantile rage" (Wagner, 1991, p. 249).

Allyson, twenty-five, is a white mother of two children, whose seven-
year-old son was removed from the home because of abuse (Wagner, 1991).
She lives with her daughter Jenni, three, and has a history of alcoholism and
of multiple hospitalizations for depression.

> Consistently deprived of the mirroring and confirming experiences
> that would allow for an internalized cohesive sense of self, Allyson
> faces mothering with a split-off and painfully needy self. She looks to
> her daughter . . . to gratify her needs. When Jenni is unable to gratify
> those needs, Allyson regresses to narcissistic rage. . . . Allyson is un-
> able to be empathically connected to either of her children. Out of her
> own inability to find inner soothing and self-love, Allyson is unable to
> provide these to her children. (Wagner, 1991, p. 251)

Allyson made progress during her therapy, using the supportive therapist
"as a selfobject" (Wagner, 1991, p. 258). In this approach, the primary emphasis was directed toward repairing and rebuilding her own sense of self
and learning ways to soothe herself and regulate her emotions (developing
the ego function of management of needs and feelings). The underlying assumption in this approach is that when this is accomplished, the mother will
internalize the good selfobject (the therapist) and incorporate the therapist's
positive regard for her into her own personality. Only then will she be able to
serve as a good enough selfobject for her children. Because the clinician
"provides mirroring and soothing functions, and helps the abusive parent-
patient anticipate and regulate her needs, she is able to internalize, or trans-
mute, the therapist's selfobject functions into self-functions" (Wagner, 1991,
p. 258).

We now turn to the cognitive and behavioral theories. In contrast to
psychodynamic theories, these theories focus primarily on intellectual
thought processes and observed behaviors, generally dismissing unconscious conflicts and motivations and affects from their approaches.

COGNITIVE AND BEHAVIORAL THEORIES

Cognitive and behavioral therapies have been developing at a rapid pace.
For some clinicians, they are the mainstay of their practice; others may use

them within a psychodynamic context. Many times cognitive and behavioral approaches are combined, and practitioners offer clients a cognitive-behavioral treatment.

Cognitive Theory

Cognition is "the process of obtaining, organizing, and using intellectual knowledge" (Kaplan et al., 1994, p. 1669). In Chapter 2, I discussed the ego function of cognition and the importance of intellectual functioning, judgment, appraising, and reasoning in coping with daily problem solving in life. It was noted that some people have chronic serious deficits in cognitive functioning, such as those impaired by schizophrenia or mental retardation, and that others may develop organic impairments later in life, such as those afflicted by strokes, brain tumors, or Alzheimer's disease. Some people may have temporary problems with cognitive functioning, such as those in emotional crisis who may be unable to apply sequential, logical thinking to their crisis, and some with chronic characterological problems may have developed deficits in functions such as judgment and logical thinking.

However, in the context of cognitive therapy, cognition is viewed in a more narrow sense. Although some people have a basic good capacity for cognitive functioning, they may show faulty reasoning about themselves and about life. Cognitive therapy was developed as a method for correcting the faulty thinking that may be the basis for dysfunctional attitudes, feeling states, and behavior (Beck, 1976). Cognitive therapy stresses that an individual's thinking is the principal determinant of emotions, motives, and behaviors. Therefore, it is the goal of cognitive therapy to reshape the faulty thinking and beliefs that produce dysfunctional behavior or symptoms of psychological distress. In other words, it is the thoughts (such as "I always fail") that produce affective distress; therefore, if the person's thinking changes (to "I can be successful") and he or she realizes that thoughts of inevitable failure are a "bad habit" of thinking, then self-esteem will improve, and will be accompanied by positive affect.

Many writers do not separate cognition and the intellectual realm from the affective, relational, or unconscious modes of being. Eagle (1987), in fact, adds the concept of the cognitive unconscious. He contrasts the cognitive unconscious to the psychoanalytic unconscious, which is a repository of "infantile instinctual wishes," whereas the revised version of the psychoanalytic unconscious incorporates the cognitive unconscious and "includes beliefs, rules, and cognitive-affective schemata" (Eagle, 1987, p. 166). Arieti and Bemporad (1978), in a similar vein, note that "motivation is not necessarily instinctual but is very often the result of complicated cognitive constructs which have become unconscious" (p. 362).

Vaillant (1993) stresses the integration of cognition and affect, noting that "the brain cannot be separated from the heart" (p. 4). He contrasts this integration with "the deliberate decision of cognitive scientists to exclude certain factors that 'would unnecessarily complicate the cognitive-scientific enterprise. These factors include the influence of affective factors . . . the contribution of historical and cultural factors, and the role of the background context in which particular actions or thoughts occur'" (Vaillant, 1993, p. 4). Noam (1996) stresses the inherent necessity for the integration of thought, feeling, and experience. "The powerful abilities to make *cognition emotional* and *feelings reflective* [italics added] has profound implications for the inner experience and the pursuit of a vital, true self" (Noam, 1996, p. 144).

Beck's (1976) theories of cognitive therapy have received great recognition, and other cognitive therapists have built their work around these major ideas.

Cognitive Therapy

In the following example, Jackie is feeling discouraged by her way of thinking about her son's birthday. In her encounter with a friend, this informal cognitive therapy alters her way of thinking as well as her feeling state.

> Jackie was about to turn thirty-nine; her son was to become thirteen. She complained to her friend Margie: "I'm almost forty, and my son is about to become an adolescent!" Margie responded: "You would be forty even if you didn't have children." As she reflected on this, Jackie didn't feel so "bereft"; she realized what she did have, rather than focusing on what she was losing. Margie reframed the situation for Jackie, and Jackie's modified "perspective" helped her change her feelings.

Beck (1976), the originator of cognitive therapy, has categorized flawed thought processes that lead to emotional difficulties. One, the tendency to overgeneralize, refers to "unjustified generalization on the basis of a specific incident. For example, a child makes a single mistake and thinks, 'I never do anything right'" (Beck, 1976, pp. 94-95). It is not unusual to find students thinking this way: "I failed this test—I don't know anything—I shouldn't be in graduate school!" In cognitive therapy, a therapist brings these habitual thought patterns to a person's attention, attempting to replace these cognitions with more positive and adaptive attitudes.

Catastrophizing, another faulty thought process, often found in anxious people, "illustrates anticipation of extreme adverse outcomes. The thinking of the anxious patient is grooved toward considering the most unfavorable of all possible outcomes of a situation" (Beck, 1976, p. 93). The following example from practice illustrates this concept.

> Carol is a bright woman who functioned well in an administrative position but sought therapy because of symptoms of anxiety. She brought up her interest in a man who seemed attracted to her. They had brief (but intense) conversations in the office but never saw each other outside of work. Carol said she was afraid of getting married to him— what if they had nothing to talk about? What if he lost interest in her? What would it be like for her to live with him? Her therapist asked: "Maybe you should date first?" Carol looked at her therapist and burst into laughter—she could see that she was catastrophizing—that is, building up a negative scenario that is doomed to failure without going through appropriate, reality-based steps in building a relationship.

Beck's (1976) model of cognitive therapy "is one of the most useful psychotherapeutic interventions currently available for depressive disorders" (Kaplan et al., 1994, p. 863). Treatment is based on the identification of a "depressive triad" of thoughts: "a negative conception of the self, a negative interpretation of life experiences, and a nihilistic view of the future" (Beck, 1976, p. 84). Patients are helped to reconceptualize their basic life assumptions.

Cognitive approaches are often used together with behavioral approaches, and the cognitive-behavioral model is cited as being helpful for a wide range of problems, including panic disorders, marital therapy, and adaptation to cancer (Kaplan et al., 1994). Beck often incorporates behavioral approaches into his therapy, such as "mobilizing the patient into more activity and positively reinforcing certain types of activity" (Beck, 1976, pp. 267-268). However, he asserts that the ultimate "goal is cognitive modification" (Beck, 1976, p. 268).

Eagle (1987) sees cognition in a broader context than Beck does and notes limitations of Beck's theory. "Beck and his colleagues write about dysfunctional cognitions and schemata . . . with little or no reference to the object-rational [relational], dynamic, and developmental contexts" (Eagle, 1987, p. 168). He adds that Beck's approach does not attempt to elicit affects and makes no use of interpretations of the therapeutic relationship, nor of intersubjectivity.

Beck (1976) finds that "cognitive techniques are most appropriate for people who have the capacity for introspection and for reflecting about their own thoughts and fantasies" (p. 216). This orientation leaves the full potential for cognitive work untapped, as often clients (such as schizophrenic patients or those with characterological problems) need help to learn how to think, how to make good judgments, and how to consider consequences of their behaviors.

The *schema* (plural *schemata*) is a concept appearing in psychodynamic and cognitive approaches; it is concerned with the organization of thought and experiences. Beck (1976) describes schemata as organized patterns of thinking and ordering of ideas, such as the depressive triad. Piaget (Elkind, 1981) refers to schemata in describing the development and organization of thought in the child. His schemata are "tied to mental operations and cognitive structures" (Elkind, 1981, p. 8). Piaget focuses on overall intellectual development and does not directly address the development of feelings or relationships, although he touches on these indirectly in some areas, such as his notion of fairness. Bowlby's (1988) attachment theory implies the development of schemata by describing how "each partner builds in his or her mind working models of self and of other and of the patterns of interaction that have developed between them" (p. 29). Bowlby's approach involves intellectual processing or cognition (working models) as well as developmental concepts of self and other.

Eagle (1987) describes a commonality present in the idea of schemata, noting that "the concept of self- and object representations is intended to refer to the implicit schemata, images, working models—whatever language one chooses to use—one implicitly has of oneself and others. Related concepts include self-image, body-image, identity, and object constancy" (pp. 170-171).

Although cognitive therapy has often been used in conjunction with behavior therapy, the latter, in its many variations, has been used as a specific intervention by itself, as well as in combination with psychodynamic therapies.

Behavior Theory

Behaviorism was introduced into psychology in 1913 by John B. Watson, who stressed that "psychology must abandon its focus on subjective 'mentalistic' concepts and instead focus exclusively on behavior" (Ashford et al., 1997, p. 65). Watson developed the concept of learning theory, which emphasizes that development proceeds from learning experiences and focuses on "studying *observable stimuli* and *observable responses* [italics added] to the stimuli" (Ashford et al., 1997, p. 66). From this perspective, concepts such as the unconscious and mental representations of self and other would be not only irrelevant but devoid of meaning. B. F. Skinner added the concept of *operant conditioning,* "a form of learning that occurs when responses are controlled by their consequences" (Ashford et al., 1997, p. 66), to learning theory.

Operant conditioning, which utilizes *positive reinforcement,* encourages desired behaviors by providing positive responses or rewards. A child completing homework might be rewarded with movie privileges. Since no simple one-to-one correspondence exists between a consequence and its effect, an individualized study of a person's motivational system is necessary, as a reward for one child (a movie) might not be a reward for another, who might dislike or be fearful of movies or prefer some other type of reward. Consequences "viewed as aversive by some may be reinforcing for others" (Kaplan et al., 1994, p. 167). Scolding is usually viewed as a negative (or aversive) experience by children. However, to some, scolding may be a positive reinforcer as it is "a form of attention" (Kaplan et al., 1994, p. 167).

Behavior Therapy

Positive reinforcement can be used purposefully or inadvertently by clinicians. A clinician may intentionally praise a client who progressively takes steps to improve a work situation. A clinician may inadvertently use negative reinforcement by appearing uninterested when a client talks about childhood conflict, and inadvertently use positive reinforcement by listening with avid attention when sexual issues are discussed. Social work students have been shown to respond positively to praise (a reinforcer) from their supervisors (Nelson, 1974). Paradoxically, some clients with depressive traits and severe superegos might find being praised uncomfortable and display a negative reaction to this reinforcer.

Mrs. Billings (discussed in Chapter 1), hospitalized for depression, was visited by her husband, who drove the long distance from their farm to the hospital. When he asked if he could take his wife out of the hospital for lunch, the interviewer encouraged this, recalling Mr. Billings saying that he should take his wife out more—"it's a help for her to eat out." From a behavioral perspective, this intervention was aimed at behavioral change. The positive reinforcing aspects of this experience might help the couple continue this behavior at home. In this instance, a behavioral approach was incorporated into a predominantly psychodynamic orientation, without the interviewer being explicitly aware that she was utilizing a behavioral intervention; this happens many times.

Systematic desensitization, which aims to "eliminate maladaptive anxiety and behavior," was developed by Joseph Wolpe (Kaplan et al., 1994, p.168). Desensitization involves application of relaxation techniques combined with gradually leading the client to the feared object (sometimes in imagery, sometimes in reality), whether it be airplanes, snakes, or other phobic situations. Bandura (1976) discusses a treatment model for agoraphobic patients (those phobic about the world outside of their homes) in which the therapist participates in activities with the patient. "Clients accompany the therapist into the avoided situation over a period of several days. The longer they are exposed to the aversive events, the more dramatic is the experience that what they dread does not happen" (Bandura, 1976, pp. 44-45). Gradually the therapist's participation diminishes and the patient's solo exposure is increased.

In a *modeling* procedure, the client learns from the therapist's purposefully modeled behavior, such as when the therapist demonstrates various ways of being assertive (assertiveness training) (Bandura, 1976). Modeling also may be more subtle, based on the assumption that the client may learn to handle situations more calmly and logically by observing the way the therapist calmly and logically approaches problem solving with the client.

In Chapter 2, while discussing the ego's executive functioning, we described a homemaker assigned to a woman overwhelmed with the care of her ten children. The homemaker did not take over and do things for her, but through modeling involved the client by engaging in household activities with her. Social work students may refer to a particular professor as a role model for them, indicating that his or her ways of responding, with empathy and caring, enabled them to further develop these characteristics in themselves. Social skills training has been utilized in recent years with many populations. Typical procedures include "instructions, prompts, modeling, behavioral rehearsal, feedback, and homework assignments" (Curran and Monti, 1986, p. 2). For example, one program with schizophrenic patients focuses on enhancing their abilities with: "interpersonal skills, nutrition and meal planning, health and hygiene, money management, prevocational [guidance], [learning how to access] community resources and social networks" (Brown, 1986, pp. 97-100). Some programs have been directed at relatives of patients to "reduce family patterns that have been implicated as factors contributing to schizophrenic relapse" (Curran and Monti, 1986, p. 3).

Social skills training has been applied in other contexts, including communication skills training for married couples (Jacobson, 1986) and the treatment of children with peer-relationship difficulties (French and Tyne, 1986). Social skills training is one aspect of a behavioral approach useful in the treatment of autistic children (Groden and Baron, 1988).

No uniformity of opinion exists on approaches among behaviorists, and a range of opinion exists on "theoretical orthodoxy" as opposed to "theoretical integration." Favoring integration, Basch (1988) comments that "by the time treatment has been completed the therapist has probably made use of a combination of dynamic, behavioral, and cognitive techniques" (p. 55). Thyer (1988) observes "behavioral approaches have had a major influence on clinical social work education and practice" (p. 127) and, citing Rubin's review of research, asserts that studies claim to show the effectiveness of " 'problem-solving and task-centered methods' " which have often been combined with behavioral work (Thyer, 1988, p. 128). Helen Singer Kaplan (1974) developed a form of sex therapy that incorporates behavioral approaches to sexual dysfunction as well as psychodynamic interventions. She recommends the "combined and integrated use of prescribed, systematically structured sexual experiences and psychotherapeutic intervention within a basic psychodynamic context" (Kaplan, 1974, p. 220). Wachtel (1977) advocates an approach combining psychoanalytic understanding with behavioral techniques that promote active intervention on the therapist's part. Marmor (1971) suggests that "all psychotherapy, regardless of the techniques used, is a learning process" (p. 26).

RESILIENCE

The observation that some children living under adverse conditions and/or who have lived through multiple stresses do not experience symptoms of psychopathology but "remain invulnerable or resilient, able to cope with the effects of misfortune and adversity" (Cohler, 1987, p. 363) is one of the conundrums of human behavior. Some resilient adults have made positive adaptations after suffering traumatic events, including physical disasters, war, concentration camps, the death of a child, marital desertion, and physical illness. Why is it that some people bounce back and forge ahead with their lives, while others seem forever scarred and frozen in their development? Interest in resilience has been increasing. Stella Chess (1989) asserts that it is important, for preventive purposes, to understand how "such individuals defy the voice of doom" (p. 180).

Resilience, a complex phenomenon, can be looked at through different theoretical lenses, applied to differing age groups, and evaluated with different measures. Vaillant (1993) states that "we all know perfectly well what resilience means until we listen to someone else trying to define it" (p. 285). To Vaillant (1993), "resilience conveys both the capacity to be bent without breaking and the capacity, once bent, to spring back. Thus, I like the definition that Emmy Werner and Ruth Smith give for resilience: 'The self-righting tendencies within the human organism' " (pp. 284-285). But, he asks, "does this merely mean survival in the face of vulnerability and multiple risk factors, or should we think of resilience only when it also permits happiness? Is it enough that the vulnerable patient survives the operation and that the orphan survives the concentration camp, or, to be called resilient, must they be able to run and laugh and feel joy as well? The reader must choose" (Vaillant, 1993, p. 285).

Resiliency has been discussed from an ecological framework, including factors in the environment and in the individual that interact to provide both risk and protection for the child (Begun, 1993; Kirby and Fraser, 1997). Kirby and Fraser (1997) stress the importance of a developmental framework to "allow for changes in resilience in individuals at different points in time and to explain the cumulative effects of risk" (p. 19).

Environmental risk factors include limited opportunities for education or employment, racial discrimination and injustice, poverty, child maltreatment, interparental conflict, parental psychopathology, and poor parenting. Individual psychosocial and biological risk factors include biomedical problems and gender (Kirby and Fraser, 1997). Environmental protective factors encompass opportunities for education; employment; growth and achievement; social support; presence of a caring, supportive adult (not necessarily the parent); positive parent-child relationships; and effective parenting. Individual psychosocial and biological protective factors include easy temperament, competence in normative roles, self-efficacy, self-esteem, and intelligence.

Other authors have utilized these or other similar factors in discussing resiliency; some have added additional factors, such as the strength of defense mechanisms (Vaillant, 1993). "I shall continue to point to maturity of defenses as the 'god in the machine' that seems to account for otherwise inexplicable resilience" (Vaillant, 1993, p. 297). However, he lists eleven other factors that are "interdependent," including temperament and attributional style, which means "how we regard our responsibility for the good and bad events that befall us" (Vaillant, 1993, p. 305). He adds hope and faith, social attractiveness, luck, and timing and/or context.

Social supports, an important contributor to resilience in ecological theory, has been described from a different perspective by Vaillant (1993). It is not sufficient for social supports to be present: "they must be *recognized and then internalized* [italics added]. Social experience is not what happens to you, it is what you do with what happens to you" (Vaillant, 1993, p. 311). The roles others play in our lives can be transforming, but "only if we can metabolize influential other people" (Vaillant, 1993, p. 180).

Temperament has been recognized as a factor in promoting resilience (Chess, 1989; Kirby and Fraser, 1997; Vaillant, 1993). Chess noted that temperaments "had been insufficiently studied with respect to their influence upon developmental outcomes" (Chess, 1989, p. 182) and evaluated nine temperamental characteristics in children: "activity level; rhythmicity; approach or withdrawal; adaptability; intensity of response; threshold of responsiveness; quality of mood; distractibility; and attention span and persistence" (Chess, 1989, pp. 184-185). Not only is temperament relevant to the way events affect children, but children's "temperamental qualities influenced their caretakers" and therefore, goodness-of-fit can "influence the quality of adaptation of children" (p. 183).

Bowlby (1988) stresses the importance of attachment in the development of resiliency. He hypothesizes that "the pathway followed by each developing individual and the extent to which he or she becomes resilient to stressful life events is determined to a very significant degree by the pattern of attachment he or she develops during the early years" (Bowlby, 1988, p. 34). Thomlison (1997), discussing childhood maltreatment, noted: "Compared with children who have no bonds of attachment, children who have a deep sense of belonging and security are widely known to function more adaptively across settings. Such attachments occur, first and foremost, because of a positive, caring caretaker from birth—a caretaker who is available in times of stress for support" (p. 57). Kegan (1982) suggests that qualities may exist within the child that may serve to recruit others in providing external supports. This ability to recruit is a critical capacity for children who must seek sources outside of their families for social support.

Paradoxically, although children need nurturance from their families, their ability to distance themselves from their difficult families can also be a protective factor. Chess (1989) asserts that under some conditions there is "a high virtue in distancing from noxious family onslaughts and underminings, in leaving behind irreconcilable conflicts" (p. 198). Berlin and Davis (1989) discuss the importance of the development of a capacity for "defensive distancing" by the children of alcoholics from their families and differentiate this from unconstructive "reactive distancing. . . . The adaptive distancer . . . tends to use some form of flight away from the pull of parental alcoholism but, unlike the reactive child, the adaptive one is more likely *to flee towards activities and relationships* [italics added] that allow some breathing room for reparative work" (p. 97).

Felsman (1989) discusses this "flight towards relationships" as a key factor in the resiliency he found in the "gamins," the street children [boys] of Colombia who are potentially "at high risk for psychopathology. . . . Darting in and out of traffic, begging in open-air restaurants, singing for change on city buses, bathing in public fountains, or sleeping together curled up among stray dogs, these young ragamuffins manage the often-tangled course of human growth and development with little or no support from the traditional institutions of family, school, church, or state" (p. 56). In describing their substitute social support system, the special place of peer relationships in their lives is emphasized. Other researchers who have studied disadvantaged children have also observed a similar tendency to rely on peers.

We will continue to examine resiliency from a developmental perspective throughout the life cycle. The lack of uniformity in evaluating resiliency complicates this task. Is social functioning a sufficient criterion? "Personal success may be attained at the cost of spontaneous enjoyment of life" (Cohler, 1987, p. 406). Children of parents with psychiatric disorders, for example, may "feel pressured to maintain maturity and responsibility for themselves and others, which may have later costs in terms of continuing adjustment" (Cohler, 1987, p. 406). Noam (1996) suggests that "we need to end idealizing the self's complexity, the linear movement from limited ability to great capacity, and instead focus on the continued struggles between strengths and weaknesses to the end of life" (p. 138).

CONCLUSION

This chapter has extended the discussion of psychodynamic theories to include object relations and self psychology, adding the perspectives offered by cognitive and behavioral theories, and concluding with a discussion of the complexities of resiliency. The central concepts of attachment and loss as well as the dialectical conflicts between separation/individuation and maintaining connectedness are present throughout the life cycle. We move through life sometimes toward others, sometimes away, needing solitude; we may move from reliance on family to attachments to friends, then perhaps develop allegiance to our own newly formed families, maybe reaching back in our new lives to include the families we grew up with.

Luck (one of the factors contributing to resilience, according to Vaillant [1993]) is also a major factor contributing to the experiences of loss in our lives; we may lose attachments through death, serious illness, or being abandoned. We can also lose attachments because attachments can be frightening; we may run away from them and push people away because intimacy can bring anxieties in its wake such as fears of loss of self-identity or of being controlled. Husbands and wives may fight over money or visiting in-laws, not necessarily because these are "burning" issues; periodic fighting may be the only way they know to keep the "distance" between them that they need, as the porcupines need, to keep from feeling "wounded" by the other and to remain safe.

Being connected to a community can be a source of strength and joy but may prove distressing, as the individual struggles between wishes for autonomy and connectedness to a group. The Mahlerian concept of separation-individuation has its parallel in community life as the individual experiences an ongoing dialectical tension between social conformity and personal freedom. The issues of community involvement are examined in the next chapter. Our psychological development and sense of well-being are affected by what happens to us directly and indirectly in the world around us. The social aspects of the biopsychosocial world is the focus of attention in Chapter 4.

LEARNING EXERCISE

1. Choose a case and discuss it from the vantage points of the various theories presented in this chapter. Think about it in terms of both assessment and intervention issues.

SUGGESTED READINGS

Article

Bowlby, J. (1988). Developmental psychiatry comes of age. *American Journal of Psychiatry, 145*, 28-37.

Books

Applegate, J. S. and Bonovitz, J. M. (1995). *The facilitating partnership: A Winnicottian approach for social workers and other helping professionals.* Northvale: Jason Aronson Inc.

Jackson, H. (Ed.). (1991). *Using self psychology in psychotherapy.* Northvale: Jason Aronson Inc.

Mack, J. E. and Hickler, H. (1981). *Vivienne: The life and suicide of an adolescent girl.* New York: A Mentor Book, New American Library.

Mahler, M., Pine, F., and Bergman, A. (1975). *The psychological birth of the human infant.* New York: Basic Books, Inc.

Mitchell, S. (1988). *Relational concepts in psychoanalysis.* Cambridge: Harvard University Press.

Wachtel, P. L. (1977). *Psychoanalysis and behavior therapy: Toward an integration.* New York: Basic Books, Inc.

Chapter 4

Social Systems and the Community

A thousand fibers connect us with our fellow men; and among those fibers, as sympathetic threads, our actions run as causes, and they come back to us as effects.

Herman Melville

INTRODUCTION

In the two preceding chapters we discussed the psychological development of individuals, giving only minimal attention to the social and political context of their lives. I utilized Heinz Hartmann's (1958) definition of adaptation as "primarily a reciprocal relationship between the organism and its environment" (p. 24), but I did not discuss the dimensions and complexities of the environment, nor how environmental factors can affect an individual's psychological being; the present chapter addresses this interaction.

We constantly absorb and filter the impact of the world around us, and our values, conflicts, frustrations, and stresses, as well as the innermost sense of our identities, are intertwined with our experiences in and relationships to our human and nonhuman environments.

Physical, economic, social, cultural, technological, and ideological influences are constantly impinging upon us. Computers, for example, a major technological advance in recent years, have had a dramatic impact on our economy, employment, education, and recreation. Some observers have noted that computers have even found their way ever more deeply into our unconscious as objects of "anxiety-filled dreams" (Kelley, 1998). In 1909, the book *10,000 Dreams Interpreted* by Gustavus Hindman Miller, "featured dream objects like absinthe, reapers and saltpeter," and now "dream lexicons are filled with cars and airplanes;" it would not be surprising if "control panels and File Not Found messages will be regularly showing up in the collective subconscious" (Kelley, 1998, p. E1).

We begin this chapter by introducing the ecological perspective, with its focus on the interactions of people and their environments, which include physical environments (landscape and weather, urban and rural settings, and housing as well as homelessness), and social environments (communities, support networks, economic issues, employment, education, and organizations).

The final section introduces the social problems of discrimination, violence, the increasing use of prisons for social control, the "warehousing" of the mentally ill, and the impact of the addictions on society. We also examine loyalties, conflicts, competing interests, and ideologies in relation to individuals, families, communities, and organizations.

An ideology can be a driving force in the lives of people: strong emotional energies are invested in such issues as antigun control (or gun control), abortion, and involvement in religious groups, cults, or political movements. Ethnic and racial hatreds can fuel discrimination and violence in this country as well as others, such as Rwanda, the former Yugoslavia, and Northern Ireland. Selected social policies are also discussed, such as laws prohibiting racial discrimination (or denying antidiscriminatory protections to homosexuals).

These subjects are not readily categorized, as these systems often overlap in reality. Housing projects, for example, part of the physical environment, also constitute a social environment, and social problems of discrimination and violence are often found there. From a social policy perspective, inadequate funding for low-income housing perpetuates the housing crisis and homelessness. Conflicting ideologies and values relating to segregation versus integration, as well as the expenditure of public funds on poor people, can affect the formulation of social policies related to low-income projects and the needs of the people who live there.

Policies or social issues will change between the writing of this chapter and your reading of it; the world will not sit still. Although current events inevitably change, what we need to understand and appreciate is the complex intertwining of people, environments, social issues, ideologies, and organizations, and how we all are affected both by the stability and the precariousness of the world around us.

THE ECOLOGICAL PERSPECTIVE

Germain (1991), in her ecological approach to social work, emphasizes that person-environmental relationships are "characterized by continuous reciprocal exchanges or transactions, in which people and environments influence, shape, and sometimes change each other" (p. 16).

The complex and problematic interactions between the fragile ecosystem of the Galapagos archipelago and its residents illustrate this perspective.

The Galapagos Islands, a major inspiration for Darwin's theory of evolution, remained until recently a protected and studied enclave, large parts of which are protected as a national park, a Marine Resources Reserve, and a UNESCO World Heritage Site. Today, major changes threaten to upset its "fragile environmental balance" (Lemonick, 1995, p. 80). Many of the competing interests and ideologies affecting this microcosm are also reflected, in different ways, in our own society. The islands are described in "idyllic" detail.

> The giant tortoises known as *galapagos,* which gave the islands their name, still amble across the scrubby landscape, sea-lion pups and Galapagos penguins gaze unafraid at scuba divers, marine iguanas crawl over volcanic rocks along the shore, and strolling tourists have to detour around blue-footed boobies (a type of seabird) busily performing courtship rituals. Puerto Ayora, the islands' largest town (pop. 8,000), comprises a tranquil collection of quaint hotels, craft shops and seafood restaurants. (Lemonick, 1995, p. 80)

The competing interest groups in the Galapagos include those concerned with preserving the archipelago's pristine environmental status and others who feel economically oppressed by environmental restrictions. One group seeking change includes residents opposed to prohibitions against sea cucumber fishing. During a melee over this conflict, the entrance to the Charles Darwin Research Station was blockaded, some workers were held as hostages, scientists were "harassed," and the tortoises were threatened (Lemonick, 1995, p. 80).

Another protest involved residents seeking greater local control, who seized both the research station and the airport for two weeks, complaining that their demands were being ignored (Lemonick, 1995, p. 80). Adding to the systemic complexities is the large influx of tourists. Many tourists and tour operators respect the environment. However, some ships dump waste directly into the sea (Lemonick, 1995, p. 81).

The dramatic increase in tourists (and the money they spend) has led to a dramatic increase in immigrants looking for tourism-related jobs. This results in a strain on the waste management and water systems as well as on the fabric of society itself (Lemonick, 1995, p. 81). Many residents resent the new immigrants and have accused them of importing and establishing an illicit sex and drug culture (Lemonick, 1995, p. 81). In addition, people have allegedly brought with them many off-islands species of plants and animals, endangering local life-forms. The now-huge goat population, for example, is decimating larger plants and also consuming plants that form a vital part of the tortoises' food supply (Lemonick, 1995, p. 82). Fishermen have been overfishing illegally, posing a threat to the sea life.

The competing conflict groups include: the national government (wanting to control excessive exploitation of the Galapagos Islands, yet wanting to retain the tourist income); the local government (seeking greater autonomy); the conservationists (concerned about maintaining the ecological system while acknowledging the islanders' need to make a living), as well as the "natives," the flora and fauna, and the tourists themselves. The local governmental group has threatened violence. Although solutions have been suggested, resolution has been difficult as issues of political control, political autonomy, economic gain, and ideologies about conservation are pitted against each other. Exploring systems issues, many of these core conflicts will be seen, in myriad forms, at the heart of systemic problems.

On the Galapagos Islands, the physical environment and its animal and plant life compete with human needs or, perhaps, attempt to reach some sort of accommodation with them. Other situations exist in which the physical environment is a significant and perhaps controlling factor in human destiny.

THE PHYSICAL ENVIRONMENT

The physical environment, such as the landscape, available natural resources, weather, the presence of active volcanoes, or proneness to earthquakes can affect human feelings and behavior in many ways.

Visitors to Iceland, for example, are often moved by the stark beauty of the country, but they may feel overwhelmed by the barrenness of much of the landscape, the absence of vegetation, and the paucity of animal life. Iceland became a training ground for the first moon astronauts to help them acclimate to living in a "moonscape." Presently, active volcanoes, geysers, hot springs, and a tendency toward earthquakes are all part of the environs. One Icelandic native expressed her belief that the untamed nature of her country is what motivated its people to become interested in trolls, fairies, and the Icelandic sagas.

The physical environment can have special meaning and significance to people based on their cultural values. To Native Americans, "working in harmony with natural forces is a way of life" (Attneave, 1982, p. 65). Animistic beliefs hold that the spirit or soul inhabits everything in nature. "Not only animals but plants, rocks, mountains and bodies of water exist as personalities or as vehicles of expression for the spiritual forces of the universe" (Attneave, 1982, p. 65).

The physical environment often plays a positive role in the mental lives of humans. According to Germain (1991), Searles asserts that "human beings not only must respect the natural world, our life-sustaining environment, but must remain in touch with its *restorative and healing forces*" [italics added] (p. 30). Germain describes "the sense of serenity and wonder felt by those fortunate enough to experience mountains, seashore, and countryside—and the powerful influence of wilderness therapy and organized camping for persons of all ages and varying states of physical and mental health" (Germain, 1991, p. 30).

Studying the physical environment of the individual requires sensitivity to issues such as personal space, crowding, and privacy (Gutheil, 1992). Living in a house (or an institution) with no physical privacy or storage space of one's own can have negative psychological effects. "Some [physical] environments have a welcoming quality . . . and encourage the development of ongoing interpersonal relationships. . . . Other environments work against the formation of relationships . . . such [as] jails and hospitals" (Gutheil, 1992, p. 392). In some psychiatric facilities, the "spatial arrangements are so different from normal experiences that they induce stress and may elicit behavior that appears bizarre" (Gutheil, 1992, p. 392).

Robert Caro (1983), in his biography of Lyndon Johnson, depicts the hill country of Texas where Johnson grew up, because he felt that to understand Johnson, one had to know his special environment. "The hill country was a trap—a trap baited with grass" (Caro, 1983, p. 8). Initially, new settlers to this area were impressed by the richness of the flourishing grass.

> The tall grass of the Hill Country stretched as far as the eye could see, covering valleys and hillsides alike. . . . To these men [the settlers] the grass was proof that their dreams would come true. In country where grass grew like that, cotton would surely grow tall, and cattle fat—and men rich. In country where grass grew like that, they thought, anything would grow. How could they know about the grass? (Caro, 1983, p. 11)

What the new farmers did not know about the grass was that the soil was thin, the roots shallow. Brush, which had been thinned by fires, grew back, blocking out the grass. Grazing increased. "The cattle ate the grass—and then there was no longer anything holding . . . the soil" (Caro, 1983, p. 21). Floods complicated matters. Succeeding on such land "required . . . a pragmatism almost terrifying in its absolutely uncompromising starkness" (Caro, 1983, p. 26). In fact, the Johnsons "were . . . particularly unsuited to such a land" (Caro, 1983, p. 26). They lost their agricultural investment and lived a life of genteel poverty, with the father being regarded as a failure by the family. These economic circumstances and resulting family interactions played a large role in Lyndon Johnson's psychological development (Caro, 1983).

Climatic conditions can have serious effects on the physical and mental health of individuals. In this country, the most dangerous kind of "extreme summer heat and humidity . . . have become more frequent . . . over the last half century" (Stevens, 1998, p. A1). Almost 600 people in Chicago died in 1995 from extreme heat and humidity. Research has "shown that extreme summer heat has more impact on people's health than any other kind of severe weather, and that the elderly are most vulnerable" (Stevens, 1998, p. A1). The absence of warmth and sunlight has also received recent attention; some people develop depressions reactive to seasons—a condition termed seasonal affective disorder (SAD) has been distinguished in recent years (Kaplan et al., 1994). These patients generally respond to light therapy.

Physical disasters, such as floods, tornadoes, hurricanes, earthquakes, and volcanic eruptions, can have a profound impact on people's lives and psychological states. In 1980, for example, Mount St. Helens unexpectedly erupted, causing a large loss of life, homes, and other property. The economy, which had had a high unemployment rate before the eruption, suffered greatly. "There was a rise in the reports of child and spouse abuse, other violent crimes, and even murders, which had been a very rare occurrence heretofore" (Mt. St. Helens, 1980, p. 1). A disaster crisis counseling unit was established.

> The cumulative effects of continued fear about the volcano's activities, the depression spurred by altered living conditions and a sense of loss, and the stress created by a badly shaken local economy, make the bolstering of the social services community a necessity. (Mt. St. Helens, 1980, p. 12)

Concerns have also been raised about pollution, both in the oceans and in local water supplies; overfishing; deforestation; air pollution; and global warming; conflict exists between groups about disposal of radioactive and other toxic waster material. "Abandoned, uncontrolled toxic dumps and poorly controlled landfills used for hazardous wastes are found in or near some rural and urban communities, especially poorer ones" (Germain, 1991, pp. 60-61).

Finally, on the microscopic or submicroscopic level, "new viruses and drug-resistant bacteria are reversing human victories over infectious disease" (Lemonick, 1994, p. 62). The agents of other diseases such as tuberculosis are developing new strains that do not respond to antibiotics. Systemic events, such as rapid increases in transportation of products and air travel by people, facilitates the rapid spread of disease. The behavior of people can also contribute to this problem (Lemonick, 1994).

> Human behavior just makes the situation worse. Patients frequently stop taking antibiotics when their symptoms go away but before an infection is entirely cleared up. This suppresses susceptible microbes but allows partially resistant ones to flourish. People with viral infections sometimes demand antibiotics, even though the drugs are useless

against viruses. This, too, weeds out whatever susceptible bacteria are lurking in their bodies and promotes the growth of their hardier brethren. In many countries, antibiotics are available over the counter, which lets patients diagnose and dose themselves, often inappropriately. And high-tech farmers have learned that mixing low doses of antibiotics into cattle feed makes the animals grow larger . . . [however] bacteria in the cattle become resistant to the drugs, and when people drink milk or eat meat, this immunity may be transferred to human bacteria. (Lemonick, 1994, p. 67)

The international AIDS epidemic has created innumerable systemic problems, including disability, death, loss, a dramatic increase in the number of orphans (especially in Africa), and the infection of unborn children. In the United States an increase in the number of children being diagnosed with AIDS, as well as children testing positive for HIV (the causative viral agent of AIDS, acquired immunodeficiency syndrome) is taking place. In addition, many children in the United States have also lost their mothers to AIDS. In 1998, 67,000 of these children were under age eighteen (of whom more than 50 percent were age twelve or under); most were children of color (Day, 2001). AIDS is discussed further in Chapter 12.

The physical environment encompasses both urban and rural settings. Urban problems such as overcrowding, lack of or poor housing, and crime are frequently addressed in the social work literature. Kaplan and colleagues (1994) assert that an increase in psychiatric illness occurs as people move from suburban areas to inner cities.

On the other hand, less attention has been paid to rural problems.

Rural Social Work

What is rural America? "Many still believe that farming is its primary occupation, with strong support from mining, fishing, and forest-products industries" (Davenport and Davenport III, 1995, p. 2076). However, while farming and these natural resource-based industries remain significant, they are being upstaged by manufacturing and services. In fact, "most growth in the rural economy has been in the service area" (Davenport and Davenport III, 1995, p. 2076). Rural areas have been classified by "specialization of their economic function" by sociologists in the U.S. Department of Agriculture, who formulated the seven following categories (Davenport and Davenport III, 1995, p. 2077). Although some overlap occurs, the populations of most rural counties belong primarily in one or two groups, which include farming-, manufacturing-, and mining-dependent counties; specialized government (with military bases or state universities); persistent poverty (especially in the Mississippi Delta, parts of Appalachia, and many Native American counties); federal lands; and destination retirement communities. This variety "dispel[s] the myth of one rural America" (Davenport and Davenport III, 1995, p. 2077).

The population in rural America is not homogenous; it includes such groups as the Missouri Amish, Louisiana Cajun, North Carolina Hmong, New Mexico Pueblo, Mississippi African American, and Southwestern Tex-Mex. In addition, many refugees are being placed in rural areas (Davenport and Davenport III, 1995).

Social workers in rural areas are usually employed by public agencies, such as child welfare, mental health, and corrections settings. "They tend to work in relatively isolated, small local and county offices and confront a host of complex problems. Specialized services common in urban areas generally are not available" (Davenport and Davenport III, 1995, p. 2081). Germain addresses the complexity of rural problems. "The incidence and prevalence of malnutrition, substandard housing, maternal and infant mortality, unemployment and underemployment, poverty, water pollution, and increase in divorce are greater than in urban communities" (Germain, 1991, p. 60).

The decline of family farms has affected rural life and has many economic and social ramifications, which were reflected in an unusual case of two young Amish men in Pennsylvania, who were brought to trial on charges of distributing drugs—behavior very much out of character for members of the sect (Remnick, 1998). Some observers thought the decline of farming led more Amish into greater involvement with the outside world, hence exposure to greater "temptations," including drugs. The trial produced a great deal of interest, because the Amish are a law-abiding religious sect with many strict prohibitions, for whom the use of modern conveniences, even zippers, are "violations before God" (Remnick, 1998, p. 28).

It is characteristic of many rural areas that their residents develop a sense of community, leading to the development of mutual support systems. These include social networks and "natural helpers," the latter being relatives and friends, "first-line purveyors of informal mental health, social, and health services" (Patterson et al., 1988, p. 272), whom others seek out. This array of social supports can be of assistance to rural social workers, who often have minimal resources available.

Conversely, while some people benefit from a sense of community solidarity and social supports, others who do not conform to community expectations may be excluded from these supports. Homosexuals, for example, can have a more difficult time coming out in rural areas than in larger cities. A tragic murder highlighted this dilemma, when a thirty-nine-year-old gay man was murdered in the rural South. Although his gay friends stated that violence against gays had not occurred in Sylacauga, Alabama, before, they felt that homosexuality was not accepted there (Firestone, 1999).

Until his death (by beating and burning), the victim lived with his disabled parents who did not know of his sexual orientation (Firestone, 1999). "The closets that gay people build in small, severe towns like this one are thick and difficult to penetrate, and Billy Jack Gaither's was locked even tighter than most" (Firestone, 1999, p. A1). But he was known to the small number of local gays, who were also fearful of exposure. A friend believed he would have left his hometown but for his concern for his parents; the relative anonymity of Birmingham evidently attracted gays from small towns in the area, "because the slightest indication of homosexuality in a town like Sylacauga would invite harassment, or worse" (Firestone, 1999, p. A9).

Social workers in rural communities, especially those used to urban living, can face special problems relating to privacy and confidentiality and to the maintenance of professional boundaries in the community in which they may both serve and reside. "Transplanted [social work] urbanites . . . refer to 'life in a goldfish' bowl. Everyone seems to know what everyone else is doing, and one's personal life affects one's professional life more than it does in urban settings" (Davenport and Davenport III, 1995, p. 2082). Attendance (or lack of attendance) at local church services might be noticed; not using the services of the only community plumber because he is a client and seeking such services out of town could cause hard feelings. Value conflicts may arise between rural residents "who tend to be more conservative and traditional, and social workers, who tend to be more liberal and nontraditional. . . . Social workers urging anti-gun legislation and anti-hunting rules may quickly lose community acceptance" (Davenport and Davenport III, 1995, p. 2082).

In recent years, rural social work, which had been out of the mainstream of social work practice and education, has been developing its own voice and sphere of influence. The Rural Social Work Caucus has been influential, sponsoring conferences and institutes on rural social work; several graduate schools of social work as well as undergraduate social work programs have developed rural curricula (Davenport and Davenport III, 1995).

Housing

Housing is a basic human need that many of us take for granted. As students, you might not be comfortable with your housing—you might be living in an apartment with five or six other students and may feel stressed by "overcrowding" or a lack of privacy. You could be living with your parents (which you might or might not prefer) because you cannot afford to live in your own apartment. Your parents might be quite pleased with this arrangement, or they may be wishing for the "empty nest syndrome" they had been counting on experiencing. You may feel safe in your neighborhood or you might be afraid to walk alone in it.

Where we live and how we feel about it are important aspects of all our lives; our psychosocial assessments of clients must incorporate this dimension of experience. Today, housing problems are widespread, related to both the spiraling costs of housing and the lack of moderately priced housing. During the past two decades, when an increase in the gap of income distribution resulted in a dramatic increase in the number of families and children living at the poverty level, a shortage of moderately priced housing developed, which has had a special impact on families with young children (Giovannoni, 1995). "The result of this imbalance in housing supply and demand has been an increase in the number of people living in substandard, overcrowded conditions, and worst of all, homelessness" (Giovannoni, 1995, p. 433).

Urban renewal has led to relocations for many people, often with great emotional cost. "As Fried . . . pointed out in 'Grieving for a Lost Home,' as many as one-third of the people who left their homes and communities because of urban renewal showed signs of clinical depression two years after relocation" (Cohen and Phillips, 1997, p. 480).

Various governmental programs over the years have assisted people with housing, including low-interest mortgage loans; subsidizing housing developments for those with middle and low incomes; the establishment of rent controls; and the establishment of the U.S. Department of Housing and Urban Development (HUD) in 1965. The decline in governmental financial aid for housing needs as well as a trend toward eliminating rent controls have contributed to the present housing crisis.

Public Housing Projects

Public housing projects have been a major source of controversy over the years. Public housing projects are often slums that the federal government helped to create in its effort to eradicate slums (Belluck, 1998b). Currently, there is a massive governmental effort to raze many projects that have been "crippled by flawed policies and mismanagement and overwhelmed by poverty and crime" (Belluck, 1998b, p. 1). This nationwide razing effort includes 100,000 apartments in the most blighted projects. The goal is to move some tenants into alternative housing developments that are not so large where families with different income levels can live together and to move others to privately owned buildings. The Robert Taylor project in Chicago is the largest housing project in the United States and is one that will be demolished (Belluck, 1998b), requiring the dispersion of isolated people, most of whom are black with annual incomes below $5,000, to other neighborhoods where new neighbors may have long preferred to have them elsewhere. But already a pattern is emerging of tenants from housing projects being moved mainly to poor black neighborhoods, some as rundown and unsafe as the high-rises they left" (Belluck, 1998b, p. 26).

Looking at the problems of the urban poor in a comprehensive way and providing a network of services to ameliorate complex and interacting social problems is a growing trend. For example, recognizing that the economic and employment situations of the residents of the Robert Taylor Housing project are desperate, the Housing Authority is also offering them vocational and educational aid. The vast majority are out of work, so that it also becomes important to enhance economic self-sufficiency (Belluck, 1998b, p. 26).

Programs have also been developed in the private sector to link social services with housing developments where tenants continue to live. One program, in an impoverished section of the South Bronx, offers programs to tenants which include on-site counseling and referral services related to economic (and rent payment) issues, employment and training, and mental health and family issues (Cohen and Phillips, 1997). The tenants were also aided in developing their own tenants' association and becoming involved with community organizations. Cohen and Phillips (1997) reported positive results and felt that this program had built a sense of community for the tenants; this is critical, as "a sense of community can be extremely fragile in low-income, urban neighborhoods where residents have experienced steep economic decline and abandonment" (p. 480).

Housing projects have been built for the elderly and for the disabled with special features, such as handrails and access for wheelchairs. Recently, a special housing complex, GrandFamilies House, was built in Dorchester, Boston, to house grandparents raising their grandchildren (Dowdy, 1998). Grandparents in poor neighborhoods had a special need for this housing, as many "found themselves falling through . . . the social-service safety net. . . . Some were prohibited from bringing grandchildren into elderly housing complexes, so they searched for affordable housing [which was] . . . in short supply" (Dowdy, 1998, B8).

Funded by both public and private sources, this project contains special facilities for both children and the elderly (Dowdy, 1998). The local YWCA pledged to provide "support programs for the elderly, and after-school enrichment programs" (Dowdy, 1998, p. B8).

Homelessness

Homelessness is the catastrophic outcome of failed social policies relating to housing, including lack of rent controls, inadequate funding, as well as the deinstitutionalization of the mentally ill.

The scarcity of affordable housing is one of the major factors leading to the dramatic increase of homelessness in the United States. Although precise statistics are not available about the homeless population, there is nevertheless "widespread agreement that the number of homeless Americans has grown significantly since 1980" (First et al., 1995, p. 1331). It is difficult to obtain a precise account of the problem due to the lack of clarity about the definitions of homelessness. Is a person homeless only if living on the street or in a shelter? First and colleagues (1995) cite other types of arrangements "homeless" people make (by virtue of which they may or may not be considered homeless): they may move in with other people; they might reside in "welfare hotels," utilize "migrant farmworker housing," or live in "single-room occupancy hotels" (First et al., 1995, p. 1331).

Three major groups have composed the homeless population during the past decade: "single men, single women and mothers with children" (First et al., 1995, p. 1331). In urban areas, most of the homeless are men; a high proportion of the homeless groups are African Americans. It is estimated that about one-third of homeless people are mentally ill (Kaplan et al., 1994).

The homeless are an "embarrassment" to the cities in which they are quite visible and where a shortage of shelters and housing exists. Sometimes they are removed for "cosmetic" purposes, without substantive comprehensive assistance to them. These issues were reflected during a major controversy that developed in San Francisco, when the mayor infuriated homeless advocates through the forcible removal of large numbers of street people from Golden Gate Park; the situation was further exacerbated by a plan to shift the homeless from tourist areas to shelters and to crack down with arrests (Nieves, 1998). It is estimated that there are 16,000 people on the streets on an average night, double the 1988 figure. Paul Boden, director of the Coalition on Homelessness, feels it is a "myth" that people move to San Francisco to be homeless (Nieves, 1998, p. A21).

> About a third are mentally ill, a third are drug addicts (or some mixture of the two) and the rest have been displaced from their homes through personal misfortunes like rising rents or loss of income. While the numbers of the homeless are rising all over the nation, largely because of a decrease in Federal benefits and public housing, Mr. Boden said, San Francisco's problem is exacerbated by its soaring housing prices, the highest in the country. (Nieves, 1998, p. A21)

In addition, there has been an increase in deaths of homeless people in San Francisco over the past year, "an increase that has alarmed and frustrated advocates for the homeless and city health workers" ("Homeless," 1998, A16). There were 154 deaths reported during that time; the average age was forty-two. Deaths resulted from multiple causes including drowning, asthma, suicide, and being hit by cars. However, "substance abuse was the leading killer" ("Homeless," 1998, p. A16). It is estimated that both in

San Francisco and across the nation, about one-third of the homeless are mentally ill.

Homeless Mentally Ill

During the deinstitutionalization process of the late 1950s, state psychiatric hospitalizations declined "from more than 560,000 beds at that time to roughly 100,000 beds today" (Kaplan et al., 1994, p. 203). Unfortunately, although many civil libertarians felt that returning mentally ill people to the community would be more humane than locking them away from society, the comprehensive services needed for maintaining them in the community have not been provided. This aid "has not been given to the extent that the planners and the supporters of deinstitutionalization would like, primarily because of the lack of adequate funding on the federal, state, and local levels. It is scandalous that funding for aftercare community services for the mentally ill continues to decline; unless that trend is reversed, deinstitutionalization will remain a failed public policy" (Kaplan et al., 1994, p. 204).

Many people with mental illness have become incarcerated in prisons. "Many of the incarcerated homeless mentally ill are arrested for minor crimes that are survival strategies . . . or for behavior directly produced by psychosis" (Kaplan et al., 1994, p. 204). The homeless mentally ill suffer mainly from schizophrenia and schizoaffective disorder; many have histories of alcohol or other substance abuse, complicated by multiple physical problems.

> The homeless mentally ill are not simply undomiciled. They are often totally disaffiliated and have few, if any, links to the community. They are unemployed, socially isolated, and out of contact with their families. Homeless women may be more likely than are men to have intact social skills and social networks. In general, the homeless mentally ill are difficult to treat because of their high levels of withdrawal and suspicion, psychopathology, homeless life-style, or negative past experiences with the mental health system. (Kaplan et al., 1994, p. 204)

As mood disorders are studied in greater depth, it has been observed that depression and bipolar affective (formerly called manic-depressive) disorders can lead to homelessness. It is becoming increasingly evident that a close association exists between depression and homelessness (Holloway, 1999). Dr. Fieve, who pioneered the use of lithium, has asserted that intensive outreach work in finding people with depressive disorders could substantially cut down the number of homeless ending up in shelters (Holloway, 1999). Because bipolar affective disorder is not easy to diagnose, many patients remain untreated. During the depressive state, a patient may feel very tired and therefore often becomes dysfunctional. Dr. Fieve added that "you've probably lost your job because of excessive absenteeism and poor performance. . . . This is where homelessness sets in. Your family can't deal with you," and you are most likely to leave home (Holloway, 1999, p. 3).

Homeless Families

During the 1990s, families have been observed to be the "fastest growing segment of the homeless population" (First et al., 1995, p. 1331). Four major factors contribute to the rise of homeless families: substantial decreases in income for poor people; decreasing availability of low-cost housing; federal cutbacks in providing housing for people with low incomes and cutbacks in welfare benefits; and the need to move from housing that is unsafe as well as dealing with family conflict and abuse (First et al., 1995). Homeless women often report physical and/or sexual abuse (Goldberg, 1999).

Homeless children who are with their parents "constitute from one-half to two-thirds of the homeless family population" (First et al., 1995, p. 1332). Typically, these families are headed by a single mother with one or two children; the average age of the children is six years. These families move often and frequently "have lived marginal, low-income lifestyles before experiencing homelessness" (First et al., 1995, p. 1332).

Children in these families suffer the negative effects of homelessness (First et al., 1995). "Although the number of children affected by homelessness may be questioned, the effects on children are indisputable. Their physical health is impaired, their school attendance sporadic, and in one study by the Institute of Medicine (1988) 43 percent of homeless preschoolers examined manifested serious developmental delays" (Giovannoni, 1995, p. 437). In addition, they tend to have "high levels of anxiety and depression and . . . [other] emotional and behavioral problems" (First et al., 1995, p. 1332).

Runaways and Homeless Youths

It is difficult to know exactly how many youths run away and how many are homeless, as authorities are not always notified of runaways, and some runaways are difficult to find (Bass, 1995). However, it is estimated that in the United States "there are 1 million to 1.3 million runaways and homeless youths each year and that 500,000 of these youths are homeless" (Bass, 1995, p. 2060). In Massachusetts, approximately 3,000 teens between ages ten and nineteen are homeless and lack adequate shelter, foster homes, and appropriate services (Hart, 1998). The lack of adequate facilities for this population in Massachusetts reflects the general picture throughout the country.

Many runaways and homeless youth have "experienced physical and sexual abuse, drug and alcohol abuse by both parents, family violence, mental health problems, and school problems. . . . Twice as many homeless youths came to agencies from foster homes or group homes than from their own families" (Bass, 1995, p. 2062). Recently, the words "push out" and "throwaway" have been coined to refer to youths who leave home because their parents (or legal guardians) have encouraged them to leave, have abandoned them, or have abused and neglected them. Nearly 25 percent of the youth who are considered runaways are, in fact, "throwaways" (Loppnow, 1985, p. 516). Adolescent runaways are discussed at greater length in Chapter 9.

Homelessness, the "shame of our cities," is a complex problem with social and psychological roots. It is imperative that skilled clinical services be available to the homeless, when appropriate, along with social services offering help with housing, education, and employment. One of the underlying issues affecting both the existence of homelessness and the lack of adequate attention to this population is the lack of financial resources allocated to this problem. Economics, a major societal issue, is discussed in the following section.

THE SOCIAL ENVIRONMENT

Economic

Economic factors are one of the most compelling aspects of life affecting (and being affected by) human behavior. On a very basic level, survival depends on having sufficient economic resources so that one does not starve or become homeless. Severe forces of nature, such as hurricanes, floods, earthquakes, and crop failures and ensuing famine, can destroy the economic base of communities or even whole countries. Political turmoil can cause economic chaos; and economic crisis can produce political turmoil. The Great Depression of the 1930s in this country produced untold hardship for millions and ultimately resulted in the New Deal programs (such as Social Security) of the Roosevelt administration. In contrast, the serious economic problems in Germany fueled the rise of Nazism, leading to the massive destruction of Europe and its peoples in World War II.

The political and economic interdependence of countries can produce turmoil when changes occur in the existing balance. Hunger and malnutrition, serious enough to permanently impair the physical and mental health of a generation of North Korean children, was brought to light by international aid groups in 1998 (Rosenthal, 1998). Researchers assert that this hunger "is linked to the collapse of the Soviet Union, which had long been North Korea's main supplier of food, fuel and fertilizer" (Rosenthal, 1998, p. A12).

At the microlevel, each social worker's ability to provide services to a client, whether environmental (such as a foster home), or therapeutic (such as clinical services) are related to available financial support. Managed care, with its major influence on health care and mental health services—usually of a restrictive nature—is based on the economic profit motive. In families, tensions can escalate about both the availability of money and its distribution.

In addition to objective concerns about money (such as whether it is available for families in poverty or whether one overspends with credit cards), subjective preoccupations can exist (such as the need for money for a sense of security or status, as a basis for self-esteem, or as a representation of love). In therapy, clients often have more difficulty talking about money than about sex. Therapists may experience discomfort "intruding" into the private world of a person's finances, especially when this involves issues about paying (or not paying) fees. In therapy (as in life), issues about paying, receiving, and "not having enough" money can be tied to emotional issues about being nurtured and loved.

Addictions, such as to drugs or gambling, can wreak havoc with a family's finances. It is common for people in the manic phase of bipolar affective disorder to overspend, often in inappropriate ways (such as Dr. Jamison's 1996 account of buying all the snakebite kits in a drugstore during one of her manic phases). These buying sprees can often bankrupt a person and/or family, and add a heavy burden of guilt to the depression following this phase. "In order to truly comprehend the frustrations and anger experienced by many clients, the economic realities they confront must be appreciated and shared on an emotional level" (Longres, 1995b, p. 291).

The United States is overall a prosperous country; many live in comfort, but, at the same time, an increase in the gap of income distribution has resulted in a dramatic increase in the number of families and children living in poverty. "During the 1980's poverty in America increased, but disproportionately among children, especially children of color and very young children. . . . By 1990 . . . the proportion of poor children under age 18 had increased to 21 percent and of children under six to 23.6 percent—almost one child in four" (Giovannoni, 1995, p. 435). The U.S. Bureau of the Census, in 1995, reported that "40 million Americans, 15 percent of our population, were living below the poverty line" (Zastrow and Kirst-Ashman, 1997, p. 467).

The infant mortality rate of the poor is almost double the rate of the affluent (U.S. Bureau of the Census, 1995). The poor have less access to medical services and receive lower quality care from health care professionals. The poor are exposed to higher levels of air pollution, water pollution, and unsanitary conditions. They have higher rates of malnutrition and disease. Schools in poor areas are of lower quality and have fewer resources. As a result the poor achieve less academically and are more apt to drop out of school. They are more apt to be arrested, indicted, imprisoned, and given longer sentences for the same offense. They are less likely to receive probation, parole, or suspended sentences. (Zastrow and Kirst-Ashman, 1997, pp. 467-468)

Poverty is found "disproportionately [in] racial and ethnic minorities and [in] women and children" (Longres, 1995b, p. 288). However, many families headed by men are also touched by poverty (Giovannoni, 1995). "Poor families headed by men are actually more common than poor families headed by women, since they include both married-couple and single-parent families" (Longres, 1995b, p. 288). Many low-income families often have one or more family members working (Longres, 1995b), but the wages they earn and the high rents they pay place them at the poverty level.

Employment

Employment is not only a major source of income but can contribute to self-esteem and personal satisfaction; for many, it serves as an "organizing principle" in life. A positive work experience can provide "an outlet for creativity, satisfactory relationships with colleagues, pride in accomplishment, and increased self-esteem. Job satisfaction is not wholly dependent on money" (Kaplan et al., 1994, p. 58). Lack of employment can produce serious psychological stress.

The effects of unemployment transcend those of loss of income; the psychological and physical tolls are enormous. The incidence of alcohol dependence, homicide, violence, suicide, and mental illness rises with unemployment. The person's core identity, which is often tied to occupation and work, is seriously damaged when a job is lost, whether it is through firing, attrition, or early or regular retirement. (Kaplan et al., 1994, p. 58)

Employment issues pertain to people at all levels of society. Job availability, satisfaction, downsizing, layoffs, and retirement affect both executives and factory workers. For example, high unemployment existed in the late 1970s and early 1980s among steel workers and automobile workers; in the 1970s, school teachers and PhDs in the liberal arts and social sciences were affected by lack of employment opportunities (Zastrow and Kirst-Ashman, 1997). An entire community that is economically based on one industry, as is common in rural areas, can prosper or be devastated by the success or failure of that industry (Davenport and Davenport III, 1995).

Women, the elderly, those with disabilities, and minorities (including people of color, immigrants, and homosexuals) often face job discrimination, which calls for remediation by legal action, advocacy, and/or legislation.

People with special needs may require vocational intervention: those with developmental and physical disabilities and/or with mental illness may benefit from specialized training, job placement, and social supports.

Members of minorities, especially those with low socioeconomic status and those living in impoverished inner-city communities, face serious unemployment problems. In a study focusing on clients overwhelmed by poor socioeconomic conditions, the authors noted that although life was very difficult for the women and the children, nevertheless, "the most overwhelmed persons were minority males who were often jobless, homeless, moving from mother to girlfriend to girlfriend, back to mother. . . . How to help them conquer 'uselessness' is a tall order but one that is a pressing national poverty question" (Hopps et al., 1995, p. 6). In the past, black males found work, but now " 'economic restructuring has broken the figurative back of the black working population'" (Hopps et al., 1995 [citing Wilson], p. 7).

In today's economy, lack of education can produce unemployment (or underemployment), as many jobs have become "high tech," for which people with inadequate educational backgrounds cannot compete. An effort toward vocational rehabilitation involving the education and vocational training provided to the residents of the Robert Taylor housing project in Chicago was undertaken, which was discussed earlier.

Attention has been directed on both local and national levels to the multiple problems faced by inner-city children and their families, including poverty, housing, and employment (Chaskin et al., 1997; Delgado, 1997; Ewalt, 1997). There have been many plans for community improvement through federal legislation (the Empowerment Zone program) or private funding (such as the Ford Foundation [Neighborhood and Family Initiative]). Because of the multiple issues and interactions among social factors, most programs aimed at revitalization take a comprehensive approach.

> The interrelationship among a number of social problems, such as joblessness, lack of education, low income, poor housing, and inadequate health care, is broadly acknowledged and has provided much of the impetus for efforts to address multiple social needs by integrating strategies. (Chaskin et al., 1997, p. 437)

Some community revitalization programs have focused primarily on creating jobs and/or businesses, building toward comprehensive services later; others have included employment objectives as part of a basic comprehensive plan. Delgado (1997) has argued that some programs see communities from a "deficit perspective" and in so doing have "ignored community assets in the search for revitalization strategies" (p. 445). He refers to the significance of "the presence and role of small businesses in the life of communities of color" (p. 447). Focusing his discussion on the establishment of beauty parlors "as economic settings and sources of support for Latinos and other women of color" (p. 448), Delgado asserts that small businesses in the Latino community can have multiple advantages.

> Latino small businesses can provide access to services for disempowered groups in their role as urban sanctuaries (residents can patronize a business without fear of being rejected because of their ethnic or racial background), as providers of culture-specific items and services, and as providers of information related to the homeland. Their accessibility to the community (geographical, psychological, cultural, and logistical) makes these institutions excellent settings for collaborative activities. (Delgado, 1997, p. 450)

An increasing need exists for employees with a high degree of literacy who are capable of technological work in today's economic marketplace. Business executives have observed that many young people today do not have the "basic competencies to perform even rudimentary tasks in industry, much less to hold positions requiring more technical ability or knowledge" (Richman and Bowen, 1998, p. 95). This brings us to a consideration of public school education and its role in the life of children and their preparation for the future.

Public School Education

Public school education is a matter of national concern and a subject of considerable debate, regarding such topics as quality of education, the preparation and adequacy of teachers, funding responsibilities, segregation in schools (and issues of school busing), school vouchers, dropout rates, and the serious lack of teachers and equipment in inner-city schools. "Too often these schools have become as impoverished as their surrounding communities" (Dupper and Poertner, 1997, p. 415).

Academic failure has been associated with "higher mortality rates, higher incidence of suicide, and more frequent admissions to state mental hospitals" (Richman and Bowen, 1997, p. 95). More than 70 percent of children growing up in poverty "experienced severe academic problems during their early elementary grades. These problems include poor cognitive development, decreased language ability, inadequate social skills . . . and little impulse control" (Dupper and Poertner, 1997, p. 416). Another recent concern has been the presence of violence in the schools, often with tragic outcomes.

Positive school experiences, by contrast, can enhance self-esteem and mastery, increase skills and the potential for employment opportunities, and also be an important factor contributing to resilience. Given the importance of supportive relationships to children's development, it has been observed that a positive school experience can act as a "protective function" by providing a setting "for supportive relationships" (Kirby and Fraser, 1997, p. 25).

Programs that are school based (or school linked) have been established in some communities to enhance children's educational experiences, to provide supportive services to families, and to serve as a link to other community programs (Dupper and Poertner, 1997; Winters and Maluccio, 1988). Dupper and Poertner (1997) discuss a number of school-linked family resource centers, established throughout the country, that provide multiple services to children and their families who live in impoverished neighborhoods. The Wallbridge Caring Communities program in St. Louis is one example.

> The Wallbridge Caring Communities program . . . is based in an inner-city school and a nearby church. The program expands the use of school buildings to create opportunities for life-long learning and to incorporate Afrocentric culture. Family crisis intervention, substance abuse counseling, afterschool tutoring and recreational activities . . . are available. . . . Teachers serve as the frontline staff in identifying children and their families who may be in need of services. . . . (Dupper and Puertner, 1997, pp. 417-418)

A good education develops the capacity to read—a necessity for the acquisition of knowledge. From a developmental perspective reading can open the door to ideas, feelings, experiences, sources of inspiration, and aid in the development of fantasy. Although one (usually) reads in solitude, one is not alone in perusing a good book, as the voice of the author (and the characters created) can be good company. Vaillant (1993) suggests that reading may be an important source of resilience worthy of further study.

The life of Frederick Douglass, who grew up in slavery in the American South and became a prominent figure and great orator during the Civil War and Reconstruction periods, demonstrates how reading developed both his ideas and oratorical skills (McFeely, 1991). Douglass taught himself to read, then taught his fellow slaves to read (secretly on Sunday afternoons) when he was returned to plantation life. During part of his adolescence he lived in Baltimore and developed his oratorical skills in his spare time. As Frederick Douglass begins his oratorical self-education, we can see, in the following passage, his human spirit triumphing over the oppression of his slave status.

> With fifty cents that must have been the product of passionate hoarding, and with the wonderful nerve—the overcoming of all fear of embarrassment—that a twelve-year-old is capable of, Frederick went into Knight's bookstore in the neighborhood, and bought his own copy of *The Columbian Orator.* Seldom has a single book more profoundly shaped the life of a writer and orator. . . . Alone, behind the shipyard wall, Frederick . . . read aloud. Laboriously, studiously, at first, then fluently, melodically, he recited great speeches. With the *Columbian Orator* in his hand, with the words of the great speakers of the past coming from his mouth, he was rehearsing. He was readying the sounds—and meanings—of words of his own that he would one day speak. He had the whole world before him. . . . *The Columbian Orator* was a book of liberties, of men exhorting mankind to a sense of higher callings, and what was more, it did not ignore that denial of liberty that was slavery. (McFeely, 1991, pp. 34-35)

Maya Angelou (1997), the famous black writer and poet, often refers in her autobiography to the value of reading in her life. It was both a solitary activity for her and one that she shared with her brother Bailey. She had a painful childhood, during which she and Bailey (at ages three and four) were sent by their parents from California to live with their grandmother in Stamps, Arkansas. The bond between these two "orphaned" children was intensely close and loyal; reading was a further bond between them.

In the following excerpt, Maya (age eight) and Bailey are now reunited with their mother in St. Louis, but Maya and Bailey have grown apart; reading seems to be a source of comfort (as well as fantasy) for her, and the themes of the books resonate with her life experiences. From her description, she did not feel alone, as she had the company of her fictional friends (Angelou, 1997).

> When spring came to St. Louis, I took out my first library card, and since Bailey and I seemed to be growing apart, I spent most of my Saturdays at the library (no interruptions) breathing in the world of penniless shoeshine boys who, with goodness and perseverance, became rich, rich men, and gave baskets of goodies to the poor on holidays. The little princesses who were mistaken for maids, and the long-lost

children mistaken for waifs, became more real to me than our house, our mother, our school or Mr. Freeman. (Angelou, 1997, p. 76)

A source of strength in Maya Angelou's childhood in Stamps was the solidity of the black community to which she and her grandmother belonged; being part of a community, with its social networks, support systems, and organizations, affects a person's psychological well-being and family life.

Communities and Organizations

Communities can be defined in different ways. They may be physical entities, in terms of geography and location, such as a small town or a neighborhood. However, as Germain (1991) notes, people residing near one another physically may not feel they are a community in terms of relatedness or common purpose, and residents may feel socially isolated from one another. Conversely, people may feel part of a community even though they do not reside in close proximity, for example, a religious or cultural community, an artistic community, and gay and lesbian people who form "network communities that provide a safe communal haven to members" (Germain, 1991, p. 39).

People participate in multiple communities, such as neighborhood, work, and cultural communities, etc. When undertaking a psychosocial assessment it is important to realize that people incorporate aspects of their community and cultural identifications into their own sense of self and that "through processes of internalization, environments and culture become 'part' of the person's self-concept" (Germain, 1991, p. 37), as well as that the community groups to which a client belongs can have differing (or opposing) goals and value systems, which may cause conflict for the individual.

Belonging to a community of "like" people does not guarantee homogeneity, or a lack of conflict about "rules" and "standards." In the lesbian "culture," women "fall along a continuum from conservative to liberal in their philosophical approaches to life" (Tully, 1995, p. 1591). Differences exist in the degree of integration with mainstream "culture" that lesbian women seek and in the degree to which they seek to remain separate and apart. Some lesbian separatists choose to "separate themselves from all that is male by forming women-only communes. The extreme separatists tend to isolate themselves from all that they view as patriarchal, and the more moderate separatists live and work in proximity to men where they interact openly as lesbians within the larger social culture" (Tully, p. 1591).This important issue of separation and integration confronts other minority groups; the current controversial issue of interracial adoption is an example of this.

Issues stemming from community affiliations can have a great impact on a client's emotional state. Some clients may belong to groups that are very controlling of all aspects of their lives, such as cults; others may drift, belonging to no group, experiencing aloneness or disconnection. Being part of a community can be a source of strength and joy but may prove distressing at times, as the individual struggles with wishes for autonomy, on the one hand, and connectedness to a group, on the other. The Mahlerian concept of separation-individuation has its parallel in community life, as the individual experiences an ongoing tension between social conformity and personal freedom.

Informal Support Systems

Informal support systems of various kinds exist in communities and organizations, including self-help groups and social networks, in which natural helpers may participate (Germain, 1991).

Self-Help Groups

Self-help groups—people with common problems who meet to provide mutual support and informal education—have proliferated in recent years. "There are now several thousand local chapters in the United States. At least six million people participate each year . . . " ("Self-Help I," 1993, p. 1). One of the oldest and best-known groups is Alcoholics Anonymous (AA). The largest number of these groups, in which both patient and family groups deal with disabling and chronic illness, centers around medical problems (Germain, 1991). The National Association for the Mentally Ill (NAMI), composed of mentally ill people and their families, has a large membership. Examples of other self-help groups include: The National Association for People with AIDS, the Scoliosis Association, Mended Hearts (for heart-attack victims), Compassionate Friends (for parents who have lost a child), Gamblers Anonymous, and Parents Anonymous (for abusive parents) ("Self-Help I," 1993, p. 2). Self-help groups also have recently proliferated on the Internet.

The multiplicity of self-help groups has been thought by some to be a "modern search for community. In an environment in which families, churches, and other traditional institutions may have come to seem inadequate, these groups are a new way of establishing a common life—a type of affiliation that is especially useful in crisis" ("Self-Help I," 1993, p. 2). Germain (1991) views self-help groups as a "preventive force and a stabilizing influence [which] can complement formal services" (p. 74). Often these groups meet without professional people, although professionals may initiate them or serve as consultants.

Self-help groups can focus on social change, rather than primarily on helping people cope with problems (Germain, 1991). They may have an educational focus, raise funds, or become politically active.

Self-help groups such as "food co-ops, day care co-ops, [and] neighborhood improvement associations . . . " (Germain, 1991, p. 75) may also affiliate with one another and become *resource-exchange networks* (Germain, 1991). Such groups "are a significant force for the empowerment of impoverished or devalued communities" (Germain, 1991, p. 75).

Sometimes conflict occurs between mental health professionals and self-help groups; in one instance, former psychiatric patients formed "radical self-help groups originally designed to assert their rights and challenge the established system" ("Self-Help II," 1993, pp. 1-2). However, generally an increase in cooperation and mutuality between professionals and self-help groups has taken place. "The absorption of AA techniques into alcoholism treatment is one example of a trend toward the adoption of self-help practices by professionals" ("Self-Help II," 1993, p. 2).

Although a lack of systematic research into the effectiveness of self-help groups exists, informal evidence suggests satisfaction and improvement on the part of many participants. However, certain "limitations and dangers" of these groups have also been noted ("Self-Help II," 1993, p. 3).

> Groups will not work for people who are paranoid or who believe themselves to be unique. Leaders may be well-meaning but incompetent. Perhaps the greatest danger is that a self-help group will perversely undermine its members' confidence by insisting that they define their lives solely in terms of the issues discussed by the group, excluding other forms of community and disabling themselves for life outside its confines. In that situation the group works mainly to preserve itself (or the power of a leader) at the expense of the self-respect and freedom of its members. ("Self-Help II," 1993, p. 3)

Shulman and Gitterman (1986) discuss a variety of *mutual aid groups* that are facilitated by social workers, who may provide direction and a "mediating" function for the group. The concept of "mutual aid in groups, one of Schwartz's major contributions . . . shifts the source of the helping from the group leader to the members themselves" (Shulman and Gitterman, 1986, p. 3). This approach has included work with: bereaved children (Vastola et al., 1986); adolescents in a residential setting (Nadelman, 1986); parents of sexually victimized children (Jones, 1986); men who batter their wives (Trimble, 1986); institutionalized schizophrenic women (Poynter-Berg, 1986); and Hispanic parents of children with cancer (Schaefer and Pozzaglia, 1986).

It has been suggested that a group member receiving help may also be helped by participating in the process of helping others. "Skovholt explained that helping enhances the helper's sense of effectance and competence, and maturity is enhanced by being able to give as well as receive" (Lee and Swenson, 1986, pp. 368-369). Lee and Swenson (1986) assert that mutual aid groups present "a needed balance in an 'age of narcissism'" (p. 374).

Social Networks

Social networks are informal interpersonal connections that serve as a source of support and aid. Networks can include any combination of family, friends, neighbors, co-workers, coreligionists, natural helpers, etc.

> Social networks serve as coping resources for dealing with life stressors. They facilitate mastery of the twin tasks of problem solving and management of feelings by providing emotional support, information and advice, and tangible aids, and by undertaking action. They may also serve a primary preventive function in effectively staving off an imminent stressor. In carrying out these functions effectively, informal systems also contribute to the member's self-esteem and relatedness and may enhance the sense of competence and self-direction. (Germain, 1991, p. 76)

Many studies have pointed to an important link between social support and a person's overall health in the physical, social, and psychological spheres (Germain, 1991; Richman et al., 1998). In one study of women with metastatic breast cancer, those receiving weekly supportive group therapy (in addition to chemotherapy) lived twice as long as a control group receiving only chemotherapy (Spiegel, 1990).

Supportive experiences in organizations may be a factor promoting resilience (Kirby and Fraser, 1997). People have been enabled to cope with extremely stressful situations, such as internment in a concentration camp, through group support (Schlossberg, 1981). During World War II, "the degree of relatedness between the soldier, his immediate fighting unit, and their leader" afforded soldiers "the strongest protection against overwhelming terror" (Herman, 1997, p. 25).

Natural Helpers

Natural helpers are people in a community who are not professionally qualified or assigned to perform a service (such as a doctor or a social worker) but are informally recognized and accepted for their ability and interest in helping others; they are persons in the social milieu who have "unique wisdom, resourcefulness, and caring qualities" (Germain, 1991, p. 81). Such helpers can meet the needs of neighbors with chores, baby-sitting, medical care, etc., by involvement as a mediator in problem-solving or as an advocate. In rural communities, natural helpers have been found to be an asset to others (Germain, 1991; Patterson et al., 1988); in the Hispanic community, folk healers often play key roles in the lives of people (Germain, 1991). "The Puerto Rican *espiritista* is likely to make use of seances and role playing to rid the ailing individual of evil sprits as well as to call on the person's protective spirits for help in the cure" (Ramirez, 1998, p. 174).

In another example of natural helping, seventeen firemen of Engine Co. 16 in Chicago have been working with the children of the Robert Taylor Housing Project (Fedarko, 1997). These firemen, most of whom are black, do more than fight "the high-rise infernos that ravage the Robert Taylor Homes" (Fedarko, 1997, p. 72).

> Children account for nearly two-thirds of these projects' population, and many of them have fathers who are either missing, in prison or dead. The firemen, therefore, stand among a handful of male role models in this urban wasteland. On their days off, they drop by to tutor children in chess and math and to encourage them to stay in school. Most important, they offer discipline, tenderness and inspiration to a community where such things are in terribly short supply. (Fedarko, 1997, pp. 72-73)

Pets can be important natural helpers, in their capacity as companions to people who live alone, such as many elderly, and they can also be significant aids in the treatment of children and adults with psychiatric and physical disabilities (Germain, 1991). A variety of pet-facilitated therapies are being utilized (Brickel, 1986). Dolly, a Seeing Eye dog, acted as a pet therapist, aiding her owner, a blind clinician, in her play therapy with children (Ceconi and Urdang, 1994, p. 186). The "human-animal bond" has been receiving increasing recognition in social work practice (Netting et al., 1987).

> Pets . . . may serve as adjuncts to therapists in clinical settings to relieve the client's anxiety. As companions, animals may assist in minimizing loneliness and may provide opportunities for tactile stimulation. In addition, touching a pet has been shown to affect the cardiovascular system. As nonjudgmental companions pets can provide informal emotional support. (Netting et al., 1987, p. 61)

Informal networks can play a vital role in the life of an organization, as well as a community.

ORGANIZATIONS

Organizations permeate our life on both formal and informal levels. In this section, employment organizations and the impact they have on the psychosocial well-being of its employees are highlighted. Emphasis is given to the impact social work agencies as organizations have upon clients and social workers. "Irrational interactions [within organizations] are expected rather than ignored. Systems theories emphasize constant assessment and adjustment" (Zastrow and Kirst-Ashman, 1997, p. 31).

Many current social issues are reflected in places of employment: affirmative action; decisions affecting "spousal" benefits to partners of homosexual employees; time granted (or not granted) for family care; the provision of day care (sometimes for both children and elderly parents) in workplaces; and deciding whether office romances are to be tolerated and how to differentiate this from sexual harassment.

Clients may bring up employment problems related to: interpersonal relationships at work (with administrators and/or peers), feeling their work is not recognized and appreciated, feeling inadequate (and perhaps like an "imposter") in fulfilling their positions, wishing for and/or fearing promotions, and feeling dissatisfied with present job and/or confused about vocational goals. Problems at work can stem from psychodynamic conflicts, from organizational stress, or a combination of both. Kaplan and colleagues (1994) discuss some of the psychodynamic conflicts that can be found in the work setting.

> People with unresolved conflicts about their competitive and aggressive impulses may experience great difficulties in the work area. They may suffer from a pathological envy of the success of others or fear success for themselves because of their inability to tolerate envy from others. (Kaplan et al., 1994, p. 797)

Some employees (including social workers) may feel stressed about job demands and be "burned out" by "physical, psychological, and emotional exhaustion"; this type of stress can result in "job dissatisfaction, tension, anxiety, irritability, procrastination, frequent absences from work, and a decision to leave the job" (Queralt, 1996, p. 289).

In a court case in Japan, a judge decided that the family of a man who committed suicide, purportedly due to overwork, should be compensated, and he "blamed [the] man's suicide on . . . working 80-hour weeks and ordered the government to compensate his family"; these suicides are increasing and "the phenomenon is so common that there is even a term for them: 'karojisatsu'" (Japan, 1999, p. A5).

Interpersonal tensions in organizations can become quite intense; issues of jealousy, competition, status, the acquisition of power, and interpersonal conflict can affect both individuals and the collective functioning of the organization. (Although we are stressing work organizations here, power struggles as well as other interpersonal conflicts can occur in churches, social clubs, organized crime associations, theater groups, therapy groups, and any organization of any size.) It has been reported that major difficulties erupted in the English department at Duke University (Scott, 1998).

> The upheaval at Duke offers a glimpse into the arcane world of an academic department, one in which a complex mixture of ideological, generational and personality differences among its 40 members led to explosive skirmishes over hiring and tenure, graduate-student admissions and the distribution of departmental tasks and perks. . . .
>
> But Duke's difficulties also reflect tensions in English departments nationwide at a time when many have been struggling to redefine their mission [a conflict between the use of classic literature and literature being used to highlight political issues and promote social change]. (Scott, 1998, pp. A1, A17)

Social Work Organizations

Social work organizations (from state bureaucracies to group private practices) are "embedded in social and physical environments. They affect and are affected by political, economic, and cultural forces" (Germain and Gitterman, 1980, p. 138). These forces have considerable impact on the clinical work offered to clients, as well as the well-being of social workers. Today, managed care is a major issue affecting medical, psychiatric, and social work practice (Geller, 1996; Strom-Gottfried, 1997; Urdang, 1999). Many social agencies now place emphasis on short-term services and quantitative outcome studies. "Social workers are confronted by an increasing emphasis on accountability, more for quantity, than for quality of service" (Gitterman and Miller, 1989, p. 152); agencies "have been forced to reinvent themselves and operate more like businesses" (Jarmon-Rohde et al., 1997, p. 31).

As funding and bureaucratic problems, which have long beset the child welfare field, continue "with crushing caseloads, low wages and high turnover, social workers in child protection face a looming crisis" (Beaucar, 1999b, p. 3). An example of this chronic, so-called crisis was seen in New York when the city's child welfare system was mandated to receive direction and supervision from the state's Office of Children and Family Services (Swarns, 1999, p. A19). Workers from the state office were not making required visits to many group foster homes.

Meanwhile, the overwhelmed workers in the Manhattan regional office lacked the manpower to comply with their own legal obligations, which include inspecting group homes, investigating abuse in these homes, reviewing child-abuse deaths and monitoring city operations. *Some say they fell ill from the stress.* [italics added] (Swarns, 1999, p. A19)

Conflict and competing interests of staff and administration often exist within organizations (Gitterman and Miller, 1989).

Different positions in the hierarchy develop different priorities and publics to please. Executives are concerned about funding, organizational stability, regulatory issues, and external politics. Clinicians are concerned about client problems and available services and all are concerned about their respective prerogatives and personal interests. These interests are often in conflict, competing with other priorities and creating tension inherent in organizational life. (Gitterman and Miller, 1989, p.154)

The interpersonal climate of the agency also affects clients, clinical staff, and social work students placed there. The analytic work of psychoanalytic candidates undergoing their training can be affected by administrative requirements and restraints (Kernberg, 1965).

Alfred Staunton described a psychiatric hospital as a "small society with established hierarchical categories"; he observed that conflict or lack of clarity about staff responsibilities can be *"transmitted to patients, whose symptoms may be exacerbated as a result"* [italics added] (Kaplan et al., 1994, p. 189). In an agency "where staff morale is low . . . the informal system may support scornful, punitive or uncaring attitudes towards clients" (Germain and Gitterman, 1980, p. 143). Negative attitudes can also be directed at social work interns.

The impact of the emotional climate of agencies on supervision was explored in a study of the self-perceptions of beginning field instructors (Urdang, 1994). Most of the beginning instructors reported external and internal stresses affecting them; however it was the interpersonal climate of the agency that was decisive on how this was experienced. One instructor, Brett, reported experiencing external and internal stresses in the agency which were exacerbated by a tense interpersonal climate.

Brett, whose agency had been in a struggle for "survival," felt tension due to the push for "productivity." He feels his clinic "is one of the hardest places I've been at. There is a certain competitiveness here. It's like who shot J. R.? You get blamed for stuff." Brett also complained about the agency's rigidity and authority. "The agency is like fiefdoms—the directors like shoving their responsibility and power— The director of X has to give his approval for pictures to be hung, so it is very rigid and compartmentalized." (Urdang, 1994, pp. 95-96)

Many [of these systemic problems] impacted on his student, such as removing cases [from her] for financial reasons. He felt he "tried to keep her away from office politics, but I couldn't." Her anxiety level around these issues "was tremendous," although this diminished. Brett was also open with his student about the tensions, intervened actively on her behalf in several situations, and encouraged her to talk with him about what was happening. (Urdang, 1994, pp. 98-99)

Although Rose reported experiencing a number of external and internal stresses in her agency, she found they were alleviated by a supportive interpersonal climate.

After discussing a number of serious systemic issues, Rose [another beginning instructor] concluded that her unit was "a very unique bunch of individuals, and it is one of the reasons that I am still here . . . we do an amazing job of trying to take care of each other ourselves." She also felt that the group has the ability to "process the dynamics" of how systemic issues impact on their own work. (Urdang, 1994, pp. 97-98)

SOCIAL ISSUES

Four major social problems are discussed in this section: *discrimination, violence, imprisonment,* and *substance abuse.* Immigration, another critical social issue, will be discussed in Chapter 5.

Discrimination and Prejudice

Prejudice is distinguished from discrimination, although a close relationship exists between the two processes. "Prejudice is a positive or negative attitude, opinion, or prejudgment concerning a person or group usually formulated on the basis of selective perception and held without sufficient evidence or justification" (Queralt, 1996). Although a person may be prejudiced positively toward another, the term usually has negative connotations. A person, for example, might have negative, stereotyped attitudes about all black people or all old people.

Discrimination, however, while often stemming from prejudice, involves "an unjustified negative or hostile *action* toward a certain group or individual" (Queralt, 1996, p. 170). In discrimination, one is acting upon a prejudice or sometimes simply from economic considerations to exclude or deprive or harm a person in some way. Some places of employment or housing developments, for example, exclude ethnic minorities. The vicious murder (referred to previously) of Billy Jack Gaither, a gay man, was an example of discrimination being carried to its ultimate destructive end: the enactment of a *hate crime*. Gay men in small towns have often felt both prejudice and discrimination against them (Firestone, 1999). Political pressure is mounting to include crimes against homosexuals in hate crime legislation.

Hate crimes are forms of violence that target individuals or organizations "because of their racial, ethnic, religious, or sexual identities or their sexual orientation or condition of disability" (Barnes and Ephross, 1994, p. 247). This type of crime includes: "arson of homes and businesses, harassment, destruction of religious property, cross burnings, personal assaults, and homicides" (Barnes and Ephross, 1994, p. 247). The United States has made many legal and social advances (such as major civil rights legislation passed during the Johnson presidency) in combating discrimination and ensuring equal rights. Although evidence exists of greater acceptance of diversity among Americans (including a high degree of intermarriage and the election of minorities to high positions of political power), some groups are dedicated to promoting discrimination and hate crimes. Studies have reported the increase of hate crimes in recent years (Barnes and Ephross, 1994).

The Southern Poverty Law Center, in 1998, reported that nearly 500 hate groups or branches had engaged in racist actions in the previous year (Sack, 1998, A1). Usually when there is a strong economy, as in the 1990s, hate crimes tend to decrease, but the good economy did not curtail the development of hate groups (Sack, 1998).

> The increase comes mostly from growth in the number of chapters of pre-existing groups like the Ku Klux Klan and in the number of churches belonging to the Christian Identity movement, which cites biblical foundations for white supremacy and anti-semitism. . . . Mr. Potok [the editor of the report] said the proliferation of hate-group Internet sites and of racist rock music seemed to be fueling the increase. (Sack, 1998, p. A1)

During the July 4th weekend in 1999, a twenty-one-year-old man shot a number of minority individuals in Indiana and Illinois, killing two and wounding twelve (Belluck, 1999). At the end of the weekend, after a police chase, he shot himself. He was an active member of the World Church of the Creator, and "represented the kind of recruit that the World Church of the Creator and groups like it are increasingly trying to attract: young, educated, energetic, articulate" (Belluck, 1999, A7). As reported in *The New*

York Times: "In the last few years, hate groups, which once appealed primarily to older white men in mostly rural areas with little education and blue collar jobs, and which later attracted young ruffians called neo-Nazi skinheads, have begun to broaden their constituencies and increase their influence inside the political and legal systems" (Belluck, 1999, A1, A7).

Prior to this event, former President Clinton, referring to the threat of "'primitive' hatreds," advocated that the hate crimes law, already in existence, be expanded by Congress (Seelye, 1999). He proposed an expansion of the definition of hate crimes under federal law to "include incidents based on a person's sexual orientation, sex or disability. . . . Current law . . . requires that the victims be participating in one of six Federally protected activities when the crime occurs. . . . The proposed legislation would eliminate . . . [this] precondition" (Seelye, 1999, A18).

The political difficulties of passing hate crime legislation was illustrated in Texas, allegedly complicated by the fact that the state's then-governor, George W. Bush, was planning to run for president. The bill in question is named after James Byrd Jr., a black man who was killed by being dragged along a road by a car driven by white men in East Texas (Lyman, 1999). Some Democrats alleged that Republicans loyal to the governor intended to kill the bill in committee to "spare Mr. Bush a difficult choice: supporting it and alienating conservative Republicans who object to the inclusion of protection for homosexuals or vetoing it and offering Democrats a juicy issue to batter him with in the 2000 Presidential race" (Lyman, 1999, A1). This bill was ultimately signed into law by Texas Governor Rick Perry in May 2001 (Shannon, 2001).

Discrimination exists against many groups, including: women, the elderly, immigrants, the mentally ill, and the physically disabled. The political process has been important in advancing the rights and liberties of minorities; the disadvantaged groups themselves have often led the way. Women's advocacy for equal rights to education and employment have been active social issues for the past thirty years. NOW (the National Organization for Women) has had a serious impact on legislation, the political process, and other social changes that have advanced the interests of women. Lesbian and gay organizations "have gone from being outcasts of the left to being an expected presence in politics, or at least in Democratic coalitions" (Lacayo, 1998, p. 35). There is also "a small, careful movement within the G. O. P." toward supporting gay issues (Lacayo, 1998, p. 36). Hispanic voters are being taken seriously as a voting bloc (Beinert, 1998); the disabled have more political clout now than they have ever had (Rosenbaum, 1999).

Legislation has dramatically enhanced the rights of minorities. When black people gained the legal right to vote, it was a major civil rights victory. Vernon Dahmer, a black man who lived in Hattiesburg, Mississippi, was killed on January 10, 1966 (in his house which was set on fire), by members of the Ku Klux Klan (Cohen, 1998). Mr. Dahmer was an active leader in black voter registration, the major factor precipitating his murder. His death received national attention, and some members of the KKK were convicted and received life sentences for this crime. However, Sam Bowers, the Klan's Imperial Wizard for Mississippi, who was accused of masterminding the murder, was not convicted. Ellie Dahmer, the widow of Vernon, accumulated evidence for thirty years to have him retried and was finally successful.

> One thing that is different . . . is black voter registration—a gateway to jury service. Up from fewer than 100 in 1960, black voters today number more than 18,000 in Forrest County—about 30 percent of the total. The attacks by Bowers and other Klansmen on civil rights workers only served to accelerate their efforts to win full participation for blacks in public life. In that sense, whatever happens in court to Sam Bowers, he and his kind have already lost the great struggle of their lives. Vernon Dahmer won. (Cohen, 1998, p. 74)

Discrimination can be experienced in multiple ways by people who are members of more than one minority group; prejudice also can exist between minority groups. Gay men, for example, may belong to ethnic and cultural groups, which can cause conflict for them in terms of competing value systems and actual prejudicial and discriminatory behaviors. "Black and Chicano gays may fail to find acceptance either among white gays or in their own communities" (Berger and Kelly, 1995, pp. 1072-1073).

In addition, people who are different or behave differently from others in their minority group may face special problems; deaf people who refuse to use sign language may not be accepted in the deaf culture; black people can have conflict with other black people based on the lightness or darkness of their skin color; tensions can exist between people of different social classes who belong to the same racial or ethnic group.

In working with clients, the history of discrimination or prejudice they have experienced as well its impact on them in terms of feelings of self-identity, relationships with others, and actual and/or felt loss of social and economic opportunities should be explored. People who do not have "minority" status may also have experienced social prejudice because they were "different." People may not have gone to church when others did, or may *not* have discriminated against minorities when this was the norm, and so may have been ostracized by their social groups. In one study of a suburban Chicago high school, many of the students saw themselves as losers. Carol M. Lieber, who directs high school programs at Educators for Social Responsibility in Cambridge, Massachusetts, has commented:

"In these big high-powered suburban high schools, there's a very dominant winner culture . . ." she said. "But . . . high school life is very different for those who experience it as the losers. They become . . . alienated and without any real connection to any adult." (Lewin, 1999, p. 26)

Issues of discrimination will be discussed throughout the book: women's issues, men's issues, and gay and lesbian lifestyles in Chapter 10; issues of race, culture, ethnicity, immigration, and social class in Chapter 5; discrimination against the physically ill and disabled will be addressed in Chapter 12; toward the elderly in Chapter 10; and toward the mentally ill in Chapter 13.

Violence

"It is well documented that the United States has the highest rate of assaults and murders compared with any other nation in the world and that most of these incidents occur among the poor" (Levy and Wall, 2000, p. 402). Violence affects people in all age groups and socioeconomic levels: infants can be victims of parental murder and physical and/or sexual abuse; children often live in fear of school violence and may live in neighborhoods plagued by murder and gunfire; many women (and sometimes men) are victims of rape (especially in prison) and domestic violence; immigrants frequently bring a personal history of trauma with them (such as torture, political imprisonment, massacres); the elderly are often victimized by criminal behavior, as well as by physical and sexual abuse (committed by family members or staff of custodial facilities).

Community violence is common in urban life (Guterman and Cameron, 1997). "Recent studies indicate that 80 percent to 90 percent of children living in urban settings are direct victims of or witnesses to significant acts of violence in their neighborhoods, school, or communities" (Guterman and Cameron, 1997, p. 495). More children have been killed by handguns in the past fifteen years than the total of U.S. soldiers killed in the Vietnam war (Guterman and Cameron, 1997). While economically disadvantaged African-American, Hispanic, and other minority children and teenagers are especially affected by this violence, large numbers of young people in upper middle-class and suburban communities "report substantial direct experiences with violence in their communities" (Guterman and Cameron, 1997, p. 495).

The presence of violence in inner cities has received much attention, but the problem continues. Parson (1995), a clinical psychologist working with inner-city children, comments:

> Though American inner cities are not officially designated as military theaters of war, the violence and carnage that exist in some inner-city

communities today can be equated to the devastation and tragedy of loss and death on the battlefield. These "killing fields" or "combat zones" expose children to painful losses, unspeakable terror, and violence—in the streets, parks, playgrounds, in the school, and in the home. Paradoxically, these potentially traumatic locations are the very places society once viewed as bastions of tradition, safety, and values. Traumatic harm to children's minds and bodies from random violence and from witnessing parental murder [the subject of Parson's paper] is expected to increase. (Parson, 1995, p. 273)

Most violence toward children takes place at home. "Intrafamilial abuse, neglect, and domestic battery account for the majority of physical and emotional violence suffered by children in this country" (Perry, 1997, p. 126). While child sexual abuse may or may not be accompanied by acts of violence, it is included here as it is a major physical and psychological violation of the child. Although it has been difficult to obtain precise statistics on its prevalence, it has nevertheless been observed that childhood sexual abuse is a major problem with serious consequences.

Attention has been paid in more recent years to the frequent occurrence of physical abuse of women by their husbands or boyfriends (Longres, 1995b). Zastrow and Kirst-Ashman (1997) state that "it is estimated that two to six million women are beaten by their male partners each year in this country. . . . Of all women treated in hospital emergency rooms, 22 to 35 percent are there to receive treatment for injuries incurred during domestic violence incidents" (p. 371). Women who are homeless often report physical and/or sexual abuse as major factors causing them to leave home (Goldberg, 1999). It has recently been reported that physical abuse of partners occurs in gay and lesbian couple relationships (Carlson and Maciol, 1997).

The police have traditionally tended to dismiss reports of domestic violence as private matters but are now taking this problem more seriously; many police departments offer special training to enable officers to handle domestic violence situations (Zastrow and Kirst-Ashman, 1997). However, although new laws and procedures are in place, they are not always enforced (Zastrow and Kirst-Ashman, 1997), nor are the procedures always effective. In one case, a woman and her two-year-old daughter were killed by her estranged husband. The woman, thirty-three, filed for divorce, told police she was abused by her husband, and that he had threatened to kill her (Verhovek, 1998). She had: "obtained a protective order . . . and moved to a secret location. She strictly followed the procedure . . . for visitation with the husband . . . . after she returned to pick up her child, [she and her daughter were] shot . . . . The system had failed her" (Verhovek, 1998, p. A12).

Physical and sexual abuse can have significant psychological impacts on individual adults who have been abused as children and dramatically affect a child's ongoing development (Glodich, 1998; Kilgore, 1988; Osofsky, 1997). In discussing inner-city children with "traumatic ego pathology," Parson (1995) lists many emotional problems, which include "sleep disturbance, disturbed attachment behavior . . . concentration and attending deficits . . . learning disabilities . . . phobias . . . depression, and low self-esteem" (p. 276). Cohler and Zimmerman (1997) comment that "children in urban areas regularly confront violence and personal abuse perhaps even more destructive to personality development than the senseless bombing of the war [WWII] was to their counterparts fifty years ago" (p. 360). The effect of trauma on the values of children has been cited by Garbarino and Kostelny (1997). Unless some positive experiences can intervene *"traumatized children are likely to be drawn to groups and ideologies that legitimize and reward their rage, their fear, and their hateful cynicism"* (Garbarino and Kostelny, 1997, p. 40).

The massacre at the Columbine High School in Littleton, Colorado, did not take place in the inner city, but in a suburban setting; most school shootings have taken place in either suburban or rural areas. Many commentators feel these violent acts by youths were caused by multiple interacting factors, including the psychological difficulties of the youths, family relationships, socialization problems, the availability of guns, and the prevalence of violence in the media. "The message from studies of adolescents who kill others or themselves is that no single factor can explain their actions" (Goode, 1999b, p. A24).

Although guns are not generally considered the major motivation for murder, the fact that they are so accessible in our society is emphasized by many. Dr. Mann, a researcher at Columbia University, is cited as saying: " 'When vulnerable kids crack, the weapons that are at hand make the consequences of that vulnerability more serious' " (Goode, 1999b, p. A24). The two gunmen at Columbine High School had four guns with them during their attack (in addition to planting many explosives) (Brooke, 1999). In the Jonesboro, Arkansas, school murder of four girls and one teacher in 1998, the two boys (eleven and twelve years old) were armed with three rifles and seven other guns, which they took from their families' homes (Labi, 1998). In the case of the woman (cited previously) who was murdered by her husband, she had given her husband's gun to the police. However, the husband purchased another weapon after getting a permit from an adjacent county (Verhovek, 1998).

Intense public debate is taking place regarding gun control both nationally and on the state level, where many laws have been enacted (Verhovek, 1999). The National Rifle Association (NRA), a powerful lobbying group, has been active in opposing this legislation, citing a constitutional right to bear arms. Many Republicans and some Democrats in Congress are very reluctant to promote gun control (Seelye, 1999). Former President Clinton "is as aware as anyone of the political risks in taking on the gun lobby. In 1994, after he forced a ban on assault weapons through Congress, the Democrats lost control of the House and Mr. Clinton ascribed the loss to the gun lobby's campaign against those Democrats who had supported the ban" (Seelye, 1999, p. A20). Since President Bush took office, " 'we've seen his administration slowly chipping away at every gun violence prevention measure opposed by the gun lobby,' said Representative Carolyn McCarthy, D-NY" (Nakashima, 2001, p. A23).

Violence is a major problem in the United States, with multiple causations, consequences, and suggested solutions. We return to this subject throughout the book, discussing violence in the context of the family as well as its effects on the development of children and adults throughout the life cycle.

Imprisonment is one solution to violent crime; however, many people in prison have not committed violent crimes.

Imprisonment

The United States has large numbers of its citizens—more than that of other industrialized nations—incarcerated in its prisons (Singer et al., 1995). Currently, 1.8 million Americans are in jails and prisons (Butterfield, 1999a). It is estimated that this will increase to two million people, which is close to twice the number imprisoned ten years ago (Egan, 1999a). Paradoxically, this should not have been happening: the economy in the United States had been improving, and crime had dramatically decreased during the previous six years; the major reason for this increase in the prison population is the incarceration of drug offenders: 60 percent of inmates in federal prisons and 22 percent of those in state prisons and local jails are there for drug offenses (Egan, 1999a).

Some authorities refer to the criminalization of the mentally ill (Butterfield, 1998, p. A1). The term *transinstitutionalization* has been coined to describe "the movement of people from state hospitals to nursing homes and also to jails" (Solomon and Draine, 1995, p. 25). About 16 percent of the prison population (or 283,800 inmates) are mentally ill, a fact confirmed by a recent study (Butterfield, 1999c).

Incarceration of the Mentally Ill

Earlier in this chapter we referred to the homeless mentally ill and noted that a significant number have been imprisoned. "Many of the incarcerated homeless mentally ill are arrested for minor crimes that are survival strategies . . . or for behavior directly produced by psychosis" (Kaplan et al., 1994, p. 204). It appears that jails have replaced mental institutions as repositories for many mentally ill people since the 1960s (Butterfield, 1999c).

The president of the National Mental Health Association, Michael Faenza, has observed that "the criminal justice system is just a revolving door for a person with mental illness, from the street to jail and back without treatment" (Butterfield, 1999c, p. A10). Professor Kay Redfield Jamison has asserted that even if psychological services are provided to mentally ill prisoners, the prison setting hinders treatment. " 'Inmates get deprived of sleep,' she said, 'and isolation can exacerbate their hallucinations or delusions' " (Butterfield, 1999c, p. A10).

In addition to the incarceration of adults with mental illness, a relatively greater increase has occurred in the incarceration of teenagers with severe mental illness as a result of the relatively greater cuts in available psychiatric inpatient facilities for them (Butterfield, 1998).

One of the major paradoxes in the present state of inadequate treatment of the mentally ill is that this situation is accompanied by a knowledge explosion regarding treatment methodologies and medication research. Model programs offering comprehensive services to patients and families are presented at conferences; papers are written describing differing philosophical approaches to treatment from psychodynamic to behavior modification to family therapy. And yet in reality, for large numbers of patients, we have retrogressed rather than progressed in our humane treatment of their persons and their illness. Butterfield (1998) reports that the use of jails as repositories for the mentally ill goes back to the nineteenth century, when their dehumanizing treatment of patients as no better than recalcitrant animals was decried by Dorothea Dix (p. A26).

Although the number of women in prison is relatively small compared to the population of male prisoners (under 10 percent), the rate of female imprisonment has been increasing at twice the rate of male imprisonment (Singer et al., 1995).

> The majority of incarcerated women are sentenced for nonviolent offenses—crimes such as prostitution, fraud, or drug offenses . . . come from impoverished backgrounds, are addicted to drugs or alcohol, and have emotional and mental health problems. . . . The crimes these women commit are often a reaction to negative life events, a response to crisis or to prolonged disadvantage . . .
>
> Women who have co-occurring substance abuse disorders are particularly vulnerable to arrest and tend to serve longer jail sentences. (Singer et al., 1995, pp. 103-104)

Dual diagnosis (of major mental disorder and substance abuse) is found in both women's and men's prisons. "There are 3,000 seriously mentally ill prisoners at Rikers Island [jail in New York City] at any one time but only 97 beds for mentally ill drug abusers, who make up a large proportion of the offenders" (Winerip, 1999a, p. A21).

Substance Abuse and Imprisonment

Many people are incarcerated primarily for drug offenses; however, the current U.S. policy of "war against drugs," utilizing criminalization and imprisonment, is being reexamined. Although White House drug policy director General Barry R. McCaffrey has spoken of federal spending of $18 billion in 1999 to combat the problem, he has also spoken of expanding "alternatives to jail for drug users, based on studies showing that prisoners who get treatment are less likely to commit new crimes than those who do not" ("White House," 1999, p. A19). McCaffrey would like to "reduce the prison population by 250,000 through promoting options for treatment" (Wren, 1999, p. A16).

Arizona, with votes of large majorities of its citizens, was the first state to require treatment rather than imprisonment for people convicted of drug offenses. In more than forty states, judges and prosecutors are being given the authority to decide when offenders can be referred to treatment rather than to prison (Egan, 1999a).

Arizona has reported good results: 77.5 percent of offenders tested drug free after the treatment program. This program "saved Arizona $5,053,014 in prison costs in the 1998 fiscal year" (Wren, 1999, p. A16). After deducting program costs, the net savings was $2.5 million.

Substance abuse affects individuals and society in multiple ways. It has had a major impact on the child welfare system.

> The drug abuse epidemic of recent years has had a profound impact on the safety and protection of children and young people, and it has placed new demands on the child welfare system. An increasing number of women of childbearing age have become involved with alcohol and drugs, prenatal alcohol and drug exposure has affected a growing population of infants, a greater number of young children have been exposed to parental substance abuse, and significant percentages of young people are using and abusing alcohol and other drugs. Alcohol and other drugs have increasingly become factors in child maltreatment and are a primary reason that children and young people enter out-of-home care. (Liederman, 1995, p. 430)

Although some advocates are pushing for a more enlightened treatment approach to people with drug problems, "institutional incentives" exist throughout the country to continue the policy of incarceration (Egan, 1999a, p. 16). The Corrections Corporation of America, the largest private company involved in the correction field in the United States, is making large profits in the building of prisons. Unionized prison guards and some rural communities may also have a vested interested in the continued growth of the prison industry (Egan, 1999a). "Unions representing prison guards are the fastest-growing public employee associations in many states" (Egan, 1999a, p. 16). In California, in 1998, for example, union members received pay increases of 12 percent, enabling experienced prison guards to earn as much as $51,000 annually (Egan, 1999a).

It is obvious that prisoners have families and children. However, the fact that literally millions of children have a parent in prison or on probation has been recognized only recently (Butterfield, 1999a, p. A1). Having a parent in prison places a child at very high risk of criminality in adolescence and adulthood (Butterfield, 1999a).

Children of prisoners tend to be poor, and their families are often beset with abuse, neglect, and drug abuse; separation from the imprisoned parent creates additional stress (Butterfield, 1999a).

Currently interest is growing in working with children of prisoners, in setting aside hospitable family visiting space within prisons, as well as offering parenting classes and other programs to both incarcerated mothers and fathers. Research suggests that supporting family relationships reduces recidivism and has a positive effect on children (Butterfield, 1999a).

CONCLUSION

When we walk free, and life feels good to us, we may not be aware of the multitude of factors contributing to our sense of well-being. If the events in our lives gradually or suddenly shift, and we are no longer comfortable, we may wonder more deeply about the forces at work in the world in which our lives unfold. In this chapter, attention has been focused on the physical and social environments in which we and our clients live; we need to appreciate that social and political processes are constantly at work in our lives, even if we are unaware of them, as we might be unaware of the intricacy of our body's chemistry.

Although this book places emphasis on the psychological development underlying human behavior, it does so within a biopsychosocial framework, and, therefore, the environmental and social influences that impact on psychological and physical well-being or malaise are given attention. Social justice and social action are within the tradition of the social work profession, and we need to address these issues when relevant.

However, from a clinical perspective, we must not lose sight of the psychological and social needs of each individual client. "Correct" social policies will not end all personal pain and dysfunction. As we look at people with an array of social problems, including homeless mentally ill individuals, runaway (or "throwaway") teenagers (often from failed foster home experiences), people with violent impulses they cannot control, their traumatized victims, and the great reliance people place on illegal and prescribed drugs to cope with stress and inner distress, we can see that skilled clinical work is needed.

Perhaps we need more skills than in the past, because we see people with serious, complex disturbances, many of whom flee from the help they need (often with attachment disorders so severe that they may not know how to relate to the human support they so badly need). We must learn how to reach behind the "rejecting" facade and not feel rejected, to care about others without complying to wishes for inappropriate physical or social contact or for "merger." We must exercise caution so that we do not automatically or blindly follow an empowerment agenda with individual clients before determining what it is they are seeking, are capable of coping with, and is consistent with meeting what may be more fundamental needs.

Finally, as we carry out biopsychosocial clinical assessments of clients, we cannot assume that a particular social condition or racial or ethnic background has affected a person in a particular way—such an approach leads to stereotyping the very people social work tradition has committed us to treating as individuals. One minority person may have grown up with essentially positive social responses from others; another may have incurred multiple traumatic experiences because of his or her status. We must inquire into and understand the subjective experience of social events as well; this is the message of the constructivist approach, which we examine in the next chapter, within the contexts of diversity and culture.

LEARNING EXERCISES

1. Interview a person, who is not a client or a family member, with the purpose of understanding that person's perceptions of his or her involvement in groups, organizations, and the community, on both formal and informal levels. How does this individual describe himself or herself racially, ethnically, and culturally, and how does he or she feel these affiliations affect his or her life? Is this person involved in the political process on any level, and what are his or her thoughts about this? Integrate this material with your understanding of relevant course concepts.

2. Select three newspaper articles related to social and/or interpersonal issues. Discuss the issues, the underlying values, and the interrelationship of the relevant forces at work.

SUGGESTED READINGS

Articles

Delgado, M. (1997). Role of Latina-owned beauty parlors in a Latino community. *Social Work, 42,* 445-453.

Dulmus, C. N., Rapp-Paglicci, L. A., Sarafin, D. J., Wodarski, J. S., and Feit, M. D. (2000). Workfare programs: Issues and recommendations for self-sufficiency. *Journal of Human Behavior in the Social Environment, 3*(2), 1-12.

Dupper, D. R. and Poertner, J. (1997). Public schools and the revitalization of impoverished communities: School-linked, family resource centers. *Social Work, 42,* 415-422.

Newhill, C. (1995). Client violence toward social workers: A practice and policy concern for the 1990's. *Social Work, 40,* 631-636.

Weinreb, L. and Rossi, P. H. (1995). The American homeless family shelter system. *Social Service Review, 69,* 86-107.

Books

Caro, R. (1983). *The years of Lyndon Johnson: The path to power.* New York: Vintage Books.

Lee, J. A. B. and Swenson, C. R. (1986). The concept of mutual aid. In A. Gitterman and L. Shulman (Eds.), *Mutual aid groups and the life cycle* (pp. 361-377). Itasca, IL: F. E. Peacock Publishers, Inc.

Chapter 5

Culture and Diversity

. . . we are all much more simply human than otherwise . . .

Harry Stack Sullivan

INTRODUCTION

In the winter of 1999, three-day-old twins were brought to a public adoption center in Bogotá, Colombia, by their U'wa tribe parents because they wanted their children to live (Kotler, 1999). The alternative, prescribed by their tribe, was to leave them in the woods (or throw them into a river) to die, because twins, according to tribal beliefs, are an evil omen. However, when the center attempted to place these children, a major custody battle ensued. The tribe fought to halt the adoption, stating they wanted time to consider changing their customs and might accept the twins back. But social workers and child care advocates opposed this solution; they feared for these children among people who might have "discarded them in the wild" (Kotler, 1999, p. A11). Following extensive negotiations, the government agreed to give the twins back to the U'wa tribe after the tribe " 'agreed to place the rights of these two children above their cultural beliefs'" ("Twin Babies Spared," 1999).

This case raises a number of important issues: (1) How far can "culturally diverse Colombia . . . go in protecting minority practices" seen as unacceptable by the majority (Kotler, 1999, p. A11)? (2) To what extent do human rights take precedence over cultural values? (3) How did these parents make their decision (brave and humane by our standards, but rebellious and perhaps "dangerous" by the tribe's standards)? How did they come to deviate from such strong cultural constraints, asserting their autonomy in the process? Did they act solely on their own; did someone outside their tribe offer guidance? However they arrived at this solution for the survival of their children, their *will* prevailed (at least temporarily) over long-established custom. But their autonomy was not absolute; when they returned to their tribe, they were removed from the community to be "cleansed of impurities linked to the birth. For four years, they cannot visit other houses or share food with neighbors" (Kotler, 1999, p. A11).

In this chapter we shall look at the ways culture influences the individual, and how individuals adapt to, conform to, rebel against, or sometimes re-shape culture to their own ends. The concept of culture "incorporates all the symbolic meanings—the beliefs, values, norms, and traditions . . . shared in a community and [that] govern social interactions among community members or between members and outsiders" (Longres, 1995b, p. 74). While cultures can be viewed at the macrolevel, such as the cultures of Japanese people or Native American people, they can also be observed at the micro-level, as developed by small groups, such as communes, cults, or fraternities and sororities. Many institutions and organizations are said to have their own internal culture.

People can belong to more than one culture and one race; many in the United States, for example, are multicultural. Tiger Woods, the famous golfer, brought this issue into prominence when he explained that he did not think of himself as African American. "I'm just who I am" (White, 1997, pp. 33-34). He is the child of a black American father and a Thai mother and refers to himself with a name he made up: " 'I'm a Cablinasian,' which he explained is a self-crafted acronym that reflects his one-eighth Caucasian, one-fourth black, one-eighth American Indian, one fourth Thai and one-fourth Chinese roots" (White, 1997, p. 33). A dramatic increase has occurred in the number of multiracial children in the United States since 1970; the U.S. Bureau of the Census reports more than 2 million such children today (White, 1997).

The clash of values between cultures as well as within cultures is high-lighted in this chapter. In Pakistan, for example, then Prime Minister Sharif, in September 1998, produced tensions by increasing the legal role played by Islam (McGirk, 1998). "Even in the best of times, the implementation of . . . Islamic law led to quarreling among the country's 72 Muslim sects and subsects over the 'pure' interpretation of the law" (McGirk, 1998, p. 56).

The issues of diversity discussed in this chapter include ethnicity, race, social class, and culture. Diversity related to gender and sexual orientation is discussed in Chapter 10, to disabilities in Chapter 12, and to mental illness in Chapter 13.

Immigration issues are presented to highlight understanding of the psychological adaptations people make as they move from one culture to another. "Immigration from one country to another is a complex and multifaceted psychosocial process with significant and lasting effects on an individual's identity" (Akhtar, 1995, p. 1052).

Two recently created cultures that played a dominant role in the lives of their members are discussed: one, the Heaven's Gate sect, had a tragic (according to my viewpoint) outcome, resulting in mass suicide (a triumphant new beginning, from their viewpoint). The other, the culture of the deaf, is an ongoing, cooperative, and supportive group of people, seeking to empower themselves and one another in their shared world of deafness.

Diversity and culture affect social work practice in many ways, sometimes unrecognized: diagnostic assessments; the nature of treatment as well as the therapeutic relationship; and the need for resolution of complex value conflicts that can confront us.

In discussing culture in this chapter, three major approaches are addressed: *cultural sensitivity, cultural competence,* and *constructivism.* Applying concepts of cultural sensitivity, the social worker emphasizes the common human needs of all clients, applies a basic casework approach, but at the same time recognizes that people may have different values and perspectives and is open to learning about the client's culture (Lee and Greene, 1999). The culturally competent clinician learns about the client's specific culture to develop "culture-specific concepts . . . and techniques from within the specific context" (Lee and Greene, p. 23).

However, although being culturally competent may help the clinician understand behaviors that may appear inexplicable without knowledge of the client's cultural background and values, the danger exists of "stereotyping" the client and assuming that culture is the explanation for every clients behavior. Cultural competence may also lead us to believe that clients accept all tenets of their culture and that, in fact, they participate in only one culture.

The constructivist stance is an approach to exploring culture that permits the clinician to be sensitive to cultural issues while at the same time individualizing each client, exploring the meaning of their culture to them, understanding their perceptions of their problems and the help they anticipate, without imposing a prescribed treatment agenda. My point of view is that a combination of cultural sensitivity, cultural competence, and a constructivist framework is more effective in working with people from cultures both diverse from and similar to our own, with a continual awareness of the conflicts culture can pose for the individual, the client-worker relationship, and treatment approaches.

CONSTRUCTIVISM

In a *New Yorker* cartoon titled: "Theories of Everything," a father, a mother, and their teenage son and daughter are sitting on a couch; they are not talking to each other, but their thoughts are revealed (Chast, 1998, p. 42). The father is thinking: "Everything's gone downhill since 1964." The mother thinks: "Everything is *my fault.*" The daughter, glaring at mother, thinks "Everything *is* your fault." And the young teenage boy thinks: "Everything would be perfect if I had a dirt bike." This scene portrays four individuals living within the same family context, but their preoccupations, interpretations, and the meanings (or theories) they have constructed are different.

It has been argued that our psychological theories are not "objective truths"; they have been constructed by people who view the world through their own values and perspectives. "Every theory is a social construction. By this we mean that all theories are of necessity a product of their time and place and culture" (Berzoff et al., 1996, p. 10). Furthermore, observers play an important role in what they observe; the "act of observing" inevitably affects what is being observed (Lee and Greene, 1999, p. 24).

The judgment of normality, within a constructivist perspective, is also seen as culturally constructed—"normality is always in the eyes of the observer" (Berzoff et al., 1996, p. 11). What, for example, is "normal sexuality," and who defines this? Whether homosexual marriages should be legalized is a reflection of a present debate on the subject of sexual normality. Sophie Freud (1999) points out that "different sexual practices have been viewed as perverse in different historical periods. Masturbation was held responsible for a wide range of mental illnesses in the eighteenth and nineteenth century" (p. 336).

Culture is not static. Becker views "culture as always a work in progress" (Saari, 1999, p. 223). He asserts:

> "People create culture continuously. Since no two situations are alike, the cultural solutions available to them are only approximate. Even in the simplest societies, no two people learn quite the same cultural material; the chance encounters of daily life provide sufficient variation to ensure that. No set of cultural understandings, then, provides a perfectly applicable solution to any problem . . . [so people] . . . must . . . adapt their understandings to the new situation. . . . Even the most . . . determined effort to keep things as they are would necessarily involve strenuous efforts to remake and reinforce understandings so as to keep them intact in the face of what was changing" (Becker, 1986, p. 19). (Saari, 1999, p. 223)

Approaching cultural understanding from a constructivist perspective affords one the opportunity to approach each client with an open spirit of inquiry; we cannot assume we know all about the client's culture or that we have the right prescription for the client. We must listen to the client's story (or narrative) and understand how clients perceive their problems and their ideas about solving them. "The therapist's questions should bring the conversation to the *edge of what language experience reveals,* so that further questioning involves the formulation of what has not been said or thought before [by the client]. The therapist is a respectful listener who does not *know too soon* nor *understand too quickly*" (Goolishian and Winderman, 1988, pp. 140-141).

This resonates with Winnicott's idea of the development of individualized theories, related to each case, as he "entered the 'swampy lowlands' of messy, confusing difficulties that elude objectively derived solutions, challenge existing theory, and are characterized by uncertainty, ambiguity, and unpredictability" (Applegate and Bonovitz, 1995, p. 18). A patient discusses the importance of her therapist understanding her world.

> Reflecting on her treatment, a patient told me, "when you understand the way my mind works without saying it should work another way, when you find the logic in my responses, that lets me experience more than I've known before (the shame . . . the terror . . . even the chaos)— about how my mind works." (Schwaber, 1997, p. 52)

Constructivism, as a theoretical perspective, has incorporated an emphasis on cross-cultural issues and has been applied to individual treatment (Lee and Greene, 1999). Some authors "have discussed from a social constructivist perspective the importance of culture in one's development of self" (Lee and Greene, 1999, p. 27). Steier has asserted that "an individual's 'self' is socially constructed as a 'person-in-a-culture'" (Lee and Greene, 1999, p. 27). In a multicultural society people may develop more than one set of values and beliefs; we must look at a person-in-multicultures. In addition, an awareness of one's own cultural background and biases becomes an important ingredient in preparing to understand and accept the culture of another.

In striving to be a culturally competent clinician, one may assiduously read all about a specific culture, then unwittingly impose this knowledge on a client in a stereotypical way. The constructivist message is to refrain from imposing definitions but rather to uncover the "culturally embedded, unique meaning" of the way the client interprets the dilemma and the way to solve it; the "explanatory model of the client's problem is influenced by the culturally distinctive way of organizing information around the problem situation" (Lee and Greene, 1999, pp. 30-31).

To illustrate: Lia Lee is a Hmong child who developed epilepsy when she was three months old and living in California with her immigrant family. Her family realized she had *quag dab peg,* which means " 'the spirit catches you and you fall down'" (Fadiman, 1997, p. 20). The constructivist question is asked: how did the parents perceive this problem? It is learned that, for the most part, the family wanted the spirit to be cured. On the other hand, as they informed their social worker, they viewed the condition as an "honor" and considered their daughter to be "an anointed one . . . in their culture" who might become a "shaman" in the future because she had "these spirits in her." Among the many professionals who had dealt with the family, only the social worker had thought to elicit the family's notion of the *"cause of their daughter's illness"* [italics added] (Fadiman, 1997, p. 22).

Belonging to multiple cultures can be a source of stress, especially when the value systems of each conflict. This is illustrated by the problems faced by religious individuals who happen also to be homosexual; homosexuality is considered taboo in many religious systems. For example, a group of Muslim men who are also gay held their first conference in New York on May 29, 1999, sponsored by the Al-Fatiha Foundation (Sachs, 1999a). The group was formed to: "create a community for homosexuals based on a shared religion. . . . 'In many instances, religion is the source of inner conflict'. . . . Our mission is to help individuals reconcile their homosexuality with their religion, in whatever way they want to do it"; members do not wish to establish a gay mosque as they feel it would further isolate them and would be in conflict with Islam's emphasis on community (Sachs, 1999a, p. 22).

Diversity exists in multiple forms. It can be invisible, in terms of a person's private thoughts, hidden physical symptoms, or "closeted" actions; at other times it is highly visible, apparent in distinctive gendered and racial characteristics or physical disabilities. People "who are different" may find acceptance in some (or all) social groups, or their differences may create a real or a felt sense of alienation.

DIVERSITY

As issues of diversity are presented, we will examine the subject both from a social and a psychological perspective. The issues covered in this section include ethnicity and race, social class, immigration, and culture.

Ethnicity and Race

Are white Anglo-Saxon Protestants members of an ethnic group (Sollors, 1986)? Is a majority group considered ethnic? Or are only minorities or subgroups to be considered ethnic? It is a "widespread practice to define ethnicity as otherness" (Sollors, 1986, p. 25). The word ethnic has its roots in the Greek word *ethnikos,* which means "gentile" or "heathen" (Sollors, 1986, p. 25). In the middle of the nineteenth century the concept of "ethnic" evolved to mean " 'peculiar to a race or nation.' " Sollors expresses reservations about the use of this concept: he cites Cohen as stating that to " 'many people, the term ethnicity connotes minority status, lower class, or migrancy. This is why sooner or later we shall have to drop it or to find a neutral word for it, though I can see that we shall probably have to live with it for quite a while'" (Sollors, 1986, p. 39).

McGoldrick and colleagues (1982) stress the importance of understanding people's ethnicity in the practice of family therapy, and Levine (1982) notes that "ethnocultural factors are more powerfully played out in family relations than in any other arena" (p. xi). McGoldrick (1982) adds that ethnicity "is a powerful influence in determining identity" (p. 5), and notes that "an ethnic group has been defined as 'those who conceive of themselves as alike by virtue of their common ancestry, real or fictitious, and who are so regarded by others' (Shibutani and Kwan). Ethnicity describes a sense of commonality transmitted over generations by the family and reinforced by the surrounding community" (p. 4).

Race is considered one aspect of ethnicity, and this controversial concept can lead to stereotyping and prejudiced thoughts and actions. Objecting to a rigid use of racial categories, Spickard and colleagues (1995) argue that the increase of diversity of racial groupings "suggests a deconstruction of the very notion of race; in this country there were "43 racial categories and subcategories on the 1990 census form" (p. 581). There had been a movement by various groups, such as the Association of Multi-Ethnic Americans, to alter the categories of the U.S. census and other governmental organizations either "to include a multiracial category or to allow a person to check more than one box" (Spickard et al., 1995, p. 582). According to a U.S. Census Bureau Population Division statement of April 2000: "Instead of allowing a multiracial category as was originally suggested in public and congressional hearings, the OMB adopted the Interagency Committee's recommendation to allow respondents to select one or more races when they self-identify" ("Racial and Ethnic," 2000). According to the Texas State Data Center, Department of Rural Sociology, at Texas A&M University, "the combinations of the six racial groups used in the 2000 Census result in 63 separate racial categories and, if these are divided into those of Hispanic and those not of Hispanic origin, there are 126 combinations of race/ethnicity" ("Comparing Race/Ethnicity," 2001).

In a book written about the impact of culture and class on psychotherapy, the authors chose to leave the word "race" out of their title (Pérez Foster et al., 1996).

> It is especially important that we confront the fact that the division of the world into black and white is a delusion of civilization. People are not black or white. Where the line is drawn is politically and psychologically motivated. The fact that "race" is the only ethnic grouping in this culture that does not allow for the possibility of dual identity belies its delusional rigidity. While "race" clearly has powerful psychological meanings that are discussed in many of the chapters in this

volume, we felt it was important not to lend it continuing scientific re-
spectability by using it in our title. (Pérez Foster et al., 1996, xvi-xvii)

I chose to retain the words ethnicity and race in this book because of the
strong positive sense of identification many people have with these designa-
tions, and also because I did not want to bury the strong negative emotions
that can be evoked by these words. Although some people of a given ethnicity may not feel that their primary identification is as a member of that ethnicity (or they may have multiple ethnicities), it nevertheless remains an
emotionally charged and meaningful concept to many. From a negative perspective, the intensity of ethnic loyalties and ethnic hatreds fuels (and has
fueled) many wars and serious conflicts, such as the recent upheavals in
Bosnia and Serbia and the large-scale massacres in Rwanda. More constructively, ethnicity can help develop identification and a positive sense of community. The negative and positive usages of ethnicity are not mutually exclusive.

The concepts of ethnicity and race are used here within the constructivist
perspective, which urges understanding of the meaning of ethnicity and race
to each individual client and family. Clinical social workers should assess
not only how clients feel about their cultural identities, rituals, values, etc.,
but how they relate to others outside their racial, ethnic, and cultural groups.
Sollors (1986) cites Barth as stating that it is " 'the ethnic boundary that defines the group, not the cultural stuff that it encloses' " (p. 27). How people
relate to outsiders is particularly relevant when client and therapist are of
different ethnicities and races.

America has come a long way in its development of human rights and improvement in race relations. But tensions continue to exist, and at times explode, as in the Los Angeles riots following the Rodney King verdict; affirmative action issues fuel major political debates; hate crimes continue to
make the news. And, at the same time, children of mixed races attend school
and play together; the rate of interracial marriages increases (Spickard et al.,
1995), as does the number of minority professionals and respected political
figures.

Generally, when racial issues are discussed, black Americans are the major focus; however, Native Americans, Asians, and Hispanics have their
own unique issues, which are drawing increasing attention. This section will
focus on these four groups.

African Americans and American Blacks

The use of the term African American is generally viewed as a "progressive" term signifying an acceptance and integration of this group. In the
past, the term Negro (viewed by many as derogatory) was widely used; then

the use of black (connotating racial pride) became customary. However, while generally accepted, the term African American is not universally agreed upon (Longres, 1995a); it is also not all encompassing, in that not all black Americans have come from Africa. In this country, for example, there are groups of Haitians, Jamaicans, and Azoreans, among others. The terms African Americans, American blacks, and blacks will be used interchangeably in this book.

The black population in the United States is not a homogenous group; persons belonging to it represent different subcultures, different social classes, different political views, and vary in the extent that their self-identities and opportunities in life have been adversely affected by racial, prejudicial, and discriminatory experiences. Black persons may also belong to other cultural groups not related to race and differ to the degree that they feel a need to remain "separate" from the mainstream culture or to be integrated into it; to the degree they are comfortable with white friends (or spouses); and the degree to which they may be looked down upon or look down on others for "acting white."

Antiblack racism and slavery. Blackness does not provide a cloak of invisibility; skin color is readily apparent (unless the person has very light pigmentation) and often subjects the individual to overt or subtle rejection.

Ralph Ellison (1980) discusses the issue of invisibility from a different perspective; the individuality of the black person is often rendered invisible by the white observer who sees only a stereotype and not a person. The protagonist of his novel declares himself to be an invisible man:

> No . . . not a spook like those who haunted Edgar Allan Poe; nor am I one of your Hollywood-movie ectoplasms. I am a man of substance, of flesh and bone, fiber and liquids—and I might even be said to possess a mind. I am invisible, understand, simply because people refuse to see me. Like the bodiless heads you see sometimes in circus sideshows, it is as though I have been surrounded by mirrors of hard, distorting glass. When they approach me they see only my surroundings, themselves, or figments of their imagination—indeed, everything and anything except me. (Ellison, 1980, p. 3)

Antiblack racism, in this country, has its roots in the slave system that was maintained for 200 years. Slavery in the United States was an oppressive, brutal, dehumanizing experience in which black people were stolen and kidnapped from their homelands, brought to this country on slave ships notorious for their inhumane conditions, and sold at auction to white Americans, without any regard for the needs of the black people or for keeping family members together. This was justified in the minds of many as an economic necessity and on the premise that black Africans were an inferior race.

Recently an increase has occurred in the publication of books describing the slave experience. "A proliferating number of popular and scholarly books about slavery are stripping away whatever is left of the velvety romance of benign slave holders presiding over docile slaves. And they are emphasizing efforts of the enslaved to escape or rebel and the punishments they faced that ranged from branding to amputation" (Carvajal, 1999, Section 4, p. 5).

A powerful book written about slavery and its psychological impact is William Styron's (1993) *The Confessions of Nat Turner.* It is a fictionalized account of a true event: a major but unsuccessful slave rebellion that Nat Turner led in 1831 in southeastern Virginia. Although Styron received the Pulitzer prize for this work, a good deal of controversy nevertheless surrounded his novel, which was published at "one of the most explosive moments in the history of race relations in America" (Horwitz, 1999, p. 83). Black critics raised questions about Styron's depiction of Nat Turner and asked whether a white author was capable of understanding the slave experience. In addition, controversy exists among historians about the facts of this case, the details of which still remain murky. Although acknowledging that the details of these excerpts may be historically incorrect, I chose to include them here because the emotional impact of the slave experience appears to "ring true" to historic accounts from other sources.

Nat Turner was tried and hanged. In the following scene, Nat is talking to his court-appointed lawyer, and the white lawyer's self-righteous deprecatory attitude is apparent. Gray, the lawyer, is talking to Nat about the fate of his coconspirators: ". . . out of this whole catastrophic ruction only round one-fourth gets the rope. . . . Mealy-mouthed abolitionists say we don't show justice. Well, we do. . . . That's how come nigger slavery's going to last a thousand years" (Styron, 1993, p. 25).

Slave experiences ranged from abject misery and brutality to some physical comfort and comparatively benign conditions; Nat and his mother were house slaves who lived comfortably with a humane master. Although lacking freedom and denied basic legal rights, Nat was not a field slave who toiled long hours at physical labor and lived in slave quarters. He was aware of this distinction (Styron, 1993). One evening he becomes aware of his own troubled feelings when, in the dwindling light, he sees "a line of Negro men trooping up from the mill . . . wearily playful . . . as they move homeward with the languid, shuffling, shoulder-bent gait of a long day's toil. . . . I turn away (could there have been a whiff of something desperate and ugly in that long file of sweating, weary men which upsets my glowing childish house bound spirit?)" (Styron, 1993, pp. 125-126).

Marse [Master] Samuel was kind to Nat and was proud of Nat's intelligence and ability to read. Marse Samuel explains his strongly held view that " 'the more . . . enlightened a Negro is made, the better for himself, his master, and the commonweal. But one must begin at a tender age, and thus . . . you see in Nat the promising beginnings of an experiment" (Styron, 1993, p. 124). Marse Samuel arranged for Nat to have special training in carpentry and promised him that, when he was older, he would have his freedom and would be apprenticed to a carpenter in Richmond.

However, the land of the plantation becomes infertile (common in the area due to overcultivation of cotton). Marse Samuel and his family leave for richer land, and Nat is left behind, with promises that his next owner will carry out the arrangements for his freedom. This is not to be: suddenly Nat is a slave in the full sense of the word and lives with a series of masters, most of whom cruelly exploit him. It is not the exploitation that fuels his rage; it is the betrayal by Marse Samuels. In the following passage, Nat recalls being sold at a slave auction by his second master, Reverend Eppes. He remembers "crying out; 'But you can't do this! You and Marse Samuel had a written agreement. You was to take me to *Richmond!* He *told* me so!' . . . But the Reverend Eppes said not a word, counting bills, each golden second climbing from penury to riches . . . as . . . he verified his booty. . . . 'You can't!' I shouted. 'I've got a trade, too! I'm a carpenter!' " He then "experienced a kind of disbelief . . . close upon madness, then a sense of betrayal . . . then . . . hatred so bitter that I . . . thought I might get sick on the floor. . . hatred for Marse Samuel, and the rage rose and rose in my breast until . . . in my mind's eye I saw him strangled by my own hands" (Styron, 1993, pp. 246-247).

In this last passage, we see the impact of total abandonment on Nat and the failed promises of Marse Samuel; Nat becomes engulfed in a nightmare world. He screams and pleads for recognition of his rights; his pleas are not only unheard but silenced. He is helpless and powerless; his despair turns into the rage, which ultimately fuels his motivation for a slave rebellion. Perhaps more recent racial "insurrections" and riots are fueled by similar feelings of betrayal, despair, utter powerlessness, and "soul murder."

> The situation of Black slaves brought to this country was devastating not only because their immigration was forced . . . but also because they were psychophysically manhandled by the "host" population. They were used as targets of projection and, in an act of collective "soul murder" (Shengold, 1989), brainwashed to believe in their inherent racial inferiority. Effects of the intergenerational transmission of this trauma (Apprey, 1993) are still evident. (Akhtar, 1995, p. 1055)

The Civil War freed the slaves, but many white people, especially in the South, retained oppressive power and disdain for the personhood of the black person. Lynchings, for which there was no legal recourse, were common; Jim Crow laws were passed in the South: "The system prescribed how African Americans were supposed to act in the presence of whites, asserted white supremacy, embraced racial segregation, and denied political and legal rights to African Americans" (Zastrow and Kirst-Ashman, 1997, p. 216).

Maya Angelou (1997), who spent a large portion of her childhood in Stamps, Arkansas, in the 1930s, discussed random lynchings as well as the many ordinary humiliations experienced by black people in her community. One degrading incident occurred in a dentist's office. Annie (her grandmother), whom she called Momma, brought Maya to a white dentist in town, knowing that he did not treat black patients but in hope that he will relent in her case for two reasons: Maya was in severe pain, and the dentist owed Annie a favor, as she had lent him money in the past when he was in difficulty.

> Momma said, "Dentist Lincoln. It's my grandbaby here. She got two rotten teeth that's giving her a fit." . . . "Annie?" . . . He was choosing words the way people hunt for shells. "Annie, you know I don't treat nigra, colored people." . . . "Seem like to me, Dentist Lincoln, you might look after her, she ain't nothing but a little mite. And seems like maybe you owe me a favor or two."
> . . . "It's been paid, and raising your voice won't make me change my mind. My policy . . . " He let go of the door and stepped nearer Momma. The three of us were crowded on the small landing. "Annie, my policy is I'd rather stick my hand in a dog's mouth than in a nigger's." (Angelou, 1997, pp. 188-189)

While Dentist Lincoln was insulting to Momma, she was not cowed. She realized that she could not win this battle, but assertively made her request. Momma is a very strong character throughout the book; she runs a grocery store and is a very respected member of her community. Momma does not seem to have experienced "soul murder." The main character in the *Invisible Man,* by contrast, has had his "soul murdered" by a web of events, all racially entwined, leading to a Kafkaesque world of betrayal, lack of opportunity, exploitation, and feelings of total powerlessness.

Debates continue today about the extent of the psychological consequences of racial prejudice and discrimination. Research has been conducted on the effects of discrimination on the mental health and self-esteem of individuals, with mixed findings. Self-esteem is not adversely affected by racism in all instances, as has been noted by some researchers (Zastrow and Kirst-Ashman, 1997). Mattei (1996) writes that following many years of research about the risks of being a minority person, "simple or clear conclusions remain elusive and contradictory" (p. 237).

There is no question that cultural discontinuity, ethnic or racial devaluing, and assaults present significant challenges for minority youth. At the same time we know that minority children are not *inevitably* less adjusted, nor do they invariably experience lower levels of self-esteem. (Mattei, 1996, p. 237)

Psychological consequences of racism. In assessing how the psychological consequences of prejudice and discrimination affect any given African-American individual, three major factors should be taken into account: systemic issues; resilience and other protective factors; and biopsychosocial assessment, including the person's self-perceptions about being black and the impact of minority status on their lives. These three criteria can be applied to understanding the impact of discrimination on a person of any minority.

Systemic issues. Major positive changes in political, legal (including the major civil rights legislation), educational, and employment opportunities for black Americans should be taken into account. Racial segregation in schools, for example, was declared unconstitutional by the *Brown v. Board of Education* Supreme Court decision in 1954 (Zastrow and Kirst-Ashman, 1997). The civil rights movement and subsequent legislation led to voting rights and greater protections for black citizens. Other positive developments fostered by the civil rights movement included the " 'Black is beautiful' and similar esteem-building social voices, [and] the search for heritage and legacy (memorialized in Alex Haley's 1976 *Roots*)" (Akhtar, 1995, p. 1055).

Socioeconomic status is relevant; members of minority groups with low socioeconomic status, for example, who live in impoverished inner-city communities face serious economic, employment, and housing problems. Poor, undereducated black males are especially at risk for unemployment and are disproportionately represented in the prison population. Other inner-city problems include: "drug abuse, school dropouts, births outside of marriage, and AFDC families" (Zastrow and Kirst-Ashman, 1997, p. 217).

However, many black families are part of a growing middle class, and some are represented in the upper class. "A middle class has emerged that is better educated, better paid, and better housed than any group of African Americans that has gone before it" (Zastrow and Kirst-Ashman, 1997, p. 217). Miles (1998), discussing social class differences in the African-American population, refers to several distinct African-American cultures and comments that as "one goes up the socioeconomic scale, the impact of institutional racism on ego development lessens" (p. 110). However, it should be added that the impact of systemic issues on any given individual must be examined both in terms of objective experiences, and the subjective constructed meaning of these events to the person.

Psychological and cultural resiliency. Resiliency, both on psychological and cultural levels, can play an important role in building a protective shield against prejudiced attitudes and treatment. Social organizations, such as African-American churches, have been a source of political action, as well as personal support to many of their members in black communities (Zastrow and Kirst-Ashman, 1997). The fact that a majority group may discriminate against a minority group does not necessarily mean that the latter is psychologically devastated; in fact, it can engender a sense of group cohesiveness and strength in the group subjected to such hostility.

> Afro-Americans have survived a harsh system of slavery, repression, and racism. Although there have been casualties, there have been many more survivors, achievers, and victors. The cultural heritage of coping with adversity and overcoming has been passed on from generation to generation, laced with stories of those with remarkable courage and fortitude. (Zastrow and Kirst-Ashman, 1997, citing Powell, p. 219)

Maya Angelou (1997) describes her all-black school graduation in Stamps, Arkansas. Her moving account captures the excitement, pride, and involvement of the whole community in this event, including days of preparations and celebrations beforehand. The ceremony is spoiled for her by the white school superintendent's very condescending speech; his underlying message was that the black people in the audience were uneducated laborers and that "anything higher that we aspired to was farcical and presumptuous" (Angelou, 1997, p. 180). But then Henry Reed, the class valedictorian, gave his speech and led his class in singing the Negro national anthem. "The tears that slipped down many faces were not wiped away in shame" (Angelou, 1997, p. 184).

> We were on top again. As always, again. We survived. The depths had been icy and dark, but now a bright sun spoke to our souls. I was no longer simply a member of the proud graduating class of 1940; I was a proud member of the wonderful, beautiful Negro race.
>
> Oh, Black known and unknown poets, how often have your auctioned pains sustained us? Who will compute the lonely nights made less lonely by your songs, or by the empty pots made less tragic by your tales? (Angelou, 1997, p. 184)

Biopsychosocial assessment. A biopsychosocial assessment sheds light on the psychological effects of discrimination within the context of a person's life, relationships, and opportunities. Clients' self-perceptions of their racial identity and racial conflicts vary; "some patients have only vague anxieties that are experienced as related to their ethnicity, while others are directly and deeply impacted by it" (Thompson, 1996, p. 123). The quality of family life and attachments of children are crucial factors in their adaptation and are important protective factors mediating against psychological harm from discrimination. "One's immediate environment appears to be the predominant system in shaping one's self-concept: It appears that the child who is loved, accepted, and supported in his immediate environment comes to love and respect himself as someone worthy of love" (Zastrow and Kirst-Ashman, 1997, p. 219).

Thompson (1996), who is a black woman psychoanalyst, found that one of the most intricate therapy issues was separating out a patient's racial issues from his or her personality issues. "In treating many black patients, the initial clarification of their struggles requires what I call a type of 'racial surgery,' which involves helping them discern the differences between those struggles that would be theirs regardless of ethnicity, and those that might be complicated specifically because of their race" (p. 125).

The issue of skin color is an important aspect involved in the development of racial identity and can produce discrimination not only from nonblack people but discrimination within the community of black people. "For many people of color, the factor of skin color itself is deeply intertwined with the sense of self-value" (Thompson, 1996, p. 125). In some black families preferences may exist for one child over another based on the lightness or darkness of skin, and differences of skin color can affect peer relationships and choice of marriage partners (Harvey, 1995; Williams, 1997). Williams warns against assuming that all black people place higher value on light skin than they do dark skin. Harvey asserts that therapists should not make assumptions about clients' feelings about their skin color but rather should inquire. "Skin color can be perceived as a positive dynamic in the clients' lives as well as a negative factor. Some individuals and families view their blackness as a badge of honor" (Harvey, 1995, p. 8).

In relating issues of blackness, whiteness, integration, and separation to the treatment situation, it is important that therapists be aware of these complex issues and address them with clients rather than make automatic assumptions. Differences in race can complicate transference and countertransference issues between therapist and patient, and often issues of trust must be worked through (Thompson, 1996). However, having a therapist of the same race "is not devoid of race-related impasses" (Thompson, 1996, p. 139). The discussion of racial and cultural similarities and differences affecting clinical work is elaborated in the final section of this chapter.

Native Americans

On September 28, 1999, groundbreaking ceremonies were held in Washington, DC, celebrating the opening of the National Museum of the American

Indian (Clines, 1999). This event signifies an important step both in recognizing the rights, history, and dignity of Native Americans and in acknowledging the history of oppression and exploitation perpetrated by the U.S. government.

> A century after the tribal devastation of the Indian wars, a place of honor on the capital Mall was finally extended to the nation's Native Americans today as construction began on a museum that Indian leaders vowed would celebrate their history of indominability, "even if it tells a sad story, even if it's a hard story to look at."
> With hundreds of tribal members and chiefs in attendance savoring ancient ritual and hopeful speeches, the museum, scheduled to open in 2002, was hailed as a long overdue antidote to centuries of racist stereotyping, broken treaties and federal "civilization regulations" that failed to rein in rich tribal cultures with a policy of assimilation. (Clines, 1999, p. A18)

In another act of reconciliation, the Peabody Museum at Harvard University, on May 19, 1999, returned the remains of approximately 2,000 Pueblo Indians to their ancient site in Pecos Valley, New Mexico, from which they had been excavated by archaeologists (Goldberg, 1999b). In 1990, Congress passed the Graves Protection and Repatriation Act; since then, Indian remains and other sacred relics have been returned to the appropriate tribes; the Harvard return is by far the largest. When the remains arrive in New Mexico, a mass reburial will take place that tribal leaders have said "will cap a process both solemn and full of the joy of rightful return. 'We are real grateful, happy and proud that our ancestors are on their way home,' said Pete Toya, the war chief of the Pueblo of Jemez" (Goldberg, 1999b, p. A1). This act of repatriation has a twofold significance: the respect for ancestors is very strong in Native American cultures; in addition, the historic "grave robbing" by white Americans is now being rectified.

In a different realm, Congress passed the United States Indian Child Welfare Act in 1978, stressing restraint in the removal of Native American children from their homes to help preserve their culture. The purpose was to prevent the separation of many Native American children from their families and tribes and to prevent them from being placed in nonNative American adoptive or foster care homes (Goldstein and Goldstein, 1996). "The rate of out-of-home placement for American Indian and Alaska Native children has been from 5 to 20 times greater than rates for comparable non-Indian populations" (Robin et al., 1999, p. 70). This Indian Child Welfare Act sought to reverse the long-standing practice of removing children from their cultural heritage and imposing a variety of assimilation experiences on them, against the will of their people.

The term Native Americans, although recognizing the fact that these groups were both the original natives and current citizens of this country, is not universally accepted (Westerfelt and Yellow Bird, 1999). The authors note that they "use the term 'indigenous peoples' . . . [as] a more appropriate descriptor for the aboriginal populations . . . [since] indigenous peoples . . . are not . . . from India. They are the descendants of the First Nations . . . [The term] Native Americans . . . may refer to most native born Americans" (Westerfelt and Yellow Bird, 1999, p. 146).

History of Native American exploitation. The history of the treatment of Native Americans is marked by acts of violence (including massacres), economic exploitation, and systematic attempts to destroy their culture. Space prohibits a comprehensive discussion of these acts, but the massacre of men, women, and children at Wounded Knee is one frequently cited example (Brown, 1972). Black Elk, a Native American present at the massacre, has written:

> I did not know then how much was ended. When I look back now from this high hill of my old age, I can still see the butchered women and children lying heaped and scattered all along the crooked gulch as plain as when I saw them with eyes still young. And I can see that something else died there in the bloody mud, and was buried in the blizzard. A people's dream died there. It was a beautiful dream . . . the nation's hoop is broken and scattered. There is no center any longer, and the sacred tree is dead. (Brown, 1972, p. 419)

The U.S. government removed Native Americans from lands that settlers wanted (Longres, 1995b), and advanced the doctrine of manifest destiny to justify their removal.

> To justify these breaches of the "permanent Indian frontier," the policy makers in Washington invented Manifest Destiny, a term which lifted land hunger to a lofty plane. The Europeans and their descendants were ordained by destiny to rule all of America. They were the dominant race and therefore responsible for the Indians—along with their lands, their forests, and their mineral wealth. Only the New Englanders, who had destroyed or driven out all their Indians, spoke against Manifest Destiny. (Brown, 1972, p. 8)

The Indian Removal Act of 1830 sanctioned the forced removal of tribes from their property. "The 900-mile march from Georgia to what is now Oklahoma is often referred to as the 'trail of tears.' The U. S. Army forcibly removed some 100,000 native people from the southern states, costing the lives of thousands and shattering any trust they might have placed in their

European dominators" (Longres, 1995b, p. 121). As settlers moved further west and wanted more Indian land, new policies were made for this acquisition and Indian wars declared.

Many Native Americans were placed on reservations where the land was usually very poor. According to Edward Spicer (Longres, 1995b), the policy of coercive assimilation was developed, under which Indian cultural life (such as religious rituals) was often prohibited, and Christian missionaries prevailed; children were often sent to distant boarding schools "where they could be Americanized" (Longres, 1995b, p. 122).

Mean Spirit, a novel set in Oklahoma in the 1920s, depicts the exploitation and murder of Indians by white Americans and government officials, primarily to obtain the oil found on their lands (Hogan, 1990). The "forced" attendance of Indian children at boarding schools is also described. Nola, who has seen her mother murdered, experiences constant fear and anxiety. She lives with Mrs. Graycloud and does not want to go to the Indian boarding school; Mrs. Graycloud, knowing her anxieties, wants her to stay home. In this passage, the school nurse and the man from the Indian Affairs office confront Belle (Mrs. Graycloud) and Nola.

> The agent lays down the law; Nola must be enrolled: " 'I can't let you do that,' Belle said. . . . Nola . . . only recently had . . . begun to speak after the death of her mother." Obviously unwilling to be dissuaded, the protest was dismissed with: "We've heard what's been going on . . . but we want to examine her ourselves." . . . Belle . . . interrupted. "She's anemic." Her face was tense. . . . The nurse looked in one of Nola's ears. "She seems normal and even bright for an Indian girl," she said sweetly. . . . The Indian agent signed an order stating that Nola would have to appear at school . . . or . . . be picked up by the sheriff. . . . his was an order by law. The old woman looked defiant but said nothing. . . . She was defeated. (Hogan, 1990, pp. 122-123)

Nola attended the Indian School, but was ultimately dismissed because the administration could not cope with her behavior. When she returned home, many of the Indian women came to visit her, but not because of the "shame" of expulsion; they wondered how she had outwitted the system, and whether their children might adopt some of her methods!

Current issues. In recent years, as the United States has begun to make amends to the Native American population, the outlook is brighter for this group. In the ceremonies for the new museum, for example, guests celebrated the tribes' endurance, reflected in an eightfold increase over the past century from a population of a quarter million, which itself had represented a profound decline from the height achieved before the colonial period (Clines, 1999, p. A18). There is also increasing economic prosperity; one major source of economic growth in recent years has been from gambling casinos built and run by Native Americans on their own lands, which have enabled them to develop other business interests and create employment for members of their tribes (Clines, 1999, p. A18).

On the other hand, poverty and social problems persist; "indigenous peoples [for example] are overrepresented in the homeless population" (Westerfelt and Yellow Bird, 1999, p. 145). The authors note that this is not surprising as many indigenous people who are not homeless have serious social problems.

> For example, indigenous peoples experience disproportionately high levels of poverty and income deterioration, work fewer annual hours and receive lower hourly earnings than whites, and experience higher levels of unemployment, residential mobility, and alcoholism. (Westerfelt and Yellow Bird, 1999, p. 147)

Weaver (1999) observes that health and social problems exist in many Native American communities where "people are experiencing increasing rates of mortality and morbidity due to such factors as alcohol and drug abuse, suicide, homicide, motor vehicle accidents, and child abuse and neglect" (pp. 127-128).

According to a study released by the Justice Department, Indians are crime victims twice as often as the national average (Butterfield, 1999b). Professor Sidney Harring, an expert on Indian crime, was interviewed on the subject (p. A12).

> Professor Harring said much of the violence against Indians by other racial groups was attributable to racism and alcohol, "with Indians being victimized by poor, drunken whites, people on the margins hurting each other." There are still high levels of prejudice against Indians in the West, he said, and especially on the edges of Indian reservations, where there is a climate that tolerates violence, including attacks by law-enforcement officials. (Butterfield, 1999b, p. A12)

In Oklahoma, the state with the most Native American residents, the "largest class-action suit ever" against the U.S. government has been filed by Indians; the grievance is the exploitation and economic manipulations of the government concerning Native American oil rights (Egan, 1999b, p. A1).

The Native American population is very diverse; many Indian tribes exist, and "tribal subcultures are many and varied" (Attneave, 1982, p. 56). It is a common error to assume that "all Indian populations in a region are alike, not recognizing that, even though a Navajo, a Hopi, an Apache, and someone from Laguna Pueblo may all live in the southwest desert, each has a different language and set of traditions" (Attneave, 1982, p. 56). Conflicts between tribes can exist as they have historically; for example, intense land disputes have arisen between the Navajo and Hopi tribes (Attneave, 1982).

Many Native Americans actually do not live on reservations (which are the focus of much of the mental health material written about this group) (Attneave, 1982; Gross, 1995); according to the Bureau of the Census in 1991, over 70 percent of Native Americans live in urban settings (Walters, 1999). About 50 percent of American Indians have married outside their race during the past fifty years (Spickard et al., 1995). Attneave (1982) notes that in an urban setting about 50 percent of American Indian families seeking family therapists will be "well-educated, typically middle-class people with similar problems and similar attitudes as the rest of [the] clientele" (p. 57).

The importance of utilizing and strengthening a Native American cultural identity, as well as offering culturally sensitive services, is emphasized by many writers (Angell et al., 1998; Weaver, 1999; and Westerfelt and Yellow Bird, 1999). Brave Heart (1999) discusses the emotional sequelae of the "historical trauma" of the Lakota people, including the Wounded Knee massacre, as well as the "forced removal of Lakota children from home and their abusive institutional treatment" (p. 112). She speaks of the intergenerational transmission of these traumas from parents to children, with serious psychological and social consequences, and emphasizes treatment focusing on "incorporating awareness of [this] trauma and the recathexis [reattachment] to traditional Lakota values" (Brave Heart, 1999, p. 111).

Although a strong case is made for incorporating and promoting Native American cultural values into social work interventions, objections to this dominant point of view have been made which argue that some Native Americans may wish to choose different values and follow other paths. Gross (1995) strongly asserts that the "politically correct approach" has made "it difficult . . . to derive views of Indianness that were congruent with the diversity of American Indian life and views" (p. 208). She expresses concern that only the voices of Native American social workers are heard and that one's views are disqualified if one is not an American Indian; this can "inhibit the development of a contemporary discourse on the subject of 'Indianness'" (Gross, 1995, p. 211). She warns that the "traditionalist" views of Indian identity prevail, which leaves those Native Americans with a different viewpoint unheard.

> American Indians who choose to assimilate or . . . depart from traditionalist values are left with no Indian identity references against which they might then positively regard themselves or be positively regarded by others. . . . American Indians who advocate for mineral

resources development may be defined as "bad" Indians (meaning not in harmony with nature). (Gross, 1995, p. 211)

The constructivist perspective suggests that we understand the unique meanings people ascribe to their lives, assuming nothing about their cultural orientation and wishes. In work with indigenous people, culture and cultural identity are exquisitely sensitive areas of exploration; a clinician may struggle to find a balance between not imposing further coercive assimilation practices on people who have had their cultural beliefs and values degraded and prohibited, and not imposing an indigenous value system on people who may view themselves through a different lens.

Asian Americans

The term Asian Americans cover a wide spectrum of people with different ethnicities, races, and nationalities (Segal, 1991; Longres, 1995b). The earliest Asian immigrants were the Japanese and the Chinese, who initially experienced years of serious discrimination and exploitation in this country. After Pearl Harbor, "110,000 Japanese—mostly U.S.-born citizens of Japanese origin—were forced to sell their properties and were detained in relocation camps" (Queralt, 1996, p. 194). Ultimately the U.S. government acknowledged the injustice of its actions and provided financial compensation to these former detainees.

The three largest Asian groups in the United States have been the Chinese, the Filipinos, and the Japanese (Queralt, 1996). According to the *San Francisco Chronicle*, "Americans of Chinese descent numbered 2.43 million in 2000, almost 600,000 more than Filipinos, the second-largest Asian group ... Indo Americans ... are now the third-largest Asian group, displacing Japanese Americans" (Kim, 2001). In more recent years, Asian immigrants have included people from Korea, India, Vietnam, Cambodia, and Thailand. People from Hawaii and Samoa compose the largest populations of Pacific Islanders in the United States (Ewalt and Mokuau, 1995).

Some groups, such as the Chinese, Japanese, Filipinos, and Asian Indians have been successful occupationally and economically in the United States. Asian Americans have made strong political gains, and "the number of elected Asian or Pacific Americans at all levels has grown to 2,000 in 33 states—a 10 percent increase since 1996" (Ratnesar, 1998b, p. 38).

The diversity of Asian Americans is great, both in terms of culture, current socioeconomic status, adaptation, and psychological stress. In contrasting the Asian Indian population, for example, to Vietnamese and Cambodian people, major differences are immediately apparent. Indian immigrants tend to be well educated and to speak English well (Segal, 1991). By contrast, people coming from Cambodia and Vietnam have experienced many traumas and hardships in their homelands and in the process of reaching the United States and do not adapt as easily as do Asian Indians to this country (Amodeo et al., 1996). Segal describes the Asian Indian population: "Most Indians in the U.S. are fluent in English and have had some exposure to Western values and beliefs which facilitates their entry into American society . . . are . . . a very select group. . . . Most Indians come . . . to seek educational or professional opportunities" (Segal, 1991, p. 234). These factors have led to a higher degree of integration into American society and greater freedom to settle where they choose rather than in enclaves, with the development of very few ghettos. Their professional mobility has insulated them from the hostility endured by otherwise similar groups (Segal, 1991, p. 234).

In discussing divergences within this subgroup, Mehta (1998) points out that there are "thirty-six linguistically and regionally diverse professional and cultural organizations of Indians" in the greater Detroit area alone (p. 133). Although adapting well in general, Indians, as other immigrant groups, can experience conflict in cultural values, accompanied by parent-child conflict as children become more assimilated to American values and lifestyles; such conflicts are associated with much adolescent turmoil (Segal, 1991, p. 236). "Many of these children experience a turbulent adolescence as a result of these conflicts" (Segal, 1991, p. 236)

Amodeo and colleagues (1996) present a very different portrait of Cambodians and Vietnamese. Such immigrants have experienced: "multiple traumas, including living in war-torn areas . . . being forced to witness the . . . deaths of loved ones . . . the dangers of escape . . . cultural differences . . . the transition . . . from a rural agrarian . . . to a highly technological urban society . . . family fragmentation . . . and . . . unfamiliar climate" (p. 404).

In addition to coping with conflicting cultural values, many people experience mental health problems, including post-traumatic stress disorder and survivor's guilt (Amodeo et al., 1996, p. 404). Nicholson and Kay (1999) note that the anxieties of traumatized Cambodian women often appear in physical symptoms. They add that frequently these symptoms "did not appear until after initial resettlement tasks were accomplished" (Nicholson and Kay, 1999, p. 470) and stress the need for innovative, culture-specific services for these women. Increasing alcoholism and drug abuse appear to be another consequence of the multiple stresses faced by Southeast Asian people and culturally appropriate interventions are needed (Amodeo et al., 1996).

Hispanics

More than 22 million Hispanic people live in the United States, according to the 1990 census report (Longres, 1995a). The largest segment of this population (63 percent) were Mexican; the next largest group (29 percent) came from Puerto Rico, Cuba, or Central or South America. The remaining 7 percent did not identify themselves with any subgroup. A large increase in the Latino population was occurring, due to both ongoing immigration and high birthrates in some groups. "If the present rate of growth continues, Latinos will replace African Americans by about the year 2010, perhaps even earlier, as the nation's largest racial/ethnic minority group" (Queralt, 1996, p. 186). According to the *Washington Post,* the "number of Americans who described themselves as Hispanic grew by nearly 60 percent in the 2000 Census and now total 35.3 million" (Cohen and Fears, 2001).

The conundrum of categorizing people by race and ethnicity is apparent when considering the Hispanic population. Prior to the 1990 census, for example, the U.S. government debated whether Hispanics should be categorized as a racial rather than an ethnic group, "but this idea was abandoned because Latino leaders were uncomfortable with the implications of being classified as nonwhite" (Longres, 1995a, p. 1217). Besides the fact that Hispanics have different nationalities, they also represent many racial groupings and racial mixtures. For example, some people from Argentina and Uruguay are descended primarily from Europeans. The Caribbean Island countries and Panama are populated largely by mixed European and African races. Hispanics from Mexico and Central America are often of mixed European and indigenous Indian descent.

Longres (1995a) has observed that "most Latinos are ambivalent about race: They are comfortable with mixed races, but they are inclined to celebrate European heritage over any other" (p. 1217). In the United States, there can be "interpersonal barriers among Latinos" based on race (p. 1217).

Opinions differ about the names used to designate the Hispanic population. *Hispanic* has been a recent unifying name; many in this group, however, prefer to refer to their nationalities. For example, Mexicans may use Mexican, Mexican-American, or Chicano. Longres (1995a) comments that people who are involved with political activism tend to use the name Latino, although Hispanic and Latino are often used interchangeably. Longres (1995a) questions whether Hispanics will ever accept a "pan-ethnic identity . . . let alone whether the term Hispanic or Latino will become the desired way of expressing the unity" (p. 1215).

Socioeconomic factors vary for groups within the Hispanic population (and some variability always exists within each group). Cubans, who represent the third largest Hispanic-American population, have done well economically (Jiménez-Vazques, 1995; Queralt, 1996). Many Cuban refugees arrived in 1959 following Castro's revolution, most of whom were "white, relatively well-educated, middle-class persons of Iberian Spanish extraction" (Queralt, 1996, p. 188), although many who emigrated later have a lower socioeconomic status. Because they were refugees from communism they received political asylum and aid from the U.S. government.

By contrast, Mexican immigrants, many from rural areas, are very poor and have low levels of education (Partida, 1996). Many have come to this country illegally to seek work because of the desperate poverty they experienced in Mexico. Their presence has caused resentment in the United States, and both the federal government and California have passed laws placing severe penalties and restrictions on illegal immigrants. A California law placing restrictions on illegal immigrants was declared unconstitutional by a federal court. This 1994 law had "barred illegal immigrants and their children from receiving government services like a public education and became one of the most contentious political issues in California history" (Nieves, 1999, p. A1).

Although Mexican-American men have a high employment rate (80 percent), their (frequently) nonskilled jobs are often unsteady and the pay is low. "Among the three large groups of Latinos, the highest rates of poverty were suffered by mainland Puerto Ricans and Mexican Americans" (Queralt, 1996, p.189).

Dominicans represent another significant group. In 1998, it was noted that in New York City the number of Hispanic women receiving public assistance was increasing (although a decrease had occurred in other groups). Puerto Ricans are the largest group receiving welfare, but their numbers have remained steady. The increase was due to the large influx of Dominican immigrants needing public assistance. The Dominicans "who are the city's fastest growing group of immigrants" generally "speak less English and experience higher levels of poverty and unemployment than other Hispanic people" (Swarns, 1998, A1). In 1999, a half million Dominicans lived in New York City (Williams, 1999).

A number of Dominicans, however, have done well in business, and of this group, 7 percent have established their own businesses (Williams, 1999). Dominicans have been developing very popular hair salons.

"Much like Koreans who have made nail salons their franchise and Indians, Afghans, and Pakistanis who have made cab driving theirs, Dominican immigrants have made beauty their business in New York, bringing with them their own hair-straightening techniques and home-brewed conditioners" (Williams, 1999, p. A20).

That many of the Dominican salons' customers are African American has caused tension with African-American beauty salon operators, who resent the competition. Adriano Espaillat, the city's first Dominican assemblyman, commented that no shortage of hair existed: "There's plenty of hair around for everybody. . . . Unless you're like me—going a little bald" (Williams, 1999, A20).

The Latino population has made many political gains in this country over the years, which, in turn, have affected the garnering of support for their interests. According to the Hispanic Leadership Institute, Latinos are "the fastest-growing group of voters. . . . From 1976 to 1996, Latinos increased their voter registration by 164 percent, compared with 31 percent for the rest of the nation" (Dedman, 1999, p. 22). Although many Hispanic elected officials hold office, their number "has not risen so fast" (Dedman, 1999, p. 22).

Bilingual education, advocated by Hispanics, has been a subject of congressional debate and has been a major political issue in several states, especially in California, where half of the country's 2.8 million non-English-speaking students live (Hornblower, 1998). Educational experts disagree about the efficacy of this approach; an underlying concern about reaching this population in an educationally sound manner is the very high school dropout rate across the country (30 percent) for Hispanic children.

In a recent trend in the opposite direction, many New Yorkers have been studying Spanish, as they feel they can no longer ignore the bilingual nature of New York (Bearak, 1999, p. A1).

> And non-Hispanic New Yorkers by the thousands, from mothers with babies to office workers, doctors and priests, are responding to the trend in a practical way. They are signing up for Spanish lessons—in their own homes, at work and in night schools. (Bearak, 1999, p. A25)

Diverse people constitute the Hispanic population; socioeconomic factors vary across this group, although overall many Hispanics have serious economic problems. A third of Hispanic Americans do not have health coverage (Kilborn, 1999b). Latinos "disproportionately lack insurance coverage and ready access to professional care. That is particularly true for the three-quarters who are from Mexico and Central America" (Kilborn, 1999b, p. A1).

Hispanics face problems similar to those of other immigrant groups, including culture shock, assimilation difficulties, and conflicts with their children in terms of traditional (Hispanic) and new (American) cultural values, as well as a range of mental illnesses. The clinician should be able to differentiate among characteristics that particularly may be related to belonging to the Hispanic culture and those related to living in poverty (Javier, 1996).

Although a need exists for counseling and mental health services, many Hispanics are reluctant to use these services—in part because they "do not see sharing personal problems with a stranger as being 'curative'" (Partida, 1996, p. 253). Many Hispanics rely on *curanderos* or *curanderas* (folk healers), believed to have supernatural powers, rather than physical or mental health practitioners (Kilborn, 1999b; Ramirez, 1998). On the other hand, Hispanic patients may be approached by clinicians who treat them in a stereotypical way, who may not be able to reach them "where they are," and who offer only concrete and limited services, overlooking the possibility that the patients may also be amenable to the insights of appropriately applied psychodynamic approaches.

> It is not unusual to construe cultural, ethnic, and linguistic behavior on the part of poor Hispanic individuals as abnormal or pathological. This . . . mentality results in those social policies aimed largely at . . . encouraging treatment programs that predominantly emphasize concrete and immediate solutions to complex life problems. . . . Medicaid policies that only allow limited therapy sessions . . . do not provide these individuals with empowerment opportunities. . . . A treatment intervention that emphasizes personal exploration gives this population a more powerful, respectful, lasting, and effective tool to deal with the vicissitudes of their lives. (Javier, 1996, p. 98)

Health, mental health, and social services sensitive to the needs of the Hispanic population (as well as to the cultural values and conflicts of the individual patient) warrant further development and study.

Social Class

Social class, defined in terms of *social stratification,* ranks people in comparison to others using the following criteria: "the amount of money they earn, the level of education they have completed, the prestige of their occupation, or the prestige conferred on them by others in the community" (Longres, 1995b, p. 75). Social class membership can play an important role in relationships; a professional family, for example, might be upset if a daughter marries a factory worker who has only a high school education. A therapist with a lower-middle class upbringing might feel uncomfortable with an upper class client.

Even if people belong to a common racial and/or ethnic group, they may react differently to others within their group, based on *class differential.* Brad, for example, was a college student from the African-American upper class whose parents "both held challenging high-profile positions in major corporations" (Miles, 1998, p. 104). When attending an Ivy League college, he encountered interpersonal problems with other African-American students related to class distinctions.

> For the first time in his life, Brad encountered black students from the ghetto. They instantly disliked him, accusing him of being "too white." Because they constituted the largest part of the black university community, Brad had little support. Every part of his character and his socialization were attacked by these students. . . . Soon, Brad wore dreadlocks and baggy clothes, and was dating an inner-city girl with multiple braids in her hair. Brad was seen as an embarrassment to his family. (Miles, 1998, pp. 104-105)

India has a strict caste system, with the lowest caste being the untouchables. Although legal changes now protect their rights, better employment opportunities are available to them, and they have greater political power than in the past, in the minds of many, nothing has changed. To complicate this picture, the untouchable caste is fragmented by constant jockeying for position. The *balmiki* subcaste is at the absolute bottom of the pecking order; they derive their living from cleaning and disposing of human waste. Srichand, a member of this caste, was doing this work when he was murdered on September 2, 1998 (Bearak, 1998).

> Srichand had been chosen for death by a gang of jatavs, another untouchable subcaste that, in the ancient pecking order of India, is a few notches above the balmikis. Days before, a balmiki boy had left the city with a jatav girl, a departure the balmikis took to be teen-age love and the jatavs considered a spiteful kidnapping. (Bearak, 1998, A3)

Social class issues can affect treatment relationships as well as treatment alternatives offered to clients. At times, the mental health field has discriminated against the poor on the premise that they are not amenable to psychotherapy; however, with appropriate approaches, they can benefit from clinical treatment (Javier, 1996).

> I have witnessed the growth of many of my poor patients who were able to take advantage of psychoanalytic interventions in various degrees. Many required a period of didactic approach in which they learned a new "conceptual matrix," that is, a verbal reformulation of their symptoms and the importance of their personal dynamic history. . . . They were, however, eventually able to appreciate the importance of insights for the modification of their conditions. Other poor patients came into the treatment situation with a great deal of curiosity about and desire for understanding their own internal world. (Javier, 1996, p. 99)

The social class of clients is often overlooked in undertaking a psychosocial assessment; however, the realities as well as their perceptions of their social class membership may be a significant treatment issue.

IMMIGRATION

Akhtar (1995), an immigrant from India who is also a psychoanalyst, discusses the experience of immigration, which entails many losses but also offers an opportunity for psychological growth.

Leaving one's country involves profound losses. Often one has to give up familiar food, native music, unquestioned social customs, and even one's language. The new country offers strange-tasting food, new songs, different political concerns, unfamiliar language, pale festivals, unknown heroes, psychically unearned history, and a visually unfamiliar landscape. However, alongside the various losses is a renewed opportunity for psychic growth and alteration. New channels of self-expression become available. There are new identification models, different superego dictates, and different ideals. One thing is clear: immigration results in a sudden change from an "average expectable environment" (Hartmann) to a strange and unpredictable one. (Akhtar, 1995, p. 1052)

Akhtar (1995) also discusses *internal immigration*, in which a person moves to a culturally different region within the same country and may face similar stresses.

One major factor affecting the adaptation of immigrants is the host country's attitude toward them (Akhtar, 1995). Are they welcomed or resented? Are they receiving political asylum and resettlement programs, or are they rejected and "hunted down," as illegal immigrants are? Being officially accepted by the government does not guarantee freedom from prejudice and discrimination. Do immigrants have support from family and others from their culture after arrival, or are they isolated?

Giving up one's native language for English can be a profound loss and painful transition. Freud, for example, an immigrant escaping from Nazi Germany to England in late life with his family, wrote in a letter: " 'Perhaps, you have omitted the one point that the emigrant feels so particularly painfully. It is—one can only say—the loss of the language in which one had lived and thought, and which one will never be able to replace with another for all one's efforts at empathy'" (Ahktar, 1995, p. 1069).

Developing an ability to speak as well as to feel and think in another language is one aspect of identity change. One indicator that this is happening is the "increasing dominance of the acquired language, which begins to appear in spontaneous humor, dreams, and in talking in one's sleep" (Ahktar, 1995, p. 1070).

The acculturation process is complex; people vary in the degree to which they remain embedded in their native cultures, become acclimated, or develop a new bicultural identity. Assimilation can produce stress in families, as members may be in different places along this spectrum. Partida (1996) describes family conflict in Mexican immigrants.

> Because children . . . are able to learn the new language much easier
> than the parents, they become the holders of power, knowledge and
> control, a fact that often leaves parents disempowered and feeling un-
> able to follow through with limit setting. . . .
>   The adults' incapability corrodes the child's ethnic pride and iden-
> tification. (Partida, 1996, p. 246)

Immigrants bring with them a past that may be traumatic and that might
also include troubled relationships or psychological instability prior to specific war and immigration trauma. They may, additionally, encounter stressful psychosocial problems in adaptation to the United States. It is, therefore,
not unusual to see immigrants manifest a variety of psychiatric problems,
including depression (Kinzie et al., 1996). In August 1999, for example, a
forty-one-year-old man from Sri Lanka who lived in Toronto for ten years
jumped to his death in the path of a subway train, holding his three-year-old
son, who also died. He had a history of depression (Elliott and Bourette,
1999). A spokesman for a community organization who had counseled Sri
Lankan refugees noted that: "immigrants are particularly vulnerable to depression and often do not seek help. . . . Depression . . . reaches a certain
level and then it bursts . . . adapting to a new culture and often a new social
status while trying to support a family can be overwhelming" (Elliott and
Bourette, 1999, A5).

Domestic violence can also be seen in immigrant families. A "pervasive
myth," for example, is that "domestic violence does not exist in the Asian
community"; but it does indeed exist (Masaki and Wong, 1997, p. 439). This
presents special complications for Asian female immigrants who may depend on sponsors who are their batterers. "The batterers use this as another
means of control: 'If you leave me, I'll get you deported!'" (Masaki and
Wong, 1997, p. 444). The Marriage Fraud Amendment Act of 1990 offers
special protections to women in this situation.

Many immigrants may become (or continue to be) substance abusers related to or exacerbated by the stresses of immigration and may require culturally appropriate interventions. A commonly employed intervention that
has little chance of succeeding with certain groups is Alcoholics Anonymous (Amodeo et al., 1996; Sachs, 1999b).

> People from the former Soviet Union, for example, often distrust not
> only their peers, but also people with authority. "We are talking about
> an enormous level of resistance to outside persuasion, because all the
> messages, all the lies, in the totalitarian society were delivered by au-
> thority figures," said Dr. Kagen of the Educational Alliance. (Sachs,
> 1999b, p. A25)

Immigrants, as other minority persons, may find that "knowing and experiencing more than one world not only presents significant challenges, it also offers richer possibilities—more flexibility and a different set of alternatives and choices given a supportive family and community resources. In fact, Latino adolescents who sustain an integrated bicultural identity show the best levels of psychosocial adjustment" (Mattei, 1996, p. 237).

Akhtar (1995) stresses the gains that can be made through the acculturation process, as the person's identity undergoes a metamorphosis and becomes a "hybrid" identity, with a new richness and new possibilities. However, change does not come easily, nor is it without pain and ambivalence, just as maturation through the life cycle has its upheavals as well as its joys, its regressive pulls, and its forward movements. Akhtar describes his own immigrant experiences in a poem, as seen in these excerpts.

> Like the fish who chose to live on a tree,
> We writhe in foolish agony.
> Our gods reduced to grotesque exhibits.
> Our poets mute, pace in the empty halls of our conversation.
> The silk of our mother tongue banned from the fabric
> Of our dreams.
>
> Forsaking the grey abodes and sunken graves of
> Our ancestors, we have come to live in
> A world without seasons. (Akhtar, 1995, p. 1077)

Akhtar (1995) wrote this poem nine years after his immigration. Now, twelve years later, he has written a more optimistic paper. He ponders the meaning of this contrast, while acknowledging that this paper "reveals the advance in my own mourning process" (p. 1078).

> What does including this poem in the paper indicate? Continued pain or its mastery or some combination of both? More important, why is it that I expressed my pain of loss in poetry and my pride over mastery of this loss in prose? (Akhtar, 1995, p. 1078)

This is reminiscent of the reflections of Jan Morris (1997) after her successful male-to-female sexual transformation. She wonders whether she has found "the real purpose of my pilgrimage, the last solution to my Conundrum . . . ? Sometimes down by the river I almost think I have: but then the light changes, the wind shifts . . . and the meaning of it all once again escapes me" (Morris, 1997, p. 160). Both Jan Morris and Salman Akhtar have made major pilgrimages; both are forever changed. And both continue to wonder about the impact of these changes as they contemplate the complexities of their lives.

As clinical social workers, we have the opportunity to explore with others their nuanced responses to major transitions. People who have made major journeys in life have much to teach us about change, identity, culture, loss, despair, resilience, and hope.

DEVELOPING NEW CULTURES

The concept of culture "incorporates all the symbolic meanings—the beliefs, values, norms, and traditions—that are shared in a community and govern social interactions among community members or between members and outsiders" (Longres, 1995b, p. 74). Cultures are usually discussed in ethnic, racial, and religious terms, with the recent addition of gay and lesbian cultures. New cultures, however, constantly emerge; some are relatively small in numbers of those subsumed in them but in which people's identifications and feelings of connectedness are necessarily intertwined.

One group that has come together and developed a distinctive culture is the deaf; they have developed their own language (American Sign Language or ASL) and in addition to this "a body of shared knowledge, shared beliefs, cherished narratives and images, which soon constituted a rich and distinctive culture" (Sacks, 1989, p. 136).

Other developing cultures include religious sects, cults, and gangs. One recent cult, the Heaven's Gate sect, ended with the mass suicide of its leader and members, as has been mentioned.

The Culture of the Deaf

Deafness has nearly universally been seen as a major disability. Helen Keller commented that to be deaf was more difficult than being blind. " 'Blindness cuts people off from things,' . . . 'Deafness cuts people off from people' " (Dolnick, 1993, p. 37). Alexander Graham Bell, whose mother was deaf, saw deafness as a "swindle and a privation and a tragedy" and his technological advances to help the deaf as being in the service of " 'correcting' God's blunders, and in general, 'improving on' nature" (Sacks, 1989, p. 149).

A major breakthrough in education for the deaf was associated with the founding of the American Asylum at Hartford by Laurent Clerc and Thomas Gallaudet in 1817. American Sign Language (ASL) was introduced and became the model for other schools for the deaf in the United States. These schools were mostly residential, and their students' involvement in these communities was an important factor in the transmission of deaf culture as well as lessening the feelings of isolation in its pupils. Many of the graduates would live near the schools or sometimes work there. Sacks (1989) refers to the 1840s as the " 'golden age' " of the development of deaf culture and community (p. 139).

In 1857, Thomas Gallaudet's son, Edward (who, like Bell, had a deaf mother and who learned sign language as a child), was instrumental in founding the first college for the deaf (established in 1864), later called Gallaudet College. However, during the 1860s, a serious controversy developed about educating the deaf. Gallaudet, who strongly favored sign language, was opposed by Alexander Graham Bell, who believed signing should be prohibited. Although Gallaudet College was very successful in producing academically qualified graduates, the battle to use sign language was lost upon Gallaudet's death.

Sacks (1989) asserts that for the seventy-five years following the 1880s, the "suppression of sign . . . had a deleterious effect on the deaf . . . not only on their education . . . but on their image of themselves and on their entire community and culture" (p. 139). ASL has made a strong comeback over the past thirty years, and Sacks credits the student strike at Gallaudet in 1988 as being a major factor in further increasing deaf pride and activism.

The issue at the heart of the strike was the students' request for a deaf president of Gallaudet. Although Gallaudet was "the only liberal arts college for the deaf in the world" it "in all its 124 years . . . has never had a deaf president" (Sacks, 1989, p. 125). The students' protest was successful: the hearing president resigned and was replaced by King Jordan, the Dean of the School of Arts and Sciences, who had been deaf since he was twenty-one. Although there was general jubilation at this event, some dissent occurred "since he was postlingually deaf" (that is, he was not deaf prior to the onset of language, an important distinction in deaf culture) (p. 157).

Sacks (1989), a neurologist, first visited Gallaudet in 1986 and 1987 and found it "an astonishing and moving experience" (p. 127).

> I had never before seen an entire community of the deaf, nor had I quite realized . . . that Sign might indeed be a complete language—a language equally suitable for making love or speeches, for flirtation or mathematics. . . . I had to see the absolutely silent mathematics department at work; to see deaf bards, Sign poetry . . . and the range and depth of the Gallaudet theater; I had to see the wonderful social scene in the student bar, with hands flying in all directions as a hundred separate conversations proceeded—I had to see all this for myself before I could be moved from my previous "medical" view of deafness (as a "condition," a deficit, that had to be treated) to a "cultural" view of the deaf as forming a community with a complete language and culture of

its own. I had felt there was something very joyful, even Arcadian about Gallaudet. (Sacks, 1989, p. 127)

For many deaf people, deafness is part of their identity, not something they wish to have fixed. To some, for example, the idea of a cochlear implant to diminish deafness is anathema. The editors of *Deaf Life* have expressed their opposition to implants (Dolnick, 1993): "'An implant is the . . . ultimate denial of deafness, the ultimate refusal to let deaf children be Deaf'" (p. 43).

The deaf culture does not represent all people who are deaf, although its influence predominates. People who have lost their hearing later in life "miss their earlier access to spoken communication, and they miss sound" (Luey et al., 1995, p. 179). For many of these people, "deafness is both a disability and a loss; it is something to be mourned" (Luey et al., 1995, p. 180). Not all deaf people (including those who are prelingually deaf) prefer sign language; some prefer other types of communication, including lip reading or cued speech, "which is phonetically based and uses hand-shapes to represent specific speech sounds" (Luey et al., 1995, p. 179). These preferential differences in communication can give rise to intense disputes between different factions of the deaf world.

In addition to some conflict existing between the medical and deaf communities, the latter are also in conflict with advocates for the disabled, although they "remain uneasy partners" (Dolnick, 1993, p. 43). The issue of separation or integration of deaf people with hearing people is a major point of contention; groups for the disabled have long fought for mainstreaming and integration. The deaf community asserts that, however well intended, trying to fit the deaf into the world of the hearing can in fact "imprison them in a zone of silence" (Dolnick, 1993, p. 43). Concern has been expressed about the disappearance of residential schools for the deaf and about the integration of deaf children into the public school system, where they may not have other deaf children with whom to associate.

In 1998, in what was called a revolutionary step in deaf education, New York City's only public school for the deaf determined that sign language will be used by all teachers as the foundation for learning (Lee, 1998, p. A28). "They say deaf students should be treated like bilingual students, not disabled ones. In their view, students first need a primary language—American Sign Language—before they learn a second language, in this case, English" (Lee, 1998, p. A28).

In clinical work with deaf people, comprehensive psychosocial assessment should include understanding the meaning of deafness in their lives, their degree and nature of involvement (or noninvolvement) with the deaf community, and their attitudes toward deafness as an identity issue.

The Heaven's Gate Sect

As reactions to cults are controversial, it is not surprising that defining cults is also controversial. The use of the term " 'new religious movements' (NRMs) [attempts] to avoid the pejorative connotation of the term 'cult' . . . [but] there are no universally accepted distinctions between NRMs and other religious groups" (Robbins, 1995, p. 667). Negative reactions to cults arose in the mid-1970s, and generally the term carries negative connotations. Cults are typically viewed as "small, unorthodox, possibly dangerous fringe groups whose members are influenced by a charismatic leader" (Robbins, 1995, p. 667). Negative feelings about cults dramatically increased in 1978 after the Jonestown, Guyana, mass suicides and/or murders in which over 900 people died (Lacayo, 1997). An active anticult movement has developed that includes people whose children are cultists (Robbins, 1995); cults, however, continue to proliferate.

The Internet plays an important role in the lives of cult members; it is used by cults to recruit new followers (Lacayo, 1997), and it is also utilized by cultists to communicate with each other (Markoff, 1997). "It's persuasive, far reaching and clandestine" (Lacayo, 1997, p. 46). The Heaven's Gate sect used the Internet to inform others of their religious ideology, which centers on an afterlife and their belief that a UFO would transport them to a special heaven. It has been speculated that the Heaven's Gate group received "information" on the Web that "an alien spaceship was lurking behind comet Hale-Bopp" (Markoff, 1997, p. A12); this may be related to the timing of their group suicide. In addition, the group's business, Higher Source, involved designing commercial Web pages for the Internet (Purdum, 1997).

The Heaven's Gate sect received national attention in the spring of 1997, when its thirty-nine members committed suicide in Southern California. This sect, as other cultures, had mutually shared "symbolic meanings—the beliefs, values, norms, and traditions" (Longres, 1995b, p. 74), which coincided with the coming millennium and the appearance of the highly visible Hale-Bopp comet.

The "charismatic" leader of this cult, Marshall Applewhite, left a suicide note discussing the group's action (Statements that Heaven's, 1997). In one excerpt he wrote:

> We came from the Level Above Human in distant space and we have now exited the bodies that we were wearing for our earthly task, to return to the world from whence we came—task completed. The distan[t] space we refer to is what you[r] literature would call the Kingdom of Heaven, or Kingdom of God. (Statements from Heaven's Gate, 1997, p. A12)

Some of the members had been in the sect for twenty years; others had joined more recently. They were an integrated group in terms of race, ethnicity, gender, and social class; "they were rich and poor, black, white and Latino—people who shared little more than willingness, or a need, to suspend disbelief, and in the end to participate in a common death" (Gleick, 1997, p. 31).

The Heaven's Gate group, as most cults are, was tightly organized and all aspects of life were controlled by Applewhite and his doctrines. "They woke at predetermined intervals to pray. They ate the same food at the same hours. They wore short haircuts and shapeless clothing" (Bruni, 1997, p. 1). Applewhite and five of his male followers were castrated; "shedding any signs of sexuality was integral to the cult" (Gleick, 1997, p. 32). Group members renounced "sex, drugs, alcohol, their birth names, and all relationships with family and friends, [so that] disciples could become ready to ascend to space" (Gleick, 1997, p. 34). Galanter (1982) asserts that religious sects typically have a "shared belief that members' work is devoted to some grand plan . . . the basis for the mystical manipulation of members' activities" (p. 1542).

Examining the nature of sects affords insight into the close interactions between individual and group psychology; it illuminates how cult members can accept a group belief system that supersedes their personal autonomy and takes precedence over family, friends, and life itself. From a psychodynamic perspective, it has been observed that people can be driven to join cults by their own inner needs, such as psychological turmoil and a paucity of social ties. "Their preoccupations with purpose and destiny are closely associated to a dissatisfaction with interpersonal relations, leading to loneliness and a sense of alienation" (Galanter, 1982, p. 1539).

For many, cults may provide multiple selfobjects (that is, the reliance on others to meet unsatisfied inner needs, especially pertaining to attachment and self-esteem). Research findings suggest that charismatic cults may aid some members in dealing with psychological problems, leading to remission of substance abuse, improved self-esteem, and an enhanced capacity for social relationships (Galanter, 1982).

Discussion

Cultures in the United States are many and diverse, including macro cultures, such as the Hispanic community, or micro cultures, such as sects, cults, and gangs. Many mainstream micro cultures, such as fraternities, sororities, Masonic lodges, psychoanalytic societies, and schools of social work, have their own rituals and values and can exert profound influences on members. Understanding the culture and/or cultures to which people belong, as well as the meaning their cultures have to them, is critical to clinical social work practice.

THE IMPACT OF CULTURAL ISSUES
ON CLINICAL SOCIAL WORK

Culture and diversity can impact clinical work in innumerable ways: biopsychosocial assessments can be skewed if culturally shaped responses are ignored; clients' motivation and utilization of treatment can be affected by cultural attitudes and values; a clash over values and lifestyles can develop; and transference and countertransference issues can be complicated by cultural factors (especially when not openly discussed).

Biopsychosocial Assessments

The interplay between culture and mental health is complex. Behavior can be misinterpreted if it is viewed as pathological, when it may be simply culture specific. A man's behavior may be misunderstood as delusional, for example, if he serves tea to his dead father and holds conversations with him. However, if this man is Japanese, he may be acting in accordance with his cultural belief that the dead are involved with the living and "the departed continue to be experienced as being alive" (Freeman, 1998, p. 53). In another example:

> A 39-year-old Haitian man is sent to the psychiatric emergency room by the police because "he was sitting in the park looking stoned and talking to himself." Upon assessment, the patient gave no evidence of substance abuse or psychosis. He stated that he had been in a healing trance brought on by the incantations of a *houngan* (voodoo priest). The man expressed the fear that another *houngan* wished to "put me in the coffin and make him his slave." (Pies and Keast, 1995, p. 14)

The cultural perspective informs us that "the basic Haitian mind-set is shaped within the voodoo . . . religious beliefs and practices that [remain] the central focus of Haitian life" (Bastien, 1995, p. 1149). In addition, hallucinations may be found in "normal, non-psychotic Hispanic individuals exposed to a variety of stressors" (Pies and Keast, 1995, p. 14); hallucinations are also accepted in other cultural groups, such as the Chinese, who view them as a normal event, and consider them to be "possession by ancestors speaking for the family" (Gee and Ishii, 1997, p. 232).

Nonverbal behaviors often provide diagnostic insight; however, these behaviors may be culturally determined rather than clinically significant. Haitians, for example, maintain eye contact with a person in conversation, but they "look away when they are listening. Prolonged eye contact is considered to be staring and, in the case of young children, disrespectful" (Bastien, 1995, p. 1152).

On the other hand, pathology can be overlooked by the clinician in the effort to be bias free; behaviors and symptoms may be erroneously ascribed to cultural factors (Solomon, 1992). "Thus, a therapist facing an Asian American who is withdrawn may consider such behavior typical of Asian American peoples instead of recognizing it as a sign of possible depression" (Solomon, 1992, p. 374). One complicating issue when distinguishing what is cultural and what is pathological is the fact that cultures are not constant; "they can and sometimes do change rapidly," and assessing culture's role can cause "mischief for students of psychopathology across cultures" (Westermeyer, 1985, p. 803).

Having an open and inquiring mind about cultural influences, using supervision and consultation when needed, and learning from clients can enhance understanding of cultural complexities in clinical work. Furthermore, in formulating a tentative biopsychosocial assessment, one can outline questions about puzzling cultural and psychological dilemmas that need further exploration in ongoing active interactions with the client.

Culture-Bound Syndromes

Some psychiatric syndromes can be puzzling to clinicians unfamiliar with them because they may be culture bound and found only in specific cultures or groups (Kaplan et al., 1994). Windigo, for example, is a condition that can be found among Native American Indians. It is a "fear of being turned into a cannibal through possession by a supernatural monster, the windigo" (Kaplan et al., 1994, p. 190). *Grisi siknis* has been observed in the Miskito of Nicaragua; it involves "headache, anxiety, irrational anger toward people nearby, aimless running and falling down" (Westermeyer, 1985, p. 799).

Eating disorders have been described as culture-bound syndromes mostly found in female North American Euroamericans (American Psychiatric Association, 1994; Westermeyer, 1985). This culture-bound syndrome, however, has made its way to Fiji, where an increase in eating disorders has been observed (Increase in Eating, 1999). A recent study correlates the new preoccupation with weight with the introduction of television to the islands, where traditionally having a "robust, nicely rounded body is the norm for men and women" ("Increase in Eating," 1999, p. A11). Now, identifying with many television female stars, many young girls want to look like them. Charles F. Grey, an anthropology professor, objects to assigning sole responsibility to television for these changes: "I think that television is a kind of metaphor of something more profound," he said ("Increase in Eating," p. A11). This argument also can be applied to eating disorder problems in the United States; underlying emotional conflicts are often found at the core of this disorder.

Treatment Issues

The treatment process can be affected by cultural identifications and behaviors, including attitudes and perceptions about receiving help; clash of values between the clinician and the client; and transference, countertransference, and intersubjectivity issues. The "cross-cultural clinical arena charged with its terrors, suspicions, and disavowed prejudices, provides some of the most fertile spaces for minds to collide and collude in their attempts to know each other" (Pérez Foster, 1999, p. 270).

Clients' Response to Clinical Services

Although the clinical services encountered in the United States are, generally speaking, a product of Western culture, people from many cultures can benefit from psychodynamically based therapeutic approaches, if the help offered is sensitive to each client's cultural issues. Parenthetically, it should be noted that many other cultures offer their own forms of psychotherapy and healing provided by healers, including shamans, "witch" doctors, medicine men, and *curanderos*. In this light, the idea of turning to a healer may not necessarily be foreign at all. Common elements cut across the varieties of healing, including support, acceptance, receiving directives, abreaction, and gaining strength from belief in the power of the healing person. Native healers may make use of the "techniques of confession, atonement, and absolution" (Ramirez, 1998, p. 174), which are akin in some ways to standard therapeutic practices in this country. Often in other cultures, the healer is also a religious figure, but adding spirituality to clinical encounters has recently been advocated by some clinicians in the United States.

The basic rule should be, not only for cross-cultural work but for work with any client: Start where the client is. This includes understanding what receiving help means to clients as well as their conceptions of how this help works. The impression is sometimes given that middle-class white Americans are sophisticated about clinical services, and those from minority cultures are not. The reverse may be the case; furthermore, people can be educated to participate in the role of client.

Although it is important not to assume that a person from a given culture has fixed beliefs or customs, it is nevertheless important to be aware that the person may have strong cultural values, attitudes, and behaviors that may affect their inclination to seek help. Cambodian immigrants, for example, while often suffering from loss, grief, and post-traumatic stress disorder, may have difficulty asking for help with these problems (Nicholson and Kay, 1999). "Because there is no comparable human services system in Cambodia, most Cambodians view requesting human services as an inappropriate and shameful solution" (Nicholson and Kay, 1999, p. 470).

Nicholson and Kay (1999) found that a group of Cambodian women were very responsive to a support group where cultural issues were recognized; group activities were used to engage them and help them feel "more cohesive and less isolated" (p. 474). Direct skills were taught (such as learning how to ride the subway, use the telephone, and shop); health needs were discussed, as was their interest in learning English; they were enabled to reach out to support networks in their own communities. The women brought Cambodian food to each session; having lunch together became an important ritual. One of the group therapists was an American social worker; the other was a Cambodian who translated Khmer into English during the group sessions.

Ultimately, the women were able to talk about their painful grief and loss issues, expressing feelings that they had never shared before "without . . . the somatic symptoms that had previously caused them to flee the room" (Nicholson and Kay, 1999, p. 475).

Clash of Values

Some therapists have been successful in integrating folk practices with traditional therapy. In one project, for example, physicians and medicine men collaborated to treat North American Indian patients; in another, efforts were made to incorporate methods used by Puerto Rican *espiritistas* into traditional health and mental health services (Ramirez, 1998). Buddhist monks have consulted and collaborated with mental health workers on behalf of Southeast Asians with substance abuse problems (Amodeo et al., 1996).

The clinician and client, however, can find themselves in conflict over competing cultural values. Should a therapist, for example, advocate for greater freedom for Americanized teenagers when their Hispanic or Asian-Indian families value exerting greater control and protectiveness? A therapist might have strong convictions that religious issues are private matters belonging outside therapy, whereas Hispanic clients might want their faith healers involved in their treatment.

One therapist discussed a cultural dilemma which arose in treating Mrs. P., a Jamaican woman with a panic disorder: the patient made some progress but avoided discussion of her marital problems, which were at the core of her panic (Watts-Jones, 1992). Mrs. P.'s husband had strong patriarchal expectations, traditional in their culture, and placed a number of restrictions on his wife's activities outside the home; he also refused to talk to the therapist. The therapist felt that unless the wife asserted some autonomy, she would not get well; she was torn between deferring to the client's cultural norms and confronting the way they might reinforce the dysfunctional patterns (Watts-Jones, 1992, p. 105).

> Clearly, traditional Jamaican values were a central issue. . . . My own values about gender roles . . . were in marked conflict with the client system. . . . It was important to insure that my therapeutic approach was not simply clinical imperialism. (Watts-Jones, 1992, p. 109)

Ultimately, the therapist decided to share this dilemma with Mrs. P., treating her as a collaborator in the therapy; she chose to work toward developing a more egalitarian relationship with her husband and broadening her outside activities. Marital tensions continued. Although Mrs. P. wanted to have a good marriage, she did not want, at the same time, to jeopardize the possibility of improved functioning (Watt-Jones, 1992, p. 112). Watts-Jones asserts that the decision to tackle the client's cultural norms must be made carefully and collaboratively (p. 112).

Conflicts Relating to Treatment Issues

Sometimes conflict occurs in clinical practice between a "political agenda" and a psychodynamic orientation. This tension was observed in the case of Amanda, a fourteen-year-old African-American girl who saw her mother murdered and her brother also murdered at a later date in a poverty-stricken neighborhood where murder was endemic (Frank, 1996). Amanda was an intelligent teenager with good ego functioning who was referred for counseling when her schoolwork began to deteriorate. She did not want to see the African-American social worker who was assigned to her because of her race; "her loathing of people of color was expressed in an unbridled way" (Frank, 1996, p. 69). She responded very positively to the "white, blond-haired" social worker, Adele, and "disclosed her own deep wish to be white" (Frank, 1996, p. 69). Amanda's wishes were in conflict with the agency's goals, which placed emphasis on children developing a positive racial identity.

> Adele [the clinician] . . . had to cope with veiled resentment and disapproval from her African-American colleagues that she had been assigned to work with Amanda after Amanda's refusal to work with the first therapist. . . . She was subtly admonished for not focusing on Amanda's hatred of her color. She was urged not to comply with her

patient's wish to walk along Newbury Street . . . [Boston's chic shop-ping street], where she would admire the white mannequins and re-mark on the peaceful looks on their faces. (Frank, 1996, p. 70)

Adele did go to Newbury Street with Amanda, where the teen's story and her grief slowly unfolded. Amanda expressed her conviction that her mother was killed because she was black. "If we were rich and white and didn't live in Roxbury maybe none of this would have happened to my family" (Frank, 1996, p. 72). She also thought her mother died because she (Amanda) was "bad and ugly," and later concluded that "the bad in her life was due to being black" (Frank, 1996, p. 72). She ultimately was able to integrate her losses into her life and her self-image; she wrote the following story about herself (Frank, 1996) in the guise of a little girl who had "shielded herself from . . . pain through hatred of herself, her neighborhood, and her race. . . . Eventu-ally the little girl felt her pain and her friend [the therapist] could feel it too" (p. 73). By learning to "live with her loss and the fact that she would never really understand it," she could "live with these awarenesses [and] didn't have to keep her false explanations" (Frank, 1996, p. 73).

This case highlights one of the existing tensions in social work today: the conflict between the social and political viewpoints and the psychodynamic approach. The agency was concerned about Amanda's rejection of her racial identity; they did not understand that her "racial split . . . was a defense" (Frank, 1996, p. 74). Paradoxically, however, when her grief was resolved, her distorted perceptions of herself and her racial identity were also resolved. This case discussion points out the hazards of allowing the political to override clinical considerations.

Frank (1996) asserts that she wrote this chapter "with a sense of urgency" because "psychoanalytic concepts are no longer studied in depth" (p. 74). Furthermore, Frank's chapter raises the question of clients' rights to accept or not to accept fully (or in part) their ethnic identities. If Amanda chose never to accept her racial identity fully, should she be free to make this deci-sion? The danger of the imposition of the values of others, however well in-tended, is ever present, in all forms of intervention (including the psycho-dynamic) and irrespective of the philosophy or principles underlying the intervention.

Cultural Aspects of Transference and Intersubjectivity

The self of the clinician is involved in the treatment relationship on mul-tiple levels. Although it has long been acknowledged that therapists' reac-tions to their clients are colored by the personality characteristics of each (very aggressive or very passive clients, for example, may evoke negative responses in a clinician), more recently attention has been paid to the way in which social characteristics, such as ethnic and cultural issues, may also affect the therapeutic relationship. Complex issues can arise when working with people from different cultures as well as when working with people from within the same culture.

Working with people from different cultures. Working with people who are ethnoculturally different can set off strong emotional reactions in either partner of the therapeutic dyad and "frequently provides more opportunities for empathic and dynamic stumbling blocks, in what might be termed 'ethnocultural disorientation'" (Comas-Diaz and Jacobsen, 1991, p. 392). As Comas-Diaz and Jacobsen note, a tendency exists on the part of some therapists to attribute any of the patient's comments about differences to "defense and resistance. However, in our own clinical experience we have found that this approach hinders the exploration of conflicts related to ethnicity and culture" (p. 392).

Although ethnocultural differences are highlighted by Comas-Diaz and Jacobsen (1991), this principle also applies to other types of diversity, including disability, gender, sexual orientation, etc. In the case of homosexuality, not only can relationship complications arise, but the nature of being gay can be viewed by some therapists as pathological, even though, since 1973, it is no longer classified as a mental disorder (Kaplan et al., 1994).

Working with people from the same culture. Members of minorities are often recruited to receive mental health training to enable them to help clients from their own cultures. In Israel, for example, ultra-Orthodox Jews enrolled in a three-year (nonreligious) social work program, which was very unusual, as secular education is not accepted by this group (Sontag, 1999). However, this prohibition was overlooked because these ultra-Orthodox men *(haredim)* were responding to the need for professional help with serious social problems arising in their communities.

> In addition to breaching the iron gate between the haredi world and the universities, the social work program will create a professional cadre of ultra-Orthodox social workers, who can better understand the cultural and religious norms of the haredi world. There are a few ultra-Orthodox women who are social workers, but in a society rigidly divided by sex, there was an especially great need for male professionals. (Sontag, 1999, p. A5)

Although clinicians working with clients from the same culture can provide culturally sensitive treatment, working within the same culture can also bring unique problems, such as overidentification, boundary issues, and conflicting loyalties. It can raise special countertransference issues for therapists who might have unresolved problems about their own cultural identities. Pérez Foster (1999) commented that what she found "most disturbing" were "treatment failures" with individuals from her own Caribbean background, who "somehow detected in me the probable confusion I felt at the time about my own bicultural identity" (Pérez Foster, 1999, p. 273).

Mehta (1998), who is an Asian-Indian therapist, has found problems in working with people from her own ethnicity, including the patient's tendency to attempt to control the therapist.

> A common rescue fantasy is elicited based on a pseudo-bond of one immigrant helping another in a foreign country. . . . However, there is also a rapid fantasy formation of parents' having control over the Indian therapist. . . . Nina's parents' immediate overt comfort with me as a fantasy family member and physician for their daughter gave way later to subtle derogation of the psychoanalytic framework of time and money . . . a sense of disappointment in me for being too "Americanized" in order to defend against their own personal difficulties with limit setting. (Mehta, 1998, p. 150)

A Bedouin-Arab social worker in a Mideastern country faced a literally life and death situation when he started to work with a seventeen-year-old unmarried, pregnant Bedouin-Arab woman who was a member of his village (although he had not known her previously) (Al-Krenawi, 1999). "In Bedouin-Arab society, it is common for women caught in pre- or extramarital affairs to be killed by an immediate family member in order to preserve *Ar*, or family honor, and to erase the shame that was perceived to have been brought to the family" (Al-Krenawi, 1999, p. 489). When Al-Krenawi first met with this client, he found himself in great emotional turmoil.

> I had two years' practice experience and had never encountered a problem of such complexity. I was shocked by the story and had feelings of anger toward the man who had put this woman in such a situation; but I also found that I was angry too at the woman who had violated cultural values of premarital chastity. The client's story raised many questions. . . . I felt that this case "put me in the corner." I did not know what to do. During the meeting with the client, I asked her, "how come you did that? Were you blind?" I criticized what she had done. I forgot my role as a social worker and spoke to her from my membership in the Bedouin-Arab culture. (Al-Krenawi, 1999, p. 490)

Al-Krenawi (1999) realized that he was in conflict with his professional values, knowing that he was "trained to respect the client and treat her with empathy and support" (p. 490); he decided to place his professional values above his personal beliefs. He felt that he could not "stand aside while the girl was exposed to her family and murdered, as she surely would have been—[this would be] far worse than my own moral dilemma" (p. 491). In addition to posing a moral dilemma to Al-Krenawi, his decision also posed a personal risk to him: "I would incur considerable damage to my personal and professional reputation" (Al-Krenawi, 1999, p. 491).

His interventions were successful: the woman, removed to a shelter, had her baby (who died three days later, before adoption could be effected); she returned to her community and ultimately married and had children.

Al-Krenawi feels that although his dilemmas were unique to his culture, there is an applicability to other situations, as "practitioners in many other non-Western cultures or socially marginal groups must also face cases where they must weigh the health or life of a client against the traditional values and norms of their own and their clients' communities" (Al-Krenawi, 1999, p. 494).

CONCLUSION

In this chapter we have examined together the roles of diversity and its re-lationship to human behavior and clinical work. I attempted to demonstrate that issues of race, ethnicity, social class, and culture are important variables to understand when working with people. We have seen how strong ethnic identifications and cultural beliefs can be guiding principles in life and in the formation of social relationships; and how sometimes these beliefs can take precedence over life itself. We have also observed that individuals grapple with cultural constraints and sometimes rebel and form new mean-ings for themselves. The constructivist framework illuminates how people uniquely create meaning in their lives and interpret their own cultures and ethnicities.

In keeping with the basic premise of this book, that life is complex and full of enigmas and conundrums, we have looked beneath the surface of some cultural customs and beliefs to see underlying conflicts, dilemmas, and uncertainties people face in accommodating to cultural demands and expectations. A psychodynamic approach remains important in understand-ing cultural phenomena, as inner worlds and affective lives of people are universally present, although myriad variations exist in the expression of feelings and in patterns of behavior.

Culture is transmitted first through family experiences, as psychologi-cally unformed children are socialized to adapt to the world around them.

LEARNING EXERCISE

1. In your small groups, prepare a role-playing exercise to present to the class involving an aspect of culture that affects a family and its relation-

ships. You can include, for example, a scenario depicting cultural rituals and customs and/or a situation reflecting cultural conflict among family members, such as a cultural value conflict between children and their parents.

SUGGESTED READINGS

Articles

Akhtar, S. (1995). A third individuation: Immigration, identity and the psychoanalytic process. *Journal of the American Psychoanalytic Association, 43,* 1051-1084.

Dolnick, E. (1993). Deafness as culture. *The Atlantic Monthly, 272*(September/3), 37-53.

Drachman, D. (1995). Immigration statuses and their influence on service provision, access, and use. *Social Work, 40,* 188-197.

Books

Espin, O. M. (1997). Crossing borders and boundaries: The life narratives of immigrant lesbians. In B. Greene (Ed.), *Ethnic and cultural diversity among lesbians and gay men: Vol. 3. Psychological perspective on lesbian and gay issues* (pp. 191-215). Thousand Oaks: Sage Publications.

Hogan, L. (1990). *Mean spirit.* New York: Ivy Books.

Jackson, L. C. and Greene, B. (2000). *Psychotherapy with African American women: Innovations in psychodynamic perspectives and practice.* New York: The Guilford Press.

Lee, E. (Ed.) (1997). *Working with Asian Americans: A guide for clinicians.* New York: The Guilford Press.

Pérez Foster, R., Moskowitz, M., and Javier, R. A. (Eds.) (1996). *Reaching across boundaries of culture and class: Widening the scope of psychotherapy.* Northvale: Jason Aronson Inc.

Chapter 6

The Family: Forms and Organization

No matter how many communes anybody invents, the family always creeps back.

Margaret Mead

INTRODUCTION

In her novel, *Paradise,* Toni Morrison (1999) describes a young woman named Seneca who visits her boyfriend in prison; he asks her to request money he needs from his mother. After a long bus trip, Seneca arrives at her boyfriend's mother's home to find her angry at her son, refusing to give the money that her husband had bequeathed her to "somebody who drove a car over a child and left it there, even . . . her only son" (Morrison, 1999, p. 133). Seneca defends her boyfriend; Mrs. Turtle (his mother) dismisses this with: "I've known him all his life" (p. 133). Seneca leaves but decides to return to the house to ask Mrs. Turtle if she might use the phone.

> At the door . . . she heard sobbing. A flat-out helpless mothercry—a sound like no other in the world. . . . Alone, without witness, Mrs. Turtle had let go her reason, her personality, and shrieked for all the world like the feathered, finned and hoofed whose flesh she never ate—the way a gull, a cow whale, a mother wolf might if her young had been snatched away. (Morrison, 1999, p. 134)

Mrs. Turtle has disowned her son; but she could not disown her strong attachment to him.

Ambivalent feelings toward one's family are universal, even when not inwardly recognized or outwardly acknowledged. If families break down, complex emotions often arise, including depression, rage, lowered self-esteem, feelings of betrayal, and fear of attachments, as unfulfilled needs remain, playing havoc with the emotional life of adults and children, and having serious consequences for a child's ego development.

Babies are totally helpless at birth and dependent on their families to meet their every emotional and physical need. As children grow, tensions relating to separation-individuation, limit setting, relationships with siblings, values, etc., are inevitable. However, bonds of attachment, acceptance, and support can withstand such tensions and sustain family ties, as negative and conflictual feelings are worked through and modulated. Ambivalent feelings become more difficult (or impossible) to work through when attachment and support are replaced by rejection, abuse, or abandonment. In this chapter, emotions and relationships are examined within the context of varying family structures as well as family breakdown.

Many forms and structures of family life exist today: the traditional two-parent heterosexual, single parent, stepfamilies or blended families, families headed by gay parents, and kinship foster families. Public opinion is strongly divided on what constitutes a family. Debates, legal decisions, and political referendums deal with such questions as whether gay marriages should be legalized and whether gay couples can jointly adopt children.

Vermont's Supreme Court, on December 20, 1999, ruled that "the state must guarantee the very same protections and benefits to gay and lesbian couples that it does to heterosexual spouses" (Goldberg, 1999e, p. A1). The rationale for this major legal decision was expressed:

> To extend equal rights to homosexual couples "who seek nothing more, nor less, than legal protection and security for their avowed commitment to an intimate and lasting relationship is simply, when all is said and done," the ruling said, "a recognition of our common humanity." (Goldberg, 1999e, p. A1)

Gary L. Bauer, one of the Republican candidates for president at the time, strongly disputed this decision, generating much controversy. " 'I think what the Vermont Supreme Court did last week was in some ways worse than terrorism,' " he said, holding that the decision was an example of " 'a judicial decision that attacks America's deeply held values' " ("Bauer Likens," 1999, p. A22).

The U.S. Supreme Court held proceedings related to a Washington State law which allows people, "without any defined relationship to [a] child, to petition for visiting rights and to succeed if the family court concludes that visitation would be in the child's best interest" (Greenhouse, 2000a, p. A11). This "opened the door to *a profound debate over the very definition of family*" [italics added] (Greenhouse, 2000a, p. A11). The legal case at the center of this controversy was the brief of *Troxel v. Granville* (Greenhouse, 2000a, p. A11).

Social workers today are confronted by a diversity that challenges conventional theories based on working with "traditional" families (Goldstein,

1999). "We can best learn what it means to a family to be defined as 'diverse' or 'different' from those who know firsthand what it is like to labor under such an assigned designation day in and day out" (Goldstein, 1999, p. 109). However, every family, even the "traditional" family, is unique; a constructivist stance, emphasizing the perceptions, values, and goals of each family without prejudging it, can illuminate our understanding of a family's life.

In addition to understanding the uniqueness of each family's way of being in the world, there are also universal issues to assess in all families; a key construct is the presence (or absence) of secure attachments, which extend throughout the life cycle from childhood through old age.

Secure attachments are important to children in any family structure (although they may be manifested in various forms in different cultures); they are the building blocks for developing a capacity to relate to others, as well as the development of healthy ego functioning. The nature of familial attachment is less determined by the structure of the family per se and far more by the quality of relationships within the family.

A child, for example, might develop a greater basic sense of security through attachment to an adoptive gay couple who relate in a caring, warm manner to the child, than another child might develop with two emotionally cold and distant heterosexual birth parents. Goldstein and Goldstein (1996) stress the importance of *"continuity of care"* [italics added] as being of vital importance to a child's successful development (p. 50). They stress this as a guiding principle in working with children needing out-of-home placement.

> We urge, therefore, that placements and the procedures for placement maximize a child's opportunity for being wanted and for maintaining on a continuous, unconditional, and permanent basis a relationship with at least one adult who is, or is capable of becoming, the child's psychological parent. By "psychological parent" we mean "one [or more] adults who, on a continuing, day-to-day basis, through interaction, companionship, interplay, and mutuality, fulfills the child's psychological . . . as well as physical needs. Psychological parents may be biological, adoptive, foster, or common-law parents, or any other [adults]." (Goldstein and Goldstein, 1996, p. 51)

Henry (1999), while emphasizing the importance of *parental permanency* for children, also notes that the "experience of *psychological and physical safety* [italics added] is a developmental imperative of childhood" (p. 561). Many children today are neglected and/or physically and/or sexually abused within their own families often with serious psychological and developmental consequences (Dore, 1999; Morton and Browne, 1998). To leave these children with their birth families "may be far more damaging than removal to a permanent, safer environment" (Adnopoz, 1996, p. 415).

If children are removed from the home in an attempt to protect them, this can cause further psychological harm resulting from lack of continuity or permanency. Furthermore, when children are removed, will they actually be moved to a "permanent, safer environment," or will they be moved through a system of revolving foster homes, where they may never know permanency? Deciding whether to remove children or have them remain with their families (or people they perceive to be their families) are among the most complex and profound decisions social workers must make.

Serious disruptions in family life are common today, including alcoholism, domestic violence, homelessness, and problematic (and sometimes disrupted) adoptions. Divorce, often though not necessarily associated with disruption of family life, is endemic; according to the American Academy of Child and Adolescent Psychiatry, it was estimated that, by 1997, divorce affected almost 1 million children per year (Kaplan and Pruett, 2000). Approximately "10 million children live with a parent who is separated or divorced" (Lopez, 1998, p. 60). Kaplan and Pruett have summarized some of the current research findings on divorce.

> Of those divorcing, nearly 10 percent involve custody litigation. Nearly half of all children in this country will spend time in a single-parent home (Glick and Lin, 1986). While the rate of divorce in this country has declined in the last decade, approximately half of all first marriages end in divorce (U.S. Bureau of the Census, 1992). An additional 17 percent separate but do not divorce. Postdivorce children usually live with a custodial mother who remains single for an average of 5 years (Castro-Martin and Bumpass, 1989). Many of these homes will include other family members or new male partners. Remarriage rates have been falling, suggesting that many children will remain with a single custodial parent until they leave home. The majority experience, however, is for two-thirds of divorced women and approximately three-quarters of divorced men to remarry (Bumpass, Sweete, and Castro-Martin, 1990). With divorce rates even higher among remarriages, *many children find themselves in the position of adapting to ever-changing family constellations.* [italics added] (Kaplan and Pruett, 2000, p. 533)

Leaving a damaged marriage can be a strength, and many families successfully transition from the loss of their original family to other arrangements. Nevertheless, painful psychological and social consequences often follow divorce for parents as well as their children, which include: experiencing loss and grief; transitioning to new homes, lifestyles, and new stepfamilies; and adapting to decreased financial resources. The ideals of continuity of care and permanency become transformed for many children.

FORMS AND STRUCTURES OF FAMILY LIFE

This section discusses the traditional family, single parents, blended families, gay families, adoptive families, foster families, kinship foster families, and grandparents raising their grandchildren.

The Traditional Family

The term traditional, when applied to families, is often associated today with the so-called Christian right and its concern with traditional family values (which includes opposition to a number of nontraditional issues, such as homosexuality and abortion). However, in this chapter, *traditional* has a structural rather than a value-laden meaning. The traditional family is defined as consisting of a husband (male), wife (female), and their children, although this no longer is the predominant picture of family life in this country. "Currently fewer than 30 percent of all families are composed of the traditional 'nuclear family' (that is one-time married parents with one or more children)" (Zastrow and Kirst-Ashman, 1997, p. 145).

Intermarriages

One factor changing the picture of traditional families is the increase of racial and ethnic intermarriages across many groups and cultures (Spickard et al., 1995).

> Since the 1960s the rate of intermarriage has skyrocketed; the percentage of Asian and Hispanic people who marry outside their ancestral group has increased from less than 10 percent in the post-World War II generation to more than 40 percent in the closing years of this century. American Indians have sustained a 50 percent outmarriage rate throughout the past half-century. Even outmarriage rates for African Americans, which have been much lower, have sharply increased. (Spickard et al., 1995, p. 582)

Children born of interracial parentage increase the number of Americans who are multiethnic and increase their options for choice of identity within a multicultural framework. This phenomenon increases opportunities for celebrating diversity and accepting others with greater comfort and even pleasure. "The simple understanding of race and the easy targets of racism grow more complex" (Spickard et al., 1995, p. 583).

At the same time, intermarriage may pose problems for individual families who may experience discrimination within their own extended families and their communities; furthermore, personal problems of adaptation may arise as couples are faced with issues of cultural conflict. The partners of an interracial marriage, for example, involving an Asian American and a non-Asian, "may not even be aware of the different cultural value systems that shape their perceptions of reality" (Crohn, 1997, p. 434).

> Culture shapes every aspect of how a person views the world and what he or she considers "normal" and "abnormal." It molds attitudes toward time, family, sex, monogamy [sic], and identity. Cultural rules govern how anger and affection are expressed, the ways that children are disciplined and rewarded, how strangers and friends are greeted, and the roles of men and women. Behavior that one culture defines as neighborly, another may label as seductive; what one defines as friendly disagreement, the other may see as a threat. (Crohn, 1997, p. 434)

Changing Roles of Fathers and Mothers

The women's movement is one influence that has produced major changes in traditional family life, with shifts in the power structure and in the roles of men and women, including the number of women in the workforce. In 1948, for example, "only 11 percent of all married women with children under age six were in the labor force" (Zastrow and Kirst-Ashman, 1997, p. 499); this figure had jumped to 62 percent by 1994.

Fathers now generally have more involvement in family life and child care than they have had in the past (Crockenberg and Leerkes, 2000; Ross, 1984). However, in the more distant past of the preindustrial world, men worked near home or in the home and were more involved with their children as they shared the routines of their lives together. Paradoxically, the computer age might revive this pattern, as more people work at their own computers at home.

Earlier writings on child development stressed the importance of the mother-child bond; if the father was discussed, it was generally in relation to his influence in the later stages of child development or of his importance in emotionally supporting the mother in her role. In current writings, the significance of the father in his direct interactions with his child from infancy on is mentioned increasingly (Crockenberg and Leerkes, 2000). Fatherhood also has significant ramifications for a man's psychological development; a child "affects a man's identity as a father as well as the self-identity and masculinity bound up with his paternity" (Ross, 1984, p. 382).

Another shift involving fathers in the traditional family is the increase in the number of stay-at-home fathers (Marin, 2000, p. 18). In 1993, the U.S. Bureau of the Census reported that "1.9 million unemployed men were the primary caregivers of children up to 14 years old—down from a recession high of more than 2 million in 1991" (Marin, 2000, p. 18). A number of men who are employed provide care for their children during the day while their wives work; the fathers then go to work on the night shift. For many fathers, however, there is no outside employment; their full employment is child care.

Some stay-at-home fathers often find social isolation to be a problem (as many stay-at-home mothers have), and some have experienced social disapproval and/or condescension from others. Some dads found " 'a glass wall' separating mothers from fathers in parks and school yards" (Marin, 2000, p. 18). Many fathers find support groups of other stay-at-home fathers, including Internet communications, to be helpful.

Day Care

Use of child care as a substitute for parental care in the home is increasing. These infants (and older children) are "cared for by someone other than their mother. These [services] include center-based care, child-care homes, care by relatives, and in-home care by nonrelatives" (Hungerford et al., 2000, pp. 519-520). The effects of day care on developing children, especially for children under age three, are controversial; however, "child care in the early years of life is now the norm for most children in the United States and other industrialized countries" (Hungerford et al., 2000, p. 519).

Many researchers think that no simple "yes" or "no" answer exists to the question of whether child care has deleterious effects on children. Some early research has been criticized for simplistic approaches and lack of attention to the full range of interacting variables. "This 'first wave' of child-care research was motivated by the simple question of whether child care was harmful for young children," and other variables, such as the quality of the care was not assessed (Hungerford et al., 2000, pp. 520-521).

During the 1980s, research was centered on the quality of the care the child was receiving. Two major variables were then studied: the " 'structural,' " aspects, including such factors as the "adult-child ratio; caregiver education, training, and commitment . . . ; and the 'process' variables including . . . stimulation caregivers provided, [and] the quality of their interactions with the children . . . " (Hungerford et al., 2000, pp. 520-521).

Then studies focused on the fact that children did not receive day care in a social vacuum; they had a family life and a socioeconomic context, and brought their individual personality and temperamental qualities to the day care situation. "The 'third wave' of child care research is therefore focused on the [effect of] multiple, interacting features of the child's experiences in shaping development. Much of the research conducted since 1990, but by no means all, is premised on this model" (Hungerford et al., 2000, p. 521).

So-called "cumulative risk models" (Hungerford et al., 2000, p. 522) have figured into studies of child mental health and resilience. Research applying this model and the "dual risk" model to child care suggests that if at least two risk factors are present, children will be susceptible later to emotional and/or cognitive problems.

> For example, infants living in a dysfunctional family with a depressed and/or insensitive mother or infants who have developed an insecure attachment during the first year may fare especially poorly if they also attend low-quality child care. That is, the impact of unresponsive or unstimulating care both at home and in child care may exacerbate each other. (Hungerford et al., 2000, p. 522)

On the other hand, a " 'compensatory' or 'buffering' experience [with] high-quality child care helps young children at risk overcome some of the negative outcomes associated with being reared in a punitive, uninvolved, or disorganized family setting" (Hungerford et al., 2000, p. 522). Many early intervention programs have been designed on this premise.

Although concluding that child care is a normative experience in this country, Hungerford and colleagues (2000) are cautious in generalizing about the effects of this experience on children; they prefer the questions: "Under what circumstances do children thrive or suffer in early child care, and how do different sources of influence mutually shape development?" (p. 519). They recommend further research to include study of long-term effects on children as they develop.

Zastrow and Kirst-Ashman (1997) assert that good day care, providing consistency and nurturing, is not harmful to a child. However, they express the concern that day care is not always adequate, and note that many studies on day care were done in high-quality facilities, which are unavailable to many parents.

This unavailability is related to many factors, including cost, location, hours available, type of care, and age restrictions on children. Substantial concerns exist when the single mother works outside the home (or when both parents work outside the home) and the children receive poor child care or no substitute care (Zastrow and Kirst-Ashman, 1997).

Commenting on the lack of uniformly strong standards for child care in this country, Margaret Carlson (1997) observed: "What an odd society it is that requires more training and licensing of the person who cuts your hair than the person to whom you entrust your most precious possession" (p. 30).

Many traditional families experience financial stress; both spouses often feel that they must work to make ends meet. Some families cannot make ends meet, even when both parents are working, and sometimes at least one parent is working more than one job. Some low-income families, due to a combination of low wages and high rents, find themselves at the poverty level (Longres, 1995b).

Homelessness

During the last decade of the twentieth century, many traditional families were found in the homeless population, although the largest number of families reported were composed of women and their children (First et al., 1995; Longres, 1995b). Homeless women often report physical and/or sexual abuse as factors precipitating separation from their husbands (Goldberg, 1999).

Homelessness itself can cause separation in a traditional family. "Some family shelters may not admit all members of a family because they lack space, while others do not allow men (and adolescent boys) to stay with their female companions, relatives and children" (Choi and Snyder, 1999, p. 57).

Single Parents

The number of single-parent families increased dramatically from 1970 to 1990 and today represents about 25 percent of families who have children under eighteen (Strand, 1995). Although fathers represent about 10 percent of single parents, approximately 90 percent of this group are mothers. Among these mothers, there are three times more African-American women than white women (Zastrow and Kirst-Ashman, 1997). Two primary factors responsible for the numbers of single parents are the increasing number of couples who divorce and the increase in births to mothers who were never married; this latter group includes babies born to teenage mothers. In addition, the rate of single people adopting children doubled through the 1970s and 1980s (Strand, 1995).

Single mothers vary in socioeconomic and employment status, social supports, etc. However, there is a large segment within this population who face major stresses related to poverty and employment (Strand, 1995); many single mothers and their children are found in the homeless population (First et al., 1995; Longres, 1995b).

> Poverty affects single-parent families significantly more than two-parent families. Differences in the average income levels of single-parent, female-headed families and two-parent families are striking and deplorable. Thirty-four percent of female-headed families are in poverty compared to 8 percent for two-parent families (U. S. Bureau of the Census, 1995). (Zastrow and Kirst-Ashman, 1997, p. 496)

Although rural poverty affects many traditional families, the increase of rural "poor single households is particularly devastating" (Wijnberg and Reding, 1999, p. 506); these families "often remain in poverty for a longer period of time than their urban counterparts" (p. 506).

In assessing the effects of single parenting on both parents and children, it is important first to understand how the single parent experiences being a single parent and being without a partner, as parents' feelings and attitudes about this affect their relationships to their children. Then, one needs to observe the basic quality of attachment the child has to the custodial parent and has (or had) to the missing parent. Other important considerations that can affect the parent and children include available social supports; the physical and mental health of the parents and children; adequate housing; employment opportunities (and job satisfaction); and financial status.

A spectrum of psychosocial functioning is found in this group. "Child welfare services have increasingly worked with single, often poor, inner-city mothers struggling to raise children in extreme situations. Foster care agencies and residential treatment programs regularly encounter single parents, and services are often geared to reuniting the child with the family of origin" (Strand, 1995, p. 2161). Some women who are divorced or separated from their spouses or partners report escaping from physical and/or sexual abuse, which was often accompanied by substance abuse.

Many well-functioning single-parent families are also raising well-functioning children, and the strengths and competencies of many of these families have been receiving greater recognition (Strand, 1995; Zastrow and Kirst-Ashman, 1997).

> In contrast to research that has found negative effects of single-parent families, other research portrays a more positive picture. For instance, Rutter (1983) found that children grew up to be better adjusted in single-parent families where they had a positive relationship with their parent than in two-parent families which were ridden with fighting and strife. Likewise, Hetherington (1980) found that a parent who is unapproachable, belligerent, and rejecting can cause more harm to a child than a parent who is not there at all. In summary, it appears that how the available parent feels toward and treats the child is more im-

portant than simply having two bodies present within the home. (Zastrow and Kirst-Ashman, 1997, pp. 495-496)

The question of the "missing parent" is a significant one that cannot be dismissed by stating that a "parent who is not there" may cause less harm to a child, compared to the parent who stays but has continual battles with a spouse or partner. If children form attachments to both parents, and if it is the father who is the missing parent (as in 90 percent of cases), then how does the child deal with this loss? Was the father ever known to the child, or does the fantasy of the missing father exist in the child's mind? What messages do mothers convey to their children about their fathers? Are children being caught (or triangulated) in a power struggle between their parents, forced to take sides? Children may feel confused about their possibly intense attachment to a "bad" father and may need sensitive help to work through their feelings. If overt marital tensions were present, how was the child affected? "The presence of prolonged marital conflict may play a greater role than divorce itself on child outcome" (Kaplan and Pruett, 2000, p. 536).

Conversely, these questions also apply to single fathers raising their children, in terms of attitudes and relationships to missing mothers. It is also understandable for social workers to "buy into" a negative picture of the missing parent painted by a the primary client; it is extremely important to exercise professional objectivity in these situations.

Men represent only a small group of single parents (10 percent), and their role is given minimal attention in the single-parent literature, "although it seems clear that they are vulnerable to special stressors" (Germain, 1991, p. 102). There has been recent interest by social workers in providing support groups and other services to single fathers.

Finally, we should bear in mind that not all missing parents in single-parent households are missing. Some fathers, although not part of the household, may frequently visit and, in terms of relationships, be a part of the family. One study, for example, suggested that "young black children benefit from the presence of nonresident fathers, particularly when these fathers are an 'active' presence in their lives" (Jackson, 1999, p. 156).

Teenage Parents

One large group of single parents are teenagers: children having children. Although some teen mothers and their children do well, many of these mothers, coming from backgrounds with multiple risk factors, face additional social and emotional stresses, as do their children. Although the United States continues to have the highest teenage birth rate of Western industrialized countries, it has nevertheless been noted that the number of teen births had dramatically decreased by the end of 1999 (Lacey, 1999).

The nation's teen-age birth rate fell again last year to a near-record low, Federal health officials said today, continuing an encouraging trend that spans ethnic groups, geographical areas and ages.

For younger girls, ages 10 to 14, the rate was the lowest level since 1969. African-American teen-agers recorded the lowest birth rate since 1960, when such data were first gathered, and the rate among Hispanic women also dropped precipitously, officials said. (Lacey, 1999, p. A14)

Experts have attributed this decline to a decrease in sexual relationships between teenagers and a more consistent use of birth control. This account did not discuss the actual number of interrupted pregnancies or the role abortions may have contributed to this decline. The continuing problem of teenage births and the complex difficulties they cause for parents and their children remain serious concerns.

Teenage mothers face multiple problems, including economic and housing difficulties and lack of emotional readiness for this event in their lives, which interferes with schooling and vocational attainment. Many of these teens have come from high-risk environments, and they may be involved in other risky behaviors (Wakschlag and Hans, 2000, p. 129). They are often unprepared for parenting, and their children tend to have developmental complications.

Compared to older mothers, younger mothers have been shown to be less responsive to their children, to engage in harsher discipline, and to be more depressed. . . . The children of adolescent mothers are more likely to have pre- and perinatal difficulties, to exhibit developmental and behavioral problems during early childhood and beyond, and to become teenage parents themselves. (Wakschlag and Hans, 2000, p. 129)

Teenage fathers have generally received little attention, although more recently research and services have been directed at this population (Kiselica, 1995). Many of these fathers "do not want to abandon their baby . . . [they] face the same emotional struggles and dilemmas that teenage mothers do, and many fathers want a baby for the same reasons that teenage mothers want one" (Ashford et al., 1997, p. 353).

The general assumption that most of the fathers of babies born to adolescent mothers are themselves adolescents is not founded in fact. "Perhaps surprisingly, it appears that only 20-40 percent of the partners of adolescent mothers are themselves adolescents" (Wakschlag and Hans, 2000, p. 131); in fact, it has been observed that there are "large age discrepancies" between teen mothers and the fathers, which "sometimes indicate abuse of the young women" (p. 132).

Generally, teenage mothers do not marry the fathers of their babies; when they do, the divorce rate tends to be high (Wakschlag and Hans, 2000). Fathers generally tend to be involved during the first year of the baby's life, after which their interest diminishes (Ashford et al., 1997). Some studies have correlated the father's ongoing interest in the child with the quality of his relationship to the mother. "When the relationship between the father and mother becomes distant or strained, the father's involvement with the infant diminishes" (Wakschlag and Hans, 2000, p. 132).

A close relationship also exists between the father's involvement and his employment status; those who are employed "are more likely to maintain involvement with their children" (Wakschlag and Hans, 2000, p. 132). Often the attitude of the maternal *grandmother* is a decisive factor in the father's involvement; "the support of a strongly involved grandmother can also foster father involvement with the child" (Wakschlag and Hans, 2000, p. 132).

The complex problems of adolescent pregnancy require comprehensive planning of services for both mothers and fathers, including education, job training, birth control education, parenting education, support groups, building a network of social supports, couples counseling, and early childhood intervention programs for the children. The need for mental health intervention is an important consideration, "although mental health and family interactions have generally not been a direct focus of intervention" (Wakschlag and Hans, 2000, p. 140).

Either parent may have problems, such as depression or substance abuse; many mothers have problems with depression and low self-esteem. In addition, a large number of adolescent mothers have been sexually abused, "which increases their risk for mental health problems as well as difficulties maintaining stable relationships with partners and establishing appropriate boundaries with their young children" (Wakschlag and Hans, 2000, p. 135).

Finally, teenage mothers are going through the adolescent stage during which, under the best of circumstances, some degree of conflict with parents as well as tensions relating to separation-individuation issues are inevitable. Some of these teenagers may have serious preexisting problems with their mothers; becoming a mother (which often involves bringing the child into the grandmother's household) can complicate these relationships; in some instances, the grandmother may be an important source of support; in others, she may increase the young mother's emotional as well as parenting conflicts (Woods and Holllis, 1990). It has been suggested that grandmothers be included in interventions in a "three generation approach to adolescent parents" (Wakschlag and Hans, 2000). Teenage parenthood is discussed further in Chapter 8.

The Blended Family

People who have been divorced (or widowed) often remarry and may bring children with them into their new marriages; the new family is now a *blended family,* which may also include children born to this new couple. Other terms to describe this constellation of "two families that are joined together by the marriage of one parent to another" are "stepfamilies . . . reconstituted families, and nontraditional families" (Zastrow and Kirst-Ashman, 1997, p. 496). A family may live as a blended family without being legally married; gay couples with children who live together would be an example of this.

Although positive relationships between all members can develop and warm and enriching experiences may then ensue, entering into a blended family presents spouses with greater complexities than are likely to arise in a new traditional family. Spouses must work out separation and/or divorce issues with their previous partners and mourn the loss of their earlier relationships. One divorced woman commented that if you have children you are never totally divorced; you are usually involved, for many years, with your former spouse in terms of child care, custody, and visitation issues.

Other problems involving the children include: adaptation of stepparents and stepchildren to one another; children's adaptations to (and jealousies about) stepsiblings; the accommodation of former family routines, rituals, myths, etc., to new family expectations; and possible changes in lifestyles (Germain, 1991).

> Blended families must deal with stress that arises from the losses (as a result of divorce or death) experienced by both adults and children, which can make them afraid to love and to trust. Previously established bonds between children and their biological parents may interfere with the formation of ties to the stepparent. If children go back and forth between two households, conflicts between stepchildren and stepparents may be intensified. (Zastrow and Kirst-Ashman, 1997, p. 496)

Grieving is critical in accepting the losses inherent in the divorce process; however, this may not occur for various reasons, including anger and denial; in addition, "because mourning is perceived as a threat to the new family, it is often blocked" (Scharff and Scharff, 1987, p. 378). One teenage boy (Bruce), for example, was having trouble with mourning the loss of his birth mother, from whom he was separated following a divorce. He lived with his father, stepmother, and stepbrother; he visited with his mother, who lived with a farming family, every other weekend. Scharff and Scharff

(1987) describe a family therapy session dealing with a family dispute, which Bruce precipitated, following a visit with his mother.

> Marge [stepmother] was already mad at Bruce for coming home late from his mother's . . . and for dirtying the living room with straw and mud from his boots. She and Fred [Bruce's father] were both mad at Bruce's mother for failing to supervise him adequately, whereas Bruce was delighted with the visit to his mother, feeling that he had had a great time doing farm work with her . . . without worrying about being a mess. Marge was concerned that Bruce go to school with matching clothes and clean shoes, which was not the way his mother had raised him.
>
> Although it was quite reasonable for Marge to prefer Bruce to shed his gear in the basement and behave in ways appropriate to their town-house life-style, Bruce could not keep separate the two kinds of existence when unconsciously he longed to merge them. At the moment of returning home, *he was still longing for his mother and holding on to her through bits of mud and hay* [italics added]. His "bad" behavior provoked Marge to be a "bad" mother, which emphasized the image of the "good" mother he was missing. The child was in the midst of two cultures in collision. (Scharff and Scharff, 1987, p. 379)

This excerpt poignantly illustrates the depth of the attachment Bruce feels for his mother and his difficulty in losing her. Bruce's "holding on to her through bits of mud and hay" is a vivid and moving example of the use of these materials as transitional objects, as described by Winnicott (Mahler et al., 1975).

Clinical social workers have an important contribution to make, through individual, couples, and family therapy, to those who need help with their adaptation to the complexities of blended family life.

Gay and Lesbian Families

Estimates vary as to the number of gay and lesbian families in the United States. "Schulenberg (1985) estimated that 6 million children were being raised by lesbians or gay men; Peterson (1984) estimated 14 million; and the American Bar Association, 6 million to 14 million" (Morales, 1995, p. 1085). One of the reasons it is so difficult to obtain accurate numbers is that not every gay or lesbian person identifies himself or herself as such.

The means of achieving gay and lesbian parenthood vary. Many are birth parents (and often their children have been born in a prior or current heterosexual marriage); their partners then often assume the role of a stepparent.

Increasingly, lesbian women, once they become a couple, may decide to have children through adoption or through insemination of one partner by a donor (Erera and Fredriksen, 1999). Some gay men choose a woman to act as a surrogate mother; parenthood may also be attained through adoption, foster care, or stepparenting.

A variety of family structures are found in this group, including divorced gays and lesbians living as single parents or with a partner, some sharing custody of their children with a former spouse; blended family structures, with each partner bringing children from former unions; single or coparenting of adoptive or foster children. The criteria for selection of family structure (for example, making clear distinctions between adopted children of gay couples and children who live with a gay couple but have visitation rights with a biological parent) are important in doing research; the criteria restrict the degree to which the findings "can be applied or generalized" (Parks, 1998, p. 380).

Little research has been done on gay fathers, in part because of the assumption that men are not appropriate or adequate caregivers for children; in addition, "being gay and a father has been viewed as impossible . . . paradoxical, scandalous, and controversial" (Morales, 1995, p. 1086). The majority of research studies on lesbian women have been limited to women who were "young, white, middle to upper class, highly educated, living in urban areas, and open about their lesbian identity" (Parks, 1998, p. 377). Therefore, research is largely unavailable concerning lesbians and their children representing other groupings, such as "racial and ethnic minorities, non-urban dwellers, [and] lower socioeconomic groups" (Parks, 1998, p. 377).

Latino and African-American gay fathers often experience cultural conflict about revealing their sexual identities, and "it is more unlikely for Latino gay fathers in the United States to seek support within gay networks or to move toward an integrated identity" (Morales, 1995, p. 1089). Many gay fathers of color also have concerns about encountering discrimination from their own ethnic or racial groups, generally believing "that their children need their communities and families to buffer racism. They also may view their churches and community as more judgmental and moralistic about their sexuality" (Morales, 1995, p. 1089).

Acceptance of homosexuality seems to be growing today in this country; yet homophobia as well as overt discrimination and acts of violence against this population remain. Children of gay and lesbian parents can encounter discrimination from other children and adults. Paradoxically, advances such as introducing educational programs on homosexual parenting into schools can lead to a backlash of gay bashing or various forms of rejection (Morales, 1995). Sometimes lesbian mothers are rejected by sectors of their lesbian communities that are opposed to motherhood (Parks, 1998). In one study, some mothers reported "an anti-family, anti-children slant in some parts of the gay community" (Lott-Whitehead and Tully, 1993, p. 273).

Little research has been done on the children of gay parents. The available findings do not reveal significant psychological problems in children of homosexual parents; their own sexual identity seems to be unaffected by this experience (Parks, 1998), and they "end up straight or gay in the same proportion as children raised in nongay families" (Morales, 1995, 1091). Researchers have found that when children of lesbian mothers have developmental problems they are related not to "the mother's sexuality" but to other areas of "family functioning" (Parks, 1998, p. 383).

Research suggests that gay fathers do in fact possess good parenting skills. "Compared with nongay fathers, gay fathers may try harder to create stable and nurturing homes, may maintain consistent contact with their children when they do not have custody, and are more likely to view themselves as successful fathers" (Morales, 1995, p. 1093). In studying children of divorced lesbian mothers, it has been observed that their children see their fathers more often than "children in custody of heterosexual mothers" (Parks, 1998, p. 383). In addition, relationships of children of lesbian mothers to other men and women were "found to be rich, engaging, and rooted in attitudes of acceptance and a tolerance for differences" (Parks, 1998, p. 383).

Many homosexual families develop informal social networks. In lesbian families, for example, a "major source of social support is their own lesbian community that tends to function as an extended family" (Erera and Fredriksen, 1999, p. 268).

Family law issues can cause special problems for gay and lesbian people. Legal definitions of obligations and rights in terms of custody, support, and visitation affect those who have separated from (or divorced) heterosexual spouses; these decisions also affect those who separate from homosexual partners who are coparents of adopted children or who were stepparents to their birth children. Many laws as well as some individual judges have been biased against gay and lesbian parents.

When working with gay and lesbian families, sexual orientation is only one factor among other critical issues to assess, including stability and quality of relationships; resolution of divorce; single-parenting and blended-family adaptations; attachment and loss issues; economic and employment status; physical and mental health problems; extended family and social network relationships; and cultural conflict.

Adoption

There are currently about 5 million American adoptees, according to Census Bureau reports (Caplan, 1990). In most traditional legal adoptions, a child (often an infant) is placed, on a permanent basis, with a married couple (typically infertile) who assume full parenting rights and responsibilities for that child. Today, adoptions increasingly take place in nontraditional families: by single persons or gay couples, by stepparents, when a birth parent remarries, or by foster parents or relatives who have acted as caretakers for a child.

Some children are adopted when they are older; those with special needs are difficult to place and may await adoption for years. International adoptions have been increasing, as have interracial adoptions, both of which remain controversial. Finally, the concept of the permanency of adoption has been eroded, as some birth parents challenge the legality of their child's adoption, and as a number of adoptive parents terminate the adoption, feeling unable to cope with their adopted child.

The traditional approach, which treats identifying information about birth parents as strictly confidential, is breaking down, as more adoptees search for their birth parents, and as more adoptions become open; the latter approach permits birth parents and adoptive parents to have some knowledge of each other and allows for some type of ongoing contact between them (Cushman et al., 1993).

Complicating the adoption arena are new reproductive technologies with which the development of legal and ethical guidelines has not kept pace. Bell (1986) asserts that "in many ways, embryo transfer and the other new reproductions are at the same stage as was traditional adoption 20 years ago" (p. 423).

Few adoptions were taking place in the United States at the turn of the century, although many children were in institutional or other substitute care. Under the influence of the then-prevailing concern with eugenics, many people were apprehensive about the "inadequate" parentage of these children and "doubted that the children available for adoption could be saved. Child-welfare experts cultivated this prejudice by opposing the placement of infants until their character and capabilities were proved" (Caplan, 1990, p. 35).

Increasing concern then developed for the psychological needs of the child, and in 1920 the Child Welfare League of America was founded. Several main principles were followed as adoption practice was formulated: "that the adoptive family was to replace the biological one; that the adoption be permanent; that the adoption take place as early as possible after the child's birth . . . and that the adoption be confidential" (Caplan, 1990, p. 37). Adoption laws did not exist in many states, and it was not until 1929 that every state had one.

Caplan (1990) emphasizes that supply and demand are important factors affecting adoption practices. In the 1960s, for example, when there was an abundant supply of babies, some couples adopted a number of children; some of these families had their own birth children (and no fertility issues) but adopted additional children for "humanitarian reasons" (Caplan, 1990, p. 40).

In the 1970s, social changes—including the increase in abortions, the tendency for unmarried women to keep their own children (diminishing the supply of babies available for adoption), and the increased incidence of infertile couples—affected the adoption scene: "the number of couples waiting to adopt had become significantly larger than the number of healthy infants available for adoption" (Caplan, 1990, pp. 40-41). Coupled with other sociopolitical and biological trends, this led to an increase in interracial and international adoptions, an increasing utilization of reproductive technologies, and a greater number of privately arranged adoptions (often through lawyers), accompanied by a decreased interest in social agency adoptions.

In addition, in 1971, adoptees began protesting past adoption practices, especially those withholding information about their birth parentage, and the Adoptees' Liberty Movement Association, "the largest search group" was subsequently organized (Caplan, 1990, p. 41). Through the legal and other advocacy efforts by adult adoptees, a movement has been established toward open records and disclosure of parental identity.

On one level, adoption is an excellent solution for all parties involved in the adoption triangle: the birth parents (although usually only the birth mother is discussed), who are unable (socially, financially, and/or emotionally) to raise their child yet wish for a secure home for their offspring; the child, who otherwise faces the life of being a "psychological orphan" with no permanent family; and the adoptive parents who want a child to love and to raise. For gay and lesbian people or heterosexual single people who might otherwise be childless, it is a way to have a child to nurture. Some adoptive families have the motivation and capacity to work with children with special needs.

However, on psychological and social levels, adoption, even when highly successful, can be a very complex psychological and social process for all members of the adoption triangle as issues of loss and insecurity can plague each member in different ways. It should be added that not all adoptions are entered into voluntarily by the birthparents; sometimes their rights to be parents have been terminated by the courts due to neglect and/or abuse, and adoption is mandated.

Birth Parents

Birth mothers face emotional conflicts in relinquishing their babies for adoption, often experiencing feelings of loss, guilt, pain, and grief; they may or may not have gone through an appropriate mourning process. Even with the passage of time, these emotional issues do not necessarily disappear with the relinquishment process; "they had a need to know about the well being of their child over the years" (Chapman et al., 1986, p. 204). Lifton has noted that " 'adoption may be compared to an amputation for a birthmother' " (Chapman et al., 1986, p. 205). Silverman observed that birth mothers who were "told to 'forget' denied part of themselves by shutting off their feelings" (Chapman et al., 1986, p. 205).

The profound nature of relinquishing a child for adoption requires exploration with those clients who have experienced this, even if this event was in the distant past. Variation exists in the degree of the mother's acceptance and positive adaptation; denial, perpetual mourning, and/or unresolved grief have been observed. Some birthmothers retain memories of the birth, have fantasies about the child they gave away, may wish for reunion, and observe silent rituals when it is the child's birthday or on other significant occasions.

Unresolved feelings about giving up her child may affect a woman's future relationships with men (or with the man who is the father of the baby) and can color attitudes toward later children. Many women have had their babies in secret and entered into an adoption process in which strict confidentiality was guaranteed; they may wish to retain this secret.

Many children adopted today are older children who may know their birth mothers. Birth mothers of such children may be angry at permanently losing them and may pursue ongoing legal actions to have the adoption overturned and/or may engage in behaviors that can be physically or psychologically damaging to the child, in seeking additional involvement with their children. It is not uncommon to find a birth mother replacing her lost child through another pregnancy.

Today, many birth mothers no longer feel a need for secrecy and have banded together for mutual support and advocacy. Organizations such as Concerned United Birthparents, Inc. have been formed by birth parents (McRoy et al., 1988). Their goals are to make "adoption more client-centered, to permit adult adoptees access to original certificates and identifying information, to allow birthparents visitation rights when adoptees are of a certain age, and to help birthparents resolve guilt feelings" (McRoy et al., 1988, p. 12).

Today a major trend exists toward open adoption (Liederman, 1995), accompanied by increasing political pressure for adoptees to have access to their birth certificates when they are twenty-one. A controversial proposal, Ballot Measure 58, for access to birth records was accepted by the voters in Oregon (Cloud, 1999). Some birth mothers sued the state of Oregon, "arguing that state statutes promise them confidentiality and that breaking these promises would be unconstitutional" (Cloud, 1999, p. 64). According to the Center for Health Statistics (and Vital Records), Oregon Health Division, Oregon Department of Human Services, on May 31, 2000, "Appeals to the

U.S. Supreme Court [challenging the open birth records Ballot Measure 58] failed, and the processing of orders began ("A Brief History," 2001).

Cindy is one birth mother who chose not to reveal her identity to her daughter (Cloud, 1999).

> Two decades ago, when Cindy (a pseudonym) was in college, a man beat and raped her. Devastated and uncertain, she had the baby but surrendered the girl for adoption. Last summer, after soul-searching, Cindy decided to find out what had become of her child. She gave the state where the girl was born permission to contact her if the daughter asked her whereabouts. The daughter already had, and the two began exchanging letters through the adoption agency. But Cindy held back her identity and location.
>
> A wise move, she now says. After Cindy told her daughter about the rape, the young woman . . . wanted to know how to find him [her birth father]. Cindy was horrified. Her daughter obviously hadn't grasped her pain, the nightmares—her whole life. The daughter, with the help of her adoptive mother, persisted in trying to find her father, a man Cindy had helped send to prison. Fearing he might find her and harm her again, Cindy terminated contact. (p. 64)

Although the father's legal rights have recently been recognized, it is notable that little reference is made to the birth father in the literature, and almost no reference is made to the maternal and paternal extended birth families. However, the father's needs and possible emotional loss and grieving also must be addressed; the extended family may also be emotionally affected by this event.

Birth fathers who are anonymous sperm donors for artificial insemination present special issues for their offspring. Sperm banks vary in the amount of information they give to the mother. The Sperm Bank of California in Oakland, for example, "offers a new contract, that, if signed by both sperm donor and mother, would allow a child access to his father's name upon turning eighteen. Lawyers warn, however, that such contracts are largely untested in the courts" (Smolowe, 1990, p. 76). Sweden has "enacted laws that give the offspring of sperm donors the right to learn their father's name upon reaching adulthood" (Bell, 1986, p. 429).

The Adopted Child

Many adoptions are considered successful with respect to the general adaptation and development of the child and the presence of positive family relationships. Some research findings have indicated that while the "social and emotional development of adopted children may be different," it is "not necessarily problematic" (Silverman et al., 1994). On a different note, Kaplan and colleagues (1994) observed that adopted children have a higher incidence of emotional and behavior disorders, including "aggressive behavior, stealing, and learning disturbances," than do nonadopted children (p. 49). These findings are correlated to the age at adoption; "the later the age of adoption, the higher the incidence and the more severe the degree of behavior problems" (Kaplan et al., 1994, p. 49).

In evaluating the impact of adoption on a child, it can be difficult to isolate the variable of adoption as an element of the context of the psychosocial environment in which these children live and interact. Many factors impinge on the adopted child, including preadoptive experiences; the quality of the relationship between the child and adoptive parents; adoptive parents' attitudes to adoption; relationships to the extended adoptive family; ongoing relationship (if any) with birth parents, siblings, or extended family; economic and employment status of adoptive family; cultural conflict; and the presence of physical and mental health problems in the adoptive parents and in the child. If an adopted child is having problems, there is a tendency to assume this is because of adoption issues, when adoption itself may play only a peripheral role.

It is common for adopted children to wonder about their birth parents; the two main questions asked by adoptees are: " 'Who do I look like?' and 'Why was I given away?' " (Chapman et al., 1987a, p. 81). Often their need to search for knowledge of birth parents is motivated by their concerns about identity, self-esteem, and connectedness. "Enough adoptees, men and women, have suffered from similar problems of confusion abut their identities that H. J. Sants has labeled this phenomenon 'genealogical bewilderment' "(Caplan, 1990, p. 82).

The fantasies that adoptees may develop about their birth parents can lead some of these children into identifying with these fantasized parents and acting out their (known or presumed) patterns of behavior, which can cause problems with their adoptive parents (Kaplan et al., 1994). A child, for example, through the process of identification with the fantasized image of a birth parent who engages in reckless behaviors might act out similar behaviors. Freeman and Freund (1998) emphasize that therapists who work with adopted clients must be alert to their fantasies about their birth mothers. Sometimes adoptees have kept their thoughts about birth mothers from adoptive parents to protect the adoptive parents. Although Freeman and Freund (1998) focus on the birth mother, a similar process can be at work regarding the birth father. The authors note that this material is often overlooked: "the birth parent is often a neglected party in psychotherapy with adoptees . . . often appears in the material if therapists are listening . . . to meet pressing needs at a particular time. . . . The mental representations . . . are constructed around whatever information is available" (Freeman and

Freund, 1998, p. 26). These "ghosts" serve many functions in the inner world of the adopted child; they may emerge in treatment, and their walled-off character gradually dissolve, allowing corrective revision to occur (Freeman and Freund, 1998, p. 28).

It should also be noted that such fantasies may be present even if information is available, and that fantasies of having parents other than one's actual parents are not uncommon in nonadopted children.

Huse (1989) sees the need for adoptees to search for their birth parents "in a normative context," and recommends that "adoption agencies provide all available *nonidentifying* [italics added] information to adoptees, including information about the parents, the reason for surrender, and family medical history. This information should be shared in a supportive manner and the *social worker* [italics added] should be available" (p. v). She notes that if there is mutual interest, a face-to-face meeting between the child and birth parents might take place.

One motivating factor for adoptees to learn their identity is their fear of becoming involved in incest. McRoy and colleagues (1988) note that there were "several documented cases of unwitting incest, including a son who unknowingly married his mother and a brother who married his half-sister. In 1960, Israel passed an open-records law primarily to avert such disasters" (p. 8). In addition, more is known today about genetics and its role in matters of health and disease; seeking past birth parent records can lead to learning about the birth family's medical history.

As we move away from traditional adoption to examine nontraditional forms, other complexities emerge. In interracial and international adoptions, adoptees may need to adapt to parents who are dissimilar in racial characteristics and who represent a dissimilar culture. Adoptees may need to deal with "looking different" from and perhaps "feeling different" from their adoptive families. Children who have been adopted by gay or lesbian parents may have to deal with discriminatory behaviors from other children and adults.

Perhaps the most complex adoption issues involve those children who have been removed from families they have known and who have been adopted when they are older. Many such adoptions are court ordered and the children involved are likely to have experienced problems of neglect and physical and/or sexual abuse; often they have transitioned through several different placements. Many have waited for long periods to be adopted because of "special needs," such as emotional and behavioral problems, retardation, autism, and physical handicaps, including AIDS.

Children who have been sexually abused often develop serious behavioral disturbances (including sexual acting out) that adoptive parents may not be able to deal with, resulting in termination of the adoption process *(adoption disruption)* or the finalized adoption *(adoption dissolution)*.

"Among special-needs adoption placements, the proportion of children who are victims of sexual abuse has been reported to be as high as 86 percent" (Smith and Howard, 1994, p. 491). A sexual abuse history is not always known prior to the adoption process; it can be discovered later through examining the causes of a child's behavior. "A number of children kept their sexual abuse secret for years" (Smith and Howard, 1994, p. 496).

Because of conflictual feelings relating to loss, betrayal, loyalty, and anger, children who have ties to their birth families may find it hard to accept adoption and attachment to new people; this is even more the case for the sexually abused child.

> For some children, the sexual abuse trauma seemed to intensify their difficulties in separating from birth parents. These children had intensified loyalties, fears, and other feelings stemming from sexual abuse experiences with their parents that they had never received help in working through. These feelings interfered with the children's resolution of separation issues and with the capacity to attach to the new adoptive family.
>
> For other children, the emotional demands of attaching to adoptive parents, trusting, and yielding control in some ways brought about a resurgence of long-submerged issues related to sexual abuse. Failure to resolve sexual abuse issues may affect the child by intensifying behavior problems or creating increased resistance to attachment. In addition, the adoptive parents' ability to deal with the knowledge of a child's sexual abuse and sexual behaviors also affects the child's acceptance and adjustment in adoptive placement. (Smith and Howard, 1994, p. 499)

Today, increasing numbers of children in the child welfare system have serious emotional problems, greatly taxing this system (Dore, 1999). Many are "recycled" through the foster home system and are often terminated from both foster and adoptive homes. Critical comprehensive and integrated social and mental health services for these children are often lacking (Dore, 1999; Shonkoff et al., 2000).

The Adoptive Parents

An adopted child's birth parents have often been referred to as the child's natural parents. How does this, then, define adoptive parents, who strive to become comfortable with their child who is not their child? The common fertility crisis (that is, the adoptive parents' feelings of loss, grief, and disappointment about not being able to conceive their own birth children) must be resolved before they can accept someone's else's child instead of the child they were unable to bring into the world. Adoptive parents can feel varying degrees of comfort or discomfort about their adoptive roles.

> The adoptive parent may be concerned about his entitlement to the child, possibly feeling somewhat equivocal about the completeness of his relationship to the child. There is a feeling that a social-emotional relationship is less binding, more fragile, than the relationship between biological parent and child in which the social-emotional component is reinforced by the mutual bond of blood. The problem for the adoptive parents is that of really feeling the child "belongs" to them. (Kadushin, 1974, p. 544)

Any sign that their children are having developmental problems or have curiosity about their birth parents can engender great insecurity in some parents. DiGiulio (1987) found that adoptive parents who could be comfortable with their roles and differences from the birth parents were more comfortable in helping children talk about and obtain information about their birth parents.

Parents in nontraditional adoptions often face additional complexities in the adoption process. Gay and lesbian applicants for adoptive parenthood are often denied children on the basis of their sexuality, at the discretion of child welfare personnel and judges (Crawford, 1999). Generally, single gay and lesbian adults have been having greater success in being accepted as adoptive parents; "for same-sex couples, however, it is another matter entirely" (Crawford, 1999, p. 272). Vermont's Supreme Court decision to give equal protections for same-sex couples mentioned previously (Goldberg, 1999e, p. A1) might be one step toward liberalizing adoption policy for this group.

Some who have adopted children privately (without a social agency's study and placement process) may find later that their children have unanticipated serious physical and/or emotional and behavioral difficulties; this can lead to adoption dissolution. In addition, those who knowingly adopt special needs children may find themselves overwhelmed; postplacement services from social workers have been critical in aiding adjustment and decreasing adoption dissolution.

Open Adoption: Pros and Cons

Pannor and Baran (1984) defined open adoption as a "process in which the birth parents and the adoptive parents meet and exchange identifying information" (p. 246); the former "relinquish legal and basic child rearing rights" to the latter (p. 246); all "retain the right to continuing contact and access to knowledge on behalf of the child" (p. 246). A continuum of options for implementation has developed; openness can range from the birth parents having input into the selection of adoptive parents for their child, to exchanging letters and pictures with the adoptive family (through the agency), to a face-to-face meeting with the adoptive parents.

McRoy and colleagues (1988) note a "growing controversy over openness in the adoptions practice for two main reasons. First, there is no consensus among adoption professionals as to what openness or open placement means. Second, the practice of open placement is relatively new and its impact on members of the adoptive triad . . . has not been adequately addressed by research" (p. 18). Arguments are advanced for and against open adoption, a procedure that can affect all three members of the adoption triangle.

Chapman and colleagues (1986), who advocate open adoption, see it as benefiting birth mothers, since they have found that birth mothers are greatly reassured when they have taken part in planning for the adoption knowing that they will have continuing access to information (p. 206); this experience can diminish the pain of the mother's loss. Openness can be extended to the birth father and extended birth family as well. Confidentiality can be maintained and negotiated. Barth (1994) argues that many adolescent mothers might relinquish their babies more readily if open adoption were available to them.

William Pierce (Caplan, 1990) strongly opposes open adoption, contending that it is "'very dangerous, tragic, and disastrous'" for birth mothers (p. 86). He argues that:

> You can give up your child without needing to separate from him, and "have it both ways." . . . Birth mothers don't view their child as lost, don't mourn the loss, and however positive the recognition they enjoy for their instrumental role in the adoption, they fail to move on with their lives. (Caplan, 1990, p. 89)

In addition, the birthmother may seek "a new set of parents in the adoptive parents. Often she expects to have a role in the family, like an Aunt, a baby-sitter, a sister, or a godmother, and doesn't face the fact that she has given up the child" (Caplan, 1990, p. 89).

It has been argued that open adoptions can help the child feel more secure and enhance a well-integrated sense of identity; the child may feel less rejected by the birth parents (Pannor and Baran, 1984). However, "contact with his birth mother can backfire, inflating his sense of rejection by her and raising anxieties about her taking him back or about his adoptive parents abandoning him, too" (Caplan, 1990 p. 89). There are also "risks of 'serious interference' [with the adopted child] at every stage of development. An open adoption is likely to leave him feeling more like a foster child" (Caplan, 1990, pp. 89-90).

Many adoptive parents are fearful that birth parents may reappear, and that their adoptive children might rejoin them. "This albatross is carried [by adoptive parents] well into the child's adulthood and is demonstrated through insecure possessiveness and ongoing anxiety. In sharp contrast, we witness comfort in the adoptive parents who experience openness with continued contact with the birthmother" (Chapman et al., 1987b, p. 10). Disagreeing, Pierce values the "sense of entitlement" that the adoptive parents feel in closed adoption, as opposed to "inevitable sharing of that responsibility with the birth mother" (Caplan, 1990, p. 93).

Decisions about open adoption are further complicated when older children who have ties to their birth and/or former foster families are adopted. Should all past ties be severed? Today, there is generally more openness about adoption than in the past, although people accept openness to varying degrees. Clearly a need exists for further research on the subject.

International Adoptions

Impelled by the fertility crisis and the scarcity of adoptable infants, many people are turning to transracial and transcultural adoptions within this country and also to international adoptions. Together, these adoptions comprise about 14 percent of U.S. adoptions (Vonk et al., 1999), although the majority of this 14 percent group represent international adoptions. "Children . . . are adopted from . . . Latin American, Eastern European, and Asian countries. . . . The number of children adopted from other countries has grown . . . from about eight thousand in 1989 to almost 16,000 in 1998" (p. 496).

Studies of intercountry adoptions have indicated that the majority of these children have adapted well to their new lives and new families (Vonk et al., 1999). Vonk and colleagues note that according to Tizard (1991), of the adoptees: "75-80 percent . . . function . . . with no more behavioral and educational problems . . . than other children" (p. 501).

Studies of these adoptive parents reveal a high degree of satisfaction with their adoptive children and their adjustment (Vonk et al., 1999). Little is known about the effects of intercountry adoptions on the birth parents, especially in countries such as the People's Republic of China, where the birth parents are often unknown. This is due to the government's one-child policy. Parents often abandon daughters (hoping for a son) and sons who are born with handicaps; these children wind up in orphanages, from which some are adopted. This parental anonymity impedes the gathering of genetic and birth histories as well as of birth family narratives to present to adopted children.

International adoptions remain a controversial issue both here and abroad. Critics have argued that adopted children are coming from countries that are in effect being despoiled of their homeless children and thus deprived of the possibility of providing indigenous resources for them; they are "exploited, victimized through colonialism, and perhaps prevented from finding internal alternative solutions for homeless children" (Vonk et al., 1999, p. 502).

Children placed in a different culture may also be exposed to discrimination and have difficulty integrating a racial and cultural identity (Vonk et al., 1999). European-American adoptive parents, who have never themselves experienced racism, may encounter it in relation to their adopted children; they "find themselves for the first time at the receiving end of racism or bigotry vis a vis their children" (Vonk et al., 1999, p. 504).

Vonk and colleagues (1999) emphasize the lack of research on the well-being of children who were not adopted from institutions in which they continued to live; they are not convinced that an adopted child would have done better if left in institutions: "it is difficult to argue that long-term institutionalized care produces a better outcome for an individual child than adoption" (p. 501). Additionally, nonadopted orphaned children are not immune to other forms of prejudicial discrimination in various countries (Vonk et al., 1999, p. 501).

Many adoptive parents attempt to foster cultural pride in their children, and some have taken specific steps to promote their children's cultural identities, including joining support groups of other transracial adoptive families. A wide range of services providing support, Korean culture, and even trips to Korea, are available to Korean adoptees (Lewin, 1998b). Camp Tiger, in Minnesota, is designed for adopted Korean teenagers. Campers reported that the most important part of being there was their involvement with other Korean teens. Camps and day programs have also been established for adopted children from Romania, Russia, and China (Lewin, 1998b).

The last point to be considered is whether a given international adoption is legal and carried out by sanctioned social agencies, or whether it is independent and/or illegal. In the adoptions of Chinese children described by Vonk and colleages (1999), adoptions were legally authorized and followed guidelines, including social work studies of prospective adoptive parents. By contrast, when Romanian children were initially adopted in the United States from orphanages, no regulated adoption practice existed, and many adoptions were highly problematic (Johnson et al., 1993).

Serious legal abuses, such as the kidnapping and selling of Latin American children to adoptive parents in this country, have occurred (Vonk et al., 1999). It is not uncommon for lawyers to offer money (which they never pay) to poor Mexican women to buy their children (Thompson, 1999a). In one case, three people were charged with running a Mexican baby smuggling ring and selling babies to New York couples who, unaware of the illegalities, paid $20,000 or more for each baby (Halbfinger, 1999).

> Prosecutors have not yet determined whether the 17 children brought through Agua Prieta, one of the chief smuggling points along the Mexican border, were stolen from their families, turned over for adoption voluntarily or sold by one or both of their parents.
> Several of the adoptive parents, who the authorities say were duped by the three defendants, said they had been emotionally devastated by the experience. (Halbfinger, 1999, p. A25)

According to Unicef ("Intercountry Adoption," 1999), the Hague Adoption Convention of 1993, recognizing that

> intercountry adoption may offer the advantage of a permanent family to a child for whom a suitable family cannot be found in his or her State of Origin . . . sets out the following hierarchy of options, generally held to safeguard the long-term "best interests" of the child: . . . family solutions (return to the birth family, foster care, adoption) should generally be preferred to institutional placement . . . permanent solutions (return to the birth family, adoption) should be preferred to provisional ones (institutional placement, foster care) . . . national solutions (return to birth family, national adoption) should be preferred to international ones (intercountry adoption). (p. 5)

Interracial Adoptions

Interracial adoptions are controversial; disputes regarding racial integration or separation are found in the sensitive arena of adoption. Many feel that interracial adoptions are compatible with our increasingly multicultural society. One white adoptive mother (with one black and two Hispanic daughters) deeply valued the family's diversity (Lewin, 1998b). According to the National Adoption Information Clearinghouse (1999), neither the gender nor the race of the child, per se, have a significant effect on adoption disruption.

On the other hand, race strongly influences the "adoption marketplace, as witness the bald fact that white children usually cost more than black children, and that in the world of international adoptions, Africa is almost ignored" (Lewin, 1998b, p. A18). Many people of black African descent are also opposed to interracial adoptions. In 1972, for example, the National Association of Black Social Workers asserted that "placing black children in white homes was a form of racial and cultural genocide" (Lewin, 1998b, p. A18). Opponents of interracial adoptions assert that they add to identity conflicts for children and increase the risk of social rejection and that insufficient attempts have been made to recruit potential black adoptive parents (Hollingsworth, 1998).

Adoption practices had supported placements in which adopted children and adoptive parents were of the same race until Congress became aware that "approximately 500,000 children were in foster care in the United States and that tens of thousands of these children were waiting for adoptive homes. Children wait a median of two years and eight months to be adopted, and studies indicated that African American children wait longer than other children" (Brooks et al., 1999, p. 169). The Multiethnic Placement Act of 1994 was passed by Congress, stating that it is now illegal to use "race categorically or presumptively to delay or deny adoptive or foster placements" (Brooks et al., 1999, p. 167); the law also stressed the importance of recruiting more minority families to adopt children.

In 1996, this law was replaced by a new law, Removal of Barriers to Interethnic Adoption; this altered aspects of the first law (Brooks et al., 1999, p. 170) and also imposed sanctions against violators. The requirement for recruitment of minority adoptive families remained. Although placement cannot be delayed on the basis of race, culture, or ethnicity, a provision appeared mandating that these factors might be considered "based on concerns arising from the circumstances of the individual case" (Brooks et al., 1999, p. 171). Difficult to interpret, these laws give insufficient guidance for implementation.

> Child welfare workers still will have to make decisions about the importance of race in the life of an individual child and whether there are reasons that the best interests of the child requires consideration of race. The elimination of [the first law's] provision specifying when race is a permissible factor could leave even more discretion to child welfare professionals. Child welfare professionals, like others, may have personal views that will affect the way they implement the law. (Brooks et al., 1999, p. 171)

A separate law pertains exclusively to Native American children, the United States Indian Child Welfare Act of 1978; its purpose was to "stop the practice of separating large numbers of Indian children from their families and tribes through adoption or foster-care placement, usually in non-Native American homes" (Goldstein and Goldstein, 1996, p. 47).

Racial matching, per se, might not be the principal stumbling block to rapid adoption placement, as other factors also intervene: "searches for missing parents, crowded court dockets . . . lengthy appeals, lack of resources, high caseloads . . . and the limitations of adoption assistance and other postadoption support" (Brooks et al., 1999, p. 172).

Subjective impressions of biracial adoptions can vary among adoptees and adoptive parents. Two twenty-seven-year-old women, for example, were interviewed about their perceptions of their own interracial adoptions. Each had one black and one white birth parent; both were adopted by white families as infants. "But in their strongly opposing views, they almost embody the whole debate over transracial adoption" (Lewin, 1998d, p. A19). For example, one tended to see the experience and the practice in generally positive terms, as beneficial to society, while the other in earlier years experienced much discomfort with respect to racial identity but seemed to become more accepting of her own and her family's situation when she visited Africa while in college (Lewin, 1998b, p. A19). " 'It was a turning point for me, the first time I felt part of something,' she said" (Lewin, 1998b, p. A19).

Although any adoption presents complex dilemmas, the world of foster care involves even greater complexities and uncertainties for its participants.

Foster Care

Although some foster children, such as Seneca in Toni Morrison's (1999) novel *Paradise* (referred to in Chapter 3), adapt by developing a false compliant self, many foster children do not comply and instead act out their feelings of confusion and rejection in such a manner as to incur overt rejection from the foster family, often leading to placement dissolution.

Foster children have been removed from their own birth families, sometimes at the request of their families; sometimes by courts. Often their lives have been complicated by neglect and/or physical and/or sexual abuse; they may have physical or psychological disabilities, and their parents may have problems with mental illness and/or substance abuse. "It is estimated that currently 50 percent to 80 percent of children who enter the child welfare system do so because of familial substance abuse" (Dore, 1999, p. 10).

The loss of their birth families, their homes, and their neighborhoods can be devastating. "All foster children struggle with the need to make sense of placement in the least hurtful way possible. The loss of home and family is a deeply wounding experience, and it must be explained and fully mourned before the foster child can begin to plan for the future. . . . A primary question posed by placement is: 'How come you can't stay with your own family?' " (Levine, 1990, p. 53).

Foster children often need to blame someone for their removal from their homes; often they blame themselves to retain the belief that their parents will come back for them and to deny that the parents are to blame. Foster children may have difficulty attaching to their foster families because of a pattern of insecure attachments; they may also feel that loving their foster parents is a betrayal of their birth parents. The often "punishing" rejection of the foster

parents and overt aggression directed toward them by the child can be a difficult burden for the foster parents to accept. "It is a little-understood and perverse fact of any foster parent's life that normal nurturing can become a constant reminder for some placed children and adolescents of their own parents'
failures. The very acts the foster parents believe will comfort and aid a foster
child may only increase pain" (Levine, 1990, pp. 61-62).

Children entering foster care today often have serious emotional problems related to the multitude of traumatic experiences encountered prior to
placement.

> There is informal consensus . . . that children entering out-of-home
> care now are more disturbed than in times past. . . . These highly dis-
> turbed children place great demands on the child welfare system.
> They disrupt placements and burn out foster parents and caseworkers
> alike. They require the most expensive, most intensive forms of care,
> thereby consuming a much greater proportion of system resources
> than their less disturbed peers. And, family reunification is less likely
> for youth with serious emotional disturbances, thereby insuring that
> they will age out, or more probable, break out of the child welfare sys-
> tem into the juvenile justice system, into adult prisons or jails, or into
> mental hospitals and institutions. Already studies have found that
> many adults who are homeless and mentally ill spent time in their
> early years in foster care. (Dore, 1999, pp. 7-8)

Therapeutic foster homes are in short supply. "Studies of placement
breakdown have repeatedly identified *foster parents' inability to manage
difficult child behavior as a key factor contributing to placement disruption*" [italics added] (Dore, 1999, p. 22). More intensive social work intervention with foster families is a major need; "collaboration across the child
welfare and mental health systems is imperative" (Dore, 1999, p. 23).

Kinship Foster Families

Kinship foster care, in which a child is placed with relatives, has the potential for providing better continuity of care, as the child remains in familiar surroundings with extended family members and may have access to
parents. The Child Welfare League reported in 1992 that "31 percent of all
children placed out of their birth parents' home are in relative care" (Henry,
1999, p. 562).

Kinship care is especially prevalent in communities of color and, "in
most instances, kinship foster parents are grandparents or great aunts or un-
cles" (Hollingsworth, 1998, p. 111). Some writers, opposed to prolonged
kinship care, note that it often slows down or actually prevents many chil-

dren in these placements from being adopted, but Hollingsworth asserts that kinship care is a form of permanency, even if formal adoptions do not occur.

> Thornton (1991) found that kinship foster parents were not interested in adopting the children in their care. Even when they were aware of available adoption subsidies, 85 percent of kinship foster parents stated that they would not adopt. . . .
> The reluctance to adopt formally among African American kinship foster caregivers is based in cultural definitions of family and attitudes about family relationships. For example, the reason given by 70 percent of kinship foster parents for their unwillingness to adopt was that they already considered the child and themselves as being a part of the same family and that it was therefore unnecessary to adopt and would be confusing to the child (Thornton, 1991). They were content to maintain a grandparent-to-grandchild caregiving relationship. . . . Also, 30 percent of kinship foster parents were concerned that adopting the child formally would result in conflict in their relationship with the child's biological parents. (Hollingsworth, 1998, p. 111)

O'Donnell (1999) raises concern about the lack of attention to the role the father plays in kinship care and finds in general that "child welfare literature has been conspicuously silent about fathers of color. With the exception of services for unwed adolescent fathers, the literature does not address whether or how African American fathers participate in social services intervention on behalf of their children" (O'Donnell, 1999, p. 429). Levine (1993) made a similar point, noting that only recently have Head Start programs, which have traditionally worked with mothers, "discovered men" (p. 4).

O'Donnell (1999) observed that even when children were placed with paternal relatives, "African American fathers in two kinship foster care programs seldom participated in interventions on behalf of their children and that caseworkers rarely engaged fathers in discussions that might lead to participation" (O'Donnell, 1999, p. 436); when caseworkers talked to the kinship foster family, they appeared "to have been no more disposed than the caseworker to talk about the father" (p. 437). O'Donnell (1999) contends that the child welfare system can "maximize support" to children "by reaching out to fathers . . . along a continuum of involvement" (p. 439).

> Many of the fathers themselves presented very difficult problems that would reduce their availability to the caseworker. More than one-third of the fathers was reported to have used drugs or alcohol, and the actual prevalence may have been higher. Sixteen percent of the fathers were either in jail or had a history of incarceration. Because all of the children in the study were from the inner city, it is reasonable to as-

sume that many of the fathers experienced poverty, unemployment, and unstable housing. Fathers' perceptions of and attitudes toward the caseworkers and the child welfare system also may have contributed to the low level of paternal involvement. (O'Donnell, 1999, p. 437)

Grandparents raising grandchildren. An increasing number of grandparents today have primary responsibility for the care of their grandchildren. "According to a report released by the U.S. Census Bureau in July [1999], grandparents are raising their children's children in more than 2.5 million households. . . . Approximately four million children live with grandparents" (Beaucar, 1999c, p. 12). This is due primarily to child neglect, often related to parental substance abuse (fueled additionally by the crack-cocaine epidemic). Other common causes of grandparents caring for their grandchildren include "parental death due to AIDS, incarceration, and mental illness" (Whitley et al., 1999, p. 112) and responsibility for the babies of teenage mothers (Landers, 1992).

The burden of caring for young and often disturbed grandchildren have placed many grandparents under considerable stress, especially given their advanced age; some have developed stress-related health problems (Beaucar, 1999c; Whitley et al., 1999), and many have reported financial problems. Various services have been developed to help this population: support groups (Landers, 1992; Beaucar, 1999c); community-based interdisciplinary interventions (Whitley et al., 1999); and special housing projects such as GrandFamilies House in Boston (Dowdy, 1998).

Grandparents in some states are unable to secure legal custody or foster care status, depriving them of "health care, food stamps and cash assistance to raise their grandchildren, and in 14 states [they] are being targeted for the child support payments their own children have failed to make" (Beaucar, 1999c, p. 12).

Grandparenting is one of the most prevalent forms of kinship care, especially in African American (Beaucar, 1999c; Hollingsworth, 1998) and Latino communities (Burnette, 1999). In one study of seventy-four Latino grandparent caregivers in New York City, it was discovered that "only 6 percent of Latino grandparents . . . were in the formal kinship foster care system" (Burnette, 1999, p. 23). Those grandparents who were providing "informal care" were not receiving the support and services of those in the "formal" system and lacked knowledge about available services: "targeting and coordinating efforts in local communities" on their behalf has been recommended (Burnette, 1999, p. 32).

SYSTEMIC ISSUES IN CHILD WELFARE

The child welfare field is faced by multiple pressures, including an increased demand for services for children with serious emotional problems

(Dore, 1999). Although model child welfare projects operate, this is not the prevailing picture. Funding and bureaucratic problems, long endemic in child welfare, persist, including high caseloads, low salaries for social workers, and high staff turnover (Beaucar, 1999b). The lack of "professionally educated caseworkers in child welfare agencies is a continuing problem" (O'Donnell, 1999, pp. 438-439).

Child welfare workers often experience burnout, due to clinical and organizational stressors, including: the need to make difficult placement decisions; feeling ineffectual; overidentifying with fragile and traumatized clients; and working with violent, threatening people (Dane, 2000). Child welfare workers are subject to *vicarious traumatization,* a syndrome endured by many clinicians working with trauma victims (Dane, 2000), as though they themselves are directly traumatized through exposure to the client's reported experiences. The symptoms of vicarious traumatization include: "decreased sense of energy . . . social withdrawal . . . increased sensitivity to violence, fear . . . and hopelessness" (Dane, 2000, p. 29).

The juvenile courts, which make determinations of serious child abuse or neglect and mandate protective services, are often a nexus of serious systemic problems (Liederman, 1995). "Like the child welfare system, the juvenile court system has experienced a caseload crisis and has been under intense pressure in its handling of child abuse and neglect cases. . . . Court hearings have become more frequent and more complex over the last several years, as the role of the court has grown" (Liederman, 1995, p. 431).

Managed care, with its cutbacks on mental health and substance abuse services, has had a serious impact on parents and children in need of long-term intensive services. According to a report of the surgeon general of the United States, the reduction of psychiatric hospital stays and emphasis on "short-term outpatient therapy, have not worked well for emotionally disturbed children from low-income families on Medicaid. Indeed, [the report] says, Medicaid may be simply shifting costs to child welfare and juvenile justice agencies" (Pear, 1999a, p. A26).

Case Illustration

The reported case of Matthew illustrates how one child's life and psychological development were affected by his traumatic experiences with his birth mother, the uncertainty about the permanency of his foster placement, and the systemic problems he encountered with the child welfare system (Paret and Shapiro, 1998). The fact that Matthew's birth family is "Hispanic and poor, his foster mother Caucasian and middle class" (Paret and Shapiro, 1998, p. 302), at times influenced custody decisions.

When Matthew was six weeks old, the police, who suspected that his single mother was selling drugs, removed him and his brother from their home because the house was "'filthy'" and "'unsafe.'" Matthews mother, Ms. Rivers, was no longer involved with Matthew's father "and could not even provide his [the father's] name" (Paret and Shapiro, 1998, p. 306). She promised to attend a drug rehabilitation program; the next day Matthew was returned to her. When Matthew was thirteen months old, Ms. River, feeling stressed, requested inpatient drug treatment.

> Matthew was placed with a foster mother, Ms. Smith, for the first time. At the time of placement the caseworker described Matthew as "ill, dirty, frightened, and developmentally lagging." The foster mother noted that, although it was February, Matthew was dressed in a lightweight summer jacket and wore no socks. When Ms. Smith put him in the high chair and started to prepare food, tears poured down his face, but he did not make a sound. The silent crying continued on and off for a few days. Matthew gradually responded to her care and allowed her to feed, bathe, rock, and comfort him. This fragile homeostasis often broke down; he would suddenly become angry, yell, and repeatedly hit a doll on the head with his fist. Ms. Smith thought he might be re-enacting something he had seen or experienced. (Paret and Shapiro, 1998, p. 304)

During the two months Matthew stayed with Ms. Smith, he began to develop language, was emotionally responsive, and seemed happy. He was then returned to his birth mother, who had finished her drug program. But the situation remained unstable: she was resistant to services, and "the severity of Ms. Rivers' psychological impairment and vulnerability became more evident" (Paret and Shapiro, 1998, p. 305). Ms. Rivers' own childhood had been traumatic; her mother had been schizophrenic and Ms. Rivers was a foster child with one family for ten years, when she then began a life of shifting back and forth among groups homes, shelters, and hospitals. As an older adolescent, she became addicted to drugs.

Matthew was returned to Ms. Smith when he was eighteen months old, and his unstable situation persisted for the next five years, as he moved back and forth between his birth mother and his foster mother. "Whenever Matthew left his foster mother for visits with his birth mother he regressed and was frightened, angry, and clinging upon his return. The psychological intensity of these transitions did not diminish over time" (Paret and Shapiro, 1998, p. 305). Matthew lived mostly with his foster mother for the next three years; a consulting psychologist then recommended that Matthew be returned to his birth mother.

> This consultant, Dr. Morris, described her plan as a "high-risk reunification." *Her decision was influenced by the dominant case law in the state, which was biased in favor of returning children to their biologi-*

cal parents [italics added]. She believed that the case law superseded the issues presented by other psychologists in the past, who had stressed the quality and valence of Matthew's attachment to his foster mother. . . . Dr. Morris believed that Matthew had the "resiliency" (Rutter, 1990) to handle the loss of his foster mother. (Paret and Shapiro, 1998, p. 307)

In the meantime, Matthew exhibited serious symptoms after his mandated overnight visits to his birth mother. "Matthew was having nightmares, wetting himself day and night, and was afraid to be alone in a room. In anticipation of each visit to his birth mother, he became defiant and upset, crying throughout the two-hour trip with the state social worker" (p. 307).

At this point in time, Ms. Smith requested therapy for Matthew, now four, to help him with the planned reunification. The therapist soon understood "his reactions to the actual danger and volatile realities of his life and brought these new observations to the attention of the authorities" (Paret and Shapiro, 1998, p. 309). The court then ordered the overnight visits to stop, but he continued to visit in the daytime. The case was brought for review to the psychologist, Dr. Morris, "who took account of the new information" (p. 311) but reiterated her former position. She asserted that reunification "would not be too damaging to him if his birth mother would seriously engage in treatment and create a stable home" (p. 311).

Ms. Rivers was not able to involve herself in therapy. In the meantime, Matthew's behavior deteriorated further. In addition to her inconsistent and sometimes harsh treatment of him, Ms. Rivers began making "veiled threats to abduct him, and supervised visits were ordered by the court" (Paret and Shapiro, 1998, p. 312).

Dr. Morris reversed her opinion when Matthew was five; she now approved his adoption by Ms. Smith.

> *Dr. Morris hoped that a voluntary open adoption could be arranged* [italics added]. . . . Ms. Rivers could not accept the idea of limited supervised visits and rejected this adoption plan. The agency now recommended that her parental rights be severed. . . . *It took almost two more years for the court to hear the case, make the decision to terminate Ms. River's parental rights, and complete the adoption process* [italics added]. Matthew remained with Ms. Smith during this period. (Paret and Shapiro, 1998, p. 312)

Prior to the trial, Matthew was evaluated by two "independent mental health professionals" (p. 312). Ms. Rivers' lawyer chose a psychologist *"well known for his views that children should remain with their biological mothers, especially in cross-racial situations"* [italics added] (Paret and

Shapiro, 1998, p. 312). During the evaluation, which lasted four months, Matthew was upset and again regressed. "His lack of autonomy was infuriating to him. 'I keep telling and telling, I want to stay with Ms. Smith!' he said to his evaluators" (p. 314). After the evaluations it was another six months before the judge made the decision to allow adoption by Ms. Smith; Matthew was now six-and-a-half years old. The adoption papers were signed when Matthew was nearly seven; this was initially a happy time for him, but then a resurgence of insecure feelings followed.

> Matthew was ecstatic when he learned of the judge's decision to allow his adoption by Ms. Smith. He was radiant when he told the news to the therapist, and at home he shouted out the window to the neighborhood that he was gong to be adopted. He stopped wetting and soiling, and his most dangerous behavior abated. . . . But this quiescent period did not last. He remained extremely sensitive to perceived loss, danger, or narcissistic injury, and gains could be undone quickly, suggestive of Balint's (1968) idea of a basic fault. (Paret and Shapiro, 1998, p. 315)

Basic fault is defined as a deep-seated sense of insecurity resulting from an insecure attachment to the mother, which manifests itself in development of later relationships.

Matthew made progress in continuing therapy, but his early traumas and insecurities did not just "disappear," even when the permanency of his new home was established; "his psychological wounds do not heal easily" (Paret and Shapiro, 1998, p. 322). Although he was now free of his frightening visits to his birth mother, conflict, ambivalence, and guilt about her remained; "his own survival left him with feelings of guilt about Bobby [his brother] and Ms. Rivers and what he thought he might have done to them" (Paret and Shapiro, 1998, p. 318). He also talked about missing Bobby, who had remained at home with their mother during this time.

This case illustrates the importance of establishing permanence as soon as possible. Although Matthew had a very strong tie to his foster mother and did experience her attachment and deep commitment to him, he lived in perpetual fear that he would be removed from her and returned to his birth mother and a nightmare existence. Matthew was fortunate to have one consistent, caring foster mother; many children like Matthew experience disrupted placements, with multiple families.

Matthew was also fortunate to have long-term therapy, which is often not available to foster children. His therapist also provided support and guidance to Ms. Smith, his foster mother, who often felt overwhelmed and discouraged about his behavior. "The therapeutic relationship enabled her to endure her own grief and frustration" (Paret and Shapiro, 1998, p. 321).

When foster and adoptive parents receive supportive clinical services, placements are less likely to break down.

This case also highlights the problem of overworked courts dealing with child welfare cases; Matthew's case waited for two years before a hearing could be scheduled. Blindly applied case law influenced proceedings in two instances. In the first, the law "was biased toward the inherent rights of the birth mother"; and the consulting psychologist used this as the basis of her decision to have Matthew remain with his birth mother. While family preservation programs have proliferated, many with successful results, this is not necessarily the solution of choice for all families.

The second instance of case law involved the issue of cross-cultural adoption. Matthew did have some racial identity issues, which became apparent as he grew older; these issues often seemed intertwined with his basic struggle to find his own identity in relation to his two mothers (Paret and Shapiro, 1998, p. 316).

The case of Matthew depicts one child caught in the mechanisms of child welfare and legal systems unresponsive to his needs; but Matthew is only one child who has been given a face and a voice by his therapist and foster mother. Many children become "cases" to be transferred to overworked child welfare workers and go round and round through a revolving door of foster homes and shelters. Their problems are multifaceted, and comprehensive systemic programs that recognize the individuality of each child fall very short of meeting existing needs.

CONCLUSION

Because this chapter focuses on family problems, a skewed picture may emerge of family life being stressful, tumultuous, and unsuccessful. For many, this is unfortunately the case. However, for many others, the intimacy, loving, and caring of family life is a source of strength and joy; it provides meaning and direction in life. Vaillant (1993), in discussing resilience in adults, comments that many people in his study, who had unhappy childhoods and who were riding a life trajectory of failure, were able to enter into successful marriages and enjoy a secure family life; their capacity to do so enhanced both their functioning and pleasure in life.

The need for a special connectedness propels people into marriages or other committed relationships and into subsequent new relationships if the first fails. Adults who wish to have children but are unable to often experience deep anguish; they want a child to love and feel bereft if this possibility is excluded from their lives. Rejected or abandoned children whose own "recruitment" abilities (Kegan, 1982) are still intact try to attach themselves, in whatever way works, to adults who may be able to give them love or at least a token of affection.

When working with families who have problems with their relationships, it is helpful to have a perspective of what might be; to encourage and help people overcome as many psychological and social obstacles as possible to achieve whatever connectedness they may be capable of experiencing.

Children are deeply affected by family life—emotionally, cognitively, socially, and developmentally. Attachment and the disruption of attachments in family life have been discussed in this chapter; the developmental aspects of these events are discussed in greater detail in Chapters 8 and 9. This chapter has focused on the external structures of family life; the internal structures of family life, with their own systemic organizations, including rules, rituals, and boundary issues, are addressed in the following chapter.

LEARNING EXERCISE

1. In your small groups, discuss the biography (or autobiography) you are reading. Share your impressions, up to the point you have read, of the family structure as well as the family relationships described. In what ways do you feel the family organization and relationships are affecting the person whose life is depicted? What commonalities and differences do you find among the different family groupings and their impact on the key person?

SUGGESTED READINGS

Articles

Brooks, D., Barth, R. P., Bussiere, A., and Patterson, G. (1999). Adoption and race: Implementing the multiethnic placement act and the interethnic adoption provisions. *Social Work, 44,* 167-178.

Freeman, M. and Freund, W. (1998). Working with adopted clients. *Journal of Analytic Social Work, 5*(4), 25-37.

LaSala, M. (1998). Coupled gay men, parents, and in-laws: Intergenerational disapproval and the need for a thick skin. *Families in Society, 79,* 585-593.

O'Donnell, J. M. (1999). Involvement of African American fathers in kinship foster care services. *Social Work, 44,* 428-441.

Parks, C. A. (1998). Lesbian parenthood: A review of the literature. *American Journal of Orthopsychiatry, 68,* 376-389.

Books

Hartman, A. and Laird, J. (1983). *Family-centered social work practice.* New York: The Free Press.

Kressel, K. (1997). *The process of divorce: Helping couples negotiate settlements.* Northvale: Jason Aronson Inc.

Chapter 7

The Family: Internal Structures and Special Family Problems

. . . every complex organization must have more or less effective self-righting adjustments . . .

Walter B. Cannon

INTRODUCTION

In Chapter 6 we discussed the variety of family organizational forms existing today; we now turn our attention to the internal structures of family life. From a structural perspective, each family constructs its unique world, with its own rules, rituals, and internal alliances, negotiating its external boundaries with the outside world and its internal boundaries among its own members (Minuchin, 1974). The family is a self-contained system; changes in one part of the system produce corresponding changes in another part. Members "dance" to patterned steps and movements, ever in synchrony, if not in harmony with the others. In this world of transactional forces, if a family has a need to have one member "psychologically ill," and the sick person gets better (perhaps through the "intrusion" of an outsider, such as a psychotherapist), then the family finds another member to be the "sick" one.

The structural perspective does not concern itself about what is taking place within the individual psyches of its members (as does the psychodynamic perspective). If one family member is depressed, for example, the focus will not be on understanding the origins of that depression or on treating it, but on such questions as the role the depressed person plays in the family, how the depression creates problems in family communication, and the ways the depressed person might use the depression to manipulate family members. Depression would be viewed as an interpersonal response to the structural issues within the family.

It has been argued that it is not possible to integrate the systemic and psychodynamic approaches as they are too disparate (Hartman and Laird, 1983). The object relations perspective, however, is one integrative theory, focusing on both the present here-and-now relationships of family members in a transactional way, as well as each member's internal representations of self and significant others from the past; "we intervene at the microlevel of the interior of the family and its relation to the developing interiors of its individuals members" (Scharff and Scharff, 1987, p. 13). A father in a family, for example, might (through projective identification) act out past feelings related to being rejected by his parents in such a manner as to produce these rejections in the present by his provocative behaviors to his wife and the therapist. Rather than feeling and acting rejected and responding in a retaliatory manner, as the wife might (adding to the family dysfunction), the therapist would process these feelings internally, then share them constructively within the family. In this context, the therapist would bring the past to life to illuminate the present.

Intersubjectivity, a contribution from the object relations perspective, suggests that emotions can be transmitted from one person to another; this often occurs within a family. Parents exposed to social traumas, such as the Holocaust (Rosenbloom, 1983) and the massacres of Native Americans (Brave Heart, 1998), can indirectly transmit their anxieties about these events to their children who have never had these experiences and who may have never even been told about them.

Happiness and a joy for life can be transmitted to children by parents, as can troubling emotions and behaviors; parental depressive affect can be felt by a child (who may also be affected by parental withdrawal); intergenerational transmission of child maltreatment has been observed (Morton and Browne, 1998; Zeanah and Scheeringa, 1997). Maternal emotions can affect a child even before birth; complex hormonal interactions pass through the placenta. "Mothers with high anxiety levels are likely to produce babies who are hyperactive and irritable, have sleep disorders and low birth weight, and feed poorly" (Kaplan et al., 1994, p. 39).

Social work has traditionally taken a family perspective; individuals are viewed in the context of their families and social environments. However, many opinions are held, both within social work and in other mental health professions, as to how much emphasis should be given to the individual and how much to the family. At one extreme are clinicians who believe that the family should always be the unit of attention; others feel the focus of treatment should be the individual. Some clinicians view the family and individual in a comprehensive, integrative way; Moultrup (1981), for example, has stated that it is as risky for a family therapist to fail to deal with the individual as is the reverse for the individual therapist (p. 113). A multitude of theories and approaches also exist for working with families, even within a given theoretical approach. "Family therapy was, and still is, a wondrous Tower of Babel; people in it speak many different tongues" (Hoffman, 1981, p. 9).

Families change as the ages and developmental needs of their members change; the needs of an infant are different from those of a teenager, and family relationships and social lives are affected by these alterations. The developmental perspective emphasizes the importance of the family life cycle, which is "composed of a natural sequence of stages or periods" (Longres, 1995b, p. 297), encompassing such events as parents having children, children leaving home, parents aging, etc. Emphasis is placed on the transitions the family makes from one phase to the next, and it is postulated that when families have difficulties it is because of transitioning problems (Longres, 1995b), such as having to face the felt loss of children growing up.

One strength of the developmental model is the emphasis it places on the "*normative* [italics added] sources of stress" (Longres, 1995b, p. 298); that is, all families pass through these stages. Disagreement, however, exists about this model: no unanimity prevails on how many family developmental stages occur within the life cycle or on the tasks involved in successful transitions. This model is also criticized for its inability to accommodate to the diversity found in modern family life (Germain, 1991; Longres, 1995b). Some have suggested retaining the basic life development framework but adding other frequently occurring transitions, such as divorce and remarriage (Zastrow and Kirst-Ashman, 1997).

Germain (1991) proposes the transactional " '*life course model,*' " [italics added] which she finds preferable to the life cycle model, as it highlights "life transitions, life events, and other life issues as outcomes of person(s): environment *processes* [italics added] rather than as separate *segments of life* [italics added] confined to predetermined ages and stages of experience" (p. 149). This book acknowledges the importance of looking at the processes of life transitions and transactions with the environment, but these are incorporated as an inherent part of the biopsychosocial perspective.

I follow a *life development model* from infancy through old age, as universal issues must be considered, such as pregnancy, the child's maturational development, and aging; the biological aspects of life development are critical to this approach. The fetus unfolds in given stages of organ development, refinement, and growth; the maturational experience of children involves the development of locomotion, speech, and cognition along a given course (albeit with some variations, including compensatory mechanisms when physical impairments, such as blindness, appear); puberty and menopause are given physical events, although considerable variation is displayed in their physical manifestations, timing, and adaptation. Within this framework, we also consider the diversity of the variations of the timing of life events (such as becoming a mother of a newborn at age fifteen or at age forty-five) and the diversity of family organizations (such as being in a traditional or a blended family).

From an ecological perspective, the family is in constant interaction with its environment and is affected by (and often affecting) their social and cultural context. Social supports and social networks, for example, are important protective factors for families; blighted neighborhoods and community violence are risk factors. The biopsychosocial perspective of this book incorporates the ecological approach.

Special problems and *events* within families can profoundly affect all family members and can lead to the dissolution of the family itself. These problems encompass domestic violence, maltreatment of children, substance abuse, and mental illness and are addressed following a discussion of family structure, object relations theory, and the biopsychosocial perspective. This chapter ends with a discussion of alternative approaches to "formal" family therapy, such as psychoeducational intervention for families who have a schizophrenic member, divorce therapy and mediation, and intensive in-home treatment for families at risk, found in the family preservation model.

Physical illness (such as AIDS or heart disease) and disability of a child or parent (such as spinal cord injuries or blindness) also have serious impacts on family functioning; this will be discussed in Chapter 12.

STRUCTURAL THEORY

Minuchin (1974), a pioneer in the family therapy field, views family systems as an overarching concept: "a family is more than the individual biopsychodynamics of its members" (p. 89). He focuses on how families organize themselves and interact with their members, by means of *"transactional patterns"* [italics added] (Minuchin, 1974, p. 51).

> A family is a system that operates through transactional patterns. Repeated transactions establish patterns of how, when, and to whom to relate, and these patterns underpin the system. When a mother tells her child to drink his juice and he obeys, this interaction defines who she is in relation to him and who he is in relation to her, in that context and at that time. Repeated operations in these terms constitute a transactional pattern. (Minuchin, 1974, p. 51)

Minuchin (1974) refers to universal rules governing family organization, a concept highlighted by Hartman and Laird (1983). Different levels of rules exist; a family may have rules about eating between meals or completing homework. At another level rules also define who is in charge and the roles and functions of family members. However, the most important rules relate to the existence of the family system itself. Sometimes families have behaviors that may be incomprehensible to an outsider. What is important to understand is the purpose of this behavior, rather than its origins (Hartman and Laird, 1983, p. 36). If, for example, a couple is in therapy because of continual tension and friction, "the question is not why they are fighting, but how the fighting helps to maintain the system" (Hartman and Laird, 1983, p. 299). From this perspective, the fighting "is not the problem but rather an attempt at a solution, and it leads us to the question, 'then what *is* the problem'" (Hartman and Laird, 1983, p. 299)?

Families also have rules about rules, which are called *metarules* (Hartman and Laird, 1983, p. 301). These metarules tell family members whether they are free to discuss the rules themselves and whether the rules are subject to alteration. "In a very rigid, homeostatic family, there is a powerful metarule that rules may not be commented upon or altered" (Hartman and Laird, 1983, p. 301).

Rules determine the specific organizational patterns of a family, including the family's subsystems, which help the family define and perform its functions. Every family has multiple subsystems, and each member is usually part of several subsystems "in which he has different levels of power and where he learns differentiated skills. A man can be a son, nephew, older brother, younger brother, husband, father, and so on. In different subsystems, he enters into different complementary [reciprocal] relationships" (Minuchin, 1974, p. 52). Each subsystem has its own boundaries, which are the "rules defining who participates, and how" (Minuchin, 1974, p. 53).

> For example, the boundary of a parental subsystem is defined when a mother (M) tells her older child, "You aren't your brother's parent. If he is riding his bike in the street, tell me, and I will stop him." If the parental subsystem includes a parental child (PC), the boundary is defined by the mother's telling the children, "Until I get back from the store, Annie is in charge." (Minuchin, 1974, p. 53)

Hartman and Laird (1983) emphasize that clarity and flexibility are major aspects of boundaries. Clarity provides family members with "clear and unambivalent messages" about boundary rules (Hartman and Laird, 1983, p. 271). A child clearly understands that he or she is a child in the family, not a parent; or, conversely, the child may receive the message that he or she is a *parentified* child (that is, he or she must act as a parent to his or her parents). Clarity raises the question of whether these roles are clearly defined. If individuals receive mixed messages (without clarity) about their roles, so that they do not know if they will be rewarded or punished at any given time for the same behaviors, they will become confused and perplexed in an inconsistent world.

Flexibility allows for changes in boundary formation "in adaptive ways as the circumstances and needs of the family change" (Hartman and Laird, 1983, p. 271). As parents age, for example, if flexible boundaries exist, they will allow their adult children to assume more responsibility for them.

In examining the boundary formation of families, two extremes have been observed: *enmeshment,* which is an extreme degree of overinvolvement and blurring of boundaries, and *disengagement,* in which boundaries are very rigid, and family members have poor communication and maintain distance from each other. On this "continuum . . . most families fall within the wide normal range" (Minuchin, 1974, p. 54).

Hartman and Laird (1983) suggest questions to judge a family's degree of enmeshment: "Do family members speak for each other, or do they respect the fact that the other, even a child, may have separate views? . . . Are the parents overinvolved in every aspect or decision to be made in the child's life? Does the family tolerate differences, or must time, interests, opinions, and activities be shared?" (p. 272).

Nora, a middle-aged client, was involved in a family with a multi-generational history of enmeshment. Her background is replete with rejection and severe family dysfunction; she was a parentified child, mothering her younger siblings. In her current life, her enmeshment with her daughters and their boyfriends was compounded by reality problems with housing and money.

> Nora's two adult daughters, at different times, were living with their boyfriends in Nora's house (with Nora). No clear-cut agreements had been reached between them about household responsibilities and sharing rent with Nora. The daughters and their boyfriends expected Nora to do the housekeeping and cooking without their help or consistent financial contributions. Nora's daughter Charlotte had a boyfriend who was very disturbed; they were entangled in endless fights and chaos. Nora could not confront them nor could she ask them to leave. She complained, in her therapy, of increased headaches and depression.

When Nora was bequeathed an inheritance, she had an opportunity to invest the money, which would have been to her advantage as she had no assets; but she did not do this.

> Nora inherited some money from her mother. Then, because both daughters were having a financial crisis, she lent them a substantial amount of money, which they promised to repay but subsequently showed little inclination to return. This added to her own financial cri-

sis, and her feelings about this colored her relationship to her daughters.

Nora suffered much emotional abuse at the hands of family members, including her parents, such as their coldly critical attitudes toward her and blatant favoritism toward her siblings despite her efforts to gain their approval. It was extremely difficult for her to assert herself with them. In a rather unprecedented "generous" gesture, her father invited Nora and her children on a trip to an amusement park.

> Her family's behavior there embarrassed her, and she was especially mortified by her mother's inappropriate loud comments and bizarre behavior. The fact that Nora knew the workers at the park caused her further shame. Although the invitation implied that her father would be taking care of the expenses, in the end he backed out, leaving Nora to use most of her week's salary to pay the bill. This was followed by a long stay in bed with depression.

In assessing if families are *disengaged,* Hartman and Laird (1983) include the following questions: "Do family members seem impervious to or insensitive to one another? Do they block each other's communications or avoid close contact, either emotional or physical or both? Some families, as Bowen (1985) has pointed out, are characterized by an 'emotional divorce' between the parents . . . careful observation discloses that there is little or no affect or energy passing between them" (p. 272).

Clara, seventeen, was hospitalized on an inpatient psychiatric ward for a serious suicide attempt and anorexia nervosa (an eating disorder in which individuals literally "starve" themselves into a skeletal appearance based on the premise that they are too fat). Her parents were interviewed.

> Dr. G., Clara's father, looked bored and was impatient; he had surgical patients to attend to. Mrs. G. was distraught, worried about the confidentiality of this interview, and hoped her daughter's hospitalization could be kept secret; she was chagrined at the thought that her family and friends might know of this "disgrace." Dr. G. looked annoyed as Mrs. G. spoke and said that she should keep her mind on the main issue: Clara needs to be discharged from this place as soon as possible, so that she can complete her academic year and be eligible for a good college.

Triangles are discussed by structural theorists. Bowen (1985) emphasizes this organizing concept, which is important not only in understanding families but in "understanding the microscopic functioning of all emotional systems" (p. 478). The process of *triangulation* develops when a two-person system experiences tension, so they " 'triangle in' a third person" to relieve the tension in the system (p. 478). A classic example is the mother who, feeling uncomfortable in her relationship to her husband, forms a "close twosome" with her child, while "the father is the outsider" (Bowen, 1985, p. 479). In couples or family therapy, people often make the attempt to triangulate therapists into the family system; self-awareness on the therapists' part enables them to observe and utilize this phenomenon in treatment without allowing themselves to be drawn into it.

Although triangulation is a normative concept frequently occurring in all families, it can reach extreme forms.

> In triangulation each parent demands that the child side with him against the other parent. Whenever the child sides with one, he is automatically defined as attacking the other. In this highly dysfunctional structure, the child is paralyzed. Every movement he makes is defined by one parent as an attack. (Minuchin, 1974, p. 102)

A given triangulation might become a fixed pattern, or it can shift back and forth, as different alliances develop. Observing triangles "brings to light special alliances, shifting coalitions, and scapegoats" (Hartman and Laird, 1983, p. 284). Bowen (1985) describes how during great stress "a system will triangle in more and more outsiders" (p. 479). Frequently encountered is a family "in great stress that uses the triangle system to involve . . . a spectrum of outside people as participants in the family problem. The family thus reduces the tension within the inner family, and . . . the family tension is being fought out by outside people" (Bowen, 1985, p. 479).

One major emphasis running through many family theories relates to issues of separation and individuation, or differentiation. This seems consistent with Mahler and colleagues' (1975) theory of separation-individuation, but the systemic theorists and the object relations theorists look at differentiation through different lenses. Mahler and colleagues (1975) are concerned about the child's psychological development, the growth of ego functions, and the development of self and object representations. The family system thinkers, by and large, are not concerned with the inner states of individuals or the development of their ego functions; their focus is the system and how each individual is part of the whole; efforts are concentrated at systemic change, so that the family as a whole can develop and mature.

Bowen's (1985) concept of differentiation bridges the gap between psychodynamic and structural theories (Freed, 1985; Moultrup, 1981). Bowen observed that, generally, people with higher levels of differentiation cope better than those who are more fused with others and therefore have lower levels of differentiation. He sees this concept as the cornerstone of his theory. It categorizes individuals in accordance with

> the degree of *fusion,* or *differentiation,* between emotional and intel-
> lectual functioning. . . . It can be used as a way of categorizing all peo-
> ple on a single continuum. At the low extreme are those whose . . .
> lives are dominated by the automatic emotional system . . . who are
> less flexible, less adaptable, and more emotionally dependent . . . eas-
> ily stressed into dysfunction. . . . They inherit a high percentage of all
> human problems.
>   At the other extreme are those who are more differentiated . . .
> whose intellectual functioning can retain relative autonomy in periods
> of stress . . . more flexible, more adaptable, and more independent of
> the emotionality about them. . . . They are remarkably free of human
> problems. (Bowen, 1985, p. 362)

Bowen, in his definition of differentiation, highlights the difference between intellectual and emotional functioning, which emphasizes the ego
functions of impulse control and cognitive skills. This discussion of differentiation appears removed from the concept of *identity consolidation.* Yet
Bowen (1985) approaches the concept of differentiation related to identity
more closely when he adds that "another important part of the differentiation of self has to do with the levels of *solid self* and the *pseudo-self* in a person" (p. 364). Although Bowen still places emphasis on intellectual and
emotional functioning, he observes that "the level of solid self is stable. The
pseudo-self is unstable, and it responds to a variety of social pressures and
stimuli. The pseudo-self was acquired at the behest of the relationship system, and it is negotiable in the relationship system" (Bowen, 1985, p. 366).

People with a pseudo-self develop as "dependent appendages of their
parents, following which they seek other equally *dependent relationships in
which they can borrow enough strength to function*" [italics added] (Bowen,
1985, p. 367). Bowen's description is similar to the concept of the utilization
of selfobjects, an integral concept in self psychology (Wolf, 1988). Bowen's
pseudo-self also resonates with Winnicott's description of a "continuum of
the *false self* [italics added] ranging from the healthy, polite aspect of the
self to the truly split-off, compliant, false self that is mistaken for the whole
person" (Giovacchini, 1993, p. 254).

Bowen's (1985) discussion of differentiation of self pertaining to family
dynamics illuminates many puzzling behaviors of families. A particularly
fascinating observation is that when people marry they *"pick spouses who
have the same levels of differentiation"* [italics added] (Bowen, 1985,
p. 377). In other words, people with a solid self tend to marry others with a
solid self and maintain a balance between the intimacy of a marriage and retaining an autonomous sense of self. The degree to which people need to

lean on the other to function is similar, so when both partners are "wobbly," mutual collapse, rather than mutual support, may ensue. Sometimes people may be frightened by the degree of fusion they experience within the marital bond (or any intimate relationship), and may need to fight or flee to create "emotional distance from each other" (Bowen, 1985, p. 377). In addition, the "amount of undifferentiation in the marriage" is expressed through "marital conflict; sickness or dysfunction in one spouse; and projection of the problems to children . . . as if there is a quantitative amount of undifferentiation to be absorbed in the nuclear family, which may be focused . . . in one area or distributed . . . to all three areas. The various patterns . . . come from patterns in their families of origin" (Bowen, 1985, p. 377).

Clinicians look beyond a family's presenting problems and assess their underlying needs and structure. Kressel (1997) has studied divorcing couples and has focused on the "*distinctive patterns* [italics added] by which our couples reached the divorce decision" (p. 226). Although he does not relate these patterns to previous patterns of marital interaction, he does suggest this as a further avenue for research and comments on the affinity of his typology to Minuchin's work. One divorce pattern Kressel describes is the enmeshed pattern. Poorly differentiated people are more prone to enter enmeshed relationships, where they reenact their struggles with separation and individuation.

> The hallmarks of this pattern were extremely high levels of conflict and ambivalence about the divorce decision. The parties debated . . . often bitterly; agreed to divorce and then changed their minds. . . . They maintained a common residence after the decision and may have continued . . . having sexual relations. . . . The impression was of parties psychically unprepared to let go. (Kressel, 1997, p. 227)
>
> The outcomes [after divorce] were as poor as the negotiations which produced them. The parties were bitter towards each other and dissatisfied with the terms of settlement. . . . In every instance there were significant adjustment problems with children. The more extreme forms of post-divorce turmoil—initiation of law suits, and (in one case) acts of physical violence necessitating police intervention—occurred only in this pattern. (Kresel, 1997, p. 228)

One of the ways we can learn more about a family's structure is through the "observation of repeating patterns of communication" (Hartman and Laird, 1983, p. 302).

Communication

The communication patterns of family members were one of the early issues of concern to family therapists. Virginia Satir (1967), for example, focused on the communications patterns in family life, which may be functional or dysfunctional. Questions such as whether messages to each family member were clear or mixed and whether people were allowed to talk for themselves were brought into focus.

Pragmatics of Human Communication

Watzlawick and colleagues (1967) describe the "pragmatics" of human communication, which refers to the "behavioral effects of communication" (p. 22). In marital and family relationships, as well as in other social contexts, nonverbal communication and body language as well as the "communicational clues inherent in the context in which communication occurs . . . even the communicational clues in an impersonal context—affects behavior" (Watzlawick et al., 1967, p. 22). What message, for example, do the decor, seating arrangements, and responsiveness of the receptionist in a waiting room of a social agency give to its clients? In a similar vein, Gutheil (1992) has discussed the psychological effects of physical environments, such as housing and institutions on people (discussed in Chapter 4).

A man boarding a train notices that a seat next to another man is occupied by his possessions. The initial impersonal message received by the newcomer is that there is no room for anyone. Being of brave heart, however, this passenger inquires if he might sit down. The manner of the other man's response, such as a smile, a quick removal of the possessions, and a gesture to sit, would convey a welcoming response; a glowering expression, a removal of the possessions accompanied by sighs, and an "inability" to place the possessions elsewhere would convey that the request is unwelcome and is causing trouble to the entitled possessor of the two seats. All this communication is carried out with barely a word spoken!

Watzlawick and colleagues (1967) present several axioms of communicating, two of which are discussed here. The first axiom is: *"one cannot* not *communicate"* (Watzlawick et al., 1967, p. 51). One might argue with this. "But every time I tell my adolescent son to do his homework he just stares at me as though he has heard nothing, and then he doesn't even say anything! How can you call that communication?" However, what the son *is* communicating to the father is that he has chosen to tune him out, especially about being ordered to do his homework.

Watzlawick and colleagues (1967) state that "if it is accepted that all behavior in an interactional situation has message value, i.e., is communication, it follows that no matter how one may try, one cannot *not* communicate" (pp. 48-49); this does not imply that all communication is effective or accurate or that "message sent equals message received" (p. 49). This axiom has particular relevance for viewing schizophrenic behavior.

It appears that the schizophrenic *tries not to communicate.* But since even nonsense, silence, withdrawal, immobility (postural silence), or any other form of denial is itself a communication, the schizophrenic is faced with the impossible task of denying that he is communicating and at the same time denying that his denial is a communication. The realization of this basic dilemma in schizophrenia is a key to a good many aspects of schizophrenic communication that would otherwise remain obscure. (Watzlawick et al., 1967, pp. 50-51)

A second axiom discussed by Watzlawick and colleagues (1967) refers both to the content of the communication *(the report aspect)* and how the communication should be taken *(the command aspect),* which refers to the relationship between the two communicants. Watzlawick and colleagues (1967) call a communication about a communication a *metacommunication* and state this axiom fully: *"Every communication has a content and a relationship aspect such that the latter classifies the former and is therefore a metacommunication"* (p. 54).

If a teacher tells her class that she expects them to read 100 pages by next week, the content or report aspect of this message is the specific homework assignment; the relationship or command aspect is that she is the teacher who has this expectation with which the class should comply.

In the following illustration, a social work student is making a visit to James, a patient diagnosed with paranoid schizophrenia, who is now living in a psychiatric foster home for adult patients. The student is talking to the foster mother, Mrs. McCarthy, who is indicating she is in charge (command aspect) of these two young people (the social worker and James) although this is never the overt subject (report aspect) of discussion.

> Mrs. McCarthy then went on to relate her experiences in caring for children at the G. Center . . . and mentioned the names of a couple of Social Workers, and asked if I knew them. She then commented on my age, and said, "Why you're not much older than James." I said that I would guess in fact I wasn't. She said you probably haven't been out of school that long. I then said that I had been doing social work for five years. James kind of smiled and said, well I guess that would make you about 26. I said well actually closer to 28, and then he said that was how old he was. Mrs. McCarthy mentioned that she had two children and pointed to their pictures on the wall. . . . I then said that I would have to run along, and I told James that we would plan on getting together next Tuesday. He commented that he had enjoyed seeing me again. Mrs. McCarthy . . . told me to feel free to stop in at any time. (Urdang, 1979, p. 7)

In this illustration, we can see Mrs. McCarthy's maneuvers in asserting her authority and dominance. Her comments about the social worker's age affirms that not only is she older (and by inference more experienced) than the social worker, but in addition, she also implies that he is not very experienced (has not been out of school very long). By comparing his age to James' age, she implies that he is not much more competent than James. She ends the discussion by giving the social worker "permission" to visit again. All these represent covert relationship or command messages.

In his novel, *A Man in Full,* Tom Wolfe (1999) describes Charlie Croker, a powerful multimillionaire in Atlanta who has borrowed large sums of money from PlannersBanc and is unable to pay the interest due. The bank sets up a breakfast meeting not only to confront him with his indebted state but to humiliate and humble him so that he will comply with their suggested solutions. Watzlawick and colleagues' (1967) concepts of communication are illustrated in the following excerpts from Wolfe's book.

In the first example, the "communicational clues in an impersonal context" (in this case, the physical setting) (Watzlawick et al., 1967, p. 22) play an important role in this situation. As described by Wolfe, this breakfast meeting takes place at PlannersBanc, an elegant establishment; however, an "inelegant" room, "cunningly seedy and unpleasant," exposed to the intense glare of the sun, was chosen to emphasize the "degradation" of the occasion, before a group of inquisitors who "knew exactly what the game was. The conference table itself . . . was put together in modular sections that didn't quite jibe . . . and its surface was . . . some sort of veal-gray plastic laminate. . . . in front of each of the two dozen people present, was a pathetic setting of paperware . . . and a paper plate with a huge, cold, sticky, cheesy, cowpie-like cinnamon-Cheddar coffee bun" (Wolfe, 1999, pp. 36, 38).

Charlie Crocker is used to exerting his power and influence and to being treated with due deference by others; a meeting room tastefully furnished and visible signs of hospitality would be expected by him. In this context, however, the deliberate set-up of uncomfortable physical conditions is covertly designed to humiliate him. In fact, the bankers feel he must be "humbled" to face up to his serious declining financial state and his large unpaid debt to the bank. In the following, Mr. Zale furthers this agenda through his condescending attitude toward Mr. Crocker.

Harry Zale was in charge of this meeting; in this excerpt we see the way Harry utilizes nonverbal communication, and the meeting's agenda to play on the relationship (command) aspects of this interaction: "Harry . . . just kept on writing. . . . He sighted Crocker down his nose. . . . And then he said in a high-pitched, rasping voice, 'Why are we here, Mr. Croker? . . . What's the problem?'" (Wolfe, 1999, pp. 41-42).

Impairments in Functional Communication

Another significant aspect of communication relates to its basic functional purpose; people must communicate to make their needs known, to have social contact, share ideas, etc. Some people have serious impairments in their basic communication abilities, and both the individual and the family may need help to overcome this difficulty.

Schizophrenic individuals can be incoherent or illogical and may have difficulty communicating on even a simple level. Families can learn successful ways of communicating with a schizophrenic family member and methods such as a psychoeducational approach with families are often effective (Anderson, 1983). In one such behavioral program, "all families were trained in effective interpersonal communication such as identifying and giving praise, compliments, criticism, and requests for behavior change" (Falloon and Liberman, 1983, p. 124).

The prelingual deaf have made great strides in their ability to communicate through sign language (Sacks, 1989). Controversy continues to exist about the use of sign language versus other methods of communication, such as lip reading (see discussion in Chapter 5). Early intervention programs aimed at teaching parents of deaf children alternative ways of communicating with them are often effective. One deaf man spoke of his hurt feelings because his hearing parents refused to learn sign language.

Some people become *aphasic*—that is, they have lost their ability to use speech which can result from various illnesses, including strokes. "For those who cannot produce intelligible speech there are alternate methods of communication, such as sign language, speech boards, and speech synthesizers" (Olkin, 1999, p. 197). One stroke patient seemed to understand what a social work student was saying but could not respond verbally. It was painful for the social worker to think about "how he was locked into himself." When she introduced a pad and pen into their sessions, he wrote his responses to her and was happy to be able to communicate; his family learned how to communicate with him in this manner.

Emotional Issues Blocking Family Communication

Specific emotional problems the family may not be able to face, such as illness, learning that a child is gay or that a family member is abusing substances, can block communication, as illustrated in the following example.

Madge, fifteen, and her parents came to the mental health clinic because she recently developed school phobia, experiencing anxiety and panic whenever she went to school. The clinical social worker, based on her understanding that school phobia was usually precipitated by separation-anxiety, explored this possibility with the family, but no significant losses, crises, or traumas were identified. Utilizing a behavioral component recommended in the treatment of school phobias, it was suggested that Madge make a gradual reentry into school. For several months, this went on in a halting fashion; feeling stuck, the therapist asked the family if anything had been left out. Was anything else happening?

> At first the family said that nothing else was happening. Then, after a pause, the parents said, well, maybe there was something they should mention. Madge's mother was about to have a hysterectomy. Although the mother's condition was benign, the affect of extreme anxiety attached to this was experienced as though a life-threatening event were about to occur—and no one was talking about it. According to the family history, Madge's mother lost her father due to divorce when she was fifteen; Madge's father lost his mother due to cancer when he was fifteen. Madge, now fifteen, was at an age of great emotional risk according to the parents' unexpressed worldview. Madge did not know what a hysterectomy was, nor did she know that retaining the uterus was not vital for life.
>
> When the subject of the hysterectomy was brought into the open, the nature of the operation was discussed with Madge, who also learned she could visit her mother in the hospital as well as talk to her on the telephone. After this session, the symptoms of school phobia quickly vanished, and Madge flourished in school and in her social life. A follow-up interview after the surgery revealed a successful medical outcome, good functioning, and an optimistic outlook for all members of the family.

The family had not been discussing their fears about the mother's medical problem but were nevertheless communicating their anxiety; the intersubjective transmission of affect was evident and became encapsulated in Madge's school phobia.

The issue of family secrets is frequently encountered; family rules do not permit discussing them, which can add to the anxiety of family members. "Deaths, alcoholism, mental illness, suicide, divorce, incest, illegitimacy, illness, adoption, business failures, deviance of any kind, battles over money are all examples of toxic issues which may become skeletons in the family closet" (Hartman and Laird, 1983, p. 248); as noted in this case, often when family secrets are discussed, "the reality is discovered to be far less devastating than were the fantasies" (p. 248).

Family Rituals and Myths

Family rituals are organized patterns of dealing with daily life as well as with holidays, birthdays, transitions (such as graduation), etc. The father, for example, reads to his son before bedtime, then the mother comes in and kisses him good night. "During the child-rearing years, creating and maintaining rituals on a daily basis are an integral part of family life" (Sameroff and Fiese, 2000, p. 13). Rituals provide a sense of security and can afford pleasure to both child and parents.

In divorcing families, rituals can be disrupted; in blended families, "as familial patterns realign" (Kaplan and Pruett, 2000, p. 533), rituals from each family may compete for attention and can be a source of anxiety and dissension. Parks (1998) expresses concern about the lack of public rituals "recognizing lesbian family formation," which she feels is another "dimension of invisibility" facing these women (p. 385). Although many lesbian families develop their own private family rituals, according to Parks (1998) "it is the public component that is critical to the sense of validation and legitimacy such rituals are intended to bestow" (p. 385).

In child welfare work, rituals are sometimes used to help children deal with transitions (Hartman and Laird, 1983). The enactment of a claiming ritual is followed by some adoptive families, when adoptions are finalized; this is celebrated by "an exchange of vows, the expression of sentiments by extended family members, a party, pictures, and gifts" (Hartman and Laird, 1983, p. 324).

Families construct their own interpretations of life, including the development of special beliefs and stories, defined by David Reiss as the "family paradigm," which is the family's "fundamental assumptions about the world in which it lives" (Hartman and Laird, 1983, p. 105). Rituals follow from paradigms; telling "family stories" is one avenue for expression of family beliefs. "Family stories may be examined by their thematic content, on the one hand, and by the process of storytelling itself, on the other" (Sameroff and Fiese, 2000, p. 12). Foster children usually have no consistent family story to tell, as they may never have known their family and/or may have had several disrupted placements. Child welfare workers often help children create a life book, where they can assemble whatever pictures and stories of their past that exist.

Myths, sometimes used synonymously with the term *family stories* emphasize the family belief system. Mythical processes are often seen in family stories of "heroic or villainous figures, disruptive events, and identifications" (Germain, 1991, p. 134). Myths may or may not be based on facts; however, "their thematic content and process can play themselves out in the current situation—for good or for ill" (Germain, 1991, p. 134). A boy, for example, who did not know his father may have heard about how "perfect" he was, and so might internalize and perpetuate this myth of the father (which may or may not be accurate). Woods and Hollis (1990) state that myths can serve defensive functions in families. "Myths may be perpetuated to avoid or to deny painful feelings of self-blame, as they often are in families that exclusively attribute their miseries or misfortunes to one family member" (Woods and Hollis, 1990, p. 322).

The Intergenerational Family

Some grandparents live with the nuclear family; their involvement is immediate and continuous. Other grandparents have actual custodial care of their grandchildren, and their involvement is primary. However, even if grandparents are not involved with the family or are no longer living, they may still exert strong influence on the family. "Boszormenyi-Nagy and Spark (1973) speak directly to the need for an awareness of multigenerational patterns" (Moultrup, 1981, p. 122). They highlight issues of "merit and indebtedness"; children develop a sense of rules and expectations from their parents, which they then transmit to their own children. Children may subsequently feel some conflict in meeting these obligations if they conflict with the expectations of their peers.

An *intergenerational transmission of child maltreatment* [italics added] has been observed (Morton and Browne, 1998; Zeanah and Scheeringa, 1997). If children receive "insensitive parenting" (Morton and Browne, 1998, p. 1098), they will introject an image of themselves as unlovable and deficient; they subsequently will be unable to develop caring, consistent relationships with their own children. Mitigating circumstances can prevent this transmission, which include: supportive substitute care when growing up, current involved and supportive spouses, and the development of self-awareness about the abusive experience (often with the assistance of therapy) (Morton and Browne, 1998).

Bowen (1985), in discussing multigenerational transmissions, stresses the concept of the family projection process, in which "the parents and the child play active parts in the transmission of the parental problem to the child" (for example, a mother denies her inner feelings of helplessness and overprotects her child, who feels and acts more helpless) (p. 127). Bowen (1985) states that this transmission continues through "multiple generations" (p. 384) and emphasizes the dominant role of differentiation in this process. The child who is targeted in the family projection process *"emerges with a lower level of differentiation than the parents and does less well in life"* [italics added] (Bowen, 1985, p. 384); over generations, the offspring of this child will have children "with lower and lower levels of differentiation" (p. 384). Moultrup (1981) comments that differentiation cannot be meaningfully conceptualized within the limits of a single generation: "It is rather a combination of issues involving the separation of selfs and the accounting of multigenerational obligations" (p. 124).

OBJECT RELATIONS FAMILY THERAPY

Object relations family therapy has many similarities to structural theory, with its emphasis on the internal organization of families. However, object relations diverges from structural theory in its concern with the inner object world of each family member and the interactions of these inner worlds of object and self-representations with the outer world of present family interrelationships. "Object relations family theory provides the theoretical framework for understanding, and the language for working with, the dynamics of both the individual self and the family system" (Scharff and Scharff, 1987, p. 14).

The utilization of the therapist's countertransference reactions is one of the foundations of treatment. Although Scharff and Scharff (1987) do not use the term intersubjectivity, their description of utilizing the therapeutic self appears synonymous with this concept. They note that, in a similar vein to Bowen's family projection process, the family will project feelings onto the therapists as they have done with other family members (projective identification); the therapists then process and utilize their reactions to these projections with the family and observe that "we are open to being used in the way family members are used, and yet we remain able to move outside of that to comment upon what is happening to us and thus to allow the family a new experience of such phenomena" (Scharff and Scharff, 1987, p. 9).

Other features differentiate object relations from structural therapy: object relations therapists deal with the past, rather than focus only on the here and now, as many structural therapists do. "In our view, *the past does still exist and is constantly reenacted in the present relationships*" [italics added] (Scharff and Scharff, 1987, p. 10); insights are shared with the families; therapists choose not to rely on directives and homework (a frequently utilized technique of structural therapists) but value the development of the family's self-awareness. They also encourage the expression of affects, whereas many systemic therapists "do not encourage emotional catharsis" (Scharff and Scharff, 1987, p. 10).

Fraiberg and colleagues (1975) have talked about ghosts in the nursery; some parents cannot see their children as individual "objects" but relate to them through the veil of past memories. Object relations therapists are concerned with these ghosts who haunt present relationships; the goal is to bring the ghosts out into the light and banish them. Symptom removal is not the primary objective; personal growth and the development of enriched interpersonal relationships are the aim.

WORKING WITH FAMILIES:
THE BIOPSYCHOSOCIAL PERSPECTIVE

The psychodynamic biopsychosocial perspective is an excellent vantage point from which to understand both the individual and the family; it enables clinicians to look *outward,* at clients' families within their physical and social environments and culture, as well as look *inward* at the individuals' anxieties, conflicts, and ego structure, and the interactive interrelatedness of these. With a constructivist perspective, clinicians search for the meanings of the unique problems of their clients and examine how they choose to involve themselves in working together with clinicians. Woods and Hollis (1990) stress the interrelationship between individual and family work.

> Individual and family dynamics interplay. . . . Whatever affects one part of a system necessarily affects the other parts to some degree. Positive shifts in a family's structure or climate can result in profound personality modifications of individual members. Changes in an entire family can occur after one member has been in treatment and makes changes. Because of this, we need not despair if we cannot gather the entire family together. When possible—whether we are seeing one family member, a subgroup, or an entire family—we search for the most accessible aspect of the system, the part that will be most responsive to intervention. (Woods and Hollis, 1990, p. 370)

Within the vast scope of social work, people seek assistance for many reasons; they may want to feel less anxious or depressed or to improve their family relationships. However, many seek services (or are referred and/or mandated for services) because of problems in living without wishing to change themselves or their family relationships; they may be in trouble with the law; wish to adopt children; need help with living arrangements for elderly parents; or learn that a family member has cancer. The problem focus itself is a major determinant of the type of service necessitated.

However, whatever the specific problem, people come with their unique personalities, ego structures, and family dynamics. Although the focus of intervention may not be on these dynamic issues, understanding both individual psychodynamics and family structure and family dynamics within the clients' social and cultural context is essential for offering appropriate assistance.

The Paul Norris case is presented to illustrate the psychodynamic biopsychosocial perspective in action in family-focused clinical work.

Case Illustration

Paul Norris, five, was referred to the mental health clinic with problems of anxiety, sleep disturbances, and bouts of vomiting for which no physical basis was found, resulting in several hospitalizations for dehydration. Mrs. Norris, thirty, his mother, found his behavior difficult to control. The biopsychosocial assessment illustrates the major features of this case.

> Mrs. Norris had been separated from her husband since Paul, her only child, was two-and-a-half years old; since then, no contact has been made with Mr. Norris, whose whereabouts are unknown. Mrs. Norris, herself an only child, and Paul live with Mrs. Norris's mother, sixty-one, and stepfather, forty-six, in comfortable housing and are supported by AFDC (Aid to Families with Dependent Children). Both of Mrs. Norris's parents work, and Mrs. Norris's primary role is mother and homemaker.

Mrs. Norris, although receiving public assistance through AFDC (which would place her at the poverty level), lives in comfortable middle-class circumstances. Paul has a room of his own and a backyard to play in.

Mrs. Norris' personality characteristics, physical health, relationship to Paul, social life, and how she views herself in the world, were explored:

> Mrs. Norris is intelligent, verbal, and has a good capacity to relate. She has many ego strengths and functions well on a daily basis, although she suffers from moderate anxiety and has passive-dependent characteristics. Her feelings toward her son are very positive, but she has difficulty controlling him. She has no social life, and all her activities center around the home; she plays bingo once a week, and her stepfather makes it clear that he will not baby-sit for her while she is "running around." On most Sundays, she and her mother go to flea markets. Mrs. Norris was emphatic with the clinician that she has no wish to change this and is very comfortable as a "homebody."
>
> Mrs. Norris has many physical ailments, some of which appeared to be psychosomatic in nature. She has received many secondary gains from her symptoms, both in the past and now. Secondary or *epinosic* gain refers to "secondary advantages accruing from an illness, such as gratification of dependency yearnings or attention seeking" (Campbell, 1989, p. 298). Her anxieties about her illnesses are being communicated to Paul constantly on both verbal and nonverbal levels; the fact that illness can bring secondary gains is also being transmitted to him.

Mrs. Norris is deeply embedded in her family, and the family is very enmeshed, with separation being a major source of anxiety. Looking at Mrs. Norris from a life-cycle perspective, the clinician observed she is an adult who might be expected to be involved in an intimate partner relationship, to have friends, and perhaps to have an interest in outside employment or other activities in addition to her age-appropriate involvement with parenting. Her present lifestyle is more reminiscent of a teenager still under parental domination, although, in fact, teenagers usually engage in social life more active than her presently restricted one. Mrs. Norris has difficulty asserting herself in the mothering role and in dealing with her mother about who has control of Paul.

Paul is the identified patient; how is he viewed by the clinician?

> Paul is an intelligent, responsive boy who is somewhat manipulative and slightly bossy; his mother reports temper tantrums. He is anxious, has sleep problems, and a number of fears, such as going into crowds. He appears to have mild motoric awkwardness and awkwardness in drawing spontaneously. Psychiatric evaluation raised question of primary skill deficits, and diagnostically he was thought to exhibit emotionally triggered cyclic vomiting. Medical evaluation ruled out a physical basis for his vomiting; asthma has also been diagnosed. He has no playmates and his life is centered exclusively around the home.
>
> Paul is caught in a power struggle between his mother and grandmother and manipulates both of them. His grandmother overindulges him; when Mrs. Norris objects, she is told: "Why not—how much longer do I have to live?" This guilt-provoking statement does not seem to have any basis in fact, as Paul's grandmother is in very good health. Mrs. Norris's stepfather has a positive relationship with Paul and seems to be a steadying force.
>
> Paul's father, from Mrs. Norris' description, was not very involved in caring for Paul when they lived together. Although totally absent for the past two-and-a-half years, he is often "present" in Mrs. Norris's verbalizations of resentment toward him, which Paul is often privy to. There are myths relating to Paul's father, which are frequently repeated and narrated with a very negative attitude. His paternal uncle has engaged in illegal activities, some of which were reported in the newspapers. Mrs. Norris has commented that "Paul has the Norris blood in him."

Paul is enmeshed in a family with a very caring but very anxious mother, continual power struggles for control of Paul, and negative myths about his father. Mrs. Norris had maintained a marriage (albeit strained) living apart from her parents for several years. How did this present situation come about?

A sketchy picture of the marital situation revealed poor communication, serious sexual problems, and an unplanned pregnancy. When Paul was two, Mr. Norris suggested that they move in with her parents "for convenience."

Shortly after they did this, Mr. Norris left and was not heard from again. It can be hypothesized that when Mr. and Mrs. Norris married, they found in each other "spouses who have the same levels of differentiation" (Bowen, 1985, p. 377) and in their case consequently were unable to provide each other with needed emotional support.

Did the abandonment by Mr. Norris cause an emotional regression in his wife? Did she need to retreat into her family to protect herself from being hurt again? Or was a pattern of enmeshment and hostile-dependent relationships already present as well? The family history sheds more light on the present dynamics of the family.

> When Mrs. Norris was a baby, her father became ill, developing many disabilities and requiring much care. His condition deteriorated, and he died when she was two and a half (Paul's age when he and his mother were abandoned by Mr. Norris). Shortly after her father's death, Mrs. Norris's mother met her present husband (fifteen years her junior; thus they were about thirty-three and eighteen, respectively). When they married a year and a half later, Mrs. Norris was sent to a boarding school in another state. She lived there from the time she was four until she was seven. Although her mother did maintain contact, Mrs. Norris felt abandoned, desolate, and lonely, and often cried. She developed a serious throat condition from which she "nearly died" when she was seven and was then removed from the school and returned to live with her mother and stepfather, where she remained.
>
> She went to public school and had some friends. Developing visual problems, she was allowed to discontinue high school and kept house for her parents, who worked. She did have a period of working (in the same factory as her mother), where she met Mr. Norris and then married him.

In reviewing her history, issues of separation, abandonment, and loss are prominent. Although the loss of her husband was an emotional crisis, her history of loss goes back much farther and is deeper. Moultrup (1981) has observed that many family therapists focus only on what is happening in the transactions of family members in the present; often the past "is thought of as that which no longer exists" (p. 120), but the past sheds light on Mrs. Norris's needs, losses, and early patterns of enmeshment with her family. Her history of somatizing psychological distress and the secondary gains of illness emerge. A serious physical illness allowed Mrs. Norris to escape from her institutional life; an eyesight problem enabled her to avoid school and start her pattern of being the family homemaker. Her somatizing tendencies as well as anxiety about her health have been transmitted to Paul.

Treatment

A combination of individual and family therapy modalities was the treatment intervention chosen. Mrs. Norris was responsive to the social work clinician, and she talked freely about herself and her anxieties, primarily fixated on her health. However, she was not seeking therapy for herself; her goal was to help Paul, and most of her attention was directed to this issue. The clinician observed that Mrs. Norris had very positive feelings toward Paul, although she was frustrated by his behaviors. She also had many insights into how to help him; very little direction was given by the clinician; rather she supported Ms. Norris in her role as mother and validated her own many constructive suggestions.

> Prior to her first appointment, Mrs. Norris called to say that Paul was becoming more anxious, having nightmares, and feeling fearful that there were snakes and bugs in his bed. When seen for her initial interview, she told the clinician Paul's anxiety had lessened. She had taken Paul to see a doctor for his asthma; he recommended that all his stuffed animals be removed from his room, and she had put them all in the attic. When she realized that this precipitated his major anxiety attack, she returned the animals to him, including his beloved teddy bear. The disturbance (precipitated by separation anxiety) immediately ceased.

Mrs. Norris also realized that she needed to assert herself with her mother about her own mothering role, and that she, not her mother, "was in control of Paul." As the situation improved, she commented that Paul "has only one boss now." She also "suddenly" found a friend who had a son Paul's age, whom she and Paul would visit, which she reported was enjoyable for both of them. A major breakthrough came when Mrs. Norris agreed to enroll Paul in a summer Head Start program; the separation was successful for both. Paul did very well in this program and made a good transition to public school. During the seven-month period of treatment, Paul made steady progress: no vomiting episodes of significance were reported; his general anxiety diminished; he began sleeping better, eating well, and growing.

The clinician saw Paul with his mother, during which time they would talk together or do a small activity, such as walking around the clinic grounds; Paul sometimes gathered acorns to plant in his garden.

Mrs. Norris's anxiety diminished as did her reliance on tranquilizers; talking to the clinician helped her "feel free like a bird." It was the clinician's hope that Mrs. Norris might engage herself more deeply in therapy to further her own adult development and develop a greater sense of autonomy and a social life. Mrs. Norris, however, made it clear, as she had at the beginning, that this was not her wish; she was content to be a homebody, did not want to live apart from her parents, and was not interested in outside employment, social activities, or dating.

Termination was initiated by Mrs. Norris, ostensibly relating to the progress Paul had made and her feelings that she could maintain the gains.

Mrs. Norris reapplied three months later, upon the referral of her physician, because Paul had another hospitalization for vomiting. The physician felt that Paul's problems in separating from his mother appeared to be a key issue. This next short period of treatment was rather tumultuous, with a focus on separation and encouraging brief separations and the use of a babysitter; both Mrs. Norris and Paul were resistant to this idea. After one session, Paul went home and vomited and told his mother that he did not want to see the clinician anymore and did not want to hear about baby-sitters anymore. Mrs. Norris returned to her pediatrician stating that she did not want to return to the clinic if it was going to make Paul worse. At this point, family sessions with Paul's grandparents were also being considered. Before this could happen, Mrs. Norris terminated. She had heard about a good gastroenterologist and was taking Paul there.

This case illustrates the power of separation and loss conflicts and how these past issues can be replayed in the present. It also illustrates the importance of understanding family dynamics and not viewing children independently of systemic issues. Although working with Mrs. Norris's strengths reduced her level of anxiety and encouraged her sense of competence, the progress was subverted by the needs of this enmeshed family system to prevail, which superseded the needs of one five-year-old boy to separate and for his mother to lead a more independent existence. Hartman and Laird (1983) indicate that "helping families . . . deal with separateness and connectedness is one of the most frequently faced challenges in family-centered practice" (p. 274). This challenge was not fully met in this case.

SPECIAL FAMILY PROBLEMS

Four special problems that can have a significant impact on family life are discussed in this section: domestic violence, including spouse/partner abuse, maltreatment of children (involving neglect and/or physical and sexual abuse), substance abuse, and mental illness. Sometimes these problems exist separately; many times some or all of them appear concurrently and represent multiple risk factors.

Domestic Violence

Families can be affected by violence that surrounds them externally, such as community and school violence (which was discussed in Chapter 4). Violence among family members affects families internally, leading to physical and psychological trauma, family dissolution, homelessness, and sometimes death. This section addresses partner violence.

Domestic violence was dealt with in the past as a private family event, with minimal police or legal interventions; the women's movement of the 1970s brought this problem into focus as a major social concern (Herman, 1989). Additional attention to partner violence was stimulated in 1994 when O. J. Simpson was accused of killing his wife and her friend, and investigation revealed that he had previously assaulted his wife. Extensive media coverage focused attention on the problem of domestic violence, and "within months, Congress approved the $1.62-billion Violence Against Women Act (1994), dedicating more money to the cause than ever before while creating new federal laws. Advocates say it may have passed without the Simpson case, but probably would have been pared down" ("War on Domestic," 1999).

It is difficult to obtain accurate statistics on domestic violence, as not every case of battering is reported to authorities. One estimate is "that two to six million women are beaten by their male partners each year in this country" (Zastrow and Kirst-Ashman, 1997, p. 371). Recently, discussion has focused on whether all abuse is perpetrated by males against females; males are sometimes the victims of partner abuse, and women have attacked other women within their families (Goldberg, 1999a). The Department of Justice has asserted that there are nearly five times as many females among the almost 1 million abuse victims recorded annually in the United States (Goldberg, 1999e, A1). Recent research has also discovered problems of physical abuse of partners occurring in gay and lesbian couple relationships (Carlson and Maciol, 1997).

Considerable controversy was stirred when it was reported that women accounted for one out of four domestic violence arrests in some states (Goldberg, 1999e, p. A1). Advocates for battered women and many social scientists have asserted that these women were in fact defending themselves (p. A1); other social scientists and police state that although the physical damage inflicted is not nearly as great, assaults by women are a reality and significant (p. A1). Husband abuse has also been perpetrated by wives who are much younger than their frail or elderly husbands (Kaplan et al., 1994). This issue, complicated by conflicting political agendas involving rights of men and women, needs further research.

A wide range of types of abuse and violence exists, which should be clinically assessed and treated differentially depending on the degree and chronicity of the violence, the social context, the presence (and degree) of substance abuse, and the personalities of the partners. In an extreme case of violence, discussed in Chapter 4, a woman and her two-year-old daughter were killed by her husband following a long-term abusive relationship.

Other situations are observed in which abuse is occasional, mutual, and the result of an escalation of arguing, with minor injuries resulting.

One extreme form of abuse, the *battering syndrome,* in which a constant terrorizing and domination of the partner occurs, has been identified and found to have three phases (Zastrow and Kirst-Ashman, 1997). In the first, a "building up of stress and tension" occurs, followed by "the explosion . . . when the battering occurs," and the final stage is characterized by "making up . . . he is forgiven . . . until the cycle of violence begins again" (Zastrow and Kirst-Ashman, 1997, pp. 372-373). The typical batterer may be violent only in the home situation and "can appear charming, deferential, and pathetic in the presence of professionals" (Herman, 1989, p. 4). Kaplan and colleagues (1994) have observed that batterers are often "immature, dependent, and nonassertive and . . . suffer from strong feelings of inadequacy" (p. 793).

> The typical batterer needs total control over his mate; any sign of independence is unbearably humiliating and makes him fear abandonment. He tries to establish dominance by isolation, enforced dependency, jealous surveillance, threats, verbal abuse, meticulous enforcement of petty rules, and even physical exhaustion. He often discourages the victim from working, using a car or telephone, or even having more than brief contact with anyone but himself. Often he says that he "regrets" resorting to violence but was "driven to it" when other ways of enforcing subordination failed. (Herman, 1989, p. 4)

Women who have been chronically battered often feel trapped in their situations; some are fearful of being killed. They regularly develop signs of post-traumatic stress disorder, often become preoccupied with not displeasing their partner; such a woman may sacrifice "her relationships with friends, her family of origin, and, most important, her children" (Herman, 1989, p. 5)

> Physical and mental exhaustion are even more common than anxiety and insomnia in abused women. They feel drained and numb. Anything beyond the minimum necessary cooking, cleaning, and child care is too much for them. They stop thinking about the future and become chronically depressed. In one clinical study of 100 battered women, 42 had attempted suicide. (Herman, 1989, p. 5)

Women often deny that they are being battered and may be resistant to call for help or to press charges when they do involve the police. Many police departments now take the problem of abuse seriously and offer special training to enable officers to handle domestic violence situations (Zastrow and

Kirst-Ashman, 1997). However, although new laws and procedures are in place, they are not always enforced (Zastrow and Kirst-Ashman, 1997), nor are the procedures always effective. Shelters for battered women have been developing for the past thirty years; and self-help groups have been found to be effective with this population.

Services may be offered to batterers, usually in the form of group therapy, "with an emphasis on controlling anger and abandoning rationalizations for violence against women and children" (Herman, 1989, p. 6). Trimble (1986) discusses his group work (sixteen sessions) with batterers and has found that these men struggle with issues of intimacy, loss of control over anger and aggression, idealizations of masculinity, and strong feelings of insecurity. Some men have come to his groups voluntarily and others have been mandated to receive therapy as part of their parole; some are also coping with recent abstinence from alcohol and drug use. Although battering behavior must be brought under control, sometimes by means of the legal system, the man's aggressive behavior should be assessed as part of an overall evaluation; underlying pathology may be present that may require specific treatment.

Children witnessing violence between their parents often develop symptoms of post-traumatic stress disorder (Davies, 1999) and may manifest developmental impairments often of a permanent nature (Davies, 1999; Zeanah and Scheeringa, 1997). It was reported in the National Family Violence Survey in 1985 that "over 3.3 million children witnessed physical assaults between their parents" (Zeanah and Scheeringa, 1997, p. 100). In addition, within the same families, an association often exists between domestic violence directed toward partners and physical abuse of children by both mothers and fathers (Davies, 1999; Zeanah and Scheeringa, 1997). Many children have been witnesses to parental homicide, although it is difficult to ascertain how many, as no specific national recording system exists (Burman and Allen-Meares, 1994); these children, who generally do not receive treatment for this trauma, develop "emotional scars of far-reaching proportions . . . [their] symptoms . . . have been likened to those of posttraumatic stress disorder" (p. 28).

Children can feel overwhelmed, frightened, and powerless seeing their mother "being brutalized" (Davies, 1999, p. 66). Many battered women, living a lifestyle of social isolation, may be without social supports and may become less emotionally available to their children, offering neither support nor validation for what is being experienced. In fact, one protective factor for children in this situation is the mother's ability "to maintain a positive and supportive relationship with the child" (Davies, 1999, p. 67).

Children from violent families are more aggressive with their peers, often using the *"defense of identification with the aggressor"* [italics added], and while boys tend to be more aggressive, girls tend to have symptoms of depression, "Children of both sexes exposed to chronic violence may adopt numbing and *dissociative defenses*" [italics added] (Davies, 1999, pp. 66-67).

Child Maltreatment

Many children today experience physical and sexual abuse and/or neglect, which usually leave profound psychological scars on their developing personalities and may cause developmental and neurological impairments, leading to serious consequences in their adult lives (Davies, 1999; Glodich, 1998; Kaplan et al., 1994; Kilgore, 1988; Osofsky, 1997; Wells, 1995). Public attention has focused on child sexual abuse, which appears to be increasing at a very dramatic rate. This increased awareness, as well as the enactment of mandated reporting laws, has raised the question as to whether child abuse is more prevalent now or whether the increased numbers of reported cases are an artifact of public attention. Many researchers assert that the increase is real (Wells, 1995). Public awareness and validation of abuse has helped many adult survivors come forward about their past abusive experiences and seek help; it has also led to more active reporting and intervention.

In 1992, according to the National Center on Child Abuse and Neglect, "child protective services responded to nearly 1.9 million reports of abuse to 2.9 million children" (Wells, 1995, p. 349). "Overall, three children die each day from maltreatment. Child fatalities for 1992 included 1,262 deaths" (Thomlison, 1997, p. 52). Many children who are physically abused "are very young, and in fact, more abuse and more fatal abuse occurs to children in the first year of life" (Zeanah and Scheeringa, 1997, p. 101). Infant abandonment has been increasing; mothers have been leaving their infants in public places, some of whom die before they are found (Roche, 2000; Whitaker, 2000); abandonment is discussed in Chapter 8.

Although child neglect is more frequent than abuse and produces a high percentage of fatalities, it has received substantially less attention than problems of blatant physical and sexual abuse (Nelson et al., 1993; Wells, 1995). "Even less attention has been given to families in which child neglect is long-standing or chronic" (Nelson et al., 1993, p. 661). Kaplan and colleagues (1994) report that victimization by abuse and neglect leads to 2,000 to 4,000 deaths every year.

Child maltreatment often encompasses multiple forms of abuse; for example, a child may be both neglected and physically abused. Davies (1999) asserts that psychological abuse is a "common denominator across all types of maltreatment" (p. 59); a sexually abused child "is often psychologically abused through threats of retribution or catastrophe if she discloses the sexual abuse" (p. 59). Maya Angelou (1997) writes that she was terrorized by her mother's boyfriend, who raped her when she was eight years old and threatened to kill her beloved brother Bailey if she told anyone. Most physically abused and neglected children have "insecure attachments [to their caretakers], ranging from 70 percent to 100 percent across studies" (Davies, 1999, p. 60). Other types of severe psychological abuse include chronic violent verbal rejection, extreme depreciation, and more insidious forms of undermining, verbal seduction, induction into criminality, and gross misrepresentations of reality.

Thomlison (1997) discusses "generic risk factors" (p. 54) that can predispose a family to maltreat a child, such as lack of resources, partner conflict, and occupational difficulties. However, "individual risk factors" are responsible for setting the maltreatment in motion; *"psychological distress is the primary risk factor* [italics added], associated with child maltreatment" (Thomlison, 1997, p. 54). These psychological risk factors include: "parental affective disturbances, such as depression . . . low self esteem, immaturity . . . excessive reliance on others, which places the parent's immediate needs in conflict with the child's needs . . . high levels of anxiety . . . lack of impulse control under stress and low social supports" (Thomlison, 1997, p. 54). Substance abuse is a major problem: "as many as 80 percent of maltreating parents have past or current substance abuse problems" (Thomlison, 1997, p. 54). Thomlison does not include the often-observed factor of parents reenacting their own past history of abuse.

Child Neglect

Although a lack of unanimity exists in defining neglect (Nelson et al., 1993), this classification usually implies inadequate supervision of the child, general physical neglect, including poor nutrition, and inadequate hygiene, clothing, and lack of medical attention. This child frequently "has a history of failure to thrive, malnutrition, poor skin hygiene, irritability, withdrawal, and other signs of psychological and physical neglect" (Kaplan et al., 1994, p. 790), and may have been subjected to abandonment, inadequate housing (including poor sanitation), and educational neglect (Nelson et al., 1993).

Parental characteristics contributing to chronic neglect include: being unmarried and having large families typically with insufficient resources; extreme poverty is often present (Nelson et al., 1993). "Because neglect is intricately tied to poverty and income, the poorest of the poor are at the highest risk. The rate of known neglect is nine times greater in families with incomes under $15,000 than in families above that level" (Thomlison, 1997, p. 52).

Many neglectful mothers are found to be depressed and lonely, to have a high rate of substance abuse, and to have low intelligence or a poor educational background (Nelson et al., 1993). They tend to be socially isolated, to have little interaction with their children, and to possess poor parenting skills (Nelson et al., 1993); they are inclined "to be more controlling . . . make more requests of their children and yet are least compliant with requests from them" (Nelson et al., 1993, p. 663). Nelson does not add the possibility that the mothers' low intelligence scores and poor educational attainment might result from their psychological depressions, as well as depressed lifestyles.

Physical Abuse

Debate also continues about the definition of physical abuse: physical punishment, for example, is acceptable (and expected) in some cultures; professionals do not always agree on definitions; state laws vary. "Vague definitions and lack of specific criteria are still rampant in discussions and research" (Wells, 1995, p. 348). Cultural practices can be reported as abuse; child protective workers, for example, had been inclined to report bruises on the skin of Vietnamese children as abuse, until they became "more knowledgeable about the practice of coin rubbing, a healing practice that leaves bruises" (Wells, 1995, p. 349). Although many gray areas exist in assessment, nevertheless clear-cut cases of serious and often life-threatening instances of abuse clearly require intervention.

> Severely abused children are seen in hospital emergency rooms with external evidences of body trauma, bruises, abrasions, cuts, lacerations, burns, soft tissue swellings, and hematomas. . . . Inability to move certain extremities, because of dislocations and fractures associated with neurological signs of intracranial damage, can also indicate inflicted trauma. . . . Abdominal trauma may result in unexplained ruptures of the stomach, the bowel, the liver, or the pancreas, with manifestations of an injured abdomen. Those children with the most severe maltreatment injuries arrive at the hospital or physicians office in a coma or convulsions, and some arrive dead. (Kaplan et al., 1994, p. 787)

One form of physical abuse recently receiving attention is Munchausen syndrome by proxy (Kaplan et al., 1994; Mercer and Perdue, 1993). Some children are repeatedly brought to the hospital for treatment of unusual physical symptoms for which no clear-cut medical diagnosis can be found; instead, it is discovered that a parent or other involved adult injures the child or makes the child become ill "by injecting toxins so as to cause diarrhea, dehydration, or other symptoms—and then eagerly seeks medical attention" (Kaplan et al., 1994, p. 787). The person inflicting the illness or injury denies any knowledge of how the child developed the problem; "symptoms quickly cease when the child and the perpetrator are separated" (Mercer and Perdue, 1993, p. 75). The diagnosis has been made with increasing frequency by secretly videotaping the parents' actions in the hospital.

Abuse is found in groups and cultures where traditionally it was not known and/or acknowledged. Japanese children, for example, have generally been observed to receive caring and sensitive maternal attention (Freeman, 1998); recently, however, attention in Japan has focused on more widespread child abuse being discovered (WuDunn, 1999). One question being debated is whether this is a new phenomenon or one that has been ongoing for a long time, but is just now being recognized.

> In addition to economic pressures, divorce rates and remarriages are rising, which experts say has led to abusive behavior by some stepparents.
>
> "In pediatric circles we thought there wasn't much child abuse and that we were different from the United States because our culture was different," said Dr. Seji Sakai, a child psychiatrist and director at the Center for Child Abuse Prevention. (WuDunn, 1999, p. A1)

In this country, physical abuse of children may be slight, occasional, used as punishment for a specific offense, and done within the context of a basically supportive family environment; or it can be frequent, violent, and committed within the context of a nonsupportive family culture. Children who are "retarded, epileptic, autistic, hyperactive, or dyslexic may be at especially high risk of physical abuse" ("Child Abuse—Part I," 1993, p. 3).

Children can be more "traumatized" by parental abuse than by experiencing other types of trauma, "partly because the damage begins early in life and partly because the usual source of protection and solace is unavailable. Child victims feel not only helpless, but betrayed, stigmatized, and contaminated" ("Child Abuse—Part II," 1993, p. 1). It is not inevitable, however, that *all* abused children feel this way; protective factors may include: support and comfort from family, friends, siblings, teachers (Thomlison, 1997), and the child's own coping capacities. To assess the specific effects of abuse on a given child, a biopsychosocial study is necessary, including assessment of the consistency and quality of relationships he or she has with primary caretakers and other important adults, the degree and frequency of abuse, the child's relationship to the abuser, and coping mechanisms.

Sexual Abuse

Sexual abuse of children is another area of abuse that is difficult to define, and disagreement exists about its parameters. One definition is: "forced, tricked, or manipulated contact with a child by an older person (generally five or more years older) that has the purpose of the sexual gratification of the older person" (Conte, 1995, p. 402). Although some behaviors are clearly considered abusive, such as adults engaging with children in sexual intercourse, fondling their genitals, or involving them in pornographic photography, "there are areas of ambiguity" ("Child Abuse—Part I," 1993), which can include: children observing parental nudity, adult cuddling or kissing of children which may or may not have sexualized overtones, and intruding on the physical privacy of a child in the bathroom. Ways abound in which children, from infants to teenagers, can be eroticized by older children or adults.

Detecting abuse is complicated by secrecy (for example, the child will not report it or will deny it when confronted). At the opposite pole, children, usually coached by adults, have falsified accounts of abuse; this has been observed in some parental custody cases. Recent attention has focused on establishing "criteria for discriminating between 'true' and 'false' cases of abuse" (Conte, 1995, p. 405). The question of whether recovered repressed memories of sexual abuse in adults (discussed in Chapter 2) are valid remains controversial.

Although it is difficult to obtain accurate numbers of children affected by abuse, it has nevertheless become apparent that childhood sexual abuse frequently occurs (Conte, 1995). Many sexual abuse cases are found in children under the age of seven, who "comprise approximately 40 percent of all substantiated reports of child sexual abuse" (Kaufman and Henrich, 2000, p. 201).

> In 1995, there were an estimated 15,128 substantiated cases of sexual abuse involving children under 3 years old, and an estimated 36,559 substantiated cases of sexual abuse involving children 4 to 7 years old, with many of these children having experienced abuse from early in life (U.S. Department of Health and Human Services, 1997). Moreover, given the limited verbal capacities of very young children, the sexual abuse of children less than age 3 is frequently quite severe, requiring positive medical findings to corroborate allegations. (Kaufman and Henrich, 2000, p. 201)

These figures may be higher for this young population, as well as for older children; many cases are not reported, discovered, or investigated. Often children are too frightened, ashamed, or intimidated by adults to report abuse. Most sexual abuse takes place within the child's immediate or extended family and has also been found in schools, day care centers, and group homes "where adult caretakers have been found to be the major offenders" (Kaplan et al., 1994, p. 788).

Sexual abuse has been reported more often in girls than boys, and the literature usually focuses on women survivors of sexual abuse. However, the fact that many men are also survivors of sexual abuse has been coming to light more recently; the full scope of the problem is not known, because it tends to be underreported (Cermak and Molidor, 1996). Sexual abuse not only has serious psychological effects on women but can have "repercussions in many areas of a man's life decades later" (Cermak and Molidor, 1996, p. 395). Boys who have been sexually abused can have more serious psychological problems than girls who have been abused (Cermak and Molidor, 1996; Nasjleti, 1980). Although boys are usually victimized by men, such as clergy, coaches, and other community leaders, in addition to birth fathers and stepfathers, sexual abuse of boys has also been found to have been committed by women, including mothers (Cermak and Molidor, 1996).

Psychological consequences of sexual abuse can be severe for both sexes and may present in a variety of symptoms and behaviors, although not all survivors have experienced prolonged psychological distress. Problems in intimacy and with the victim's own sexuality are not uncommon. "No specific psychiatric symptom universally results from sexual abuse. Vulnerability to the sequelae of sexual abuse depends on the type of abuse, the chronicity of the abuse, the age of the child, and the overall relationship of the victim and the abuser" (Kaplan et al., 1994, p. 789).

Children who are most vulnerable for negative outcomes are those who have been abused at very young ages; they are also likely to be exposed to more physical abuse and neglect; "their sexual abuse experiences were more likely to have been chronic and to have involved multiple perpetrators, one of whom was a parent or stepparent" (Kaufman and Henrich, 2000, p. 201). On the other hand, chronic and even brief experiences of sexual abuse by trusted community figures, especially because they are not easily shared with parents and are associated with profound shame, have been reported as devastating much later in life.

Many psychological symptoms and disturbed behaviors have been noted to be a consequence of sexual abuse: post-traumatic stress disorder, dissociative symptoms, sexual acting out (noted in the last chapter to lead to foster placement and adoption disruptions), anxiety, depression, and behavioral disturbances, including aggression toward others (Kaplan et al., 1994; Kaufman and Henrich, 2000; "Child Abuse—Part II," 1993). Many people who have borderline personalities, dissociative disorders, and substance abuse problems are adult survivors of abuse (Kaplan et al., 1994). A substantial number of health-related problems were found in sexually abused children and adult survivors (Wells, 1995).

Recent evidence suggests that "disproportionately large numbers of women on welfare were sexually abused as children" (DeParle, 1999, p. 1). Adolescent mothers often have histories of sexual abuse (Wakschlag and Hans, 2000) as do many runaways and homeless youth (Bass, 1995). In a study by the Department of Justice, a high percentage of both male and female prisoners indicated that they were physically or sexually abused as children ("High Percentage," 1999).

Another dimension of increasing prevalence is the outright commercial sexual abuse of children which includes child prostitution, child pornography, and child trafficking and kidnapping.

In assessing the impact of abuse on the child's developmental progress, the whole context of a child's life must be observed, including other risk and protective factors present. One of the most important protective factors is "the availability of a supportive parent or alternate guardian" (Kaufman and Henrich, 2000, p. 202).

Substance Abuse and the Family

Substance abuse is a major problem with serious physical, social, emotional, and economic consequences. "The scope of the problem is enormous. More than 15 percent of the United States population over 18 years of age have serious substance use problems, with about two-thirds of them abusing alcohol primarily and the other one-third of them abusing substances other than alcohol primarily" (Kaplan, 1994, p. 383). Substance abuse has been related to family problems and disorganization, and increasing attention has been paid to the negative impact of parental drinking on the emotional well-being of children.

Substance abuse has had a major impact on the child welfare system, as "alcohol and other drugs have increasingly become factors in child maltreatment and are a primary reason that children and young people enter out-of-home care" (Liederman, 1995, p. 430); "as many as 80 percent of maltreating parents have past or current substance abuse problems" (Thomlison, 1997, p. 54). It was estimated that "70 percent of the 41,000 children in foster care in New York City have a parent who is an addict" (Rohde, 1998, p. 35).

An important associated risk factor is the added presence of specific psychopathology; for some, substance abuse serves a "self-medicating" function. In one major study, it was found that "more than 50 percent of substance-abusing individuals had major psychopathology. Anxiety disorders were most prominent, followed by affective disorders, and schizophrenia" (Lester et al., 2000, p. 167). The most common psychiatric problems for women with substance abuse problems are depression, anxiety and post-traumatic stress disorder (Smyth and Miller, 1997).

It is often difficult to isolate the consequences of parental substance abuse on a child's well-being, as "most substance-abusing parents have multiple risk factors, including child maltreatment, psychiatric disorders, marital conflict, or domestic violence" (Davies, 1999, p. 70). Clinicians should assess the actual severity of substance abuse and its specific impact on parenting; whether the child becomes parentified (assuming adult responsibilities as well as responsibility for the adult); and whether the child has a supportive relationship with one nonsubstance abusing parent or other important adult (Smyth and Miller, 1997). Berlin and Davis (1989) discuss the importance of children of alcoholics developing the capacity for an adaptive defensive distancing from their families whereby they can form healthy relationships with others and enter into constructive activities.

However, substance abuse itself is an important risk factor, as "parenting ability is often severely affected" (Davies, 1999, p. 70). A mother who is "intoxicated . . . will be less able to monitor her children's activities both in and outside the home. If she is bringing other drug users into the house, she may be less aware of their interactions with her children. If she is using drugs away from the home, she may lose track of time and leave her children unattended" (Smyth and Miller, 1997, p. 129). A number of problems have been observed in children of substance abusers, including fetal alcohol syndrome, neglect, physical and sexual abuse, behavioral/conduct disorders, illnesses, injuries, depression, suicidal behavior, substance abuse, and antisocial behavior (Smyth and Miller, 1997); these children have "poorer social skills, peer relations, and academic performance" (Davies, 1999, p. 71).

Treatment of substance-abusing mothers has often focused only on treating the substance abuse, without offering comprehensive services dealing with poverty, lack of education, her past maltreatment, and difficult interpersonal relationships, as well as mothering capacities and skills (Dore, 1999). Some mothers have had to make the choice of temporarily giving up their children to enter residential treatment programs; greater emphasis has recently been placed on providing services to women that involve their children in different ways. "When programs provide treatment for the family, single mothers are spared the difficult choice between their own recovery and caring for their children" (Smyth and Miller, 1997, p. 134).

Several studies have pointed to successful results when women in recovery programs have had their children remain with them in residential treatment; a parenting component was often part of this program (Lester et al., 2000); "treating mothers and children as one unit" can be beneficial (Sun, 2000, p. 144). Some outpatient substance abuse programs have begun offering parenting groups, and social agencies sometimes offer outreach programs to children of substance abusing parents. Substance abuse issues are further discussed in Chapter 13.

Mental Illness of Parents

The mental illness of parents often has a significant impact on the emotional and developmental life of their children, who "are at risk for mental illness and other behavioral problems" (Seifer and Dickstein, 2000, p. 145).

Although genetic influences are involved in the transmission of some mental disorders, the emotional environment of the home and parental response to the child are very important variables. A given diagnosis is not a definitive statement about how a child will be affected; the entire biopsychosocial context of each family must be evaluated, including the availability of emotional supports to the child and the strengths and competencies present in both the child and the ill parent. Multiple risk factors may be present in addition to, or perhaps resulting from, the mental illness.

Many children of severely mentally ill parents experience parental abuse, neglect, and are often subject to irrational responses from their parents (Davies, 1999); this can result from "a parent's judgment and thought processes [which] may be impaired. Parents who are depressed or psychotic or have severe personality disorders may view their children as bad or as trying to drive them crazy" (Kaplan et al., 1994, p. 786). In addition, parents with a diagnosis of schizophrenia or bipolar disorder "often behave inconsistently and lack emotional attunement" (Davies, 1999, p. 68). Children with mothers who have serious and long-standing depressions may suffer from maternal withdrawal and lack of responsiveness (Davies, 1999); they are "at much greater risk for depression and other disorders over the course of adolescence than their counterparts in families where parents are not ill" (Beardslee and MacMillan, 1993, p. 249). There may also be acute, devastating, and threatening crises when severe decompensation occurs; mental health law today, while aiming at protecting civil liberties, may leave desperate families and professionals with little recourse for treatment.

Beardslee and MacMillan (1993) describe family therapy involving children of depressed parents, where the focus is helping the children adapt to the parental illness and enhance their own resiliency. The identified patient receives individual treatment, and the parents are involved in deciding with the therapist what to tell their children about the details of their depression.

> The intervention involves the entire family and has a strong educational component, with an emphasis on the expression of feelings and interactions in the family about the mother's [or father's] illness. Its main aim is to assist the family to develop a process through which the parents can help their children cope with parental illness and move forward with their own lives. . . . In general, it is designed to address poor communication and misunderstanding among family members . . . . It is also based on the clinical observation that parents are generally committed to the well-being of their children's development, even in the midst of a painful and crippling mental illness. (Beardslee and MacMillan, 1993, pp. 250-251)

The approach of Beardslee and MacMillan (1993) resonates with the biopsychosocial framework; the individual patient receives treatment, but if the patient is a parent, the needs of the children and partner are considered. It is usually in the best interests of patients to help them help their families and enhance family relationships to whatever degree this is possible for them.

Discussions of child development often exclude the father; this also tends to be so when discussing the impact of mental illness of children, as usually emphasis is on the mother who is mentally ill. Although the impact on children of their fathers' alcohol abuse and delinquency have received research attention, the impact of a father's mental illness on his children and family life also merits further study. There are many autobiographical reflections, both in fictional and nonfiction writings, on the long-term, formative, and even crippling effects of serious emotional or mental illness of a father on his children.

For many clinical social workers, the range of disorders currently defined as mental illness may not be immediately visible in clients and may in fact be camouflaged by serious social problems, such as homelessness or child neglect. Depression, for example, is often found in homeless people, neglectful mothers, pregnant teenagers, those who abuse substances, and runaway teenagers. It is imperative to look beneath the surface of social chaos and dysfunction that clients often present and to recognize underlying psychological pain and disorder so that appropriate help can be offered.

SPECIAL APPROACHES TO FAMILY TREATMENT

Families often seek help for themselves, applying to family therapists or family service agencies; they are experiencing discomfort with their relationships and have some motivation to correct this basic situation. Other situations precipitate a call for help, in which a crisis has led to a temporary immobilization or increased tension in interpersonal relationships. A medical crisis, for example, can precipitate feelings of anxiety, fears of loss, and can create economic and employment problems. Medical social workers address many of these problems as they see families facing major disabilities, such as a heart attack, cancer, or stroke in an adult, or leukemia or a spinal cord injury in a child. Most families in these crises are responsive to support, grief counseling, and help with appropriate rehabilitative services. At the same time, medical crises can also complicate pre-existing psychosocial difficulties. Family work with medical problems is discussed further in Chapter 12.

Divorce Therapy and Divorce Mediation

Divorce brings about major disturbances in family relationships, has a major impact on children, and alters basic patterns of family structure. Although some couples attempt marital therapy prior to divorce, once the decision has been made, they can benefit from divorce therapy, which can help them work through their ambivalent motivations toward divorce and decrease tensions between them so that they can reach a constructive divorce settlement, including arrangements for the children (Kressel, 1997). Divorce mediation, while having some commonalities to divorce therapy, is a separate specialization.

Divorce mediation is a new field, established approximately ten years ago; most of its practitioners are social workers and psychologists, with a smaller number of practicing lawyers. The goal is to move away from the adversarial model of divorce and to help a divorcing couple reach amicable or at least constructive agreements. Divorce mediation does not usually replace the need for lawyers; they are consulted during the process, but ideally the couple is enabled to use legal services more constructively (Kressel, 1997). Kressel (1997) sees the potential in divorce mediation but does not view it as a panacea; it is a "complex and stressful social role with difficulties that are remarkably similar to . . . [and can produce] the headaches of the divorce attorney" (pp. 178-179).

> Divorce mediation refers to a process in which divorcing spouses negotiate some or all of the terms of their settlement agreement with the aid of a neutral and trained third party. Some . . . negotiating sessions may involve separate meetings between the mediator and each of the parties, but the emphasis tends to be on face-to-face sessions. . . . The mediator's overarching objective is the establishment and maintenance of a cooperative, problem-solving orientation between the spouses. . . . The mediator's attention is directed to two principal areas: establishing a productive negotiating climate and addressing the substantive issues. (Kressel, 1997, p. 179)

A Psychoeducational Approach

A psychoeducational approach is one treatment modality that has gained popularity in work with schizophrenic patients and their families and is also utilized in other aspects of social work, such as assisting patients and their families with medical issues and helping parents with substance abuse problems to learn adequate parenting skills.

In the past, schizophrenia was viewed by many as an illness caused by parental psychopathology; the term *schizophrenogenic mother* was often applied to mothers of schizophrenic patients, with the underlying assumption that their pathology and behaviors toward the patient produced the illness. Today, with increased recognition of the prominent role of genetic and biological factors in the etiology of schizophrenia, a less blaming and more supportive approach is taken with these families; it is recognized that they must cope with a child with very disturbed behaviors, which they do not understand and do not know how to handle.

Families need support to deal with the guilt and shame they often experience when their child becomes severely mentally ill; they need guidance in ways to cope with the patient, and validation of the importance of their role in helping the patient to adapt. Families must also be helped to understand the role of stress in producing the illness and in causing exacerbations of symptoms. Kopeikin and colleagues (1983) discuss objectives in helping families prevent stress in the patient's life.

> A four-objective treatment model guides the conduct of sessions. . . . (1) identifying the two or three current, most hazardous stressors threatening the patient; (2) developing strategies to prevent stress and cope with it; (3) having families implement the strategies, evaluate them, and refine them; (4) engaging in anticipatory planning to prevent and cope with future stresses. (Kopeikin et al., 1983, p. 74)

Family Preservation Programs

Clients are often mandated to seek services, as when men who have battered their partners are court ordered to receive group counseling. Child welfare agencies can require protective in-home services for children, which can lead to out-of-home placement; mothers can be mandated by courts to receive substance abuse treatment.

Most protective work and foster placement services are provided in the home. Although the quality and consistency of home visits vary, the goal is to provide supportive psychoeducational services to the mother as well as to provide specific community services, such as helping the mother obtain welfare assistance, employment, medical care, and special day care, nursery school, and recreational programs.

One model of in-home services are family preservation programs, based on the concept of *permanency planning,* which has as its goals keeping families together and reunifying them if the child is in an out-of-home placement. Family preservation services are time limited and staff intensive, with frequent home visits, responsiveness to emergency calls, and provision of multiple community services (Whittaker et al., 1990). In the homebuilders model described by Whittaker and colleagues (1990), services are offered to families at the point when out-of-home placement is being considered for their children.

> In short, the service delivery features of intensive preservation programs are designed to engage families in service (even those families who have "failed" in other counseling attempts), to keep them in service intensively for a time-limited period, and to increase the likelihood that they will benefit from service. IFPS [intensive family preservation services] provide a combination of services designed to deal with crisis situations, to enhance family functioning, to meet both concrete and clinical service needs, and to decrease the family's isolation. Most IFPS work from family strengths and include use of extended family, community, and neighborhood resources. These services make maximum use of a variety of worker tasks and roles— counselor, parent trainer, advocate, consultant and resource broker. (Whittaker et al., 1990, pp. 3-4)

When family preservation services are successful, the goals of family permanency have been achieved, and family functioning has improved. However, it has been argued that in some seriously neglectful and/or abusive families, keeping children at home subjects them to further maltreatment and delays appropriate placement. In the last chapter, for example, we noted that a professional's preference for family reunification caused considerable suffering to Matthew, whose wished-for adoption by his foster mother was delayed for many years. Matthew's biological mother did not seem to have the capacity to cope with him, and although therapeutic services were offered to her, she did not utilize them. If an intensive homebuilders program had been provided, would his mother have had the capacity to respond to this program, or would Matthew have remained in the same predicament?

Although family preservation might not succeed in producing the desired reunification, perhaps its success can be measured differently; if a parent has the opportunity and assistance to correct child maltreatment and fails, then the need for out-of-home placement might be more apparent and may proceed with greater speed. Although most family preservation services are short term (several months), in some cases might a parent regress after services are removed; in fact, might a mother feel more deprived after all the attention that has been showered on her has disappeared?

> An immature, maladjusted, or overstressed parent who has abused a child is at risk for repeating the abuse, despite the best performance agreement prepared by a caseworker and regular supervision of the family. Parents must be given an opportunity to overcome their dysfunctions, and although many interventions are successful, some are

not. When interventions are unsuccessful, some children may die at the hands of abusive parents. (Alexander and Alexander, 1995, pp. 812-813)

In one study of disrupted family reunifications in sixty-two families, both family problems and lack of adequate services contributed to the family seeking further placement for their children (Hess et al., 1992). Looking at family characteristics that led to poor outcomes, the authors note that "the degree of parents' ambivalence about parenting, a history of two or more unsuccessful reunifications, and the length of time the child has been in placement should have strongly suggested that reunification was not an appropriate case goal" (Hess et al., 1992, p. 309).

Barth (1994) has observed that although intensive family preservation programs are effective with some families, they may not be effective with families experiencing "mental illness . . . chronic neglect . . . drug abuse, and problems with older children's behavior" (p. 516). In addition, a family's housing might not be adequate to contain a preservation model.

> Other families do not succeed in family preservation programs because the programs are too short lived. This may be particularly true for very young mothers and drug-involved mothers who experience relapses; they may look successful at termination and brief follow-up but are not adequate parents a year later. In addition, some children require more protection than can be provided by social workers, even if social workers are in the home for as many as 10 hours a week. (Barth, 1994, p. 521)

Barth (1994) advocates the provision of "shared family care," in which out-of-home care is provided to both child and parent "so that parent and host caregivers simultaneously share the care of the child and work toward independent in-home care by the parents" (p. 516). Barth indicates that in this model the gap between in-home and out-of-home care is bridged; "shared family care arrangements provide both" (p. 516). Examples of this include: foster care or residences in which pregnant teenagers can receive help and remain (for varying periods of time) with their newborn babies; children entering substance abuse treatment residences with their mothers (and in some instances, their fathers); battered women's shelters that traditionally have accepted both the mother and her children; and residential treatment programs for children in which parents may reside and/or play an active role in their children's care.

Although Barth's suggestions are very constructive and may work for many families, the necessity of permanency planning outside of the home and apart from their families may be the only viable alternative for some children.

CONCLUSION

In this chapter, we have examined the internal structures of families, including rules, boundaries, and myths. The family is a powerful system, whether existing in a stable, secure form or involved in disengaged, enmeshed, or disorganized systems. Cultural values and beliefs permeate family life, yet family theory applies to families in any culture; every family has rituals, patterns of attachment, boundaries, and so forth. It is not possible for people to be unaffected by their past and present family lives, as family members are the first attachment figures and generally interact with the child through adolescence and adulthood. The family exists outside the self and is also internalized as part of the self.

As clinicians working within a family system, we are often drawn into the maelstrom of its emotional forces with pulls and countervailing pushes. If we can manage to maintain our balance and not be swept away by these intense pressures, we can then tune in to our reactions to and interactions with family members, gaining rich insights about the inner dynamics of a family's existence.

Serious problems face families in our society; many modes of intervention become necessary, including comprehensive community programs, preventive strategies, and constructive social policies. As we examine issues such as family breakdown, maltreatment, substance abuse, and homelessness, we see over and over again the presence of individual malfunction, hopelessness, depression, and inner turmoil, hand in hand with social problems. Attention needs to be focused on enhancing individual mental health; strengthening family stability is one critical piece of this approach. However, even within a family context, the individuality of each family member must be understood and appreciated. Although a life trajectory of biological and psychological development is common to us all, the construction of reality and the inner world remain unique for each person.

The birth and evolving development of the neonate into a unique individual will be examined in the next chapter.

LEARNING EXERCISE

1. In your small groups, prepare to do a role-play, selecting some aspect of family communication, patterns of relationship, and/or specific family problem, such as divorce or maltreatment.

SUGGESTED READINGS

Article

Farley, J. (1990). Family developmental task assessment: A prerequisite to family treatment. *Clinical Social Work Journal, 18,* 85-98.

Books

Beardslee, W. R. and MacMillan, H. L. (1993). Preventive intervention with the children of depressed parents: A case study. In A. J. Solnit, P. B. Neubauer, S. Abrams, and A. S. Dowling (Eds.), *The psychoanalytic study of the child,* Vol. 48 (pp. 249-276). New Haven: Yale University Press.

Cummings, E. M., Davies, P. T., and Campbell, S. B. (2000). *Developmental psychopathology and family process: Theory, research and clinical implications.* New York: The Guilford Press.

Kiselica, M. S. (1995). *Multicultural counseling with teenage fathers: A practical guide.* Thousand Oaks, CA: Sage Publications.

McCourt, F. (1996). *Angela's ashes: A memoir of childhood.* London: HarperCollins Publishers.

Minuchin, S. (1974). *Families and family therapy.* Cambridge: Harvard University Press.

Satir, V. (1967). *Conjoint family therapy.* Palo Alto: Science and Behavior Books.

Scharff, D. and Scharff, J. (1987). *Object relations family therapy.* Northvale, NJ: Jason Aronson Inc.

Smyth, N. and Miller, B. (1997). Parenting issues for substance-abusing women. In S. L. A. Straussner and E. Zelvin (Eds.), *Gender and addictions: Men and women in treatment* (pp. 123-150). Northvale, NJ: Jason Aronson Inc.

SECTION II:
THE LIFE CYCLE

Chapter 8

Reproductive Issues, Infancy, and Early Childhood Development

But what am I?
An infant crying in the night:
An infant crying for the light,
And with no language but a cry.

Alfred Tennyson
"In Memoriam," *liv. Stanza 5.* 1850

INTRODUCTION

This chapter focuses on children from conception through the preschool years and emphasizes their physical, cognitive, and emotional growth and maturation, as well as their age-specific needs, behaviors, and problems. The prominent role of attachment is stressed, and children's development, as they interact with their families within their social and cultural contexts, is viewed transactionally.

From the moment of conception, a transactional interrelationship exists between the mother and child. Even if the father is absent or not involved, the mother's feelings and attitudes about the father color her reactions to the child. And once the child is born, the father's (or partner's) presence (or absence) is also relevant. Many times, as noted earlier, fathers and partners are actively involved in caretaking and may be the primary caretaker.

Although family organizations, internal structures, and problems (discussed in Chapters 6 and 7) are not related extensively to the discussion of the child's developmental issues in this chapter, it is important to keep these concepts in mind. Because the child's early evolution is so eventful and complex, developmental details are the focus; space does not allow further elaboration of the range of possible family and cultural configurations that are possible.

REPRODUCTION

Conception

For some, to conceive a child is a profound decision; for others it is an unplanned consequence of sexual activity, which may be accepted with positive feelings, may be viewed fatalistically, or may be accompanied by negative feelings. However, it may be assumed that *ambivalence* is common to all, as a readjustment in relationships and lifestyle is inevitable. Major physiological alterations occur in the mother's body, accompanied by psychological shifts; for men, the anticipation of fatherhood can produce strong, sometimes conflicting emotional states. Both parents typically experience changes in self-concept and identity. Becoming a parent is a developmental phase with the potential for psychological growth (Benedek, 1970; Cohen and Slade, 2000; Elson, 1984; Zayas, 1987). This phase may also be accompanied by psychological regression.

Conception, in a "natural" pregnancy (that is, one not manipulated by reproductive technologies), occurs following sexual intercourse when the egg is fertilized by the sperm in the woman's fallopian tube. After four to seven days, the fertilized egg moves to the uterus, where it may successfully implant itself in the uterine wall and begin to grow; if this does not happen, the fertilized egg will be expelled. The developing embryo is referred to as a fetus after the first eight weeks. The gender of the child is genetically determined at the moment of conception, as are a multitude of physical and intellectual endowments.

Genetics

We are in the midst of a "knowledge explosion" in genetics, with new research findings, practical medical applications, and an accompanying host of moral, ethical, and legal dilemmas. In January 1999, it was predicted that in a few years, scientists will probably have completed "deciphering the human genome, the 100,000 genes encoded by 3 billion chemical pairs in our DNA" (Isaacson, 1999, p. 42). However, it was only a short time later, in June 2000, that this was accomplished (Wade, 2000). Although many scientists felt more work and refinement of the findings was necessary, this was nevertheless considered a major breakthrough. Wade (2000) looks for this knowledge to radically alter medical practice.

> Biologists expect in time to develop an array of diagnostics and treatments based on it and tailored to individual patients, some of which will exploit the body's own mechanisms of self-repair.

The knowledge in the genome could also be used in harmful ways, particularly in revealing patients' disposition to disease if their privacy is not safeguarded, and thus resulting in discrimination. (Wade, 2000, p. A1).

Increased genetic knowledge of fetal development has led to the development of new reproductive technologies and interventions to correct fetal defects. Tests (such as amniocentesis, to examine cells contained in the fluid surrounding the developing fetus) are performed on the fetus to determine the presence of certain genetic disorders; certain congenital conditions (such as spina bifida, nonclosure of the developing spinal column) have been experimentally treated in the womb (Golden, 1999a). Pregnant women may face the difficult decision of whether to abort a defective fetus, such as one with Down's syndrome (a form of mental retardation more commonly found in pregnancies of older mothers). Genetic testing, performed prior to conception for people with genetically transmissible disorders in themselves and/or their families, can provide knowledge of probabilities of genetic transmission to a child.

A couple at risk for conceiving a child with genetic problems can experience many disturbing emotions, including anxiety, sadness, and anger at the partner with the genetic vulnerability; genetic problems can also affect the whole family. Rauch and Black (1995) point out that a "genetic diagnosis is always a *family* diagnosis"; therefore, risks may be encountered, such as the discovery that an adverse gene could be transmitted or the disclosure of family secrets such as incest which may lead to guilt or recriminations. Families may also gain greater cohesion (Rauch and Black, 1995, pp. 1112-1113).

Genetic research has enabled parents to choose the sex of the child, a procedure critical in preventing the conception of children with sex-linked illnesses, such as hemophilia, but which becomes more controversial when parents choose a sex for purely social reasons (Kolata, 1998; Lemonick, 1999).

The infertility of many couples today has been a major factor accelerating developments in reproductive medicine.

The Fertility Crisis

The expectation that one can decide to be (and when to be) a parent can be tragically dashed when a couple discovers fertility problems, a situation reported to be of "epidemic" proportions in this country. Infertility often creates psychological distress; the introduction of fertility treatments and reproductive technologies may create additional distress due to their biological, psychological, social, and legal complexities. Fertility treatments can be expensive, time consuming, and emotionally draining, and may produce a pregnancy with multiple fetuses.

Approximately six-and-a-half million couples in this country have fertility problems, "and about half of them seek treatment for it" (Hilts, 1999, p. A12). Fertility treatments are becoming more technologically advanced, and many couples, utilizing them, have successfully delivered healthy babies. For some fertility problems, procedures are fairly straightforward and not especially time consuming. For others, procedures are complex, costs are high, repeated disappointments are experienced, and the quality of marital life may be negatively affected for many years, taking a high emotional toll on both partners. Additionally, fertility drugs can affect the mother's mood (Cohen and Slade, 2000). Jill Smolowe (1997), a journalist, wrote of her difficult experiences going through fertility treatments.

> I found every moment of that battle against biology a nightmare. The first salvo was Clomid. . . . I swallowed the pills. But rather than stimulating more eggs, the drug plunged me into a deep depression that left me unable to . . . think of anything but babies. (Smolowe, 1997, p. 46)

Smolowe's (1997) fertility treatments were not successful; she then turned to adoption, concluding, in China, when "a tiny hand reached up and touched my cheek. I was, at last, a mother" (p. 46). The solution of international adoption, discussed in Chapter 6, is reached by many who have struggled unsuccessfully with the fertility crisis.

Reproductive Technologies

One of the most successful reproductive technologies is in-vitro fertilization (IVF), in which doctors remove eggs from a woman's ovary, fertilize them with sperm (from her partner or a donor) in a petri dish, and then surgically place the fertilized product in the woman's uterus. Louise Brown, an English baby conceived in a petri dish, achieved fame when, in 1978, she became the first test tube baby to be born (Lemonick, 1997). Since then, "more than 33,000 babies have been born in the U.S. thanks to in-vitro (literally, 'in glass') fertilization" (Lemonick, 1997, p. 42).

In vitro fertilization has aided conception in postmenopausal women. "With IVF, hormones and another woman's [donor's] egg, even a postmenopausal woman can give birth" (Lemonick, 1997, p. 45). More than 100 women over the age of fifty in the United States as well as many in other countries have successfully given birth. In 1996, Arceli Keh, a sixty-three-year-old woman in California, made news when she gave birth.

It is possible to freeze embryos after IVF to be used successfully in future pregnancies. However, the existence of frozen embryos sometimes leads to complex legal and ethical dilemmas. Divorcing couples have fought over custody rights regarding the disposition of their frozen embryos. One forty-one-year-old Boston woman, for example, sought to become impregnated with her frozen embryo against her former husband's wishes. She stated that it would in effect be a "forced abortion" not to be allowed to do this (McKim, 1996, p. A1); the husband objected to the enforced responsibility (p. A20). "What exactly is a frozen embryo, property or person? And while case law holds a woman responsible for the fate of a fertilized egg inside her body, who should have the last word about an egg fertilized outside her body?" (p. A20).

Such a ruling was upheld by the Massachusetts Supreme Court in April 2000; it added that "as a matter of public policy, we conclude that forced procreation is not an area amenable to judicial enforcement" (Goldberg, 2000, p. A14); this opinion "is expected to influence court decisions around the country in a nascent area of law" (p. A14). Legal disputes will probably increase, as approximately 150,000 frozen embryos currently exist (Goldberg, 2000).

Women unable to use their own eggs for fertilization sometimes use donor eggs from other women. How does one select which eggs (or rather, whose eggs) to use; is this always anonymous? Calvin Trillin (1999) underscores this complex and painful dilemna in a humorous vein:

> Plowing through *The New York Times* on a recent Sunday, I read in the Metro Section that infertile couples in the market for smart-kid genes regularly place advertisements in the newspapers of their own Ivy League alma maters offering female undergraduates $7,500 for a donated egg. Before I could get that news comfortably digested, I came across an article in the Magazine section describing SAT prep courses for which parents spend thousands in the hope of raising their child's test scores enough to make admission to an Ivy League college possible. So how can people who have found a potential egg donor at an Ivy League college tell whether the donor carries genuine smart-kid genes or just pushy-parents genes? (p. 20)

Dilemmas regarding artificial insemination were discussed very briefly in Chapter 6. How anonymous should the father be? Is his genetic background known? Do children have the right to know him or know about him? Similar questions can be asked about the female donor of an egg.

A heterosexual couple using artificial insemination from an anonymous donor because the father is infertile, may experience special psychological problems (Landau, 1998); many such fathers harbor the sense that the "donor is the 'real' father" (p. 79). In some cases, they feel inferior, assuming that the donor (not to mention the child) is "more gifted than they are (most of the donors are medical or graduate students)" (Landau, 1998, p. 79).

For lesbian couples or single women seeking artificial insemination, the donor may be known and involved in the life of the women. In many other cases the donor is anonymous and remains so. Differences of opinion exist regarding utilization of sperm from anonymous donors; to some, this is preferable; others feel that ignoring the "donor's existence may cause the donor offspring to feel like only half a person" (Landau, 1998, p. 81).

Little is known about the psychological reactions of the sperm donor. There is some indication that they may eventually experience "regret, concern, and fear for the children . . . they will never know" (Landau, 1998, p. 80). Similarly, how do egg donors feel about their donations in later life?

The psychological sequelae of artificial insemination have received little study. Many families are inclined to some degree of openness (rather than keeping this a family secret), with emphasis on sharing this fact with relatives, including the child, and of obtaining genetic history and some personal information about the donor. Baran and Pannor (Landau, 1998) advocate the right of the child to the truth, and thus full disclosure of identifying information about the donor, who is not reducible to the sperm he has contributed (p. 85): "The donor father is a real person, not a teaspoon of sperm. The donor offspring is a genetic product of two parents, with the right to know the truth" (p. 85). The question of the right of birth mothers to privacy in the adoption process, raised in Chapter 6, can also be raised in relation to the privacy of donors of eggs and sperm.

Pregnancy

Pregnancy is typically divided into three trimesters (each of three months' duration); the developments during each trimester have important consequences for both the fetus and the mother.

The First Trimester

The first trimester produces many dramatic and rapid changes in the newly developing embryo, as previously undifferentiated cells change into specific tissues and organs. The baby is especially vulnerable during this stage to certain diseases developing in the mother as well as her ingestion of drugs and alcohol; these can irreparably affect fetal development. By the second month, the embryo appears generally human in form.

The mother is also undergoing major physiological changes during this time; dramatic changes are occurring in her hormonal system, as her body adapts to the state of pregnancy; she may feel morning sickness and mood changes. There is a 25 percent chance that a pregnancy may result in miscarriage during this trimester (Cohen and Slade, 2000).

The Second Trimester

During the second trimester, the baby's further growth, organ differentiation, and maturation continue; eyes and hair develop, for example, and regulation of the baby's heartbeat progresses. The mother usually becomes visibly pregnant and can begin to feel the baby moving inside her. Morning sickness of the first trimester tends to diminish, and the hormonal surges are modulated, triggering less emotional lability. The baby often feels more real to the mother, and this feeling is enhanced for many by the recent availability of medically indicated ultrasound pictures of their babies.

Psychodynamic theorists speak of the mother developing a greater emotional connection to the baby during this stage; her "emotional investment is drawn away from the outside world and refocused inward toward her baby and the transformations taking place inside her. . . . not only is she becoming a mother physically, she is now evolving into one psychologically" (Cohen and Slade, 2000, p. 22).

The Third Trimester

By the third trimester, the baby's body is almost completely formed, the internal organs undergo further differentiation, and the nervous system and brain go through major development. An important achievement is the baby's weight gain; the mother also gains the most during this period, often causing her to feel more physically uncomfortable, especially during the last month. Psychologically, the mother is becoming more prepared for the baby's birth.

Reactions of Fathers and Other Partners to Pregnancy

Fatherhood generally receives little attention in the literature on children, and even less is written about the experiences of becoming a father. In general, this is a positive experience: "incipient fatherhood is an exciting, compelling, and profoundly moving experience" (Cohen and Slade, 2000, p. 24). However, many fathers also feel anxiety related to changes in the marital relationship, assuming financial and other responsibilities, worries about the wife's pregnancy and health, and confusion about parental roles and involvement with the new child (Cohen and Slade, 2000). Becoming parents can also stir up "sleeping" conflicts about the parents' own childhood and relationships to their parents; this may present an opportunity to work through these conflicts and reach a higher level of integration (Benedek, 1970; Cohen and Slade, 2000; Elson, 1984; Zayas, 1987).

Lesbian couples often choose to have children; as one option, one partner becomes pregnant through artificial insemination. The partners may have to endure social stigma. Kaplan and colleagues (1994) note, however, that "if the relationship between the two women is secure, they tend to bond strongly together . . . against that prejudice" (Kaplan et al., 1994, p. 25).

Multiple Births

Increased fertility treatment has led to a 55 percent increase in the number of twins born since 1980, according to the National Center for Health Statistics (Steinhauer, 1999a). Pregnant women carrying twins are placed in a high-risk category, receive close medical attention, are prone to more medical emergencies, and may need to limit their activities; twins are more likely be born prematurely and may have medical complications (Steinhauer, 1999a). Raising twins can create stress, and many parents of twins meet together for support. "In the first year, many parents said if the house hadn't burned down it was a successful day," Dr. Junior said. "But then there is something so magical about watching these two beings share a budding relationship together" (Steinhauer, 1999a, p. A25).

Multiple births, in general, are increasing; Lemonick notes a fourfold increase "in the past quarter-century" (Lemonick, 1997, p. 37). National attention was focused on the McCaughey family of Iowa, when the mother, after fertility treatments, gave birth to septuplets in 1997. Although other births of septuplets have been recorded, this is the first time the babies have lived more than a brief period. Parents who have multiple fetuses must often make the painful decision whether to follow the medical recommendation to abort some of those fetuses to "increase the chances of carrying at least one fetus to full term, reduce risk to the mother, or reduce the often overwhelming burden of caring for multiple infants" (Cohen and Slade, 2000, p. 32). The McCaugheys refused to consider this option. For them, it was not an issue as they adamantly rejected abortion. " 'That just wasn't an option,' Kenny told reporters. . . . 'We were trusting in the Lord for the outcome.' By conventional medical standards, the McCaugheys were taking a huge gamble; by their own, they were simply living their faith" (Lemonick, 1997, p. 36).

In a study and editorial reported in a 1999 issue of the *New England Journal of Medicine,* it was observed that fertility drugs do increase the likelihood of pregnancy, however, "the drugs should be used cautiously to avoid the possibility of multiple births" (Hilts, 1999, p. A12).

Risk Factors in Pregnancy

The mother's nutrition, exposure to infections and radiation, utilization of alcohol and drugs (including prescribed drugs), and psychological distress can affect fetal development (Davies, 1999; Garbarino, 1982). Teenagers, women who are older, and/or those carrying multiple fetuses are at special risk for health problems for themselves and/or their babies.

Maternal malnutrition can slow the rate of fetal growth, impair brain development, and give rise to neurological problems; some infectious diseases, such as German measles, contracted during the first trimester by the mother, can cause multiple birth defects, including blindness (Garbarino, 1982). Babies born to mothers with HIV infections often become HIV positive as well (Zastrow and Kirst-Ashman, 1997).

Women should receive prenatal care to safeguard their health and that of the fetus; lack of "early and regular prenatal care has long been associated with poor reproductive outcomes, particularly low birthweight, neonatal death, and postpartum complications" (Cook et al., 1999, p. 129). Many pregnant women in this country do not receive adequate prenatal care (Cook et al., 1999), and 21 percent do not receive this care until after the first trimester (Perloff and Jaffee, 1999). "Rates of late entry into care are even higher among teenagers and members of racial and ethnic minority groups" (Perloff and Jaffee, 1999, p. 117).

Maternal Substance Abuse

Maternal substance abuse can have serious consequences for the developing fetus; *fetal alcohol syndrome,* for example, is present in many infants whose mothers' alcohol intake was absorbed in utero (Kaplan et al., 1994). Kaplan and colleagues (1994) note that "Microcephaly, craniofacial malformations, and limb and heart defects are common. . . . The risk . . . is as high as 35 percent (p. 409).

Some states regard maternal substance abuse as a form of child abuse and have arrested or imposed legal penalties on offending mothers. The Supreme Court, in February 2000, agreed to hear a case tried in South Carolina involving a hospital's policy of reporting illegal drug use by pregnant women to the police. "The case is an appeal on behalf of 10 women who sued after being arrested as a result of the policy, some while they were still weak and bleeding from childbirth," presenting "the Supreme Court a narrow but important aspect of a legal and public policy debate that began in the peak years of the crack epidemic of the 1980's: the extent to which a state may intervene to protect fetal health, and the circumstances under which pregnant women may be held criminally responsible for behavior that endangers their fetuses" (Greenhouse, 2000b, p. A12).

A petition, produced by organizations supporting this appeal, including the National Association of Social Workers, stated that a great deal of research supports the notion that "intrusion of the criminal justice system on health care practices aggravates exponentially the already strong reluctance to seek medical attention and treatment" (O'Neill, 2000a, p. 7). Issues of treatment versus punishment for substance abusers have been addressed in Chapter 4, and its relevance to maternal substance abuse was discussed in Chapter 7. When children are born with birth defects from substance-abusing mothers, "they will have special needs that substance-abusing or recovering mothers will be ill-equipped to meet on their own" (Smyth and Miller, 1997, p. 133). This point advances the argument in favor of ongoing supportive intervention rather than punishment.

Loss of Baby During Pregnancy

The loss of a baby due to miscarriage is often a very painful event. "Women experience much greater grief following pregnancy loss than is commonly recognized" (Cohen and Slade, 2000, p. 30). Abortions can also be distressing to the mother and her partner, no matter the reason for the procedure, and may be followed by grief reactions. Abortions are chosen for many reasons: to save the life of the mother; in cases of rape and incest; to prevent the birth of a fetus with serious physical defects; and for social, economic, and psychological considerations. "Grief following abortions for fetal anomalies has been shown to be as intense as grief following spontaneous perinatal losses" (Cohen and Slade, 2000, p. 32). Aborting some fetuses in a multifetal pregnancy can be accompanied by "powerful feelings of guilt, anxiety, and sadness" (Cohen and Slade, 2000, p. 32).

Although the Supreme Court legalized women's right to abortion in the *Roe v. Wade* decision, bitter and strong political and religious debates continue between pro-choice and pro-life forces; abortion clinics have been bombed; harassment of abortion clinics' medical personnel has also taken place, culminating in several murders.

Birth

In the past, the process of giving birth was a high-risk procedure, accompanied by a high mortality rate for both the mother and child. Abraham Lincoln, for example, with great sorrow, attended the funeral for his sister (who raised him) and her newborn child. Today, with advances in medicine and prenatal care, mortality rates for mothers have dramatically decreased, and infant mortality has declined, although not consistently so. Cook and colleagues (1999) note that despite progress, "nearly 30,000 infants in this country die because of low birthweight (LBW). . . . LBW infants who do live have a high probability of . . . chronic and costly disabilities. . . . This unnecessary loss . . . is even more pronounced for the children of low-income women. . . . Infant mortality and morbidity rates often approximate those of Third World countries" (Cook et al., 1999, p. 129).

The Delivery

Options mothers can choose for delivery include: obstetrician-assisted childbirth in a hospital, which could be by natural childbirth (with or without anesthesia), or utilization of a midwife at home or in birthing centers. In the past, fathers (and partners) were excluded from the delivery room. This is no longer the case; today many partners choose to be present, providing support and/or coaching assistance. Women frequently take prenatal classes (often with their partners) to prepare themselves for childbirth.

The surgical procedure, *caesarian section,* has been increasingly utilized for obstetrical complications, such as prolonged labor, certain breech presentations, fetal distress, and Rh incompatibility. In debates about this subject, concern has been voiced that caesarians may be overused or used other than for strictly medical reasons, which include the doctor's fear of malpractice suits (a frequent occurrence in obstetrical practices) and the doctor's convenience.

Natural childbirth has developed its own subculture, with a distinct philosophy, set of procedures, and commitment of participants. Women attending classes are given support, education, and practice exercises to help them experience birth in a natural way, without anesthesia and with their active physical assistance. The enthusiasm for this method is embodied in sentiments such as those expressed by Ina May Gaskin, president of the Midwives Alliance of North America. "Natural childbirth is 'hugely empowering,' Mrs. Gaskin said '. . . . After a natural birth, you have so much power you feel you could do anything.'" (Grady, 1999b, p. A1).

But this commitment may also have a downside. Sometimes women enrolled in natural childbirth programs feel social pressure to have a successful delivery. When a social worker asked one mother how her delivery went, she burst into tears, saying she had failed! She had been in pain, asked for anesthesia, and so "let everyone down."

On the other hand, in a recent survey of 750 hospitals in this country, it was found that women increasingly prefer to forego the challenge and are willingly opting for the use of analgesia during labor and delivery (Grady, 1999b, p. A1). The development of newer, safer, and lighter anesthesias, such as *epidurals,* are used by many doctors and requested by large numbers of their women patients, who, with this medication, can remain awake and participate in their deliveries. This trend is opposed by many adherents of natural childbirth, who assert that women electing this procedure are forfeit-

ing a transcendent experience as well as running the risks of using unnecessary medications (Grady, 1999b, p. A1).

Cultural attitudes and customs can affect attitudes about childbirth practices. The Hmong, for example, attach a great deal of meaning to the placenta, which they formerly buried under their huts in their native Laos
(Fadiman, 1997). The Hmong word for placenta signifies "jacket . . . one's
first and finest garment." Upon death, a Hmong's soul "must travel . . . until
it reaches the burial place of its placental jacket, and puts it on. Only after
the soul is properly dressed . . . can it continue its dangerous journey . . . to . . .
where it is reunited with its ancestors and from which it will . . . be sent to be
reborn as the soul of a new baby. If the soul cannot find its jacket, it is condemned to an eternity of wandering, naked and alone" (Fadiman, 1997,
p. 5).

In one California hospital, where many Hmong women received medical
attention, some requested to take the placentas home with them. Sometimes
doctors agreed, "packing the placentas in plastic bags or take-out containers
from the hospital cafeteria;" most, however did not comply, concerned either that "the women planned to eat the placentas" or that this could lead to
the "possible spread of hepatitis B, which is carried by at least fifteen percent of the Hmong refugees in the United States" (Fadiman, 1997, p. 7).

Emotional Reactions to Birth

It is not uncommon for mothers, after the baby is born, to go through a
period of postpartum depression, which may last for several days. In this
"normal state of sadness," women may experience "dysphoria, frequent
tearfulness, and clinging dependence" (Kaplan et al., 1994, p. 36). This is
attributed to a combination of factors, including dramatic hormonal changes
in the mother's body, feeling stressed from childbirth, and anticipatory worries about coping with parental responsibilities. Sometimes the initial depression does not diminish but persists or deepens, or a depression develops
when the baby is one to three months old. These depressions can be related
to many factors, including an earlier history of depression, anxieties about
mothering, a reawakening of conflicts from the mother's own parent-child
relationships, or current stressors, such as marital problems or social isolation. In a small number of cases, the depression may reach psychotic proportions. "Hippocrates described postpartum disorders in ancient Greece,
and recent studies in rural Africa have found rates of partpartum depression
just as high as that of the industrial West" ("Postpartum Disorders," 1989,
p. 2).

It has been observed that fathers may also experience mood changes,
both during pregnancy and after birth (Kaplan et al., 1994). They may experience conflicts about being a father, changes in their marital relationship,

and the burden of additional responsibilities. Some fathers experience phys-ical symptoms similar to those of pregnancy and childbirth, which can in-clude "nausea, fatigue, back pain, and even abdominal pain" (Ashford et al., 1997, p. 136).

> In certain tribal societies, the father behaves as if he were giving birth. While his wife is delivering the infant, the father goes to bed and may even complain of labor pains. This custom symbolically establishes the man as father of the baby and gives him legal rights as the parent. (Ashford et al., 1997, p. 136)

Perinatal Loss

Perinatal loss, which is a baby's death upon delivery *(stillbirth)* or after a brief life, is a trauma for parents. In the past, the mother would be tranquil-ized, isolated, and rapidly discharged. "The less contact the mother had with the baby the better, and the less spoken about the baby the easier for her to forget and get on with her life" (Zeanah, 1991, p. 12). Now, it is recognized that parents need an opportunity to mourn and to become involved with their dying or dead children, such as naming them, holding them, and holding memorial services (Zeanah, 1991). *Pathological grief reactions,* manifested months or sometimes years following the baby's death, have unique features due to the nature of this loss, and individual psychotherapy is recommended (Condon, 1986).

Abandoned Babies

Current media attention has focused on discarded babies, that is, babies who are found in public places, such as parks or hospital parking lots (per-haps where mothers wanted them found); others, usually dead, have been found in dumpsters or garbage dumps. Houston, Texas, in 1999, experi-enced "an unprecedented rash of baby abandonments"; the number jumped from an average of two to three cases a year to thirteen cases, including three babies who died (Yardley, 1999, p. 14). The Department of Health and Hu-man Services found that there were 105 abandoned children nationally in 1998, of whom 33 died (Whitaker, 2000). Texas was the first state to pass legislation to encourage women to leave babies in a safe place. Other states have started working on legislation or establishing programs to make it safe, rather than punitive, for new mothers to seek agencies or hospitals where they can leave unwanted babies.

Many more mothers have abandoned their newborn children in hospital maternity wards; in 1998, 31,000 infants had mothers who were usually drug addicted or HIV infected and who left them in the hospital (Whitaker,

2000; Yardley, 1999). Congress created the National Abandoned Infants Assistance Resource Center in 1998, to address the problem of "these new-borns, called 'boarder babies,' [who] frequently languished in hospitals for months as officials struggled to find foster homes for them" (Yardley, 1999, p. 14).

Implications for Clinical Social Work Practice

Couples with genetic problems or needing fertility treatment using repro-ductive technologies, or who have experienced losses of pregnancy often benefit from clinical social worker services as they work through their unique struggles with these difficult problems. Sometimes mothers and their partners have particular psychological (or psychosocial problems) re-lated to becoming parents or to other aspects of their lives for which clinical services can be utilized appropriately. Many mothers-to-be (and their part-ners) are amenable to accepting referrals for social work services.

Many women, such as those carrying children who are at high risk for birth defects and illness (such as HIV) and others from poor and disadvan-taged environments, may find themselves facing social and economic barri-ers to good prenatal care and may have other (sometimes multiple) risk fac-tors for parenting. This group may benefit from outreach efforts by social workers (Cook et al., 1999).

THE EVOLVING CHILD

A four-year-old girl commented: "I used to be a little baby. Then I closed my eyes, and when I opened them up—all of a sudden, I was a kid!" The first few years of life are awesome to watch, as a "little bundle" evolves into a thinking, talking, walking little person, deeply attached to his or her par-ents but busy exploring the world and becoming increasingly autonomous. In this section, children are discussed from a developmental perspective, en-compassing their psychological, physical, cognitive, and social develop-ment.

The First Year of Life

Babies, even when welcomed with joy, are "newcomers" to their parents; their coming together and developing a synchronous way of relating is a ma-jor task of infancy. *"In the early weeks, therefore, parents and infants face a task of mutual adaptation initiated by the parents"* (Davies, 1999, p. 123).

The neonate has many capacities and competencies soon after birth, in-cluding the ability to recognize sound and visual patterns and a capacity for social communication (Thomas, 1981). The beginnings of "state modulation" are present, which represents the capacity to "remain alert and attentive," on the one hand, but to be able to block out stimuli to prevent the interruption of sleep, on the other (Davies, 1999, p. 122). This is basic to developing *self-regulation,* leading to the regulation of body rhythms involved in such activities as eating and sleeping and ultimately to the regulation of emotions. *"Emotion regulation is the keystone of social-emotional development during infancy"* [italics added] (Crockenberg and Leerkes, 2000, p. 62). Children can adequately develop these innate self-regulatory capacities only within "secure attachment relationships" (Crockenberg and Leerkes, 2000, p. 62).

The infant's *temperament,* including the *emotional reactivity* of the child, influence early transactions between parents and infants, which, in turn, affect patterns of self-regulation. Some children, for example, with a greater sensitivity to stimuli, react with more intense emotion than placid children. A child who cries frequently and loudly might elicit angry reactions, causing the mother to withdraw or handle the child roughly, whereas the same mother might respond more gently to a placid child. The mother's "rough" handling may increase the child's reactivity and retard the development of self-regulation.

In addition, children with special needs, such as those born drug addicted or those who are premature, require more time to self-regulate. Premature babies are initially "ill-equipped to deal with the sensory environment outside the womb," unless they receive special remediation (Sameroff and Fiese, 2000, p. 15). The development of the premature's central nervous system lags by the "number of weeks of prematurity"; this, combined with the illnesses and interventions experienced by them, make them "easily overstimulated, more reactive, and unsettled for a longer period" (Davies, 1999, p. 125).

Massage therapy is one program found to be effective with premature infants. Infant massage has long been used for normal babies in many countries, notably in Africa and Asia; in India, "infant massage is a daily routine that begins in the first days of life" (Field, 2000, p. 495); it has been adapted for high-risk infants in this country. Research done at the Touch Research Institute has found that massage therapy done with some high-risk infants, including those with regulatory problems, premature births, drug exposure, and exposure to HIV, showed good preliminary results in terms of such measures as weight gain, lowered irritability, improved sleep, fewer medical complications, and increased motor development (Field, 2000). Some evidence suggests that "beneficial effects for the caregivers who provide the massage also may accrue" (p. 499) with enhanced caregiver-child interactions. In an experimental program, teenage mothers from inner-city neighborhoods are learning massage methods "to build parenting skills" (Drummond, 1998b, p. 54).

> For much of this century, the prevailing thought was that pre-term babies should not be touched, since the slightest shock could prove fatal. . . . Slowly, the medical establishment has been warming to the idea that massage helps sickly babies. (Drummond, 1998b, p. 54)

Nevertheless, very few nurseries in this country provide massage to such infants.

Attachment

During the first eighteen months, the child's attachment to parents or other primary nurturing figures is essential for physical growth, ego development, and a developing sense of well-being, as well as actual survival; this is emphasized by many theorists, although their perspectives and language may differ. Erikson (1963) refers to the development of "basic trust vs. basic mistrust" (p. 247). Mahler and colleagues (1975) term the early union of the mother and child "symbiosis"; Winnicott (Grolnick, 1990) stresses the holding environment provided by the good enough mother; and Bowlby (1988) posits deep instinctual needs for attachment as the foundation for a "secure base."

Bowlby's attachment theory has been supported by Main (1995), along with Ainsworth, whose longitudinal studies observed and assessed the degree of attachment found in the interactions between mothers and children. Mary Ainsworth, who began her studies of patterns of attachment in children in the 1960s, originally studied babies ranging from nine to twelve months by observing them for seventy-two hours in their homes. The ratings of her observers were then correlated with ratings from observers of the experimental program of the Strange Situation (Davies, 1999), as described by Karen (1990). At one year of age the infant was separated from its mother in the lab and observed; a stranger was present with the infant "during two intervals . . . during another the baby was alone. . . . Ainsworth spotted three distinct patterns in the babies' reactions. One group . . . protested . . . on separation, but when the mother returned, they greeted her with pleasure . . . relatively easy to console"; this group Ainsworth categorized as securely attached (Karen, 1990, p. 36).

The other two groups had either insecure-avoidant attachment or insecure-ambivalent/resistant attachment behaviors. Infants with insecure-avoidant attachments initially appeared self-reliant, did not seem to be affected by the mother's leaving, and tended to ignore their mothers when they returned. During home observations, their mothers often "ignored and actively rejected" these infants (Davies, 1999, p. 19). Parents often characterized these infants negatively and inaccurately, making comments such as "he's just crying to spite me"; the mothers were angrily "intolerant of the infant's distress and tended to reject or punish the infant for being distressed" (Davies, 1999, pp. 19-20).

> Avoidant babies develop precocious defenses against feelings of distress. Distress is split off from consciousness, and the defense mechanism of *isolation of affect* [italics added] emerges. Avoidant infants tend not to show distress in situations that are distressing for most infants; rather they appear somber, expressionless, or self-contained. (Davies, 1999, pp. 19-20)

Children who developed insecure-ambivalent/resistant attachment patterns reacted with intense feelings upon separation from their mothers in the strange situation, and their behavior reflected the paradox of an intense wish for attachment but little expectation of attaining it (Davies, 1999, p. 22). These babies were upset and angry and could not be comforted by their mothers. The mothers of the ambivalent infants were described as:

> *inconsistently responsive* [italics added] to their infants' attachment-seeking behavior. Ainsworth notes, "The conflict of the C babies [ambivalent/resistant] is a simple one—between wanting close bodily contact and being angry because their mothers do not consistently pick them up. . . . Because their mothers are insensitive to their signals C babies lack confidence in their responsiveness" (Ainsworth, 1982, p. 18). The infants' heightened affect and ambivalent behavior reflects their anxious uncertainty about how their parent will respond (Ainsworth, 1982, p. 18). (Davies, 1999, p. 22)

Infants seek their parents as a source of comfort, when they are frightened. However, what happens when parents are not only *not* comforting, but in addition are the *source* of the fright? Main (1995) has added disorganized attachment to the attachment classifications. "Any parental behavior that directly alarms an infant should place that infant in an irresolvable paradox in which it can neither approach . . . shift its attention . . . or flee. . . . The great majority of parentally maltreated children (about 80 percent) in high-risk samples have been found to fit the disorganized category" (Main, 1995, p. 426). In addition, this pattern of attachment has also appeared in children whose mothers themselves had disorganized or dissociated states.

> Battering parents are . . . directly frightening. . . . *Frightened* parental behavior may also alarm an infant and leave him without a strategy . . .

especially likely if the parent withdraws from the infant as though the infant were the source of the alarm and/or appears to be in a dissociated or trancelike state. We have . . . observed dissociated, trancelike . . . and fearful behavior in some parents of disorganized infants who . . . seem to suffer from still partially dissociated experiences of loss or abuse. In these cases disorganized behavior may appear as a second-generation effect of the parent's own traumatic experiences rather than as a direct effect of physical or sexual abuse [of the child]" (Main, 1995, pp. 426- 427)

Main's observations of the mother's reactions to her own trauma affecting the inner security of her child was "the first research" that demonstrated the "intergenerational transmission of secure and insecure attachment" (Karen, 1990, p. 37).

Criticisms of Ainsworth's work relate to issues of research design and lack of studying cultural differences. In the original research, repeated, detailed observations were made (many at home) of mother-child interactions over time. These observations were then correlated with the child's response in the experimental *Strange Situation* setting. Since a high degree of validity existed between the data sets, much of the recent research has utilized observations *only* from the *Strange Situation* to classify a child's attachment behaviors. Question has been raised about the reliability of these observations and whether one can draw valid conclusions from them about the quality of the child's attachment.

The *Strange Situation* applied to examine the effects of day care on the developing child may give inaccurate results, as these babies may have adapted to daily separations from their caretakers and therefore "the Strange Situation may not be sufficiently stressful to activate the attachment system" (Hungerford et al., 2000, p. 523).

The *Strange Situation* has been demonstrated to have consistent results with samples of children from middle and lower classes, those who were black or Caucasian as well as interracial and interethnic babies; however, with infants living under high-risk conditions, the attachment classifications were inconsistent; it has been postulated that stress on the caregivers at different points in time, would affect their attachment behaviors to their children (Davies, 1999).

Japanese children were often classified as having anxious-ambivalent/resistant forms of attachment because of their extreme reactions to separation from their mothers. However, Davies (1999) reports that Takahashi (1990) questions this, as Japanese infants are rarely separated from their caregivers even for sleeping and bathing, being suddenly separated in this experimental situation produced such great distress that this procedure may not be a valid measure of their attachment security.

Although attachment behaviors can vary cross-culturally, strong research evidence supports the fact that children need secure, consistent, responsive caregiving. *"The growing evidence of empirical studies points to quality of attachment as a fundamental mediator of development"* (Davies, 1999, p. 27).

Multiple attachments. Attention has shifted from a primary focus on mother-child interactions to the early involvement of fathers, siblings, day care providers, and extended family with the child. Grandparents play a dominant role in the life of many children (sometimes being the primary caretakers); children in blended and stepfamilies often develop multiple attachments. Children frequently form bonds with many people "that are selective and provide comfort and security" (Frankel, 1994, p. 89); however, research supports the idea "that there is a hierarchy of attachments, with the mother most frequently at the top" (p. 89).

The role of siblings as figures of attachment affecting child development has received insufficient attention (Lieberman, 1984); a recent legal case revolved around the rights of siblings, when removed from their own home, to be placed together in another home (Glaberson, 1998). The lawyers, in the case of Hugo, hope to "persuade the United States Supreme Court to change children's rights law in this country" (Glaberson, 1998, p. A1). Hugo and his six-year-old sister "are so close that, when Hugo has difficulty making himself understood, Gloria sometimes speaks for him. . . . They are, for each other, all that remains of their original nuclear family" (Glaberson, 1998, pp. A1, A12). The dispute that is being adjudicated arose because Hugo's foster mother had already adopted his sister and now wanted to adopt him, but a maternal aunt also claimed him (Glaberson, 1998, pp. A1, A12).

Today, with the increase of multiple pregnancies, the exclusive mother-infant bond no longer is so exclusive, as a baby is not alone with mother, who may have two, three, or more infants simultaneously. Further research is needed on the impact of being a twin or multiple other on the development of internalized object relations and the quality of early infant-caretaker interactions. It is known, for example, that twins often develop their own private language with each other, which is not immediately comprehensible to their parents.

Psychobiological Aspects of Development

The interrelationship between attachment and biological function and development is most apparent in the first year of life. A child deprived of adequate nurturing may not thrive; a premature child or one affected by maternal substance abuse may lack an adequately mature nervous system. Erikson (1963) illustrated the psychobiological connection succinctly when he noted: "the first demonstration of social trust in the baby is the ease of his feeding, the depth of his sleep, the relaxation of his bowels" (p. 247). Eating and especially sucking are important reflexes that must be exercised and satisfied during early infancy; Freud named this stage the oral phase, as previously noted.

Debate, over the years, has focused on breast-feeding in terms of advantages and disadvantages to both mother and child. Recent medical research supports breast-feeding being advantageous to the child in terms of digestion and the mother's transferring to the child her immunity to certain diseases. If a mother is comfortable with breast-feeding, psychological advantages may exist for both mother and child in the enhancement of intimacy and attachment. However, a child gains security primarily from being held, talked to, and cuddled during the feeding process, whether breast- or bottle-fed. Many mothers are not comfortable with breast-feeding or are biologically unable to do this due to physical problems or because the child is adopted, but often provide their children with excellent nurturing. Paradoxically, a mother who breast-feeds but remains uncomfortable with this, holding her child rigidly in an emotionally unresponsive manner, can precipitate anxiety and attachment problems in the child.

Freudian theory has been criticized for its emphasis on instinct theory. Freud's concept of early infancy as the oral phase has been jettisoned by many clinicians (including some psychoanalysts) as misleading or irrelevant. Although Rutter (1975) concedes that "the oral area is a particularly sensitive one in infants, and undoubtedly infants not only get pleasure from sucking but also tend to suck objects as a form of exploration and satisfaction," he nevertheless asserts that infants get satisfaction from other sources of exploration and finds that "sucking does not seem to be due to an innate desire" (p. 64). Rutter (1975) stresses the importance of attachment in the first year of life, which "does not primarily depend on sucking and feeding" (p. 64).

It can be argued that although attachment is fundamental, strong biological urges exist for oral satisfaction, including sucking, that must be satisfied. An infant will suck its thumb not necessarily due to hunger but as a method of self-soothing. Putting substances in one's mouth (such as cigarettes or chewing gum) as well as eating and interest in food seem to be important to people throughout the life cycle; it is not unusual for people to overeat or chew their nails when they are nervous; and obesity (not due to medical problems) as well as the major eating disorders are centered on fixations on food, which go beyond mere satisfaction of hunger. People who talk incessantly have excessive oral needs, and the uncontrolled drinking of alcohol has an oral component. Although strong psychological determinants of these acts are present, the physical appetites and their underlying drives should not be relegated to insignificance. In fact, the close correspondence between physical and psychological need, one fueling the other, may make it more difficult for a person to combat this duality of forces.

The Neurobiological Aspects of Development

Neurobiology and emotional relatedness, affect, and the regulation of affect are closely interconnected (Shapiro and Applegate, 2000). Although it has long been observed that early emotional reactions to events often remained "fixed" in a person's personality and later functioning, the mechanisms have not been totally clear. Now, with the recent advances in neurobiology and neuroscience, it has been learned that feelings aroused by the nurturing the infant receives "become 'hard-wired' into neuronal structure, thus explaining their persistence in later development" (Shapiro and Applegate, 2000, p. 9).

Freud, who was originally a neurologist, theorized that affect regulation "might be regulated by processes within the person," and "hypothesized neurobiological phenomena not yet discovered" (Shapiro and Applegate, 2000, p. 11). Hartmann also theorized about "biopsychological regulatory mechanisms," and Bowlby's concepts of the "neurobiology of attachment" formed the foundation for much of the research of present-day neurodevelopmental aspects of "caregiver-infant interactions" (Shapiro and Applegate, 2000, p. 11).

When born, the infant's brain is not fully developed, and the "wiring of the brain is incomplete" (Shapiro and Applegate, 2000, p. 14). Although orderly neurobiological progressions occur in brain and nervous system development, this progression in the young child is particularly dependent on the nurturing that the child receives. And so, while the brain is "thought to remain plastic and responsive to new experience throughout life," during the early years the "neuronal organization and structure of the brain is still in its formative stages" (Shapiro and Applegate, 2000, p. 15). The child's experience with caretakers, including attachment and stimulation, affect neuronal wiring in three major ways (Shapiro and Applegate, 2000). First, Shapiro and Applegate (2000) describe a sequence of events starting in early childhood in which "interconnections are constructed between brain systems," which are charged "with either positive or negative affects," depending on the quality of the child's experiences at the hands of caregivers; the abundance of the connections is "dependent, in part, on the quality of stimulation . . . the child receives"; second, because the brain as it develops is subject to a " 'use it or lose it' " principle, the opportunity to form connections may be lost if stimulating experiences are not made available (p. 15); third, this sequence constitutes a "critical period" for "indices of . . . competence such as affect regulation" (p. 15).

Intelligence, a genetic endowment, is also affected by the emotional supplies the child receives. It is not uncommon for children diagnosed with low intelligence to show remarkable intellectual gains when removed from a neglectful or abusive environment to a nurturing one. Children with insecure and disorganized attachments tend to show "low self-confidence, deficient cognitive regulation, and an abnormal disequilibrium of thought under cognitive stress . . . . [and some children are] adversely affected by an insecurity that curbs exploration" (Edelstein, 1996, p. 106).

The Development of Intelligence

Jean Piaget made major contributions to understanding the acquisition of intelligence and knowledge in children. He was not concerned with theories of attachment, nor how emotionality affected and was affected by cognition; for these reasons he has been criticized and rejected by some present-day psychologists. Piaget was intrigued with the way in which children developed and constructed their cognition and understanding of the world in a step-by-step procedure. It was his hypothesis that children must essentially complete each stage of learning, before they could move on to master the next stage, which is also a point of dispute among psychologists, who have argued that children sometimes skip stages or go through them in a different order (Thomas, 1981).

Piaget conducted experiments with children, asking them to manipulate physical objects, solve puzzles, and answer questions related to subjects such as spatial relations, mathematics and logic, reasoning, physical causality, and moral feelings and judgments. He observed how their intelligence progressed from a concrete and self-centered understanding of the world to a more abstract understanding, in which different ways of viewing a situation were possible and attention could be focused on other people's perspectives and feelings. He frequently used his own children as subjects, for which he was further criticized; however, he applied his experiments to different cultures and to children all over the world.

An important Piagetian concept is *assimilation,* whereby children learn new information by comparing a new object to one that is familiar. A pear, newly introduced to a child, is different from a known apple, but it is like an apple in that it is a fruit, it is sweet, and it can be eaten. Assimilation continues throughout life. A new social work student, for example, expressed anxiety because she did not know what to say in an interview. When she realized that she had many conversations with people, it enabled her to feel more comfortable talking to a new "classification" of people (clients) by means of the familiar activity of conversing. She actively assimilated her past experiences of interacting with people, to her present task of interacting with people in a professional situation.

Piaget also introduced the concept of *accommodation,* a process by which children, encountering a strange phenomenon, adapt to the new idea or experience. A social work student, now reasonably comfortable with interviewing, is suddenly confronted with psychotic patients as clients. The student might protest: "they don't make sense; they can't relate! I don't know how to talk to them." The ability to adapt to this new experience, to change one's conception of the world (or psychotic clients) and integrate it into one's learning, is the process of accommodation.

Assimilation and accommodation usually act together, and the mechanism that regulates this process is *equilibration,* which "leads to expanded forms of thought and broader levels of assimilation. It thus insures that new accommodations become integrated within existing forms of thinking" (Elkind, 1981, p. 5). As the social work student gets to know psychotic patients, it then becomes apparent that they too are people who also talk and interact but in a different way. So the student who has gone through the phase of assimilation in realizing that clients are people and that conversing can be applied to clinical work now has reached a higher level of development (accommodation) as this newly acquired skill (clinical interviewing) is adapted (through the process of equilibration) to psychotic patients who communicate in a different way.

Piaget's Sensorimotor Phase

During the first two years of life, cognition evolves through infants' sensorimotor experiences, such as sucking, visual and auditory sensations, and an increasing sense of the awareness of their own different physical states. "The first law of dawning psychological activity could be said to be the search for the maintenance or repetition of interesting states of consciousness" (Piaget, 1995, p. 202). First, a lot of "hit and miss" activity occurs; then the baby begins to realize that a sequence of events takes place which leads to certain predictable outcomes (or *causalities*). In the following excerpt, Piaget describes how the baby experiences assimilation.

> With all this activity, a baby naturally hits upon lots of new elements. Not always does he successfully find the breast: his mouth sometimes finds his hand, the pillow, the covers, or something else. The assimilation of the world to the self is the phenomenon most typical of psychic behavior in its beginnings. . . . A foreign body with which the mouth of a baby comes in contact is not interesting in itself but only from the point of view of its place in the baby's scheme of things, that is, as something suckable that activates sucking. Thus, the object is assimilated by the schema of sucking. (Piaget, 1995, pp. 202-203)

Sensorimotor knowledge exists before language develops and is the foundation for all future cognition. Behavior, which was originally reflexive, evolves into voluntary movements as the baby begins to achieve eye-hand coordination. Babies become more interested in the world around them, responding to toys, mobiles, and people. A beginning sense of causality develops as the child makes certain predictions from observing causal events; the baby is hungry, the baby cries, and the mother comes. The baby smiles and laughs at the mother, and the mother will smile back; the toy telephone will make funny noises if the buttons are pressed, and the baby will press the buttons with delight.

Developmental Landmarks

The child's growth during the first year of life is remarkable in terms of gains in weight and height, brain and central nervous system maturation, and beginning adaptations to the external world. The child will begin its journey from relatively helpless infant to active, socially interactive, and inquisitive explorer.

During the first three months of life, the infant is "settling in" to the world, developing regulation of body rhythms and emotional states, forming reciprocal interactions with parents, and, at about six weeks of age, begins to smile, a "magic moment" for parents; laughter, another wonderful interactive highlight, follows shortly. Over the next several months, the baby is basically happy, outgoing, and experiences pleasure in itself and in the world. Parents (even unrelated others), unless deeply self-absorbed or frozen in emotional responsiveness, respond with affection and joy to the radiating happiness and the tender and trusting affection of this baby.

During the second half of the first year, the child enters the *practicing phase* (Mahler et al., 1975), in which locomotion and the joyful exploration of the world are primary occupations. Crawling and walking, while generally requiring extra parental energy and attention to "keep up" with the child and to provide damage control (for the child and household possessions), is usually a source of pleasure and pride to parents. Yet this very beginning, these very first steps, marks the beginning of the child becoming more autonomous. Mahler and colleagues (1975) quote the philosopher Kierkegaard in this connection:

> The loving mother teaches her child to walk alone. She is far enough from him so that she cannot actually support him, but she holds out her arms to him. She imitates his movements, and if he totters, she swiftly bends as if to seize him, so that the child might believe that he is not walking alone. . . . And yet, she does more. Her face beckons like a reward, an encouragement. Thus, the child walks alone with his eyes

fixed on his mother's face, *not* on the difficulties in his way. He supports himself by the arms that do not hold him and constantly strives towards the refuge in his mother's embrace, little suspecting *that in the very same moment that he is emphasizing his need of her, he is proving that he can do without her,* because he is walking alone. (Kierkegaard as quoted in Mahler et al., 1975, pp. 72-73)

But in the other unhealthy mother, the situation is very different:

There is no beckoning encouragement, no blessing at the end of the walk. There is the same wish to teach the child to walk alone, but not as a loving mother does it. For now there is fear that envelops the child. It weighs him down so that he cannot move forward. There is the same wish to lead him to the goal, *but the goal becomes suddenly terrifying.* (Mahler et al., 1975, p. 73)

Mahler and colleagues (1975) also note Anthony's observation that the psychotic mother " 'fills these moments with apprehension so that the child not only has nowhere to go, but he is afraid to get anywhere' " (p. 73). This statement also reflects the impact of the child's *attunement* to the emotions and moods of the mother, which can directly affect developmental progress. Mahler and colleagues (1975) have observed that the first unassisted steps the child takes are "away from the mother or during her absence; this contradicts the popular belief . . . that the first steps are taken toward the mother" (p. 73). Generally, mothers in Mahler and colleagues (1975) study helped their children "move away, that is by giving them a gentle or perhaps less gentle push, as the mother bird would encourage the fledgling" (p. 73); however, once the child began to move further away, "it was as if suddenly the mother began to worry about whether the child would be able to 'make it' out there in the world" (p. 73).

Case Illustration

The following excerpt illustrates the development of Carl, a "normal" five-month-old boy, observed by a social work student who made monthly home visits from the time Carl was seven weeks old until he was eight months old. This report highlights Carl's physical development, his emotional responsiveness, socialization, and his mother's sensitive attunement to his needs and interests (Urdang, 1964).

Carl is now five months old. He sleeps from eight at night until eight in the morning and naps from about twelve-thirty until three in the afternoon, usually sleeping on his stomach. He uses about ten diapers a day. His mother puts two diapers on him at night. In the evening she sometimes removes the diaper for a while, and he likes that. He can get out of his infant seat and is trying to crawl although he cannot quite get up on his knees. He cannot roll over yet. He grabs things he sees. He is teething and chews on everything he can reach. He scratches things because he likes to hear the sound. He screams to hear his own voice, and his pitch has gone up. He recognizes more people now and is much more responsive. The cat fascinates him, and he likes to try to imitate the sounds it makes. I watched Mrs. S. bathe him and observed that he enjoyed it. (Urdang, 1964, p. 11)

Special Problems

Two of the special problems affecting some infants include maltreatment or other traumas and physical disabilities. The loss of the primary caretakers, addressed in Chapters 6 and 7, are later discussed in Chapter 11.

Maltreatment and Other Traumas

As noted in Chapter 7, many children have been subjected to physical and sexual abuse and neglect, often resulting in developmental, psychological, and neurological impairments. Child abuse is the major cause of infant mortality during the first year of life. There is "something deeply disturbing about the juxtaposition of violence and infancy" (Zeanah and Scheeringa, 1997, p. 97).

Serious neurobiological effects of violence in infants and young children are possible. "Profound and perhaps permanent brain changes can result following violent trauma in the first 3 years of life" (Zeanah and Scheeringa, 1997, p. 107).

> Essential to understanding the neurobiology of violence is this: The brain's impulse-mediating capacity is related to the ratio between the excitatory activity of the lower, more primitive portions of the brain and the modulating activity of higher, subcortical and cortical areas. Any factors that increase the activity or reactivity of the brainstem (e.g., chronic traumatic stress) or decrease the moderating capacity of the limbic or cortical areas (e.g., neglect, alcohol) will increase an individual's aggressivity, impulsivity, and capacity to display violence. A key neurodevelopmental factor that plays a major role in determining this moderating capacity is the brain's amazing capacity to organize and change in a "use-dependent" fashion. (Perry, 1997, pp. 129-130)

Infants can be affected by witnessing parental violence, both directly by experiencing fear and indirectly through their reactions to the mother's response to this assault; in addition, many parents who are involved in partner violence also tend to abuse their children (Zeanah and Scheeringa, 1997, p. 110). Two of the most frequently observed disorders in infants exposed to violence are attachment disorders and post-traumatic stress disorder (PTSD) (Zeanah and Scheeringa, 1997, p. 110). In research with infants experiencing PTSD, it was discovered that "in addition to the classic triad of reexperiencing, avoidance/numbing of responsiveness, and hyperarousal, the investigators also found that new fears and new aggression were present in infants after the traumatic event that had not been present before" (Zeanah and Scheeringa, 1997, p. 111).

The role of traumas other than maltreatment, such as car accidents and hospitalizations occurring in infancy, can also be very significant in terms of the child's personality development (Gaensbauer, 1994). Gaensbauer's observations support the findings of Zeanah and Scheeringa (1997) that symptoms of post-traumatic stress disorder can be found in young children, "even prior to the onset of language fluency" (Gaensbauer, 1994, p. 123).

Terr, in 1988, observed that young children who might not be able to give verbal reports of trauma nevertheless could act out their trauma, and asserted that for children, even younger than twenty-eight months, "traumas create powerful and lasting visual images. She hypothesized that the child's enactments or behavioral memories derive from these 'burned in' visual imprints rather than from verbal memory" (Gaensbauer, 1994, p. 124). Gaensbauer (1994) observed that when children express themselves in nonverbal ways they often "give evidence that salient sensory and somatically based elements of a preverbal traumatic experience have been encoded and retained in memory over extended periods of time" (p. 125).

Many children, as noted in Chapter 7, also suffer from chronic maternal neglect, which can be related to maternal depression. Children with mothers who have serious and long-standing depressions may suffer from maternal withdrawal and lack of responsiveness, which can lead to attachment disorders and developmental delays, including cognitive and neurobiological impairments.

Physical Disabilities

Some children are born with physical disabilities such as blindness, deafness, or motor handicaps. If a child cannot gaze at its mother's face and see her smile, will attachment be thwarted? If a deaf child cannot hear language, will cognitive development be impaired? And if a child cannot crawl or walk, will the practicing subphase and the achievement of autonomy ever be negotiated? The concept of the plasticity of the brain suggests that the brain has sufficient flexibility and adaptability so that other pathways will be developed to permit developmental progress (Thomas, 1981).

The course of development of disabled children might be different from children without handicaps, but nevertheless they can achieve good developmental progress, dependent upon the nature of the actual deficits and given that they have the average expectable environment. Early prevention programs (discussed next) are often of valuable assistance to parents of disabled children, providing support, rehabilitative services, and guidance.

In Chapter 5, we discussed how deaf children, utilizing sign language, developed good cognitive abilities. In discussing the development of blind children, Thomas (1981) observed: "just as a deaf child is capable of normal language development, so a blind child is capable of normal affective and social development . . . can hear, smell . . . be aware of kinesthetic stimuli; the child can grasp, learn to cuddle and kiss" (p. 588).

Illness, physical disabilities, and developmental disabilities, such as retardation and autism, are discussed in Chapters 12 and 13.

PREVENTIVE PROGRAMS

The federal government provides financial aid to states (as part of the Individuals with Disabilities Education Act passed in 1987) to provide early intervention services to infants, toddlers, and their families (Gilkerson and Stott, 2000). Although this program is optional, all fifty states provide services through this program, mostly to children with developmental delays or who have medical or psychiatric conditions which would probably lead to developmental delay. Although all programs have a multidisciplinary staff and a family-centered approach, some conflict exists about the degree to which the focus should be on parent-child relationships.

Historically, early intervention programs focused on educational and rehabilitative services, directed toward "the amelioration of developmental deficits through child-focused, stimulation models using primarily developmentally prescriptive, Piagetian, or behavioral approaches to develop training programs or recommendations for families that would enable them to teach their children at home" (Gilkerson and Stott, 2000, p. 461). Emphasis was given to empowerment of the families as they collaborated with the staff. Current research added emphasis to the importance of the child's relationships with the family and to the "relational processes in promoting the development of children with disabilities" (Gilkerson and Stott, 2000, p. 463), although this is not accepted as an emphasis in all programs.

Gilkerson and Stott (2000) advocate a holistic approach, which blends a strength-based, family-centered approach with an infant mental health perspective.

Infant mental health helps us focus on how people understand, respond to, and make meaning of their own experiences. It offers the possibility for holding the pain as well as the hope. The crux of early intervention rests on how individual practitioners respond to individual children and families. (Gilkerson and Stott, 2000, p. 469)

Specialized programs for infants who are at risk for serious psychosocial problems exist under various auspices. One model, based at the Infant-Parent Program at San Francisco General Hospital, works with clients who are "psychologically and socioeconomically disadvantaged"; many belong to minority groups (Seligman, 1994, p. 482); problems include: "parental psychopathology that impedes parenting, disorders of attachment, inorganic failure to thrive, parental drug abuse, and infant characteristics, including developmental disabilities, that place special stress on the caregiving system" (p. 483). Some of the children were placed in foster homes due to abuse and neglect.

Seligman incorporates home visiting and the provision of concrete services, within a psychoanalytic framework, with an emphasis on the development of a therapeutic relationship with parents, and the encouragement of parental self-reflection. Seligman's work, as well as much of the work done in infant-parent psychotherapy, is based on the work of Selma Fraiberg, whose insights about the "ghosts in the nursery" led to understanding how parents' relationships to their children can be dominated by their own conflicts about being parented (Seligman, 1994).

The parents in Seligman's project (1994) often had characterological problems and sometimes low-level psychoses and, combined with their seious social problems, required "extraordinary efforts" from clinicians. These families had had:

> few, if any, positive experiences with social agencies or psychotherapy. . . .They have felt that the fragile capacity for hope . . . has been betrayed. . . . These disappointments have often repeated those suffered in their earliest relationships . . . and these new parents are now reenacting these painful relationship patterns with their infants. The infant-parent therapist is often attempting to enter a system of . . . relationships that is dominated by . . . an overall sense that . . . intervention will make no difference. (Seligman, 1994, p. 485)

Persistent efforts to reach out to families, rather than giving up on those who have difficulty keeping regular appointments, is an important principle of this program. Supportive and concrete services were provided to the families (as seen in the homebuilders model in Chapter 7 of this book), such as making referrals for other needed services or actually driving clients to appointments. These efforts were often necessary before other types of psychological work could be carried out; these procedures actually "enhance such work; a number of crucial interpretations are made in irregular situations, such as while driving parents and infants to appointments or while watching television at families' homes. Interpretation is thus integrated with an array of other intervention tactics (Seligman, 1994, p. 485). Seligman's observations are also similar to Kanter's (1990) utilization of Winnicott's holding environment as an underlying basis for engaging in case management activities with clients (discussed in Chapter 3 of this book).

The development of the therapeutic relationship, which in itself is a "corrective attachment experience" (Lieberman et al., 2000, p. 483), is seen as the key factor in helping the parents understand how their past relationships are alive inside them now and how they are reenacting aspects of these relationships with their therapists and with their own infants.

Utilizing "nondidactic developmental guidance" with parents encourages them to think and reflect about their children's needs and experiences. "The infant-parent psychotherapist might ask the mother what she thinks of her child's interest in the toys rather than giving direct instruction in play techniques" (Seligman, 1994, p. 489). However, in the following illustration, we can see a behavioral suggestion (not identified as such) was made to the mother, Paula, with good results. Paula had difficulty responding to her infant Naomi, showing "a kind of emotional blankness, rather than malevolence" (Seligman, 1994, p. 490). When Naomi was a year old, the therapist brought her some washable crayons and a pad, as her mother had been upset about Naomi marking the walls.

> She [Naomi] opened them with pleasure and presented them to her mother. . . . Paula was . . . unresponsive and effectively mute. The therapist then wondered *what it would be like if she sat on the floor with Naomi, and just kind of did whatever she did.* [italics added] . . . Soon, the two of them were scribbling together with glee. Paula then spontaneously said that no one had ever done this with *her* as a child. . . . She became tearful and pleased at the same time. (Seligman, 1994, p. 491)

If the interactions between mother and child begin to change, benefits can be experienced by both; the elation, joy, and welcoming of a mother by her child can produce joy in a mother, if she is open to this. "Adaptive changes in behavior and intrapsychic life can be synergistic, especially when *the infant's special ability to support and reinforce parental responsiveness is at work*" [italics added] (Seligman, 1994, p. 489); when this happens "the self-righting tendencies of infant-parent caregiving systems can take hold, and progressive changes may occur unusually rapidly" (p. 489).

The Toddler

The first birthday finds the child beginning the *toddler phase,* characterized by major developments in language and speech, greatly increased locomotion and motor skills, the development of play, and major advances in
cognition, including the formation of mental representations. The toddler
begins the *practicing subphase,* with pleasure in walking and exploring the
world, then goes through the dramatic *rapprochement subphase,* with ambivalence about independence/dependence, and is on the road to object constancy, with internalized representations of mother and of self at the end of
toddlerhood (Mahler et al., 1975).

Toilet training is one of the major developmental achievements. Normal
struggles with parents about this, relating to autonomy, reflect similar struggles in other areas of the toddler's life, such as feeding and dressing oneself.
Erikson (1963) characterizes this phase as the achievement of "autonomy
vs. shame and doubt" (p. 251). The child begins to form a sense of self-
identity, and "mine" as well as "I do it" are frequently used words and
phrases.

Although children struggle to attain self-sufficiency during toddlerhood,
the attachment to parents remains a primary need; the intensity of these two
opposing wishes are at the root of many "emotional storms" and tantrums of
this period. Children begin to use soft and cuddly objects, such as teddy
bears, as transitional objects, which Winnicott described as an important
stage in the psychological separation from their mother; they can be comforted by an object that is like their mother, but not their mother, and one
which they can control (Mahler et al., 1975; see discussion in Chapter 3 of
this book).

Language Development

Language, which begins during the latter half of the first year with exuberant babbling and extends to a few words toward the end of the first year,
increases dramatically by eighteen months. However, language develops at
different rates, and some normal children may say only a few words by the
time they reach age two (Rutter, 1975). Children have actually been communicating with their parents from early infancy in nonverbal ways, and
language greatly enriches the level and depth of communication. "The so-
cial-affective exchange occurring between infants and caregivers provides
the foundation for the social or pragmatic aspects of communication"
(Prizant et al., 2000).

Language has many developmental purposes, including facilitating children's engagement in social communication; enabling them "to process and
organize experience," by telling stories about their experiences; and provid-

ing "a way of sharing [their] inner life in an active way" (Davies, 1999, p. 178). Language aids children in understanding people and the world around them and assists toddlers with self-regulation, as they learn to use words instead of action.

Stern (1985), observing that language can be used as a "transitional phenomenon," described the "crib talk" of a two-year-old girl whose "goodnight" talking rituals with her father and her "monologues" after he left her room were recorded (pp. 172-173).

> The important features of her monologues were her practice and discovery of word usage. . . . But even more striking . . . is that it was like watching "internalization" happen right before our eyes and ears. After father left, she appeared to be constantly under the threat of feeling alone and distressed. . . . To keep herself controlled emotionally, she repeated in her soliloquy topics that had been part of the dialogue with her father. Sometimes she seemed to intone in his voice or to recreate something like the previous dialogue with him, in order to reactivate his presence and carry it with her towards the abyss of sleep. This of course, was not the only purpose that her monologue served . . . but it certainly felt as though she were also engaged in a "transitional phenomenon," in Winnicott's sense. (Stern, 1985, p. 173)

Cognitive Development

Brain development progresses rapidly during the child's first two years; in the toddler period, the major cognitive event is the "integration of perceptual and cognitive functions" and the beginnings of "self-awareness" (Davies, 1999, p. 171).

The child remains in the latter part of the sensorimotor phase during the second year, moving into the *preoperational phase* during the second year, and progressing in this phase until age seven (Piaget, 1995a). During this time, language, symbolic play, and drawing skills are elaborated; a child's thinking at this stage tends to be concrete, and an *egocentric view* of the world emerges. Egocentricity refers to children's cognitive inability to see (and understand) things from another's perspective or point of view; they are convinced by their own "prelogic" logic; what makes sense to them *is*.

A three-year-old child insisted to her grandfather that the moon was moving, denying his assertions that the moon looked as though it were moving because their car was moving; the moon was not moving. The grandfather attempted to explain this in different ways, but the child insisted: No! The moon was moving! She could see this happening, and this was her final conclusion! Piaget (1995a) comments that the child "takes his own immediate perception as absolute," and cites his observation that "most of the boys in Geneva go on believing till they are 7-8 years old that the sun or the moon follows them on their walks because they always happen to be above them. They are greatly perplexed when they have to say which of two boys walking in different directions is being accompanied by these heavenly bodies" (Piaget, 1995b, p. 100).

Piaget (1995b) asserts that many adults remain "egocentric in their way of thinking" (p. 95).

> Such people interpose between themselves and reality an imaginary or mystical world, and they reduce everything to this individual point of view. Unadapted to ordinary conditions, they seem to be immersed in an inner life that is all the more intense. . . . Our discovery that other people do not spontaneously understand us nor we them is the gauge of the efforts we make to mold our language out of the thousand and one accidents created by this lack of adaptation and the measure of our aptitude for the simultaneous analysis of others and of ourselves. . . . (Piaget, 1995b, p. 95)

The toddler's sense of reality is developing, and toddlers can have difficulty distinguishing what is real from what is unreal. They have a sense of *animism*; that is, inanimate objects can be alive, so if an arm of a chair falls off because it is broken, the child may think this action hurts the chair; if toddlers trip on a rug, they may think the rug has tripped them. They engage in magical thinking and may believe that if something has happened, the cause was their action. If, for example, the mother dies, it was because he or she was bad that Mommy disappeared.

Piaget introduced the concept of object permanency, which raises the profound puzzle of whether an object out of sight continues to exist for the child. He observed that infants will not look for, nor attempt to retrieve, an object (such as a ball) when it rolls away from them. When they reach the age of eighteen to twenty months, they have developed the sense of permanence and will look for and/or reach for the missing object. Is Piaget's concept of object permanence the same as Mahler's concept of object constancy, and does it take place at the same time?

Mahler and colleagues (1975) observed that children develop an early sense of permanence of physical objects, but only later (at closer to three and a half years) do they develop a sense of mother's permanence. The later acquisition of object constancy relates to the mother being so affect laden for the child; more intense feelings are attached to the mother than to physical objects. "The mother, an 'object' in the psychoanalytic sense . . . is far more than an 'object' in the merely physical-descriptive sense. We expect that repeated contact and high arousal make for differences in the rate of acquisition of a concept of permanence" (Mahler et al., 1975, p. 110).

Piaget's (Elkind, 1981) famous principle of *conservation* asks: does an object change in size (or volume) if its shape or container changes? Children in the preoperational stage have difficulty with this idea and tend not to understand aspects of this until they are about six or seven years old. In a famous experiment, Piaget poured equal amounts of water into containers of the same size, and children agreed that the same amount existed in each container. Then, when he poured the water from one of the containers into a taller container, the children said that the taller container had *more* water. The logical capability of understanding this was not accessible until a later age.

As children navigate their perplexing *Alice in Wonderland* world without a white rabbit as a guide, they need parental guidance to help them find a path through the maze of daily reality. Good enough parents offer this assistance; however, this passage becomes overwhelming and incomprehensible when the assistance is not only unavailable but the guides, through their own confusions, depressive withdrawal, or maltreatment, add uncertainty, unpredictability, and fear.

The Development of Play

The infant's beginning exploration of objects continues on a more advanced level into the toddler phase. Toddlers generally love exploring the contents of drawers, pulling things out, and taking things apart. They love sandbox play, in which they put sand in pails, pour it out, and, with great delight, pour water into their creations.

Play becomes more social, and they enjoy playing and exploring with others. "When young children want to engage another human being . . . they ask, 'Do you want to play with me?'" (Colarusso, 1993, p. 241). Children enjoy pretend games; one three-and-a-half-year-old served pretend soup to her parents' guests, asking each guest which ingredients they would like in their soup, as she poured it into her doll dishes and watched with pleasure as they drank this soup and expressed their satisfaction with it.

Play begins to take on symbolic meaning as the child's imagination develops (Davies, 1999). One of the earliest types of symbolic play occurs when the toddler substitutes one object for another. Davies describes a boy, age sixteen months, who, when playing with cooking utensils, "stepped into two pots and said, 'Shoes'; about a year later, a more 'dramatic substitution' occurs when the child makes believe he is 'someone else'" (Davies, 1999, p. 183).

Play, the development of imagination, and use of symbolic representations serve many psychological functions for children, enabling them to understand how the world works, anticipate events, work out difficult experiences, and cope with emotions. One three-and-a-half-year-old girl, being prepared by her parents for upcoming back surgery, was told she would be awakened during the operation and asked to wiggle her fingers and toes. When her grandfather visited, she put a rubber tube on his arm representing an IV, told him to lie down on the bed, close his eyes, then she rubbed his back, told him to "wiggle your fingers and toes," and when he succeeded at this, she said he could "wake up and have some presents."

Toilet Training

One of the major developmental events for the toddler is toilet training, in which a clash of will between parent and child often ensues; one toddler commented: "I can't want to try." Although this subject was minimally treated (if at all) in several recent texts on child development and human behavior for social workers consulted by the author, this subject received recent attention on the front page of *The New York Times* (Goode, 1999a). A conflict erupted between John Rosemond, a writer of parenting books, and T. Barry Brazelton, a pediatrician, concerning "forced" training as opposed to a more relaxed model. Rosemond stated that it is " 'a slap to the intelligence of a human being that one would allow him to continue soiling and wetting himself past age 2' " (Goode, 1999a, p. A1). He advocates a method called " 'naked and $75,' " based on the notion that children dislike getting soiled, which involves placing a potty near the child and "removing his clothing" (Goode, 1999a, p. A17). When they soil themselves, they are reminded that they could have used the potty, then are put on the potty, cleaned up, and reassured, resulting, within a few days, in self-initiated use of the toilet (Goode, 1999a, p. A17). The seventy-five dollars, he added, is for carpet cleaning.

Brazelton, by contrast, advises against forcing toilet training, which can cause ongoing difficulties; he firmly suggests that parents refuse to be stampeded and that they allow the child to make the choice (Goode, 1999a, p. A1). Brazelton has given this advice in his television ad for large-sized Pampers for older children. Rosemond accuses Brazelton of a conflict of interest; Brazelton responds that he held this view long before he became affiliated with Pampers (Goode, 1999a).

A large-scale study carried out in Philadelphia revealed that while nearly 100 percent of children were toilet trained by a year and a half in 1957, today less than a quarter of that age group have been trained, and that 40 percent were not yet trained by three years (Goode, 1999a, p. A1).

Pediatricians have been anecdotally reporting more toilet-training problems, which include withholding, chronic constipation, and urinary and bowel accidents at later ages (Goode, 1999a, p. A1). Bruce Filmer, an associate professor at Thomas Jefferson Medical School in Philadelphia, noted that an increasing number of children had been referred for both daytime and nighttime bladder-control difficulties (Goode, 1999a, p. A1).

Toilet training is not a simple a matter for parents and children; some very basic issues about autonomy and control are involved, based on complex physiological and psychological processes involving the child's bodily sensations and feelings, which the parents are now trying to regulate. Children are often more aggressive and angry when parents begin training too early "because they face the frustrating situation of the parent's exerting control over *an internal body function*" [italics added] (Davies, 1999, p. 190).

Freud asserted that instinctual feelings about bowel movements, retention, and control, culminating in conflicts about toilet training, were major concerns during this period, which he called the anal phase. "Pleasurable and unpleasurable sensations are associated both with the retention of feces and with their expulsion, and these bodily processes, as well as feces themselves and fecal odors, are the objects of the child's most intense interest" (Brenner, 1974, p. 24). As with Freud's other instinctual theories, issues of anality are downplayed if not altogether ignored; emphasis is placed on the larger contextual issues of autonomy and control that are played out between children and parents.

Although Rutter (1975) agrees that the child's "attempts to gain control of his bowels and bladder are important sources of interest and exploration for him," he adds, "there are no good reasons for regarding the anus as the main focus for sexual interest" (p. 70). I would argue that physical sensations relating to bowel activities are important; young children obtain pleasure from smearing their feces, and pleasurable physical sensations are associated with bowel activities. Although disturbed bowel activities occur within a psychosocial context involving attachment issues, conflict, and aggression, they also have a strong physiological component.

It is not uncommon for childhood disturbances to be accompanied by toileting problems such as bed-wetting or encopresis; some adult psychotic patients, in a regressive state, play with their feces or smear them on walls. Some adults obtain pleasure by giving themselves frequent enemas (not medically prescribed) and become quite anxious when they cannot do this. Some mothers are excessively preoccupied with their children's bowel habits; giving their children regular enemas can be a source of excitement to them. Buxbaum and Sodergren (1977) refer to cases "where the mothers or caretaking people had for different reasons a pathological and therefore pathogenic interest in the processes of elimination" (p. 211).

> Sphincter control is one of the areas in which a partial symbiotic relationship between mother and child can develop. The child remains dependent on the mother's ministrations beyond the usual time. However,

the mothers promote this dependency in order to satisfy their own needs. One patient reported that his mother did not allow him to flush the toilet until she had seen the results, and she wiped him until he was 9 years old. A woman patient reported a similar procedure, which was followed by an enema if the mother thought she had not defecated a sufficient amount. She finally locked the mother out of the bathroom when she was 16 and gave herself the enema if she needed it. She continued to do this into her adult life—it remained her form of sexual satisfaction. (Buxbaum and Sodergren, 1977, p. 210)

Relationships to Parents

Toddlers' relationships to their parents can be stormy at times: the precursor of adolescence. The tasks of toddlerhood are enormous as children become more autonomous, explore their strange world with its "illogical" logic, communicate when they understand more than they can say, and separate (to a degree) from parents for whom they feel intense attachment and fear losing. Parents often feel great pleasure at their toddler's developing personality, loving overtures, inquisitive mind, and charming language; parents can also feel frustrated and angry at their tantrums, their refusals to let parents dress them (especially when an appointment must be kept), their messy eating, and the continual need to baby-proof possessions while constantly keeping an eye on the unsteady toddler who has a poor sense of what is dangerous. One loving father, referring to the impossible places his son climbed, remarked: "I think he is trying to kill himself."

Parents may have difficulty finding a balance between limit setting, and permissiveness, between providing closeness and allowing for appropriate autonomy. The toddler needs ongoing help in self-regulation, and, to the extent that good enough parents can provide a holding environment that is secure, structured with firm limits, and consistent, the child will thrive.

On the other hand, being confronted with insecure attachments and violence, and having no adults to rely on can be especially threatening to a toddler.

This unreliability can be particularly devastating to toddlers, whose increased ability to function autonomously rests on the parent's ability to encourage and applaud their strivings toward mastery, while remaining a constant and reassuring source of support and mirroring. Such young children may increasingly doubt their own competency, and may gradually come to avoid contact with potential sources of help, instead of seeking out trusting and helpful relationships.

Conversely, young children who experience violence may evidence their distress by desperately clinging to a parent or caregiver, unable to tolerate the peril of repeated loss. In this case, one may see behaviors that include anxiety, clinginess, inconsolability, sleep disturbances, toileting problems, and temper tantrums related to difficulties in separation. For the young child who is learning to actively master his or her own aggressive impulses . . . exposure to uncontrolled hostility on the part of others may unleash a wave of regressed, disorganized, and unchecked aggressivity. (Marans and Adelman, 1997, p. 207)

The Preschooler

From ages three to six, children make great strides in socialization, cognitive abilities (including logic and reasoning), language, locomotion and motor coordination, self-regulation and impulse control, identity and gender identity, and can say with confidence: "Now I am a kid!" Their world expands, and extended family, friends, and preschool activities (if available) are important parts of their lives. Preschoolers love to tell stories that include descriptions of their daily activities: "I went to the doctor today and he said to walk across the room, and then he looked at my back and then I put my pants on and went home."

The Development of Language

Language continues to develop rapidly, and, by age three, children have the ability to ask questions. This capacity "to ask 'why' and 'what' gives him power over his own learning," and when parents answer, this furthers the opportunity to add words to his vocabulary (Davies, 1999, p. 238). Children develop " 'private speech,' talking to themselves a great deal, saying out loud what older children and adults say to themselves in silent thought" (Davies, 1999, p. 239). This often takes place when they are playing; they seem to use this speech to gain self-direction and to assist in gaining "self control, as when a child repeats parents' limit-setting words to himself: 'Don't run in the house, Amani' " (Davies, 1999, p. 240).

Bretherton (1996) stresses the importance of the dialogue between parents and children in "guiding the child's construction of internal working models through joint talk about past and future"; it can also "facilitate a child's memory productions" (p. 16). Stern (1985) asserts that "language is potent in the service of union and togetherness" (p. 172) and highlights the importance of language in developing the child's "ability to narrate one's own life story, with all the potential that holds for changing how one views oneself. . . . It involves thinking in terms of persons who act as agents with intentions and goals that unfold in some causal sequence with a beginning, middle, and end" (p. 174).

Case Illustration

Children can have difficulty developing language for many reasons, including general developmental delays or specific physical problems, such as hearing disabilities. However, psychological conflicts were at the root of Susan's speech and developmental problems when she was referred for a social work evaluation at three years and ten months of age, with a diagnosis of "delayed articulation ability," and "a poor speaking environment in the home," in the sense of speech not being sufficiently encouraged. Mother reported that Susan's speech is not clear, and she doesn't make sentences. She does have "private speech," as she "jabbers as she plays . . . usually baby talk." Susan was lagging in speech development; generally, by age three, children are speaking distinctly by four, they use sentences.

> Susan, a pretty girl, was attractively dressed, somewhat hyperactive, and had indistinct speech, and a marked tendency to control her parents. Her mother, Mrs. B., thirty, and her father, Mr. B., thirty-two, had been married thirteen years and adopted Susan when she was five days old. Their biological son is one year old, is developing well, and talks: "says several things plain." The parents function at a high level and seem comfortable financially, although Mr. B. works long hours as a store manager, six days a week. Mrs. B. is a homemaker and has no outside activities or interests, other than attending church. They report a positive marital relationship and socialize with friends, but, Mrs. B. emphasized: *"We never leave Susan."* No medical or psychiatric problems were reported in the family; the only concern expressed was related to Susan's speech problem.

The B.s adopted Susan from a lawyer because Mrs. B. was unable to conceive. The B.s know nothing about Susan's parental or genetic history. Susan's developmental landmarks were within normal parameters: She talked at nine months (which is on the early side), walked at twelve-and-a-half months ("maybe she was a little slow with coordination"), and has always been affectionate; she had an initial problem with colic, which cleared up, and she has always been a good eater. She was toilet trained at two; "it was real easy."

As the parents discussed Susan, two major factors stood out. Mrs. B. has difficulty separating from Susan and has difficulty setting limits. Susan's pediatrician wrote: "Susan never learned to mind her parents; she runs them instead of their controlling her."

> The parents commented that they talked a great deal to Susan as she grew up . . . "that's about all we did . . . we stayed with her, talked to

her, devoted all our time to her . . . she was like a toy, I guess." The B.s are aware of a difference in their feelings toward Susan and the baby . . . if the baby cries, they let him. "It is easier to say no to him than to Susan . . . why, I don't know." Mrs. B. "can't stand for her to be crying . . . I feel sorry for her." For the first six months of her life, a nineteen-year-old girl took care of Susan. "She was real good with the baby." Mrs. B. continued her secretarial job. After that, Mrs. B. "never left her." Until this past summer, Susan did not play with other children. "She did not want to leave me at all."

The parents also reported that since Susan was two and a half years old, she has been sleeping in her parents' bed.

Sometimes they try putting her in her room; but she wakes up and cries. For her to go to sleep, one of her parents would lie down with her in bed; sometimes for a half hour. She sleeps soundly if someone is with her . . . "if she feels someone's body close to her, she is o.k. She seems to think we will leave her." During the day, she naps on the couch in the living room; the mother states she usually works in the kitchen and living room while Susan naps. Sleep problems first occurred when Susan was sixteen months old while on vacation with her parents for two weeks and sleeping in the same bed with them during a visit with relatives. When returning home, Susan persisted in this; at first, her parents would let her sleep in their bed then transfer her to her room. She began objecting to the transfer: "woke up at night crying . . . it did not work."

Although preschoolers want to remain close to mother, they venture into the outside world from "a secure base" and enjoy playing with children. Sometimes the toddler needs a "gentle push" out of the nest (Mahler et al., 1975, p. 79), but Mrs. B. cannot do this. Why is there a "desperation" in her need to be with Susan and to never let her feel she has been abandoned?

Mrs. B. and her brother, two years younger, lived with their mother and father. When Mrs. B. was about two or three, her mother's night-gown caught fire, and she died from burns and pneumonia which set in. Her father left home right after this incident, and Mrs. B. and her brother were raised by an aunt and uncle who had four children of their own. She felt "they wanted me . . . they were like parents to me." Mrs. B.'s father married about a year after his wife's death, but he had minimal contact with his children. Mrs. B. married when she was sixteen and completed high school after her marriage.

Losing a mother at age two is a very traumatic event due to the intensity of the child's attachment at that age as well as the child's lack of the cognitive and verbal skills to process this event. Mrs. B. also lost her father who abandoned his children at that time. His abandonment may have been motivated by an intense grief reaction, rather than overt rejection, in the usual sense. We conjecture that this terrible loss was "encoded" in Mrs. B.'s neurophysiological system, while perhaps only a dim awareness of the actual memory remained.

Although other factors may have contributed to Susan's difficulties (including the birth of her brother and the possible ambivalence her parents may have felt about adopting a child), the issue of Mrs. B.'s abandonment seems primary. The fact that Susan was adopted facilitated Mrs. B.'s identification with her as she was also an "adopted" child of her aunt (whether or not this was a legal fact). Susan's difficulties began before her brother was born; they seem to have come to a head when Susan was at the same age that Mrs. B. suffered the loss of her own mother. The intergenerational transmission of the loss of her grandmother, whom she never knew, was a major family dynamic.

The Use of Play

Play continues to be of central importance as the child develops symbolic thinking, engages in exploration and discovery, and copes with developmental anxieties. In the following illustration, Nathaniel Hawthorne's five-year-old daughter, Una, watches her grandmother die. Hawthorne is critical of Una's behavior relating to her grandmother's death, feeling she is unsympathetic and callous, in fact, "fiendlike" (Herbert, 1993, p. 169). Hawthorne does not seem to realize that Una is attempting to master this difficult situation through play. Hawthorne was deeply attached to his mother and looked to Una for comfort she could not provide.

> Not only does the child speak bluntly of death, but she is also fascinated by the slow failure of his mother's body. Nathaniel is appalled by this specter of annihilation, while Una "takes a strong and strange interest in poor mother's condition, and can hardly be kept out of the chamber—endeavoring to thrust herself into the door, whenever it is opened." On the day following Nathaniel's paroxysm of sobbing, Una playacts the deathbed scene in heroic detail: "She groans, and speaks with difficulty, and moves herself feebly and wearisomely—then lies perfectly still, as if in an insensible state. Then rouses herself, and calls for wine. Then lies down on her back, with clasped hands—then puts them to her head." As Nathaniel witnesses this performance, he is

startled to realize that the child appears to take pleasure in torturing
him. (Herbert, 1993, pp. 169-70)

The Drifters

The previously described developmental stages of childhood occur successfully in the average expectable environment; however, not all children
experience this advantage. What happens to children, to their developmental course and ego functioning, if they do not have a stable, caring, and consistent environment? One important and insightful study focused on such a
group of children. We are adding some observations from this study to this
chapter to illustrate the importance of attachment, developmental progression, and good ego functioning, and to see what happens when this goes
awry.

In *The Drifters* (Pavenstedt, 1967), we encounter children from impoverished and disorganized families with multiple risk factors. They were part of
a pilot study whose goals were to understand their special needs and those of
their families and to offer remedial services to them through a therapeutic
nursery school and outreach social work to the families. The underlying assumption was that *"only by supporting overall developmental maturation
can children be helped to attain the personality and cognitive tools with
which to build satisfactory lives for themselves"* (Pavenstedt, 1967, p. 5).
The project stressed the importance of working with children in their formative years because *"the children's early experiences are the most decisive
influence in the perpetuation of the maladaptions of these families over generations"* (Pavenstedt, 1967, p. 7).

The twenty-one children described in this study came from thirteen families and were of preschool ages (three and four); ten of the families were
white and three were black. Typically, each couple had different ethnic and
religious backgrounds. This classic study, done more than thirty years ago,
is fresh in its insights and compassion for this population.

Mattick (1967a) described these children, who initially appeared similar
to other preschoolers by virtue of their "friendly ingratiating manner. . . . On
the whole they are responsive to people. . . . However, as . . . we . . . watched
the quality of the children's interaction with people as well as their . . . play
behavior, it became apparent . . . that these children were different" (p. 55).

The children displayed a poor self-image, low self-confidence, confusion about their identity, and a tendency to devalue themselves; a low level
of enjoyment was evident, and they showed no discernible drive toward
goals (Mattick, 1967a). In addition:

> There were many signs of confusion . . . about who they were . . . rap-
> idly shifting . . . between infantile and adult mannerisms . . . referring

to themselves as "me" or in the third person.... Very few ... said *I*....
a nonspecific *her* was used ... in talking about ... anything at all. [The
failure of] clear self-differentiation and self-acceptance was demonstrated when a child was confronted with a positive statement.... The
response to ... "What nice clean hands you have!" ... would be a puzzled look. . . . A direct question such as "Who are you?" would be
more likely to bring a reply of "Nobody." ... [A number of children]
when led to the mirror . . . would claim to see the teacher only.
(Mattick, 1967a, pp. 59-60)

These children had relationships to people that were need oriented, dis-
trustful, shallow, and nonspecific; their approach to others was ingratiating
and manipulative (Mattick, 1967a).They had not yet attained the concept of
object permanence and seemed frightened by the separation and closeness
issues inherent in the rapprochement crisis. The "disappearance" of objects
or persons, or even parts of persons or of their own selves, appeared absolute:

even their own hands covered with sand brought an anguished shout or
frightened stare.... One child stared at a teacher each time she had put
on tights. . . . "But where's you legs, her gone?" . . . It took several
months in nursery school before the children could express . . . their
preoccupation with the problem of separation, loss and abandonment.
(Mattick, 1967a, p. 68)

Much time passed before the team appreciated the centrality of the issue
of separation and its significance for relationship building with such children (Mattick, 1967a).

The children had poor language skills and had difficulties conceptualiz-
ing, symbolizing, and problem solving. Their ability to carry knowledge
from one situation to another (the ego function of integration) was limited.
They did not know how to play, received little encouragement from their
parents to explore and play with toys, and internalized their parents' devalu-
ations and expectations that they would not succeed. Creative work brought
home from school might be responded to scornfully by a father as junk; a
gift to one child might be appropriated by a sibling without parental protection of the recipient's property rights or emotional needs (Mattick, 1967a,
p. 79).

Although appearing uninterested in many aspects of what was happening
around them, the children paid a great deal of attention to self-selected outside stimuli that they felt were needed to protect themselves. "Auditory and
particularly visual *hyperalertness* [italics added], with excessive focusing

on the actions of adults, existed alongside their striking unresponsiveness to large segments of the external world" (Mattick, 1967a, p. 62).

The children were very responsive to a nurturing and well-structured nursery school experience. Three major teaching approaches were emphasized: the establishment of a structured, predicable environment; providing a "corrective relationship" in which the children could feel supported, learn to play, and regulate their emotions; and providing opportunities for "actively experiencing the environment" (Mattick, 1967b, p. 171).

The thirteen families in the study were seen as "disorganized" to varying degrees; the parents had unmet developmental needs which took "precedence over the needs of the children" (Bandler, 1967, p. 231). Active outreach intervention was provided to families through home visits with a focus on educating the parents through methods such as modeling and discussion. The relationship with the caseworker was a critical aspect of the work and served as a bridge that enabled the parents (often socially isolated) to move back into the community. For some, attendance at family nursery school parties was a new experience that helped further their socialization.

Overall, the children responded positively to the program, becoming "more alive and they showed pleasure in their activities"; they also showed a greater capacity for learning and becoming involved in age-appropriate activities (Mattick, 1967b, p. 200).

The needs of disadvantaged preschoolers are very apparent today and "have become increasingly complex in the past decade," related to multiple environmental, economic, health, and family risk factors (Edlefsen and Baird, 1994, p. 566). Edlefsen and Baird recommend that integrated preventive mental health services be offered to children and their families within the preschool setting.

Psychosexual Development

During preschool years, awareness of gender identity (which began at age two when children learned whether they were a boy or a girl) increases but now becomes more sophisticated and complex. Children tend to engage in behaviors that are gender related; girls may be more interested in dolls or having their fingernails polished, whereas boys are often immersed in play with toy cars and fire engines. The extent to which these patterns are influenced by socialization and parental gender stereotypes has been debated; some assert that the sexes are equal in constitution and physical endowments. Recent research supports the presence of many physiological differences in gender development but suggests many ways each sex can make adequate adaptations and take on opposite sex roles; women can be competent doctors, construction workers, and astronauts; men can become good nurses, preschool teachers, and stay-at-home dads.

Some children are conflicted about their gender identity; feelings that they should be the opposite sex may be persistent and troublesome to them. Some may undergo sex change surgeries when they become adults (discussed in Chapter 10).

Preschool children develop sexual feelings, become interested in their genitals, and may find that masturbation is pleasurable. Many enjoy games of sexual exploration with other children or make overtures to adults (Davies, 1999). The child's developing attachment to the parent of the opposite sex, accompanied by sexual feelings and competition with the parent of the same sex, was termed the Oedipus complex by Freud (and sometimes referred to as the Electra complex in girls) and is one of the most strongly debated topics in psychoanalytic theory.

The Oedipus complex, based on the ancient myth of Oedipus, who unknowingly married his mother and killed his father, postulates that children during the oedipal phase work through their conflictual feelings; eventually these wishes are given up and an identification is formed with the same-sex parent. During this process, the child's superego, or conscience, emerges. The boy during the oedipal stage (out of fear of retaliatory anger by the father) develops *castration anxiety;* the girl develops *penis envy* (because of alleged feelings of inferiority and jealousy related to a lack of a penis). The concept of penis envy is especially objectionable to many feminists, some of whom have rejected Freudian theory based on their belief that Freud viewed women as being inferior.

> From the time Freud (1897) first proposed [the Oedipus complex], scholars both within and without psychoanalysis have debated its existence, questioned its importance, and refuted its universality. Even such contemporary analysts as Kohut (1982) have argued that the oedipal situation is not inevitable, that conflict between generations need not occur given adequate parenting, and that, in any event, its roots are not primarily sexual or aggressive. (Tang and Smith, 1996, p. 563)

Freud, in his early theory development, thought that the root of neurotic conflict was sexual trauma in the patient's childhood. Further analytic work revealed that this so-called trauma never took place; the patient instead had a sexual wish or fantasy which produced so much guilt that it was repressed; the aim of analysis was to bring this unconscious material to consciousness and help patients accept and work through their conflict. This led to Freud's formulation of the Oedipus complex.

While some regard this theory as a major insight, others are appalled, insisting Freud was mistaken to downplay or ignore the supposedly actual trauma that occurred—that many women who were victims of childhood sexual abuse were wrongly treated by analysts and that the problem of sexual abuse was kept undercover much longer than necessary. Some attribute to Freud the motivation that he knew about childhood sexual abuse but was silent about it for his own political ends.

A recent controversy concerns recovered memories of childhood sexual abuse and whether they are actually the return of repressed memories of sexual abuse which has occurred or are distortions of memories and represent unconscious fantasies, wishes, and/or are related to suggestions of a therapist (Chapter 2 of this book). To the degree that such memories may be fantasies, Freud's theory of the Oedipal complex is relevant.

Many parents and nursery school teachers have reported expressions of normal sexuality in preschoolers (Berzoff, 1996b; Davies, 1999; MacFarlane et al., 1986). One mother reported the following conversation between her daughter and her husband (Berzoff, 1996b):

> Four-year-old Lilly, who had been dressed for bed, suddenly began to take off her nightgown in a kind of strip tease before her father, saying, "Bosom Dance, Bosom Dance." Her father responded, "Lilly, put your nightgown back on! What are you doing?" Lilly replied, "Daddy, you know I've been thinking that a 3-year-old couldn't marry you but I bet a 4-year-old can!" (Berzoff, 1996b, p. 35)

In this instance, the father is helping Lilly "regulate her emotions" and is setting limits on her behavior. He is not being "seduced" into sexual acting out with her. However, when "a parent is very needy and has trouble with boundaries in the family, he or she could easily misinterpret the child's Oedipal/Electra behavior as sexual attraction and might act on this misinterpretation in a way that leads to sexual exploitation of the child" (MacFarlane et al., 1986, p. 24). This statement could be amended to state that this behavior may indeed represent sexual attraction—that is, the child may be experiencing erotic feelings.

One psychological dilemma for sexually abused children may be that the actual eroticization experienced through this act can leave them feeling confused and guilty. It is not uncommon for social work students to tell a sexually abused child: "It is not your fault—what Daddy did was wrong!" But if the child experienced erotic pleasure from this act, the guilt might intensify if not recognized and the child's feelings would seem validated. If Daddy was wrong (and bad), so is the child. At the same time, the child needs to understand the inappropriateness of this sexual involvement and not bear the burden of responsibility for it.

Sexual acting out of children can present problems for their therapists who may find the children's "sexualized behavior arousing; this causes discomfort and guilt, and may lead to avoidance of the sexual material. . . . If a therapist responds to a child in a sexual manner or fails to set appropriate limits, then he or she may be viewed as similar to the child's parents" (MacFarlane et al., 1986, p. 202).

Moral Development

According to Freudian theory, as the Oedipal complex is resolved, the superego (the conscience of the child) evolves. Objections to this construct emphasize that the development of moral thinking starts at a much earlier age, and children have been progressing in knowing right from wrong based on the approval of parents and other important people in their lives. During the preschool years, they develop a "more internalized sense of right and wrong" (Davies, 1999, p. 259). The topic of moral development is expanded in the following chapter.

CONCLUSION

This chapter has followed the child's evolution from conception through birth and infancy to becoming a preschool "kid," with a developing personality, intelligence, and social skills. Biological, psychological, and social factors in concert affect children, as they, in turn, affect their social environment. Attachment to consistent, warm, and caring nurturing figures is the foundation of healthy physical and psychological development—as essential to survival as is the air we breathe and food we eat.

Emphasis has been placed on looking at children through a developmental lens; it is through the study of the multiphysical, cognitive, psychological, and social abilities and demands of each stage that we can evaluate children's progress and understand their given capabilities and vulnerabilities. Individual case studies are needed to determine if a given child has passed through each stage successfully or whether developmental lags have occurred.

When delays do occur, many children compensate later; some children, however, develop severe maturational delays, which can be due to illness, physical disability, or developmental disabilities such as retardation or autism. In the case of the children in *The Drifters* (Pavenstedt, 1967), the disorganized families in which they were raised and inadequate parental nurturing led to serious ego deficits, including problems with separation, identity, and high levels of anxiety and hyperalertness. Intensive early intervention through a therapeutic nursery school and outreach work with the families enabled the children to overcome these deficiencies and gain a sense of mastery. Early intervention services have been emphasized by many writers; the sooner a child at risk receives rehabilitative services and/or caring nurturance, the self-righting tendencies of development will assert themselves.

Resilience, discussed in Chapter 3, is related to the capacities of people to adapt to the nonexpectable environment, to survive, and to function well; in examining parent-child interactions, another perspective on resilience emerges. Some people, such as Susan B.'s mother, are resilient. She survived the death of her mother and abandonment by her father and was able to sustain a stable marriage, to hold a job, and develop friendships. However, when she become a parent, and her child became a toddler (as she was when her own mother died), holes appeared in the protective armor of her resilience; parenthood brought her in touch with early trauma that had been safely buried. Family dynamics, such as the family projection process and the development of enmeshed or disengaged relationships, are generally related to the parents' early attachment difficulties, which may emerge when a new family is formed, experiences a new level of intimacy and relives the developmental vicissitudes of the past through the mirror of their own children's experiences.

A psychodynamic developmental approach to studying children and their families provides us with insights that one can find only by going beneath the surface of presenting symptomatology, enabling us to provide constructive and healing experiences to children and their families so that they can continue their interrupted maturational journeys. Children have an enormous capacity to love, to give, and to forgive; if parents can tune in to this, they can be well rewarded. Helping families reclaim the happiness and joy of close relationships which was excluded from their lives can be a major achievement.

LEARNING EXERCISE

1. Select a family with an infant or young child (other than a family member or a client). Observe the child and have an interview with the mother about the child's development, skills, interests, etc. Relate your observations to course material.

SUGGESTED READINGS

Articles

Shapiro, V. and Gisynski, M. (1989). Ghosts in the nursery revisited. *Child and Adolescent Social Work, 6,* 18-37.
Talbot, M. (1998). Attachment theory: The ultimate experiment. *The New York Times Magazine,* May 24, pp. 24-30, 38, 46, 50, 54.

Books

Akhtar, S. and Kramer, S. (Eds.) (1998). *The colors of childhood: Separation-individuation across cultural, racial, and ethnic differences.* Northvale: Jason Aronson Inc.

Davies, D. (1999). *Child development: A practitioner's guide.* New York: The Guilford Press.

Fraiberg, S. (1968). *The magic years: Understanding and handling the problems of early childhood.* New York: Basic Books.

Hughes, D. A. (1998). *Building the bonds of attachment: Awakening love in deeply troubled children.* Northvale: Jason Aronson Inc.

Zeanah Jr., C. H. (Ed.) (2000). *Handbook of infant mental health,* Second edition. New York: The Guilford Press.

Chapter 9

Middle Childhood and Adolescence

When the voices of children are heard on the green
And laughing is heard on the hill,
My heart is at rest within my breast
And every thing else is still.

William Blake
Songs of Innocence

ELEMENTARY SCHOOL YEARS

Middle childhood (ages six to twelve) is a time "when most of all the child develops (or fails to develop) mastery of his environment" (Rutter, 1975, p. 86). It is characterized by the child's increased involvement in the outside world (through school and other social activities) and the integration of intellectual and psychological capacities. Erikson refers to this stage as "industry vs. inferiority"; the child is ready for the " 'entrance into life,' except that life must first be school life, whether school is field or jungle or classroom" (1963, p. 255). The child learns to master skills, and if unable to do this, will develop a sense of inferiority. In our country, the world of the latency-aged child centers around school, which "seems to be a culture all by itself, with its own goals and limits, its achievements and disappointment[s]" (Erickson, 1963, p. 256).

Children in middle childhood develop greater self-control and mastery over their impulses, replacing impulsivity with words, thought, and fantasy; their conscience and moral sense mature; major gains in testing reality and in cognitive development are made; and involvement with peers becomes important (Davies, 1999). "Logical exploration tends to dominate fantasy, and the child shows an increased interest in rules and orderliness. . . . The ability to concentrate is well established by age 9 or 10" (Kaplan et al., 1994, p. 47).

In Freudian terminology, this period is referred to as the latency stage, because this is a period of relative emotional (and drive) quiescence between the upheavals of the oedipal period and the turbulence of adolescence. Rutter (1975), however, does not agree that it is a period of sexual quiescence.

> In fact Freud was clearly wrong about sexual latency, as it is a period of *increasing* sex interests. Sex talk and games with a sexual component are frequent, but often they are concealed from adults. Some children even develop immature heterosexual love relationships, although these usually remain largely or entirely in fantasy. (Rutter, 1975, p. 86)

Twenty-five years have passed since Rutter made his statement; it has now been observed that sexual interests and dating develop during the preteen and early teen years; it is not uncommon for fifth graders to go on dates, which is a step beyond fantasy (Jarrell, 2000). Although older teenagers seem to be practicing sexual abstinence more, indications are that the opposite is the case with younger adolescents, who seem be starting their sexual careers even earlier (Jarrell, 2000, p. 8). Although "no in-depth studies" of sexual activity of children (ten to thirteen years old) have been undertaken, middle school surveys and anecdotal information from mental health professionals, educators, and adolescent physicians point to this phenomenon.

A number of reasons have been cited for this, such as the increase in divorce, insufficient parental attention, the easy accessibility of condoms, and the fact that puberty starts earlier now than in the past. "But the most frequent explanation is that today's culture sends a very mixed message to its young" (Jarrell, 2000, p.1); concern has been expressed that these youngsters are unable to cope with "the profound feelings that go with early sex," and that this increased activity is "often of a detached, unemotional kind" (p. 8).

Piaget (1995a) observed that ages seven to eleven are the time for the development of *concrete operations,* in which children learn how to develop conceptual and representational thinking, enabling them to figure out in their heads what they had previously needed real actions to understand. The child can classify, order, and find alternatives. For a child who wants a toy, thinking has moved beyond: "It is mine" and "I want to play." It is a toy that does certain things because it has certain properties, and it costs five dollars, but in another store it costs four dollars, and both toys do the same thing.

> The school-age child is now capable of having a clear sense of right and wrong, of having empathy with the feelings of others, and of "playing by the rules." Optimally, the school-age child engages in aspects of daily living such as hygiene, dressing, and looking after possessions with greater autonomy. The capacity for operational thought

and problem solving, along with increased frustration tolerance, increases the range of potential activities and sources of satisfaction. (Marans and Adelman, 1997, p. 212)

Many of the attributes of latency are illustrated in the behavior and thinking of Derek, a nine-year-old Caucasian boy, who was referred to his school's social worker by his fourth-grade teacher because of his "difficulty in focusing and following directions in class and because of his difficulties in peer relations." During one therapy session, Derek described what happened when he and his friend got lost going to school that morning. His narrative depicts his competent problem-solving skills based on his well developed concrete operations.

> Derek missed the school bus this morning, so his mother put him and his friend on a public bus. After riding for fifteen minutes, he and his friend realized that they were going in the wrong direction and asked the bus driver what to do. He let them off at the next stop, in front of a gas station. They proceeded to look for a telephone, but neither of them had any money. Derek thought of searching for a dime in the change slot of the pay phones; after a few tries, they found a dime and called Derek's home. There was no answer, so Derek called his mother at work. She came and drove them to school. I remarked that Derek had been very resourceful and asked Derek if he knew what that meant. Derek replied with a huge grin, "Yeah, it means smart."

Derek's social worker recognized his competence, an attribute important to latency-age children and especially important to Derek, who struggled with strong feelings of incompetence. In the second grade, his teacher labeled him learning disabled but had no evaluation done; she frequently called the class's attention to Derek's academic difficulties and poor social skills. Derek developed nervous habits, such as nail biting and nose picking, which further isolated him from his peers; he became anxious about school. When asked to write down some of his worries, he wrote: "getting brain damage," but then crossed this out. His social worker felt that "deep down, Derek may be truly worried that he is incompetent, learning disabled, stupid, and a 'nerd' (a name that other children sometimes call him)."

Although Derek had problems with peers, he had a friendship with a boy in his class and several playmates in his neighborhood. Harry Stack Sullivan (1953) asserted that during the preadolescent period, children develop a special close relationship with "a *particular* member of the same sex who becomes a chum or close friend" (p. 245). Sullivan notes that this is a very important part of psychological development, and that during this time the child "begins to develop a real sensitivity to what matters to another person

. . . [and thinks about] "what should I do to contribute to the happiness or to support the prestige and feeling of worth-whileness of my chum" (Sullivan, 1953, p. 245).

School-age children may be ashamed of being in therapy because others may think something is wrong with them; their developing conscience may add to anxieties that their behavior and thoughts are bad; they are usually not comfortable talking about feelings directly (Davies, 1999). The use of "play, structured activities, and talk is an effective approach in middle childhood" (Davies, 1999, p. 346). Derek's social worker found that her "attempts to encourage him to verbalize his feelings felt like an intrusion to him." She "discovered that Derek is somewhat more expressive in his artwork than he is verbally."

> Derek drew a picture of his house; he seems to have a lot of confidence about his ability to transfer what he sees into his art. He spoke about how difficult it would be to draw the stairs, but, in fact, he went right to drawing the stairs and seemed pleased with them. What is most interesting about the drawing is the anthropomorphic features on the door and on the facade of the house.
>
> The two windows in the door even have what look like eyeballs. Derek explained that they are stickers. The doorbell is the nose and the mail slot is the mouth, grimacing. Derek pointed out to me the face on the house itself. Two upstairs windows are the eyes, a center window, the nose, and the living room window is a grimaced mouth, with gritted teeth. The face on the house appears angry or frightened. When I wondered aloud what the house is feeling, Derek quickly added smile lines to its mouth.

The social worker sensed that Derek was expressing frightening and/or angry feelings through his drawing, but when she tried to explore this directly, he immediately changed an "angry or frightened" face on the house to a happy face. She reflected later that asking Derek to discuss feelings may have made him feel too vulnerable. Changing her approach, she helped him extend the playful and imaginary aspects of his activity rather than confront him directly.

> I asked Derek to take out the picture of his house. I explained that since he had shown me that face on his house, I thought we could play a pretend game and have him make other houses and buildings that could talk to one another. I asked Derek if he knew what a speech bubble was, and he drew one for me. Derek liked the idea and knew immediately which buildings he wanted to draw.

Derek then proceeded to draw a series of houses and buildings with eyes, noses, mouths, braces, hands, missing teeth, and pockets. He developed a story about one of the buildings owing others money and the verbal conflict that ensued. Derek's story struggled through such themes as anger, injustice/fairness, disappointment, trust, deceit, and, finally, resolution. I was able to get bits and pieces of information from Derek about some of the connections to his life, but this was territory carefully tread upon because I knew that too much direct questioning might inhibit Derek's self-expression.

School

Erikson (1963) refers to school as being a culture unto itself; every classroom has a racial and ethnic composition, an interpersonal environment, and its own values, standards, and rules. Each class is part of the school community, which can be accepting, nurturing, motivating, safe from violence, or restrictive, punitive, adversarial, and unable to protect its charges from violence, harassment, and bullying. Many children adapt well to the academic and social expectations of school and achieve a sense of mastery and competence.

Many other children have difficulty adapting to school, developing academic difficulties, behavioral problems, and inadequate social skills. Sometimes these problems are corrected by such means as remedial education, child therapy, family treatment, and social skills groups. However, often these problems remain uncorrected, and the child enters a downward spiral of failure, low self-esteem, and underachievement; school dropout can ensue, with more serious behavioral and emotional problems in its wake. Ultimately, when these children become adults, they have difficulty earning an adequate income; "helping to keep students in school and to promote academic success are critical steps toward promoting greater and more competent adult role performance" (Richman and Bowen, 1997, p. 95). As we have become a technology-based society, literacy and education are even more important than they might have been in the past.

Academic failure is found more frequently among minority children and those with low socioeconomic status (SES); in fact, low SES individuals "are five times more likely to drop out of school than those in higher SES families;" these young people are at risk of "failing to achieve the entry-level abilities necessary to function as competent adults in a complex society" (Richman and Bowen, 1997, p. 96). One major problem facing inner-city schools across the country is the high rate of turnover of both its students and teachers; *mobility*—a problem associated with such diverse circumstances as eviction, homelessness (families who "live in homeless shelters, or doubled up with relatives in cramped quarters or in single illegal rooms in ramshackle buildings"), relocation, foster placement, and the impermance of living arrangements related to immigration—is one of the "least acknowledged and most intractable difficulties" (Holloway, 2000, p. A29).

The high rates of teacher turnover due to the stress of working in suboptimal inner-city conditions (Holloway, 2000) compounds the problem. Experienced teachers often choose to work with suburban schools, which may have higher rates of salary.

The highest dropout rates in the country exist in schools for Native American children; achievement test scores are also very low for this population (Belluck, 2000).

> Many are dealing with a cycle of low expectations from non-Indian teachers, a generation of poorly educated parents, broken and overwhelmed families, a society historically suspicious of governmentrun schools and a culture that may not always see the relationship between being academically rigorous and being successful on the reservation. (Belluck, 2000, p. A22)

Federal and state efforts are being directed toward this problem, and former President Clinton requested a $1.2 billion increase for Native American education, including an Indian Teacher Corps and other social and economic programs. The Friends Committee on National Legislation has reported that Bureau of Indian Affairs' (BIA) "school programs are slated for a 3 percent increase ($15.6 million) in FY2002, to a total of $504 million, barely above the rate of inflation," and that "the FY2002 request for BIA school construction is $292 million, virtually the same (0.5% increase) as FY2001 enacted levels. This would be a cut below the inflation-adjusted baseline" ("Native American Legislative Update," 2001). "Currently, most teachers in reservation schools are non-Indian, the turnover rates are extremely high and many believe that the teachers do not understand Indian culture and learning styles" (Belluck, 2000, p. A22).

National debate swirls around the issue of what constitutes school failure. Often school dropout is counted as school failure; however, the concept is more complex than this, as children may be physically present in school, but do not achieve or involve themselves in the educational process. Richman and Bowen (1997) cite Alpert and Dunham who "have postulated that the number of 'academically marginal students' or 'interior dropouts,'" as Martz has termed them, "is equal to the number of students who actually drop out of school" (p. 97). Richman and Bowen (1997) suggest that the issue needs to be reframed to emphasize "school success . . . because a focus on school success includes the entire school-aged population" (p. 97).

The school environment itself contributes to a child's sense of well-being as well as academic achievement. The ecological concept of goodness-of-fit is particularly relevant when looking at a child's school adjustment. Some schools are sensitive to their students' needs; others (and many in poor inner-city areas) are overcrowded, lack resources, and may not be able to provide adequately for children with special needs. A poor goodness-of-fit can exist in classrooms, where teachers—such as Derek's second-grade teacher—contribute to the academic and social deterioration of students through negative assessments and interaction.

For some children, like Andrea, age seven, school can be a sanctuary from difficult and chaotic family situations:

> Andrea's parents are divorced. Her mentally ill father remarried and, when his new child was born, distanced himself from Andrea. Andrea's single mother is overwhelmed caring for her and her two teen brothers, one of whom had to be hospitalized for a psychotic episode. School is a positive factor, helping Andrea develop resilience. Her first- and second-grade teachers were both very patient and supportive in helping Andrea succeed in school. The school nurse has helped Andrea's mother set limits with Andrea; she also knows that Andrea's tendency to experience psychologically triggered vomiting is part of Andrea's wish to go home; the nurse helps keep her in school.

Child maltreatment, family problems, living in unsafe environments, experiencing depression, anxiety, attention deficit disorder, and/or posttraumatic stress disorder—all of these situations can contribute to children's school problems. Preoccupation with violence can led to inattentiveness, which, in turn, can lead to poor school performance, which can dramatically affect how children feel about themselves (Marans and Adelman, 1997).

Education is a matter of national concern, and school vouchers was one major issue in the presidential election campaign of 2000. Should children be given vouchers by the state to attend private schools, including religious schools? In Florida, when the Florida legislature passed a voucher plan, a split occurred between the National Association for the Advancement of Colored People (opposed to the plan), "contending that it would reduce support for public education and violate the constitutional separation of church and state," and the Florida branch of the Urban League, which defended this program (although the National Urban League, with its headquarters in New York, opposes vouchers) (Holmes, 1999, p. 15). "While liberal civil rights groups generally oppose school vouchers, polls show that many low-income African-Americans, especially those with children in poor-performing public schools, support the concept" (Holmes, 1999, p. 15). The separation of church and state is a nationally debated topic: Should religious schools be supported with tax dollars; should prayer be allowed in public schools?

Another topic of current debate concerns homeschooling, which has been growing at a rapid rate since the 1980s when it first began to develop seriously (Talbot, 2000; Kilborn, 2000). Although data regarding the numbers of homeschoolers are difficult to obtain, it has been estimated that "1.3 million to 1.7 million, or about 3 percent of all 53 million school-age children, attend school at home" (Kilborn, 2000, p. A1). Initially, this method of schooling was adopted by some conservative Christian families who had wanted to separate themselves and their children from mainstream culture; "now it is being adopted more broadly, by parents who are disenchanted with the regimentation of schools, public and private, and the idea that a child's age, alone, marks the threshold of learning" (Kilborn, 2000, p. A1).

Controversies exist about bilingual education (discussed in Chapter 5), the qualifications of teachers, funding disparities between wealthy school districts and poor ones, as well as the allocation of funds for students with different needs within the same public school system. Should children with learning disabilities (currently about 2.6 million students) be taught in special classrooms or "mainstreamed" with "average" children? If they are mainstreamed, do teachers have sufficient qualifications to handle both groups as well as sufficient resources to cope (Ratnesar, 1998a)?

Do public schools have adequate financial resources as well as adequate personnel to handle children with serious emotional disturbances? "Because the federal government does not provide adequate funds for treating children with emotional disorders, local school districts must often bear the steep costs, experts say. Children who should be educated in alternative schools or even in residential centers are kept in the 'mainstream' because local school boards can't afford to do otherwise" (Beaucar, 1999d, p. 3).

Some parents and educators have raised concerns about the neglect of the average student.

> Across the U.S., average students . . . a group researchers call "woodwork children" because of their tendency to fade into the classroom background—are suffering from an unofficial policy of neglect as public schools overlook students in the middle in favor of the bright stars or the learning disabled. The share of public school budgets devoted to "regular education"—which almost two-thirds of students receive—plummeted from 80 percent in 1967 to less than 59 percent in 1996, according to the Economic Policy Institute. The trend has accelerated in the past decade. . . . Average students have become casualties of a spoils system in which every morsel of every school district's budget has a different interest group staking a claim to it. "If you don't have someone representing you, your needs get lost," says William

Purkey, an education professor at the University of North Carolina at Greensboro. "The average child slips through the cracks. There's no strong voice on their behalf." (Ratnesar, 1998, p. 60a)

Successful programs with disadvantaged and minority students have resulted in improved learning. The Education Trust, a nonprofit group in Washington, studied 366 elementary and high schools, located in twenty-one states, and found that many of their students showed good academic progress ("Helping Poor Students," 1999).

> The trust found that the schools that are doing well or have improved shared five characteristics: increased learning time for reading and math; money devoted to continuing education for teachers and staff members; systems to monitor student progress and provide extra help; efforts to involve parents in the day-to-day learning process, and state or district accountability requirements for teachers and the staff if students fail to show measurable improvement.
>
> "Poor kids can achieve at high levels if we teach them at high levels," said Kati Haycock, the director of Education Trust. ("Helping Poor Students," 1999, p. 24)

Debate continues about the school's role in the life of a child. Should schools assume "parental" functions? Are they "social agencies" or educational institutions? Pilot projects, often introduced by social workers, have viewed school in a ecological perspective and education in a comprehensive way, some becoming part of a link to other community programs (Dupper and Poertner, 1997; Winters and Maluccio, 1988). In Chapter 4, we referred to the development of school-linked family resource centers, which provide multiple services to children and their families who live in impoverished neighborhoods.

Social workers have had an increasing role in elementary and high schools, involved in activities such as special education evaluations, crisis intervention, sexual and physical abuse case finding and referrals, group work, individual and family work, and suicide and violence prevention. Many school social workers, however, "struggle for recognition" within their schools, and some are threatened with losing their positions as some school systems are "squeezing licensed social workers out of the schools in favor of 'privatized' services to save money" (Beaucar, 1999d, p. 3).

Special Problems of Middle Childhood

Children today are often affected by many problems including poverty, family breakdown, maltreatment (Chapter 7), and disabilities (Chapter 12).

Violence and mental health problems affecting children are discussed in this section.

Violence

There is a "trend toward children of younger ages becoming perpetrators, victims, and witnesses of violence" (Murphy et al., 1997, p. 223). Homicide is now the third most common cause of death among elementary school children (Glodich, 1998; Osofsky, 1997). School-age children are developmentally ready to engage in the wider world; as they fight against normal regressive pulls, involvement with violence may be a very "disruptive" experience, "requiring various attempts to ward off the associated feelings of fear and helplessness" (Marans and Adelman, 1997, p. 212).

> As with younger children, school-age children may respond to their exposure to violence with circumscribed symptoms, involving sleeping difficulties, nightmares, worries about burglars, bodily injury, and death. In addition, regression to earlier modes of relating to parents may be prominent. For example, increased struggles over food, self-care, school-work, or household responsibilities may be some of the behavioral phenomena that accompany children's attempts to defend against and give expression to the anxiety associated with witnessing interpersonal violence. (Marans and Adelman, 1997, p. 212)

If children continue to be upset, secondary problems can develop, such as poor school performance, which can further lower their self-esteem (Marans and Adelman, 1997). Violence has also been associated with childhood depression, post-traumatic stress disorder, and attention deficit symptoms (Murphy et al., 1997). Children subject to violence might respond with aggression to their friends, and their "identifying with the aggressor may become a chronic hedge against feeling vulnerable to attack as the child courts recognition and affiliation with the toughest figures on the neighborhood streets and becomes involved in antisocial and violent activities" (Marans and Adelman, 1997, p. 213).

Illustration of a Violence Remediation Program

Schools frequently offer violence prevention programs with a general emphasis on "teaching strategies to promote nonviolent conflict resolution" (Murphy et al., 1997, p. 223). However, this approach, with its emphasis on teaching appropriate behaviors, does not touch upon the trauma many children have already experienced, nor does it focus on their reactions, symptoms, interferences with their development, and their relationships. Murphy and colleagues (1997) describe a comprehensive program in an elementary school that offered children touched by violence a program which included three months of individual psychotherapy, then three months of group therapy, followed by three months of involvement in a mentorship program; parents, police, and teachers were included.

The children in this program had been exposed to serious problems as well as violence, including: death of parents, physical abuse, rape or sexual abuse, neglect, and the knowledge that seven children known to them had been murdered. The group goals included: providing support and helping the children accept their experiences, increasing their ability to tolerate feelings and respond emotionally to others, and developing their social skills (Murphy et al., 1997). Each group had five to eight members, and sessions were ninety minutes long.

Leaders, aware that latency children generally "fear some form of peer rejection and being overwhelmed by negative emotions," chose age-appropriate group activities, such as motoric activities, drawing, and games (Murphy et al., 1997, p. 234). Once mutual trust and acceptance were established, the children began sharing their traumatic experiences; hearing the other children speak and express their fears was a validating experience for them:

> In one group, the therapist noted that two boys who were without fathers had become friends. The first boy had ... [made] efforts to resuscitate his father after waking up to find him unresponsive in a living room chair. The second boy had addressed his witnessing of domestic violence and drug use that led his mother to ask his father to leave the family. The therapist [commented], "I have noticed you two have become friends and wonder if you have been drawn to each other because of painful feelings you share about being without your father." The first child immediately responded, "Yea, that's true, he knows what it's like. . . . Being the oldest, I have had to look after my younger brothers and sisters." The other boy, also an eldest child, nodded in agreement. The therapist then continued, "Sometimes, it feels like you don't get to be just a kid," and, the second boy responded, "I have to look after my mom, too." (Murphy et al., 1997, p. 249)

The group support enabled children to discuss trauma that they had not been ready to reveal in their prior individual therapy sessions. One boy, who told his teacher " 'I want to be dead when I grow up' " (Murphy et al., 1997, p. 239), told the group how, when he was seven, he had seen his best friend murdered. He had never told anyone about this event before; he was afraid that if he did, he would be in danger, too.

The group discussed plans for revenge and other retaliatory measures against perpetrators, and alternative ways of handling these feelings were explored. The boy who was afraid to talk about his best friend's murder had retaliatory fantasies toward the assailant: "he would want to get back at this person . . . by shooting him with a gun, too" (Murphy et al., 1997, p. 240).

> The children then mutually examined their respective revenge fantasies and their struggles over human accountability. Another spoke of wanting to beat up an uncle who had so badly beaten him. Another child spoke of wanting to run over the man who had run over his best friend. The group therapist addressed these expressions of two underlying wishes by saying, "I bet you'd like him to feel as bad as you did and to make sure he can never make you feel like that again." In response, one child began to discuss whether putting people in jail might not answer the wish for retribution, punishment, and protection. (Murphy et al., 1997, p. 240)

Latency-age children are concerned with rules and developing a moral code of behavior. Even in the average expectable environment, this is not an easy task. How much more complicated it is when antisocial "amoral" codes control their lives, and violence is a regular occurrence.

These children were helped to express their grief, which was facilitated by using exercises such as "writing a letter to the deceased or absent parent or sibling" (Murphy et al., 1997, p. 240). The latency child's concern with fairness was intensely expressed as "protests of unfairness over [their] loss" were often noted (Murphy et al., 1997, pp. 240-241). These losses were compounded by the traumatic events which frequently surrounded the losses. "Special attention is then needed to address *the interplay of trauma and grief that complicates childhood bereavement*" [italics added] (p. 241). Children often felt "shame and humiliation" over some of their losses, which was alleviated through group validation.

Parents or guardians were involved in one of the group sessions with the children; this was of "noticeable therapeutic benefit to both parents and child" (Murphy et al., 1997, p. 241), especially when the traumatic loss was mutual.

Police officers attended several group sessions, giving the children an opportunity to discuss directly their grievances about the police, which decreased the lack of trust and communication that existed between them. In one instance, a child told the officer about his upset over the way his cousin was treated by the police when he was arrested; in another instance, a child's grievance was that the police had not found the person who ran over his best friend.

Efforts have been increased to involve police constructively in solving community problems, including a national community policing initiative (Jenkins et al., 1997). One of the " 'core components' of community policing [is] the development of community partnership and problem solving. Community policing demands a relationship with the community that is built on the positive contact between patrol officers and community members" (Jenkins et al., 1997, p. 306).

Mental Health Problems

Many children experience mental health problems, including anxiety, depression, post-traumatic stress disorder, behavioral disorders, attention deficit disorder as well as developmental disabilities, such as autism. "It is estimated that 12 percent of children, or 7.5 million, suffer from emotional or other problems that warrant mental health treatment. Only 20 percent to 30 percent may be getting appropriate mental health services (Eamon, 1994). Recently, attention has focused on suicidal behavior in young children (Pfeffer, 1988); "suicide among children under 15 is still rare but apparently becoming more common" ("Mood Disorders," 1993, p. 3).

According to a recent surgeon general's report (O'Neill, 2000b), attention-deficit/hyperactivity disorder "is the most commonly diagnosed behavioral disorder of childhood, occurring in 3 percent to 5 percent of school-age children in a six-month period" (O'Neill, 2000b, p. 5). However, the highest prevalence of childhood (and adolescent) psychiatric problems are anxiety disorders.

> The most common anxiety disorders are: Separation anxiety disorder, which occurs in about 4 percent of children and young adolescents, and sometimes lasts for years and is a precursor to panic disorder with agoraphobia; Generalized anxiety disorder, which affects about 3 percent of all ages and makes children worry excessively about all manner of upcoming events and occurrences; Social phobia, with a lifetime prevalence of 3 percent to 13 percent, depending on how great the fear and how many situations induce the anxiety. (O'Neill, 2000b, p. 5)

Attention-Deficit Hyperactivity Disorder

Attention-deficit hyperactivity disorder (ADHD) has received considerable attention professionally and in the popular press. This serious problem particularly affects school performance, as ADHD children have difficulty concentrating and listening to others and are overactive and impulsive. "Individuals often have difficulty sustaining attention in tasks or play activities and find it hard to persist with tasks until completion" (American Psychiatric Association, 1994, p. 79). Hyperactivity is characterized by "excessive running and climbing in situations where it is not appropriate . . . by having difficulty playing or engaging quietly in leisure activities . . . by appearing to be often 'on the go' or as if 'driven by a motor' or by talking excessively" (American Psychiatric Association, pp. 78-79).

The cause of ADHD is not known; and the incidence is higher in boys than girls. It has been speculated that "contributing factors for ADHD include prenatal toxic exposures, prematurity, and prenatal mechanical insult to the fetal nervous system. . . . [There is also] evidence for a genetic basis" (Kaplan et al., 1994, p. 1063). Although it can coexist with other serious childhood disorders, if left untreated it can also lead to problems of school failure and poor conduct. Drugs, notably Ritalin, have been found to be highly effective in treating children with this disorder (Noble, 1999; "Study Sheds," 2000).

Ritalin was found to be more effective than behavioral therapy alone or standard medical community treatment in a recent major study sponsored by the National Institute of Mental Health ("Study Sheds," 2000). Peter Jensen, the principal collaborator of this study, emphasized the importance of "carefully monitored medication," which involved monthly visits with the research team and involvement from parents and teachers. " 'In contrast, community physicians saw children in our control group only about twice a year for 10 to 15 minutes with no input from teachers,' said Jensen," ("Study Sheds," 2000, p. 20). Ritalin used in combination with behavior management therapy also had good results, especially when other psychiatric problems (comorbid conditions) were also involved.

> The researchers also found that medication combined with intensive behavioral treatment "offered consistent advantages over the community comparison group in reducing comorbid aggression, ODD [oppositional defiant disorder], [and improving] academic performance, social skills, parent-child relations, and children's anxious/depressive symptoms," said Jensen.
>
> "Using a therapist-consultant to train teachers and summer camp aides to work with ADHD children on their academic skills, behavior management, and peer relationships, combined with parental reinforcements, appears to have paid off" said Jensen. ("Study Sheds," 2000, p. 20)

One criticism about Ritalin relates to the misdiagnosis (and overdiagnosis) of ADHD; children who are not adequately stimulated in school can become restless and appear to have these symptoms, as can children with an oppositional disorder, or those from disorganized or chaotic families (American Psychiatric Association, 1994). Questions have also been raised as to whether some children (including those below age six) are being inappropriately medicated for this condition as well as for other conditions, such as depression (Goode, 2000).

ADHD can be found in very young children, in adolescents, and in adults (in whom it has only recently been diagnosed). It is particularly critical during latency years that diagnosis and treatment of this problem take place; untreated ADHD can lead to school failure, secondary behavioral problems, social difficulties, and the inability to attain a sense of mastery and competency.

> Children who do not learn to read and to gain social approval from peers by grade four and/or who develop social incompetence, impulsivity, and aggressive behavior during this period are at high risk of developing a mental disorder (Institute of Medicine, 1994). Additional risk factors for development of a mental disorder include poor parenting, high levels of family conflict, and a low degree of bonding between children and parents. (Dulmus and Rapp-Paglicci, 2000, p. 299)

Conduct Disorder

Conduct disorder, more frequently found in boys than in girls, is "the most common disorder seen in child mental health clinics" (Williams et al., 1997, p. 144) and is often found in youth who engage in delinquent behavior, but "not all individuals engaging in delinquent activities meet the criteria for conduct disorder" (p. 141). According to the DSM-IV (American Psychiatric Association, 1994), "the essential feature of Conduct Disorder is a repetitive and persistent pattern of behavior in which the basic rights of others or major age-appropriate societal norms or rules are violated" (p. 85). Those with this problem "may have little empathy and little concern for the feelings, wishes, and well-being of others" (p. 87). One subtype of this diagnosis with a poor prognosis has its onset in childhood; a second subtype has its onset in adolescence with a better prognosis.

Antisocial behaviors displayed have been classified from mild (such as lying or truancy), to moderate (such as vandalism) and severe (such as physical cruelty or use of a weapon). "Suicidal ideation, suicide attempts, and completed suicide occur at a higher than expected rate" (American Psychiatric Association, 1994, p. 87). Children with this disorder often have low academic achievement, and attention-deficit/hyperactivity disorder is common. Many factors related to other types of child and adolescent malfunctioning are also associated with this disorder, such as child maltreatment, inconsistency in nurturing, and frequent changes of nurturing figures and living in institutions (American Psychiatric Association, 1994).

ADOLESCENCE

McGrath, a photographer, reflecting on photographs of teenagers, finds them very moving and special because, by contrast with babies, teenagers are more elusive in their expressiveness (McGrath, 1998).

> It's only when children approach adolescence, and begin to become social beings, that they start to develop private, inaccessible selves—and it's just at that moment that they tend to disappear or go out of focus. They stop turning up in our photo albums, that is, almost at the same moment that we stop comprehending them. (McGrath, 1998, p. 30)

Adolescence is a time for intense privacy and intense friendships—a turbulent, joyful, optimistic time, but also a time of confusion, mood changes, and feelings of wonderment, excitement, and alarm at the beginnings of sexual development. It is time to leave the world of kids, although still feeling like one, and enter the threshold of the adult world; it is time to develop one's identity (Erikson, 1963). The adolescent has already journeyed from preschool to the larger realm of elementary school, but now the stakes are higher, as adulthood, with its responsibilities and difficult choices, beckons.

Although the universe expanded for the schoolchild, the family remained clearly at its center, and family rituals and outings were major high points. Now family events may feel boring, friends replace relatives as central figures, and the magnetic attraction of social activities, dating, and driving pull the adolescent further from home. But adolescents do not wish to sever connections to their families; they struggle to find the right distance without losing the comfort of closeness as they reenter the rapprochement crisis at a higher level (Blos, 1962).

For the family, life can be delightful and stimulating as the adolescents' mental growth and social involvement increase. Parents can also experience bewilderment and conflict as the adolescent "darts away" from them and then returns for "emotional refueling" (Mahler et al., 1975); parents may feel puzzled as their adolescent develops values and habits that may be different from their own. Although setting limits on their young child's behavior may have created tension, this tension can escalate as parents struggle to decide which limits to place on their adolescent's behavior and how to enforce them. Yet, overall, in the average expectable environment, adolescents do basically get along with their parents (Kaplan et al., 1994; Rutter, 1975) and "for the most part, are receptive to parental approval and disapproval. The majority of adolescents and their parents are able to bridge the generation gap successfully" (Kaplan et al., 1994, p. 54).

Adolescence has been divided into three periods: early adolescence (from eleven to fourteen); middle adolescence (from fourteen to seventeen), and late adolescence (from seventeen to twenty) (Kaplan et al., 1994). Adolescence occurs earlier now (physically) and is considered to last longer (due to greater time needed to achieve full adulthood in our society) than it has in the past, when it had extended from ages thirteen to eighteen.

Although adolescent turmoil is normal (Kaplan et al., 1994, p. 55), adolescents can have difficult problems and such risk-taking behaviors as drug and substance abuse, promiscuous sexual activity (putting them at risk for pregnancy and AIDS), gambling addictions, and "accident prone behavior, such as fast driving, skydiving, and hang gliding" (Kaplan et al., 1994, p. 55). Adolescents are prone to depression, eating disorders, and a high rate of suicide. Many have experienced violence, have witnessed homicide, and are victims of family maltreatment. Some have responded to this by running away, becoming homeless, and/or turning to prostitution.

Some adolescents have been subject to discrimination based on race, ethnicity, or sexual orientation; those from different cultures experience conflict integrating family values with the values of their peers and struggle with becoming assimilated or developing a bicultural identity.

A discussion of adolescent development will be followed by a focus on their special problems.

Physical Development of Adolescents

Adolescents experience biological changes, including major increases in height and weight and hormonal activity, producing primary and secondary sexual characteristics and sexual feelings (de Anda, 1995). These biological changes do not uniformly occur; girls generally reach puberty two years before boys do, and the age differential at which individual boys and girls reach puberty can be several years. As both growth spurts and sexual development are so prominent, and as peer approval is so important, early or late achievement of puberty can affect one's social standing and social image (de Anda, 1995).

> Precocious or delayed growth, acne, obesity, and enlarged mammary glands in boys and small or overabundant breasts in girls are some deviations from the expected patterns of maturation. Although these conditions may not be medically significant, they often lead to psychological sequelae. Adolescents are sensitive to the opinions of peers and are constantly comparing themselves with others. Any deviation, real or imagined, can lead to feelings of inferiority, low self-esteem, and loss of confidence. Girls are more sensitive to early physical manifestations of puberty than are boys. (Kaplan et al., 1994, p. 51)

Adolescents will sometimes go to great lengths to alter their physical appearance, including undergoing cosmetic plastic surgery. Although eating disorders (discussed in Chapter 12), seen predominantly (although not exclusively) in adolescent girls, have multiple interacting psychological factors, preoccupation with appearance (especially thinness) is a key feature. Teenage boys have taken steroid drugs to improve their physical appearance and athletic prowess; studies today find that steroid use among teenage girls is increasing, with the aim of improving physical appearance and gaining in athletic prowess (Gorman, 1998b; "Steroid Use," 1999).

> The new interest among teenage girls . . . reflects a gradual change in attitude and fashion, or teenage peer pressure, away from a preoccupation with thinness. Some teenage girls now desire to look more healthy and somewhat more muscular, but this has led some girls toward an unhealthy compulsion to be ever fitter with larger muscles. ("Steroid Use," 1999, p. A12)

Psychological Developments in Adolescence

A major psychological task of adolescence is the development of an identity (Erikson, 1963) and resolving, in greater depth, problems of separation and individuation. Blos (1962), who refers to adolescence as a "second step in individuation" (p. 12), views many adolescent rebellions and psychological storms as serving this process.

> Before the adolescent can consolidate this [identity] formation, he must pass through stages of self-consciousness and fragmented existence. The oppositional, rebellious, and restive strivings, the stages of experimentation, the testing of the self by going to excess—all these have a positive usefulness in the process of self-definition. "This is not me" represents an important step in the achievement of individuation and in the establishment of autonomy; at an earlier age, it is condensed into a single word—"No!" (Blos, 1962, p. 12)

The restive and rebellious components of the adolescent experience are related to action and acting out behaviors in many adolescents. Dugan (1989) notes that although the term *acting out* often carries a "pejorative" connotation and is seen as "pathological," this behavior "may also be an indicator of hope and potential for success in the face of adversity" and may lead to the development of "resiliency" (p. 157). Dugan (1989) contrasts acting out to the development of "patterns of inhibition, inaction, and compliance [which] are shown to foreshadow the development of a sense of helplessness and despair" (p. 158). Frequently, acting out has "communicational aspects," and can be a " 'cry for help' ' "; in fact, there is an "adaptive capacity of being able to act in relationship to others, even when such behavior results in provocation or annoyance" (Dugan, 1989, p. 158).

Adolescents can experience troubling feelings as they move toward individuation.

> Adolescent individuation is accompanied by feelings of isolation, loneliness, and confusion. Individuation brings some of the dearest megalomanical dreams of childhood to an irrevocable end. They must now be relegated entirely to fantasy; their fulfillments can never again be considered seriously. The realization of the finality of the end of childhood, of the binding nature of commitments, of the definite limitation to individual existence itself—this realization creates a sense of urgency, fear, and panic. Consequently, many an adolescent tries to remain indefinitely in a transitional phase of development; this condition is called *prolonged adolescence.* (Blos, 1962, p. 12)

The early phase of adolescence is often accompanied by a need for privacy and creating distance from parents, "represented by closed doors in bedrooms and bathrooms, and secretiveness usually initiated by self-consciousness about body change" (Newton, 1995, p. 27). As the adolescent turns to peers, it is not uncommon for them to develop "secrets with best friends and subsequently a peer group" (Newton, 1995, p. 27).

An interesting transitional phenomenon at this age is the keeping of diaries; this is more common behavior in girls than in boys (Blos, 1962). "Daydreams, events, and emotions which cannot be shared with real people are confessed with relief to the diary" (p. 94). Often the imaginary friend in the diary to which the adolescent girl writes is female, and she is usually given a name (Blos, 1962; Dalsimer, 1982); in Anne Frank's diary, her "friend" is called Kitty. This diary friend is an "imagined 'other' whom the adolescent brings to life [in] an effort at restitution for the loss at the heart of the adolescent experience" (Dalsimer, 1982, p. 521).

Diaries give their writers an opportunity to work through and reflect on their lives, conflicts, and goals; perusal of these documents offers psychologists insights into the adolescents' inner lives, fantasies, and sequences of development (Blos, 1962; Dalsimer, 1982). Dalsimer's (1982) analysis of the diaries of Anne Frank captures Anne's depiction of the unique aspects of her adolescent experience.

During World War II, Anne, from the ages of thirteen to fifteen, was confined to living in a hidden attic with her own family, a second family, and a dentist, to escape the deportation of Jews from Amsterdam to concentration camps. Although living in this "abnormal" world, Dalsimer (1982) found Anne to be a "delightful girl—bright, lively, curious, mischievous, whimsical, passionate" (p. 487). She was also a good observer of both other people and her own inner experiences.

> Even within the confines of the secret annexe, we see the familiar movement back and forth, during adolescence, between the world outside the family and the family itself. The extrafamilial world offers a refuge from the conflict that, with the onset of puberty, invades the bonds with parents; at the same time, the family becomes a refuge from the anxieties aroused in new relationships. It is this repeated movement back and forth that ultimately brings about what Blos (1967) has called the "second individuation process" of adolescence. (Dalsimer, 1982, p. 515)

Anne falls in love with Peter, the teenage son of the other annexe family.

> Like any teen-ager in love, Anne finds herself suddenly bursting into tears, thinking that perhaps Peter doesn't like her at all, or only thinks of her casually. The mood swings, the excitement, the restlessness, the exhilaration—all the characteristics of first love are recorded here. (Dalsimer, 1982, p. 507)

Anne is sexually attracted to Peter, and the intensity of her feelings frighten her: " 'I am afraid of myself, I am afraid that in my longing I am giving myself too quickly' " (Dalsimer, 1982, p. 512); then, seeming to need some external control, she asks her father about the situation in a way that almost guarantees his response: " 'Daddy, I expect you've gathered that when we're together Peter and I don't sit miles apart. Do you think it's wrong'?" (p. 512).

> As is characteristic of adolescents, Anne has found a way of externalizing the conflict which, until then, had been internal. Predictably, her father tells her not to spend so much time alone with Peter. This allows Anne to espouse the other side of her ambivalence. In defiance of her father's request that she not go to Peter's room, she declares emphatically to Kitty [her diary], "No, I'm going!" The "war that reigns incessantly within" is no longer within; it is between Anne and her father, each expressing an aspect of Anne's own conflict. By telling her father, she has drawn the lines of battle between them. At the same time, she has succeeded in reengaging him in her intimate concerns, calling upon him to be once more the authoritative and protective father of childhood. (Dalsimer, 1982, p. 512)

Although it is generally understood that adolescents rebel from authority as they seek autonomy, it is less understood (and put into practice) that they also need external limits to help them regulate their emotional states and behaviors, recapitulating their earlier needs for parental assistance in developing self-regulation—albeit now, they need this assistance on a higher level and in more complex ways.

Sexual Development in Adolescence

The adolescent develops sexually, which is a total biopsychosocial occurrence; physical changes, including hormonal activity and sexual feelings, intermingle with psychological reactions and adaptations and identity formation. To isolate sexuality as a biological phenomenon only would be an inaccurate representation of its complexity. Puberty is experienced universally in all cultures—sometimes welcomed and heralded in socially sanctioned ways, sometimes ignored or hushed. Many "hunter/gatherer and herding cultures" had "rituals" which recognized the onset of puberty, and the initiation into "adult status" (Newton, 1995, p. 25).

> As the first menstrual period began, the female child would typically be taken away from family and village and isolated in a "menstrual hut." Various activities would take place during the period of isolation, some ritual and some instructional, all aimed at ending her identity as a child, celebrating her reproductive maturation and, most importantly, teaching her the behaviors and rules for an adult female in her culture. At the end of the withdrawal period, she would return to the village in a ritual ceremony celebrating her new status as a full adult woman in the society. (Newton, 1995, p. 25)

It is not uncommon for adolescents in our culture to feel uncomfortable and awkward in their new bodies and both sexually excited as well as guilty with their newly developing sexual feelings. Sexual experimentation is common, sometimes leading to pregnancy, or sexually transmitted diseases. Excessive sexual acting out may be related to having been sexually abused (Dore, 1999); adolescent prostitution is a common phenomenon in runaway adolescents (Kaplan et al., 1994); and HIV/AIDS, associated with a propensity to engage in unsafe sex (and use intravenous drugs), is particularly seen in the population of homeless teens. (HIV/AIDS is discussed further in Chapter 12.)

There is a general decline in the number of teenagers having sexual intercourse according to Dr. Kolbe, the former Director of the Centers for Disease Control and Prevention's Division of Adolescent and School Health ("Fewer High School," 1998); "the trend toward abstinence is in sharp contrast to the 1970's and 80's, when sexual activity ballooned among teenagers" (p. A18). Dr. Kolbe could not pinpoint the factors causing this change but thought it could be attributed to the " 'efforts by parents, schools and health officials to educate young people about safe sex and the risks of pregnancy and sexually transmitted diseases like AIDS' " (p. A18).

The emphasis on sex-education programs in the schools in this country is on abstinence; more than half of these schools do not offer information about birth control (Wilgoren, 1999). When birth control information is taught, the emphasis is often on the failure rates occurring when using birth control. The subject of sex education is responsive to political forces; legislation was passed in 1996 providing $440 million in state and federal funds for five years for so-called "abstinence only programs"; in 1999, Congress appropriated another $50 million to this bill, and many parents are insisting that an abstinence message either be the main focus or an important piece of any sex education program (Wilgoren, 1999, p. A16). James Wagoner, president of Advocates for Youth, which supports a broader approach, stated:

> "Parents and adults are prepared for a far more realistic policy than are members of Congress, who seem more concerned with posturing and simple solutions to complex issues. . . . In too many school districts around the country, young people are being denied critical information about contraception that could protect their health and save their lives." (Wilgoren, 1999, p. A16)

The rate of teenage pregnancy has dramatically decreased; this has been attributed to a decrease in adolescent sexual relations as well as to an increased use of birth control (Lacey, 1999). Teenage parents were discussed in Chapter 6.

It is not uncommon for adolescents to experience homosexual feelings early in adolescence (Blos, 1962); usually, this is a stage on the way to the development of heterosexuality. However, a number of adolescents realize that their sexual orientation is gay, lesbian, or bisexual, and this realization can cause distress and confusion.

Gay, Lesbian, and Bisexual Adolescents

As heterosexual adolescents experience turmoil about their sexuality, gay and lesbian adolescents often experience even greater turmoil; this is not the expected norm. They face the possibility of rejection by their parents, peers, teachers, and social institutions; they may become socially isolated and depressed and are at high risk of suicide (Hunter and Schaecher, 1995; Proctor and Groze, 1994); they are "seven times as likely as straight kids to be threatened or injured by a weapon at school and five times as likely to skip school because they feel unsafe" (Barovick, 2000, p. 52).

The struggle with identity development is compounded for teens with a gay or lesbian orientation (Hunter and Schaecher, 1995). One helpful step is the coming out process; the decision to share with others in their lives this important fact as well as to integrate their sexual identities into their sense of self may lessen their turmoil if others are supportive of them.

> Young people grow up in a society that assumes they will be heterosexual; that is, they will date people of the other sex and eventually get married and raise their own children. In this context, the process of coming to terms with being lesbian or gay is formidable. Krysial (1987) poignantly noted that gays and lesbians are one of the few groups who do not have parents as role models. The nurturing and support that most families provide in the development of children is usually absent when the sexual orientation points toward homosexuality. (Hunter and Schaecher, 1995, p. 1056)

Some adolescents struggle against their homosexual feelings, denying or suppressing them, and become involved in at-risk behaviors such as, "engaging in unprotected sex with people of the same sex or the opposite sex, even getting pregnant or fathering a child, so that no one will suspect the young person's homosexuality . . . [using] alcohol or other drugs . . . [and putting themselves] at significant risk for HIV infection" (Hunter and Schaecher, 1995, p. 1057).

Gay and lesbian adults have made social and legal advances in terms of increased social acceptance and legal rulings in their favor, but violence, discrimination, and homophobia in overt and subtler forms remain; a similar picture is present in the adolescent gay and lesbian population.

Joyce Hunter (Cloud, 1997), a researcher at Columbia University who has been studying the gay and lesbian youth culture since the 1970s when few adolescents came out, finds that now teenage openness about homosexuality has undergone a dramatic change. "Lonely gay kids can find solace in two Webzines, dozens of on-line chat rooms and some 500 community support groups, usually run by social workers not affiliated with local schools"; churches offer programs to homosexual adolescents (Cloud, 1997, p. 82); 700 gay-straight clubs exist in schools throughout the country (Barovick, 2000). On college campuses, "gay equality has . . . become a '90's version of Birkenstock environmentalism for many youths. Even in certain parts of suburbia, gay is becoming more than O.K.; it's cool" (Cloud, 1997, p. 82).

In February 2000, a legal battle was waged at El Modena high school in Orange County, California, challenging the rights of students to establish a gay-straight alliance (a support group open to both homosexual and heterosexual teenagers). Opponents, including some parents, took action to prevent this group's formation due to concerns about "destructive lifestyles" and the dissemination of AIDS (Barovick, 2000, p. 52).

> Many straight kids join the[se] clubs for reasons more social than sexual. Some are simply offended by homophobia. . . . Finally, some straight kids join to learn to be proud of their families. . . . A high school freshman in the Midwest, says that in middle school, he was afraid to talk about his mother, who is a lesbian. Now, as a member of an alliance, he feels comfortable that "no one would say anything. And if they did, someone would tell them off." (Barovick, 2000, p. 52)

The recent court case related to the ousting from the Boy Scout organization of a gay Eagle Scout epitomizes the current mix of attitudes on this subject. On August 4, 1999, the New Jersey Supreme Court ruled unanimously that the Boy Scouts had violated New Jersey's antidiscrimination law when they expelled a gay Eagle Scout nine years earlier (Hanley, 1999). Contending that homosexuality is inconsistent with the Scout pledge of morality, the Boy Scouts had insisted that they had the right to bar James Dale, now twenty-nine, from scouting as they were a private organization and had First Amendment protections (Hanley, 1999, p. A1). The New Jersey Supreme Court rejected this idea as being similar to "discrimination against women and blacks" (Hanley, 1999, p. A1). Upon a later appeal by the Boy Scout organization, the ruling in favor of Dale was overturned.

Social workers deal with many teenagers who may be gay or lesbian, but are often afraid to discuss their sexual orientation; many times they are "invisible in family services" (Proctor and Groze, 1994, p. 511); those in shelters or residential care "are treated differently from other participants" (Hunter and Schaecher, 1995, p. 1060); teens "who hide their homosexual orientation do not get their needs met and their relationships are distorted, including the client-worker relationship" (Hunter and Schaecher, 1995, p. 1060). Attunement to the needs of this population is an important professional challenge for clinical social workers.

Cognitive Development in Adolescence

During adolescence, considerable growth and development occurs in the brain, which results in the adolescent's "higher and more complex cognitive ability and behavioral repertoire" (Newton, 1995, p. 33). Adolescents enter Piaget's stage of *formal operations,* in which they think more abstractly and conceptually, becoming involved in the world of ideas. Piaget and Inhelder (1995) have observed that adolescents are able to analyze their own thinking and develop theories and look at situations from multiple perspectives. "The fact that these theories are oversimplified, awkward, and usually contain very little originality is beside the point. From the functional standpoint, [adolescents'] systems are significant in that they furnish the cognitive and evaluative bases for the assumption of adult roles" (Piaget and Inhelder, 1995, p. 437).

Levine (1990), in discussing adolescents in foster placement, emphasizes how the development of formal operations processes enables adolescents to think through their family life with different perspectives, which has the potential of leading to internal conflict resolution and growth. She observes that preadolescent children (who are in the concrete operations stage of development) have difficulty dealing with the abstract, think that " 'what is, ought to be,' " and feel that they are to blame for being placed by their parents in foster care (Levine, 1990, p. 58). Adolescents, with their capacity for abstraction, "can deal with ideas and possibilities" and have the capability of comparing "their parents to other parents, and in doing so become aware of their parents' limitations. Their faith in parental infallibility erodes" (Levine, 1990, pp. 58-59).

> Placed adolescents do not compare abstract parents. They live trapped between two sets of parenting figures: their own parents, either as experienced or imagined, and foster parents. Moreover, the discrepancy between the idealized parent of childhood and the objectified parent of adolescence is usually greater for foster children than for children who are raised by their own parents. When combined with changes in the belief system inherent in an adolescent's cognitive development, being in placement frequently forces a premature and too rapid awareness of parental limitations upon the adolescent. (Levine, 1990, p. 59)

During adolescence, creativity often flourishes, idealism develops, and the adolescent becomes interested in the "world of ideas—humanitarian issues, morals, ethics, and religion" (Kaplan et al., 1994, p. 53). Piaget and Inhelder (1995) discuss the tendency for adolescents' "egocentrism" to manifest itself in a "sort of Messianic form such that the theories used to represent the world center on the role of reformer that the adolescent feels himself called upon to play in the future"; gradually, this egocentrism recedes in a process called "decentering" (p. 440). Many teenagers join the Peace Corps, do community volunteer work, and make constructive contributions to school newspapers, literary magazines, orchestras, dramatic societies, and student government.

At Midwood, a public high school in Brooklyn where academic achievement is emphasized, some students receive specialized science education, aiming for recognition by Intel, a company that sponsors a prominent national science competition annually. Midwood is one of the "most overcrowded, antiquated, ethnically diverse and, in terms of science education, unusually successful schools in New York City's public school system" (Hall, 2000, p. 54). "At a place like Midwood, which draws on a less elite population than city schools with admission exams . . . the Intel contest provides the flame that heats a new, high-tech version of the melting pot myth" (Hall, 2000, p. 54).

One downside of the Midwood program is the pressure to perform as well as some curtailment of students' other interests and social life (Hall, 2000). However, these students are given opportunities in the here and now to develop intellectually and to anticipate a future filled with opportunities, as opposed to feeling they have no future, as many ghetto children and gang members feel. These teens experience a social milieu in which academic achievement is both accepted, expected, and rewarded, and in which supportive, involved teachers are role models. This program highlights the potential for adolescent academic achievement and intellectual creativity.

Moral Development in Adolescence

Piaget observed that morality evolves along with children's cognitive thinking. In the preoperational stage, children obey the rules of the adults who care for them; during the stage of concrete operations, children follow the rules rigidly but are not able to see subtle distinctions or allow for different interpretations; in the stage of formal operations, adolescents can think about rules in terms of the needs of society (Kaplan et al., 1994).

Kohlberg, utilizing Piaget's theory, developed his own conceptual framework, in which he highlighted three phases of morality. In *preconventional morality,* the child responds to parental authority and punishment through obedience; during the phase of *morality of conventional role conformity,* the child is concerned with the opinions of others and seeks to feel validated and accepted. In the final phase, morality of self-accepted moral principles, the child has internalized a set of moral and ethical concepts, operates on this basis, and is capable of thinking through conflicting situations to arrive at a decision of how to respond (Kaplan et al., 1994).

The development of morality in individual adolescents is dependent on a number of circumstances: the moral code of their families and social environments; the overt and covert messages they receive from their families about acceptable behavior; the quality of their attachments and identifications with their parents. An important distinction is the adolescents' ability to think morally and capacity to act morally. As adolescents' respond to their own impulses and tendencies toward risk-taking behaviors, some immoral behavior may be the consequence. The development of a personal moral code is often part of the struggle to develop their own sense of identity.

Can adolescents whose behavior has been judged by society to be immoral and illegal have the capacity to make valid moral and legal judgments about the illegal behaviors of their peers? In an innovative social experiment, teenagers charged with lesser, nonviolent legal misdemeanors are being judged by juries of their peers (who had also been charged with legal misdemeanors) in about 650 youth courts throughout the country (Sengupta, 2000a, p. 32).

The Bronx Youth Court, which by mid-2000 had been operating for two years under the auspices of New York City's Probation Department, differs from other youth courts as it "judges more serious offenses—drug possession with intent to sell, robbery, weapons charges" (Sengupta, 2000a, p. 32). The peer judges are not easy on offenders: "Among the judges, jurors and lawyers are those whose own sentences included serving in Youth Court" (Sengupta, 2000a, p. 32).

This project raises tantalizing questions about both the effectiveness of peer group opinion on decreasing teenage delinquency behaviors, as well as the impact on the "court officers" themselves in terms of potentially enhanced self-esteem, feeling respect from authorities, and the internalization of a new moral code. The developmental processes of adolescence speak to the potential feasibility of such a plan due to the influence of peer groups at this age, the increased capacity of the adolescent to think through problems from different perspectives, and the move to higher levels of moral development.

Family Life of Adolescents

One typical struggle between teenagers and their families relates to familial direction, rules, and control; parents often walk a fine line between rigid overcontrol of their teenagers and not providing enough guidance or setting any limits. Parents may be struggling with their own unresolved adolescent issues, which have been reawakened by experiencing their children's adolescence, causing parent-child conflicts about authority. The Vietnam War ushered in social changes in this country including civil protest, the breakdown of authority, and the increased use of drugs. Parents and social institutions became more permissive, and children were given freedoms they may not have been ready to handle.

At present, there seems to be a general turning away from this "permissiveness" toward a greater concern with structure and limits, and parents are evidently keeping a closer eye on their college-age children. Many colleges, for example, now provide greater in loco parentis structure, guidance, and rules, often at the request of parents, and sometimes at the request of students: "Many parents are former students who worry that their children will repeat their wild college years and who have much to say about college life

. . . . Students increasingly want to talk about their varied and difficult backgrounds" (Bronner, 1999, pp. A1, A15).

Major family disruptions, such as divorce or joining a newly formed blended family, can create special stress for the adolescent who is in the midst of working out separation-individuation issues. Familial maltreatment, parental substance abuse, or mental illness can leave the adolescent emotionally vulnerable and feeling conflicted. A strong association exists, for example, between adolescent suicide and poor relationships with parents and/or actual family breakdown.

Cultural Influences Affecting Adolescents

Adolescents are affected by the broad cultural climate as well as the subcultures to which they belong. It is not uncommon for culture clashes to occur; a teen, for example, might live in a family in which drinking is prohibited but belongs to a social group in which *not* drinking is ostracized. Teens whose parents are immigrants and/or who hold strong ethnic and cultural traditions are in a particularly vulnerable situation; the influence of peer culture is great and may carry a greater pull on them than parental expectations.

In Asian cultures, emphasis is placed not on the development of individual identity but on family and collective identification; "a sense of belonging and affiliation is provided by the rigid boundaries of the kinship-based family network" (Huang, 1997, p. 176). One major conflict between Asian Indian adolescents and their parents, in this country, revolves around dating (Segal, 1991). "The parents' greatest fear [in one study] was that their children would marry non-Indian Americans and thus lose their cultural identity . . . the idea of marriage to a non-Indian is especially disturbing" (Segal, 1991, pp. 238-239).

Adolescents with different ethnic and cultural backgrounds vary in the rigidity with which they adhere to parental values or reject their cultural background; those who attain a *bicultural identity,* meaning they can be comfortable in both cultures, seem to be well adjusted and function at high levels.

Special Problems of Adolescents

Although adolescents' behavior at times can appear tumultuous, their mood swings difficult to understand, and their arguments with families intense, these events are considered within the range of to-be-expected, everyday occurrences. However, some adolescents must deal with very serious problems, such as malfunction and breakdown, depression, substance abuse, suicide and violence in their families.

Family Dissolution

The dissolution of a family is a painful process for all its members and can occur through many means, including death, divorce, and abandonment. This section will discuss divorce, homelessness, when adolescents have run away or have been thrown out of their families, and the ending of foster placement for adolescents when they "come of age."

Divorce. Although seemingly removed from the family, the adolescent still needs a secure base. Loss and its resolution are a normal part of the adolescent experience; loss accompanied by the "finality" of family breakdown makes emancipation far more painful and complex. Adolescents whose parents are divorcing may become depressed or act out. Suicide attempts by teens are not uncommon during the separation or divorce process, in part because of the message this attempt sends parents to preserve the unity of the family.

Often when divorcing, parents, due to their own preoccupations, "abdicate" their parental role (Isaacs et al., 2000, p. 182).

> We use the term abdication to describe parents' almost complete failure to carry out the usual socialization functions: taking a tender interest in the youngster's everyday triumphs, struggles, and disappointments; consistently checking curfews and actively appraising the adolescent's girlfriends and boyfriends; meeting periodically with teachers . . . and making occasional but necessary checks with the other parent. The youngster is left to make it alone. Two levels of the abdication phenomenon can be differentiated. The first is the absence per se of indispensable parental functions because of parental depression, obsessive preoccupation, or physical absence. . . . The second is more directly linked to the spousal battle. Here, abdication serves to sustain a parent-adolescent, cross-generational coalition that undermine or excludes the other spouse. (Isaacs et al., 2000, p. 182)

Adolescents can adapt to divorce, especially when parents are supportive of them and do not triangulate them into the divorce process (Isaacs et al., 2000). *Abdication* of parental involvement also occurs in families other than those affected by divorce. Many homeless adolescents, for example, have run away from group homes and foster homes (Bass, 1995), and "push out" and "throwaway" teens have been physically and/or emotionally abandoned by their families (Loppnow, 1985).

Runaways and homeless teens. It is estimated that in the United States "there are 1 million to 1.3 million runaways and homeless youths each year and that 500,000 of these youths are homeless" (Bass, 1995, p. 2060). Many runaways and homeless youth have "experienced physical and sexual abuse, drug and alcohol abuse by both parents, family violence, mental health problems, and school problems. . . . Twice as many homeless youths came to agencies from foster homes or group homes than from their own families" (Bass, 1995, p. 2062). "At the Covenant House teen shelter in Manhattan, 80 percent of the roughly 400 teenagers who stay there nightly are former foster children. Many come directly from the jails at Rikers Island" (Sengupta, 2000b, p. A25).

Many homeless youth become involved in stealing, prostitution, and drugs. " 'Some do all of them,' said Dean Wright, a sociology professor" (Hart, 1998, p. B4). Wright added that half of the runaway boys and about three-quarters of the girls engage in prostitution, most commonly with older males, and "before these teenagers are pressed into prostitution, their will to resist is often broken by forced sex" (Hart, 1998, p. B4). A large percentage of all prostitutes are teenagers—"estimates ranging up to 1 million teenagers involved in prostitution" (Kaplan et al., 1994, pp. 55-56).

> Most teenager [prostitutes] ran away from home and were taken in by pimps and substance abusers; then the adolescents themselves became substance abusers. They are at high risk for AIDS, and many, up to 70 percent in some studies, are infected with the human immunodeficiency virus (HIV). (Kaplan et al., 1994, p. 56)

Health problems, including AIDS and other sexually transmitted diseases, are a major risk faced by all homeless youths; they are less likely to be treated for alcohol or drug abuse problems and are much less likely to be reunited with their families (Bass, 1995, p. 2062). They are at risk for mental health problems; approximately "61 percent of these youths suffer from depression and . . . about 10 percent are considered suicidal" (Bass, 1995, p. 2061). Rotheram-Borus and Bradley (1991) assert that in regard to the high rate of multiple suicide attempts and long-term psychiatric disturbances, "strategies are needed to identify suicidal runaways" (p. 122). "Shelters are seeing an increasing number of youths . . . who . . . may never be reunited with their families. *In addition, once youths leave foster or shelter care, they are immediately without income, housing, and a social support system*" [italics added] (Bass, 1995, p. 2066).

Teenagers leaving foster placement. If many teenagers in foster and group homes run away or end up in the criminal justice system, does this mean that foster care per se is a malevolent institution? For some adolescents, the stability of a good foster home can be a *protective* factor in developing coping skills and resilience. For others, the foster experience can be a path to future unhappiness and poor functioning. According to the Child Welfare League of America, a quarter of adolescents terminating foster care "experience homelessness, only about half have finished high school, less than half have jobs and over 60 percent of females leaving the system have a baby within four years" (Beaucar, 1999a, p. 7). More research is needed to clarify the "differences between youth who leave [foster homes] by emancipation [they are 18 and services end] and those who leave through family reunification, running away, or incarceration" (Courtney and Barth, 1996, p. 76). In one large study, Courtney and Barth (1996) found that adolescents who were discharged from kinship foster care (discussed in Chapter 6), "seem to be most likely to either return home or make a relatively smooth transition out of foster care" (p. 82).

In most states, when adolescent foster children become eighteen, they are abandoned by the child welfare system, and "forced into the world with little else but bad memories, patchwork educational experiences and no money" (Beaucar, 1999a, p. 7). In New York City, the child welfare department gives discharged teenagers "a handful of classes in things like cooking and resume writing, a check for $750 and up to three years of modest stipends for rent" (Sengupta, 2000b, p. A1). "Teenagers moving from foster care to independence will receive extra federal assistance until they are 21 under a bill [The Foster Care Independence Act]" signed in December 1999 ("Bill Extends," 1999, para. 1). The legislation extends educational, health care, and housing assistance to those who had previously lost such benefits at age eighteen or upon completion of high school. Courtney and Barth (1996) advocate for independent-living programs for teens discharged from foster care but for flexible programs to meet the needs of different groups; "the adolescent foster care population is not singular. It consists of youths from different backgrounds who have considerably different experiences while in foster care" (p. 82).

Although foster teens are an especially vulnerable group, other programs have been established to provide assistance with independent living for an ostensibly high-functioning group of adolescents; that is, college students have been receiving more structured help with adaptation to adult living and campus life (Bronner, 1999).

Depression

Depression for many adolescents is mild, occasional, and part of their normal mood swings. However, for some, depressed feelings are more than a *transient state* of sadness; depression can be experienced as a pervasive, underlying sense of despair, loneliness, hopelessness, and emptiness; other symptoms of adolescent depression can include weepiness, boredom, physical symptoms, sleep problems, and changes in eating habits (Mack and Hickler, 1981). Depression is associated with many other adolescent problems, such as teenage pregnancy (Wakschlag and Hans, 2000), substance abuse (Slaby and McGuire, 1989), and running away (Bass, 1995); it "has been singled out as a major etiologic factor in suicide" (Braga, 1989, p. 7). There are "high rates of comorbid depression with chronic PTSD [post-traumatic stress disorder] among children and adolescents" (Murphy et al., 1997, p. 231).

Many adolescents do not ask for help with their depressive feelings but "may more easily complain of chronic boredom, lack of interest for activities and simply lack of 'drive.' These symptoms frequently alternate with temper tantrums, restlessness, defiance, acting out and 'dare devil' type of activities" (Braga, 1989, p.7).

Adolescent depression may be present in various disguised forms. Rossman (1982) uses the terms "masked depression" and "depressive equivalents" to describe how the adolescent will use "acting-out or disruptive behaviors . . . to translate depressive thoughts or feelings into action equivalents"; in addition, "failing grades, truancy, drug and alcohol use, social withdrawal and accidents" can be part of the symptomatology, and "depressed children may walk in front of an oncoming train or car or suffer multiple athletic injuries" (Slaby and McGuire, 1989, p. 23). ·

Substance Abuse

Many teenagers experiment with drugs and alcohol; for some it becomes a way of life. Substance abuse, while declining among teenagers and children (de Anda, 1995; Wren, 1998), remains a major public health problem and has many ramifications for the physical, psychological, social, and educational functioning of teenagers (Oster and Caro, 1990). Substance abuse, however, exists within a broader social-cultural context (Nowinski, 1990).

> America has become a drug oriented society; in other words, our ethics with respect to the use of mood-altering chemicals are basically permissive and sympathetic. The past two generations have witnessed a proliferation in the development and use of both licit and illicit mood-altering chemicals. We use drugs—those we obtain from physicians as well as those we obtain in liquor stores and on the street—to enhance feelings of well-being and to help us cope. Adolescents are not very different from adults in this regard. The adolescent subculture, despite differences in form, has a great deal in common with its adult counterpart; this is true across the socioeconomic spectrum. (Nowinski, 1990, p. 12)

Substance abuse may contribute to adolescents' scholastic underachievement because of its neuropsychological effects (Newton, 1995); it is often an important factor in adolescent suicide (Hoberman, 1989) and is highly correlated with fatal car crashes among teens (Nowinski, 1990); intravenous drug use can lead to HIV infection (de Anda, 1995). The three major causes of death for adolescents and young adults (accidents, homicides, and suicides) are associated with drug and alcohol use (Newton, 1995).

Teenagers use a wide range of substances. Marijuana is the most frequently used drug by adolescents; other drugs include cocaine, heroin, inhalants, amphetamines, and LSD. Ecstasy use (which is often not included in the government's drug survey) seems to be increasing, in contrast to the general decline in the use of other drugs (Cloud, 2000b). Ecstasy is considered by many to be safer than other drugs, and users find that it makes them "feel peaceful, empathetic and energetic—not edgy, just clear. . . . [Ecstasy] allows the mind to wander, but not into hallucinations" (Cloud, 2000b, p. 66). Dangers include ingesting pills that have been altered with toxic substances, and Ecstasy itself can cause dramatic increases in the body's temperature, held responsible for the deaths of "dozens of users around the world" over the past twenty years (Cloud, 2000b, p. 67). Questions have been raised about negative long-term effects on brain function.

Alcohol is the most frequently abused drug by adolescents (de Anda, 1995). In a large study of drinking patterns among college students conducted by the Harvard School of Public Health, it was discovered that although high risk binge drinking had been increasing, moderate alcohol use was declining, and an increasing number of students were abstaining from alcohol (Wilgoren, 2000).

Nowinski (1990) discusses factors contributing to adolescent substance abuse, including: the adolescent personality (taking risks, living in the present, rebelliousness); peer pressure (difficulty deviating from the adolescent "substance-using subculture") (p. 21); adolescent alienation (feeling "a disconnection from parental and societal values and ideals, traditions and rituals") (p. 21); internal and external stress, such as maltreatment, living with dysfunctional families, loss, as well as poor coping skills, insecurity, and low self-esteem.

Substance abuse among lesbian and gay adolescents is "two to three times higher than among their heterosexual counterparts" (Morrow, 1993, p. 657); this rate is related to this population going to gay and lesbian bars (when they are of age) to avoid social isolation, and the social stressors they experience in a homophobic culture (Hunter and Schaecher, 1995; Morrow, 1993).

Close associations are found among depression, substance abuse, and suicide; "few addicts, in fact, have not contemplated suicide, and many have acted on these thoughts in one way or another" (Nowinski, 1990, p. 50). One study reported that "as many as 40-50 percent of adolescent and college-aged suicides were abusing alcohol and/or drugs at the time of their death" (Hoberman, 1989, p. 67). Depression as expressed by adolescent substance abusers should be taken seriously; "and suicide risk must be thoroughly evaluated and treated" (Morehouse, 1989, p. 358).

Adolescents are accident prone, and "alcohol and drug-related fatal car crashes are more common by far among youths than any other age group" (Nowinski, 1990, p. 11). Depressed adolescents "drink or take drugs and drive. Decreased reaction time and careless driving contribute to their own injury or death and that of innocent others. Forty-five to 50 percent of fatal car crashes in this group are associated with alcohol use" (Slaby and McGuire, 1989, p. 23). Car accidents themselves (especially one-car crashes) can be intentional suicidal acts.

Native Americans as a group have a high rate of alcohol abuse, resulting in a "disproportionate toll among American Indians" (Moran, 1999, p. 52). Alcohol abuse starts early; for many Native American youths (male and female), drinking begins in the preteen years and the pattern of alcohol abuse is established for roughly 90 percent of these youths by the twelfth grade; the "frequency and amount of drinking are greater, and the negative consequences are more common" (Moran, 1999, p. 53).

Moran (1999) describes a preventive outreach effort with urban American Indian fourth and fifth graders to reach children before age twelve, when drinking presumably starts. The project used a combination of "mainstream prevention strategies with American Indian cultural practices" (Moran, 1999, p. 64). Although the results of standardized measures were disappointing, the children and parents in the study expressed positive feelings about the program. Moran (1999) recommends the use of qualitative methods of evaluation for this work, including the use of narratives, which would be a way to "tap into the oral traditions of American Indian culture" (p. 64).

An experimental program for white and African-American high-risk children between ages twelve and fourteen and their families is aimed both to reduce the amount of drinking of those who have already started and to prevent others from beginning (Johnson et al., 1998). This comprehensive program emphasized working with family resilience by using a combination of "parent and youth training, early intervention, and case management services throughout a one-year period" (Johnson et al., 1998, p. 305). In addition to enhancing family life, interventions achieved "positive moderating effects on alcohol and other drug use among youths" (Johnson et al., 1998, p. 306).

Many colleges are taking an assertive, proactive role in addressing the problem of heavy drinking on campuses, including alcohol education programs; one option that is attracting an increasing number of students is the choice to live in alcohol-free dormitories (Wilgoren, 2000).

Although our National War on Drugs has placed emphasis on the criminal justice system, efforts are increasing to offer rehabilitative and preventive services to both adults and adolescents. It is difficult to motivate substance-abusing adolescents to seek treatment, but developing their motivation is essential. "When adolescents are unmotivated for treatment but are coerced into entering a program, they usually act out or become passive participants who drink when the opportunity arises" (Morehouse, 1989, p. 357); this requires considerable clinical skill. Nowinski (1990) discusses the "arrogance" of the adolescent addict: "They are desperate, but all they reveal is indifference . . . they may become very controlling over others, very demanding, exceedingly defensive, and blaming. This is the point at which they most often enter treatment. The clinician needs to be prepared for it" (p. 50).

Cigarette Smoking

Cigarette smoking, declared a major public health problem, has been increasing among teenagers. The Centers for Disease Control and Prevention reported a 73 percent jump in teenage smoking from 1988 to 1996 (Drummond, 1998a). According to recent research, "early smoking may trigger changes in DNA that put young smokers at higher risk for cancer even if they quit later" (Golden, 1999b, p. 48). A large share of money being paid in lawsuits by cigarette companies is allocated for combating adolescent smoking (Drummond, 1998a).

Florida, in 1997, "criminalized" teenage smoking; if caught, teenagers pay fines or do community service; a third offense mandates giving up their driving licenses. Questions have been raised about the effectiveness of this procedure (Drummond, 1998a).

Suicide

Suicidality is one of the most serious mental health risks faced by adolescents; it is the third leading cause of teenage death, following accidents, and homicides (de Anda, 1995). The actual number of suicides are probably underestimated and completed suicides "are three times the reported rates . . . taboos, impact on relatives, and exclusionary clauses in insurance policies militate against more accurate disclosure" (Slaby and McGuire, 1989, p. 24). In addition, some accidents (such as one-car fatalities) and homicides (provoked by the victim) can be suicidal in nature. Males have a higher rate for successfully completed suicides; females have a higher rate for suicide attempts (de Anda, 1995).

The rates for white adolescents are higher than for African-American teenagers; however, "suicide among black teen-agers, once quite rare, has sharply increased over the last two decades, a troubling rise that might reflect the strain some black families feel in making the transition to middle-class life" (Belluck, 1998a, p. A1). Hispanic adolescent females are "twice as likely as African American and non-Hispanic white adolescent females to have made suicide attempts requiring medical attention" (Zayas et al., 2000). The ethnic group with the highest suicide rate is Native Americans; within this group, "the highest rates are found among younger Native Americans (15-24 years old)" (Ivanoff and Riedel, 1995, p. 2361).

Adolescents who attempt suicide are often depressed, have a high rate of drug abuse, and usually have multiple stressors in their lives, including families with "higher rates of conflict and dysfunction, divorce, separation, and parental death, particularly at an early age" (de Anda, 1995, p. 27). Physical abuse has also been found in some of these families (de Anda, 1995; Slaby and McGuire, 1989), and it is not uncommon to find a family history of suicide (de Anda, 1995).

Attempted suicides occur at a high rate among gay and lesbian adolescents; about "30 percent of lesbian and gay youths have attempted suicide while in adolescence, a percentage five times higher than that of their heterosexual peers" (Hunter and Schaecher, 1995, p. 1060).

In the teenage population, it is not uncommon to find the *cluster effect* after a teenage suicide; that is, others engaging in *copycat* behavior—teens in the same school or community as the "successful" suicide victim will make their own suicide attempts. Some teens enter suicide pacts with a friend, committing suicide together. In New Jersey, for example, in 1987, two sisters (ages sixteen and seventeen) in the company of two boys (ages eighteen and nineteen) committed suicide together.

> The youngsters drove into the dark garage, shut the door and locked it. They left the car idling, its windows open. Then they sat back and waited.
> The steadily burning gasoline did its job, releasing deadly carbon monoxide fumes. Within an hour all four were dead. By the end of the week they were notorious. Their multiple-death pact had traumatized their hometown, inspired copycat acts more than 700 miles away and dramatically spotlighted the painful problem of teenage suicide. (Wilentz, 1987, p. 12)

Vivienne: An adolescent suicide. Vivienne (Mack and Hickler, 1981), discussed in Chapters 1 and 3, committed suicide when she was fourteen—an act precipitated by the loss of her favorite teacher (her selfobject), when he moved across the country. "Most suicide attempts occur after a 'major disruption of a personal relationship,' either parental or romantic" (de Anda, 1995, p. 27).

Vivienne lived in a traditional family with three children; her father was a minister, and her mother was a homemaker with (unfulfilled) artistic interests. Vivienne excelled in her private school and was creative, writing poetry and keeping a diary; these protective factors, however, were not strong enough to protect her.

Vivienne was depressed, which was neither recognized nor treated; in fact, what was "most impressive from the behavioral standpoint is not what Vivienne demonstrated of her depression, but, rather how well she concealed its essential features" (Mack and Hickler, 1981, p. 97). Her emotional pain was revealed in her diaries and her poetry and, toward the end, in her letters to the teacher who had been so special to her. Her suicide was "a direct outgrowth of [her] depression, while the depression in turn derives from the structure of her personality. . . . Yet for Vivienne herself the 'terrific depressions' seemed to have a kind of independent life, to come at her as if 'from the middle of nowhere'" (Mack and Hickler, 1981, p. 94).

Vivienne had great sensitivity and an unusual ability to identify with (as well as feel overly responsible for) others. Although warmth and caring were expressed in the family, Vivienne's mother was described by Vivienne's sister, Laurel, as "often abstracted, absorbed in her own struggles. 'My mother was always sick, always tired . . . she needed attention. . . . Sometimes she got attention by making people feel guilty'" (Mack and Hickler, 1981, p. 9). Vivienne's mother tended to see Vivienne "in terms of her own personal needs, as a treasure . . . the one to whom she turned with her burdens. . . . In the last weeks of her life Vivienne felt especially the weight of her mother's problems and needs" (Mack and Hickler, 1981, p. 109). Vivienne's mother reported feelings of alienation from Vivienne as an infant.

Vivienne's suicidal wishes were related to her low self-esteem and her "inability to experience herself or her world as having enough value to make living tolerable" (Mack and Hickler, 1981, p. 136). Vivienne's *ego ideal,* "the agency of personality carrying the principal responsibility for regulating self-esteem, became a rigid taskmaster, insisting upon the most exalted standards of human conduct and intimacy" (Mack and Hickler, 1981, p. 136).

> It [the ego ideal] is built on the one hand upon the internalization of parental values and expectations, while at the same time it looks to society to provide objects and examples with which to structure more realistic aims and goals. . . . But the selection of models or examples is powerfully determined by the residual needs of childhood. . . . In Vivienne's case we have seen how deeply affected the structure of her ego ideal was by early injury to the self and by the example of parents, especially her mother, who sought to fulfill through this child, from whom she felt estranged, her own longings for perfection. (Mack and Hickler, 1981, p. 137)

Vivienne felt a special closeness to her father, but he stated that "he never really knew Vivienne or 'where she was.' Sweet and gentle, he was, nevertheless, indecisive, had difficulty handling his son, and surrendered much of the authority in the family to his wife" (Mack and Hickler, 1981, p. 109). He also felt responsible for " 'all the problems of the world,' " according to Laurel, and it was this quality with which Vivienne identified.

Other family problems existed. Vivienne's parents had problems with Laurel and with Vivienne's brother Rob, who was sent to a private school during his first three grades and lived with his grandparents, coming home on weekends. " 'I had to get him out of the house,' Paulette [Vivienne's mother] explained. 'He had problems with his father, acted out against the girls, and did nasty things behind my back' " (Mack and Hickler, 1981, p. 7). During adolescence, Laurel acted out sexually; once, there was concern that she might be pregnant.

Vivienne's early school experiences were unhappy. Laurel described how " 'we were different from everyone else. . . . We wore old-fashioned dresses that Mommy smocked herself. Other girls wore smart shifts' " (Mack and Hickler, 1981, p. 8). Vivienne excelled academically, which also "set her apart as 'different.' 'She always seemed to be the butt of playground jokes,' Laurel remembers" (Mack and Hickler, 1981, p. 8). Vivienne's mother observed that "Vivienne felt awfully isolated and alone, but she didn't let you know any of that. She developed this sarcastic wit that would be devastating. I think it alienated other children even more'" (Mack and Hickler, 1981, p. 8).

When Vivienne entered private school in the sixth grade, where the teacher who became her favorite taught, he "spotted Vivienne and another girl as two sixth-graders who had been outcasts in public school" (Mack and Hickler, 1981, p. 12). He reached out to these children, and Vivienne thrived and blossomed with his caring, empathic relationship. However, she was not only unable to maintain these gains without his presence but deteriorated emotionally when he left. His departure "had a greater significance than his loss as a person. It struck at the core of Vivienne's psychological vulnerability" (Mack and Hickler, 1981, p. 101).

Attempted suicide by Hispanic adolescent females. In examining the high rate of suicide attempts in Hispanic females, *familial factors* and *self-image* have been found to be of key significance, shaped by cultural factors but not determined exclusively by social factors; it has been observed that "the vast majority (80 percent) of adolescent Hispanic females do not attempt suicide" (Zayas et al., 2000, p. 53). Although substance abuse is highly associated with adolescent suicide, this does not hold true for Hispanic teens.

The suicide attempt typically occurs within the context of a progressive intensification in conflicts between the adolescent and her parents. An acute situation, usually an intense argument with parents regarding issues associated with autonomy or sexuality, embodied in the adolescent's involvement with a boyfriend, often triggers the suicide attempt. (Zayas et al., 2000, p. 56)

Differences in levels of acculturation between Hispanic female teens and their parents play an important role in suicidal behavior, as does being socioeconomically disadvantaged. "Fewer incidents of suicide attempts are reported among middle-class adolescent females than among girls of lower socioeconomic status" (Zayas et al., 2000, p. 56). Family dysfunction, including marital conflict and psychological problems in the parents, affect the parents' ability to help their adolescents. Families with a traditional Hispanic structure "emphasize restrictive, authoritarian parenting, especially with regard to girls . . . [which] may affect a family's capacity to respond flexibly to a daughter" (Zayas et al., 2000, p. 57).

Hispanic female teen suicidal behavior tends to be viewed exclusively in relation to the mother-daughter tie; fathers have not been studied because they are often not present in the home; those adolescents who live for a longer period with fathers in the home tend to be less prone to suicide.

Mothers who are immigrants may not have the extended family support they had prior to immigrating, and therefore "mothers of those who attempt suicide may seek their daughter's companionship . . . and become overdependent on their daughters, creating a situation in which the adolescent feels she must parent her mother" (Zayas et al., 2000, p. 58). Abdication of some maternal functions, such as providing guidance and support as well as "interruptions of mutuality" in the mother-daughter relationship, have been found in these cases (Zayas et al., 2000, p. 58).

As typical of Vivienne and many other adolescents who have attempted suicide, Hispanic females are often depressed and have low self-esteem; they frequently "perceive themselves as 'bad' and to blame for family problems" (Zayas et al., 2000, p. 59). Coping with anger is especially difficult, as an Hispanic adolescent "may be socialized by her own more tradition-bound parents to suppress her anger"; and this, combined with inadequate problem-solving skills, may be decisive factors leading to the suicide attempt (Zayas et al., 2000, p. 59). The intent of the suicide attempt is generally "intended to solve an interpersonal problem or draw the attention of others who can assist the adolescent in coping" (p. 59). Although Hispanic teens may experience interpersonal stress in peer relationships, this is usually not a factor in suicide attempts; family problems play a dominant role.

Many Hispanic mothers of suicidal teen daughters had psychological problems themselves when they were adolescents, including suicide attempts or other acting-out behavior, such as pregnancies or running away. "Often the mother's conflicts in adolescence were related to her relationship with her own mother, reflecting a possible intergenerational dynamic" (Zayas et al., 2000, p. 58). Although the mother-daughter relationship is of major importance, the role of the father also needs to be evaluated because, even if absent, fathers "remain psychologically and emotionally present in their daughters' experience" (Zayas et al., 2000, p. 60).

Homicide as suicide. Black and Hispanic men tend to view suicide as a passive response to frustration and condone a more outwardly direct approach. "Dying is regarded as more honorable if it accompanies rage and aggression rather than passive solitude. Provoking a fight and being killed as a result may be culturally more appropriate as an expression of suicidal intent, but it will be reported as homicide" (Wyche and Rotheram-Borus, 1990, p. 327). Teens with other ethnic backgrounds may place themselves at risk of being killed and this risk may be related to both male and female adolescents remaining in (or seeking) situations in which they are severely abused and battered.

Toni Morrison (1977), in her novel *Song of Solomon,* describes the black teenage hero Milkman, who is being pursued by his girlfriend, angry with him because he wishes to end their relationship; she has attempted to kill him six times. Milkman, who is depressed over family relationships, does not care if he dies. He also does not care if she dies. He lies passively in his friend's apartment as he hears his girlfriend breaking the window, coming to stab him with a knife: "He lay there as still as the morning light, and sucked the world's energy up into his own will. And willed her dead. Either she will kill me or she will drop dead. Either I am to live in this world on my own terms or I will die out of it" (Morrison, 1977, p. 129). She stabs him with a butcher knife but not fatally; she raises the knife again, but "could not get her arms down. . . . The paralyzed woman and the frozen man" (Morrison, 1977, p. 130).

Suicide prevention. Clinicians, parents, and teachers can fear that talking to adolescents about suicide may *give* them this idea, but this is not so. Rather, *not* talking about suicide can give impetus to this process if the intent is present. The teacher, who was very supportive to Vivienne did not understand the seriousness of her intent when she wrote to him about hanging herself, although he responded to her suffering. If he had responded to her threat, he might have alerted her family.

Whenever adolescents (or adults) refer to "ending it all" or are depressed or feel hopeless and alone, suicidal ideation should be discussed and clarified. In addition, if earlier suicide attempts have been made (as they were in Vivienne's case but went "unnoticed"), and if adolescents also abuse substances, have poor impulse control, a history of suicide in the immediate family, or if recent suicide has been publicized in the media or in their school, then these individuals are at risk.

Teens can make suicide attempts to get attention or retaliate against someone who has hurt them, without actually intending to die. However, any attempt should also be taken seriously, as it can lead to future suicidal acts. Asking what purpose the suicide would serve can shed light on the underlying motivation and message of this act.

Some adolescents are full of "anger and hatred" and have "fantasies of future revenge"; clinicians are usually concerned about their "aggressivity, impulsivity and potential for violence, and may overlook the possibility that they may become seriously suicidal if they lose connectedness with the treatment setting, for instance, in the aftermath of a precipitous discharge" (Braga, 1989, pp. 14-15). Hoberman (1989) observed that "while older adolescents were more likely to be described as sad or despairing, younger suicides were much more likely to display anger prior to suicide" (p. 66).

A mental health assessment is important as serious conditions, such as psychosis, can underlie the suicidal wish; family evaluation is usually a critical part of assessment. The adolescent should receive immediate help; sometimes hospitalization must be considered.

Violence

Many adolescents are exposed to violence in their homes and communities; in response, they may engage in self-defeating or high-risk behaviors, which may not only cause physical harm but can interfere with other aspects of their development (Marans and Adelman, 1997).

> Reactions [to violence] may range from staying away from school in order to avoid the potential for violence on the streets and in the classroom, to arming themselves as protection, to involvement in gang or other criminal activities. As with disturbances of neurovegetative functions, withdrawal into fantasy, social isolation, and regressive symptomatology, these responses serve the adolescent's attempts to guard against and even reverse feelings of helplessness and overwhelming fear. (Marans and Adelman, 1997, p. 215)

Homicide rates among young people are very high; it is the second leading cause of death among all fifteen- to twenty-four-year-olds (Glodich, 1998; Osofsky, 1997); a national increase in youth homicide of 153 percent between 1985 and 1991 was reported (Glodich, 1998). Black adolescent males have a homicide rate close to ten times higher than that of white adolescent males, and both black and white adolescents between ages sixteen and nineteen are "victims of violent crime more than any other age group," followed by twelve- to fifteen-year-olds (Glodich, 1998, p. 321). On an annual basis, almost "a million young people between the ages of twelve and nineteen are raped, robbed, or assaulted, often by their peers. The rate of victimization is substantially higher for Black male adolescents" (Glodich, 1998, p. 322).

Juvenile Delinquency

In 1993, the Federal Bureau of Investigation developed three classifications for delinquent behavior, according to the seriousness of the crime (Williams et al., 1997).

> The most serious of the three categories is *violent index crimes* [which] include forcible rape, robbery, aggravated assault, murder, and nonnegligent manslaughter. *Property index crimes . . .* include burglary, larceny (theft), motor vehicle theft, and arson. All other delinquent acts are categorized as *nonindex offenses . . .* [which] include forgery, vandalism, gambling, driving under the influence, drunkenness, disorderly conduct, vagrancy, and status offenses such as running away and violating curfew. (Williams et al., 1997, p. 141)

Research based on self-reports suggests that "a majority" of young people in this country "will commit at least one delinquent act by the time they reach adulthood" (Williams et al., 1997, p. 142); delinquency generally "represents a transient response to adolescence" (p. 143) and most will give up this "antisocial" behavior during adolescence. However, some adolescents have chronic delinquent behaviors; this group is "estimated to constitute between 5 percent and 12 percent of the adolescent population . . . [and] accounts for a substantial amount of the total incidence of juvenile offending" (Williams et al., 1997, p. 143). The arrests of juvenile offenders for violence has increased; the most dramatic increase has been in the "lethality of violent acts, a result of increased handgun use in violent adolescent interactions" (Williams et al., 1997, p. 141).

Conduct disorders (discussed earlier) are associated with delinquent behaviors, but not all delinquents have conduct disorders. Delinquent behavior in general has been related to family breakdown, domestic violence, parental attitudes and behaviors relating to antisocial behaviors, abdication of the parenting role, and parental substance abuse and mental illness. Many delinquents (mostly boys) "have been found to be more likely to come from families where the parents are suffering from depression" (Williams et al., 1997).

Adolescents, with their strong affiliations with peers, tend to have friends with similar values and backgrounds; "high levels of delinquent behavior are strongly correlated with high levels of association with delinquent friends" (Williams et al., 1997, p. 149). Neighborhood influences contributing to juvenile delinquency include "high population density and mobility, physical deterioration, low attachment to the community, and high crime" (Williams et al., 1997, p. 146). School failure is often a major factor; "the level of an individual's commitment to education is considered one of the best predictors of delinquent behavior for adolescents" (Williams et al., 1997, p. 148).

Gang violence. Gangs, generally developing in industrialized urban settings, now also proliferate in small cities and suburban and rural areas (Regulus, 1995). Gang members are usually adolescents of color and Hispanics; they often include young adults who remain in the gangs as leaders, using the gang as a base for illegal activities, including dealing in drugs. Recently supergangs and multigang alliances have developed, leading to gang memberships with as many as several hundred and sometimes several thousand members; smaller gangs of the past averaged from fewer than twenty to fewer than one hundred members (Regulus, 1995).

> Contemporary gangs are more violent than earlier gangs for several reasons. They have greater access to guns; intergang competition over status, turf, and criminal enterprises is more pervasive; and drug use has increased among gang youths. In addition, the more serious gang violence occurs in communities where the general youth culture has become more asocial and alienated, consequently promoting fear and emphasizing violence as a means of survival and social domination. (Regulus, 1995, p. 1046)

Adolescents who have weak attachments to their families, who lack a positive affiliation with their schools, who receive little direction and control, and who have few opportunities in their communities tend to be drawn to gangs, who socialize them into their "value orientations, codes of loyalty, and behavioral styles [which are] consistent with gang membership" (Regulus, 1995, p. 1046).

Success in stabilizing or diminishing gang activity has been related to community organization efforts and the provision of other opportunities for teens; "suppression strategies alone were unrelated to stabilization or reductions in gang problems" (Regulus, 1995, p. 1052). In Chapter 4, we discussed the development of comprehensive community strategies for dealing with such problems as unemployment and inadequate education. Work with gangs can be encompassed in this type of strategic planning; "an additional ingredient must be the inclusion of effective interpersonal engagement of gangs and gang memberships in the intervention process" (Regulus, 1995, p. 1052).

The juvenile justice system. Public debate is ongoing about the effectiveness and utilization of the juvenile justice system; it was noted, for example (in Chapter 4), that many people with mental illness (including juveniles) are sent to jail rather than mental hospitals, which are in short supply; sometimes parents are advised to turn their children over to the law, as that way services will be provided that are no longer available through the mental health system.

One of the current national debates is whether to try and sentence juvenile offenders as adults. It has been reported that discriminatory practices exist in the sentencing of minority youth (Williams et al., 1997). A new report by the Justice Department and six major U.S. foundations confirmed this finding (Butterfield, 2000).

> The report found that minority youths are more likely than their white counterparts to be arrested, held in jail, sent to juvenile or adult court for trial, convicted and given longer prison terms, leading to a situation in which the impact is magnified with each additional step into the juvenile justice system. (Butterfield, 2000, p. A1)

Another controversy concerns the execution of adults who committed their crimes when they were juveniles (under age eighteen) (Rimer and Bonner, 2000). This country

> is one of only seven countries in the world that permit[s] such executions, according to the State Department. But even many prosecutors who support the death penalty, as well as national organizations that are neutral on the issue, are expressing concern about sentencing to death those who were, according to most laws, still children when they committed their crimes. (Rimer and Bonner, 2000, p. A1)

CONCLUSION

Peter Pan, the title character of the play (Barrie, 1904), was a wonderful latency-age child living in never-never land, surrounded by his chums, ever coping with an exciting but benign environment, having fun, free from the constraints of adult supervision. Dangers abounded, but they were well known, such as Captain Hook and crocodiles, and Peter was protected by the fairy Tinkerbell. Wendy became his "child-mother," and he was not averse to her tender ministrations. Peter did not want to grow up; middle childhood was the ideal state to be in.

Peter's spirit exists in latency children who are excited about exploring their world, who enjoy their involvement in sports and computer games and being with friends. However, never-never land is not within reach of many children today; they do not have the luxury of fighting only fictional pirates; their world is populated by real dangers experienced through community and family violence, substance-abusing parents, broken homes, and schools that are fortresses rather than comforting and exciting places. If they run away, it is not to an enchanted forest but to cities where they are not welcome, to empty warehouses and vacated slum dwellings, and to friends who are also outcasts. No Tinkerbell offers them protection.

Some children and teens live under benign conditions, as Vivienne did. Vivienne's demons were internal, and her guilt and lack of pleasure in herself and in life culminated in her suicide; she had no happy future to dream about. She could not live Peter's carefree existence. Some teens deal with their demons through reckless actions and frantic activities; they may seem to be having fun, but often their behavior is driven by inner anxiety and despair; Peter's exuberance is not there.

How can we keep Peter's spirit alive in children or help them develop it if it has never come to life? We face a great challenge as we consider reaching out to our lost children and to their parents, many of whom were lost children themselves. And how can we infuse our schools, institutions, and neighborhoods with Peter's welcoming and sunny optimism?

Peter chooses to stay in never-never land, forever a boy; our children grow and become adolescents, then adulthood beckons. Peter felt he could not live in Wendy's world; if he had and grew to manhood, we would like to think that his exuberant spirit would have remained, as a spark of love, laughter, and delight that would infuse his friendships and be shared with his children.

As we turn to explore adult development, we need to remember grown-ups are just that: grown up from kids, and their child past is part of their adult present. Perhaps every grown-up, at least sometimes, wishes for a never-never land to allow them to leave their adult responsibilities behind and run free.

LEARNING EXERCISE

1. Interview an adolescent (who is not a client or a relative). Discuss their views of their lives, families, friends, school, interests, plans for the future. How do they describe their ethnic and cultural backgrounds? Do they experience any conflict or stress in relation to this? What are their thoughts about problems facing adolescents today? (It is possible to discuss these interviews in class in small groups; then have a class research project, in which findings are shared with the larger group and analyzed.)

SUGGESTED READINGS

Articles

Morrow, D. (1993). Social work with gay and lesbian adolescents. *Social Work, 38,* 655-660.

Zayas, L. H., Kaplan, C., Turner, S., Romano, K., and Gonzalez-Ramos, G. (2000). Understanding suicide attempts by adolescent Hispanic females. *Social Work, 45,* 53-63.

Books

Angelou, M. (1997). *I know why the caged bird sings.* New York: Bantam Books.

Canino, I. A. and Spurlock, J. (2000). *Culturally diverse children and adolescents: Assessment, diagnosis and treatment,* Second edition. New York: The Guilford Press.

Guterson, D. (1995). *Snow falling on cedars.* New York: Vintage Books.

Irizarry, C. and Appel, Y. (1986). Growing up: Work with preteens in the neighborhood. In A. Gitterman and L. Shulman (Eds.), *Mutual aid groups and the life cycle* (pp. 111-140). Itasca, IL: F. E. Peacock Publishers, Inc.

Osofsky, J. (Ed.) (1997). *Children in a violent society.* New York: The Guilford Press.

Chapter 10

Adult Development

When I was a boy of fourteen, my father was so ignorant I could hardly stand to have the old man around. But when I got to be twenty-one, I was astonished at how much he had learned in seven years.

Mark Twain

Until recently, adolescence was considered the final stage for the consolidation of an individual's psychological development; today, it is recognized that developmental and psychological change continue in the adult personality even into late adulthood. This chapter discusses the latter part of the life cycle, from the twenties through midlife into late adulthood. Although characteristics and tasks of each life stage are presented, it is with the understanding that this is not a rigid classification; considerable variation exists as to when and how people go through these stages.

Neugarten's (1979) concept of "off-time" and "on-time" events is relevant, as life events today can occur at unexpected times in the life cycle, differing from past patterns; many first-time mothers of infants, for example, are the same age as their peers who have adolescent children; grandparents increasingly attend college and/or may be in the role of parenting their grandchildren. Not only do older people nearing the end of the life cycle face death and the loss of their friends and relatives, but so, for example, do young people with AIDS and children living in neighborhoods pervaded by violence and homicide.

Because of social changes resulting from the recent cultural revolution centered on gender, including the advent of the women's movement, the less-well-publicized men's movement, and the increasing recognition of gays, lesbians, and transgender people, the issue of gender is addressed first to add this perspective to our understanding of the life cycle.

383

GENDER

Women's issues, including equal rights to education and employment, have been raised as major social concerns especially over the past thirty years resulting in political and legislative advances as well as influencing changes in society, family, and personal lives. Women's studies, a new field of scholarship, has affected the development of psychological theories by increasing the focus on the psychology of women. The impact on the social work field has led to new programs, such as services for battered women and rape crisis counseling. Many women feel emancipated from previous restrictions on their lives; some feel they remain oppressed by the stereotyping and prejudice they continue to experience. Some women feel stressed sorting out their priorities, establishing their own identities, and resolving conflicting demands between family and work.

Men have also been affected as they have adapted to changes in the lives and attitudes of women and as they face their own issues. A men's movement as well as an academic field of men's studies have also developed, although on a smaller scale.

Women's Issues

Women's suffrage, a major achievement of the early women's movement, was codified in the nineteenth amendment to the Constitution in 1919, ending women's political disenfranchisement. A more recent landmark was the formation of NOW, the National Organization for Women, in 1966 (Longres, 1995b).

> The National Organization for Women adopted a statement of purpose calling for attacks on discrimination in the legal system, employment, and education that had limited women's ability to control their own lives. In regard to women's role in the family, the statement declared: "We believe that a true partnership between the sexes demands a different concept of marriage, an equitable sharing of the responsibilities of home and children and of the economic burdens of their support." (Longres, 1995b, p. 204)

Career Issues

Dramatic changes have occurred in employment and educational opportunities; women are now employed in occupations that were considered traditionally "male" vocations; they work as doctors, lawyers, construction workers, police officers, pilots, etc. In one illustration of this change, one-third of the employees in Antarctica are now women; women never stayed overnight at Antarctica's McMurdo base until 1971 and never lived there through the winter until 1979.

The presence of women has also brought about important social changes to the base (Dean, 1998). When only a handful of women were at McMurdo, their reception seemed to range from being "stared at" to "leered at" to rejected (Dean, 1998, p. D1). Now, with about one-third of the personnel being women, McMurdo has become a "laboratory for watching what happens when an all-male group is gradually infiltrated by the opposite sex. . . . As more and more women join an organization . . . there is a 'tipping point' when its atmosphere changes" (Dean, 1998, p. D1). In essence, a more normal social interaction begins to prevail, and tensions appear to decline; even the amount of fighting that had gone on among the men in the past has diminished.

National attention focused on the McMurdo base in 1999 when a doctor stationed there learned that she had breast cancer, and her ability to cope, as well as the abilities of those who came to her aid, was tested. Until Dr. Nielsen was rescued by a National Guard plane, by means of "satellite consultation with U.S. doctors," she underwent "oral chemotherapy, using medical supplies air-dropped by cargo planes" ("Doctor with," 1999).

Most women, however, still are employed in fields that are filled primarily by women and usually do not pay well, including office work, nursing, child care, sales, and social work (Gottlieb, 1995). Many young mothers experience stress related to conflicts between work and family obligations; the children of more than half of working mothers are under one year of age (Kaplan et al., 1994). Critics note that employers often do not make sufficient accommodations to meet the needs of working mothers, such as facilitating arrangements for caring for children and for elderly parents (an increasing concern of adult children), offering flexibility when determining the hours of work, and providing parental leaves without pay (Kaplan et al., 1994).

Some industries do offer good day care services for mothers as well as day programs for elderly parents. It has recently been noted that, during the past ten years, "the military has so improved its child care system . . . that it has become a model for state and national programs" (Becker, 2000, p. A17). The improved programs were motivated by the military's interest in having people remain in service, as service in the military is now on a voluntary basis only. In addition, it was realized that "quality care" was essential to reduce the absenteeism resulting from parents providing child care (Becker, 2000, p. A17). Former Secretary of Defense William S. Cohen has commented: "We simply can't afford to have our service members worried about the basic well-being of their families" (Becker, 2000, p. A17).

Women's Developmental and Clinical Issues

As women's studies have proliferated, it has been argued that masculine traits have been valued and female traits ignored in the development of psychological theories (Belenky et al., 1986). Belenky and colleagues have also (1986) argued that insufficient attention has been paid to the "development of interdependence, intimacy, nurturance, and contextual thought," which are women's ways of being and knowing (pp. 6-7). Gilligan (1982) observed that "sensitivity to the needs of others and the assumption of responsibility for taking care lead women to attend to voices other than their own and to include in their judgment other points of view" (p. 13). Self-in-relation theorists (from the Stone Center at Wellesley College) see women as a group dominated by men and that they have adapted to their inferior position (Berzoff, 1996c).

Is this portrait of women universally true? Are we stereotyping women (as well as men) in these descriptions? During the past ten years, postmodern feminist psychoanalytic critiques have questioned some of these assumptions and ask whether these qualities belong to all women, to all cultures, to all ages, etc.? Citing the work of Comas-Diaz in 1994, Berzoff (1996c) notes her point of view that one's identity is more complex than that which is based only on gender, just as it is more complex than an identity that is based only on race, ethnicity, or social class. Berzoff (1996c) stresses the importance of the postmodernist point of view in clinical work; although she does not refer specifically to the social work value of individualization, this seems present in her words.

> If we are truly to understand women in clinical work, then we must be able to attend to the difference, the paradox, the ambiguity between and among them. While the concept of difference sparked the very psychology of women, it will be the appreciation of a complex multiplicity of gendered possibilities that will ultimately help our clients, both women and men, achieve their full relational potentials. (Berzoff, 1996c, p. 258)

Two points should be added to Berzoff's comments. One relates to the development of intersubjective sensitivity, involving our understanding of prejudices and biases, so that they do not negatively affect our attunement to clients' feelings. In marital therapy, for example, might a feminist therapist "favor" wives because they are "oppressed" and not see their part in a relationship difficulty?

The second point is that women's generalized anger directed toward men is often accepted as a valid expression of righteous indignation rather than its own form of sexism, and remains unexamined. Although societal injustices to women must be righted, are all men guilty of oppressing women and being insensitive to their needs? Are we engaged in a battle of the sexes? Judith Herman (1997) asserts that this is so when she comments that "the subordinate condition of women is maintained and enforced by the hidden violence of men. There is war between the sexes" (p. 32).

Do women have no hidden violence? Women are known to have rages, to commit child abuse, and to act in other violent ways. Recently, violence in both gay and lesbian relationships has been acknowledged (Carlson and Maciol, 1997). "Because of gender-based stereotypes about who becomes a batterer and who becomes a victim, it is often difficult for people to perceive gay men as victims and lesbians as abusers" (Carlson and Maciol, 1997, p. 109).

A final point is the unfounded statement that male theorists have not been concerned with intimacy and attachment. Many serious male leaders in the object relations school, including Fairbairn, Winnicott, and Bowlby—Bowlby devoted an entire book, *Attachment and Loss* (1969) to the subject—have focused on these issues. It was Margaret Mahler, a female analyst, who emphasized separation, individuation, and autonomy; but Mahler saw these unfolding within the context of warm, connecting relationships to others. She has been criticized for emphasizing autonomy, but her overarching concern with relationships has often been overlooked.

> In agreeing with Bowlby, Mahler affirmed her recognition that significant interpersonal as well as intrapsychic relationships are essential from birth to death. We wish to highlight this point for there are those who have understood Mahler as valuing independence, self-reliance and autonomy to the exclusion of object need and connection. From our readings of Mahler's writings and our talks with her, we understand separation-individuation theory as acknowledging a common human need for others as well as a need for autonomy. (Edward et al., 1992, pp. xxii-xxiii)

If indeed a battle of the sexes is going on, how are men being affected?

Men's Issues

When men's issues are discussed, they do not center on societal oppression, as women's issues often do, but rather on society's changing constructions of manliness and the issues surrounding this (Lichtenberg, 1995). Germain (1991) comments that men as well as women feel stress related to their own sexual roles. Greater recognition is also being given to men in their role as fathers; the significance of fathers (as well as the tendency by child welfare workers and others to ignore them) is discussed in Chapter 6.

Attention has also focused on the fact that definitions and roles of masculinity can vary by class, race, ethnicity, and culture (Lichtenberg, 1995).

It has been asserted that men have been acculturated to develop a "macho" image, which includes emphasis on characteristics such as aggression, domination, and physical prowess, while sensitivity, emotionality, and asking for help are frowned on; but men also have a capacity to experience intimacy (Lichtenberg, 1995). Although it has been argued that women seek psychotherapy more often than men (often put forward in support of the idea that women have more problems because they are "oppressed" by men), men are no less likely to have psychological problems but may have more difficulty asking for help.

Attention has rightly focused on unequal opportunities for women regarding education and career paths; an insidious problem, however, has been developing related to men's apparently increasing failure to make use of available educational opportunities. Colleges, which in the past were "dominated by males are becoming the place where the boys are not" (Lewin, 1998a, p. 1). In 1996, 6.7 million men were attending college in contrast to 8.4 million women. It is estimated that this differential will continue to grow in future years. It has also been observed that "the skew is much larger" in the population of part-time college students, which includes many older students and African Americans (Lewin, 1998a, p. 1).

No general agreement prevails as to why this is happening. Arthur Levine, the president of Columbia University Teachers College, stated that "we need to be concerned that higher education is losing poor and minority men, that more African-American men are going to prison than to college" (Lewin, 1998a, p. 38).

Men's violence toward women, including wife battering, rape, and sexual harassment, has come under much greater scrutiny as a result of the women's movement. Actually, male violence is directed more often toward other men than toward women (Lichtenberg, 1995), but such violence is usually between physical equals. Violence has been viewed as a consequence of insecure feelings about one's masculinity (Lichtenberg, 1995). Self-help programs and group therapy for men who are violent toward women and who sexually abuse children have been increasing. Issues addressed in these groups include feelings of sexual insecurity, unmet dependency needs, and feelings of isolation (Lichtenberg, 1995).

The fact that many men who abuse were also victims of sexual abuse themselves as children has been coming to light recently. Therefore, quite possibly, identifying with the aggressor and the need to reenact past traumatic events may be related to and interacting with the issues of power and aggression that are often attributed to sexual abusers. The full scope of male sexual abuse is not known because it tends to remain underreported (Cermak and Molidor, 1996). Although sexual abuse can have serious psychological effects on girls and women, it can also have serious psychological consequences for boys and men later in life (Cermak and Molidor, 1996; Nasjleti, 1980).

Although boys are usually victimized by men, sexual abuse of boys has also been committed by women, sometimes mothers; professionals must be aware of this often-hidden problem (Cermak and Molidor, 1996). Cermak and Molidor (1996) suggest that "feminists may have unintentionally done a disservice to the male victims" who might have been overlooked because of the primary focus on the "plight of all *female* victims . . . this oversight may have had the effect of re-victimizing these boys" (p. 398).

Gay, Lesbian, and Transgender Adults

Lesbian Women

Female homosexuality exists all over the world; "it occurs across all industrial, preindustrial, and subsistence economies" (Falco, 1991, p. 12). Although the number of homosexual people who live in the United States is not known, it is estimated that between 4 and 13 million lesbians live here (Tully, 1995). Although lesbians are often part of supportive networks of lesbian women, considerable diversity exists in this group. Furthermore, it is obvious that lesbian women may belong to other minority racial, ethnic, or cultural groups, may have physical disabilities, or may be elderly.

The complexity of problems faced by lesbians who have multiple minority affiliations has been explored: the formation of a homosexual identity in Asian-American lesbians (Chan, 1997); issues of being a lesbian and an immigrant (Espin, 1997); the complexity of being female, lesbian, and Jewish (Dworkin, 1997); and the interrelationships of self-esteem, acculturation, and lesbian identity formation in Latina lesbians (Alquijay, 1997). Feeling stigmatized as both a lesbian and a substance abuser can create special problems for women seeking treatment for addictions (Rathbone-McCuan and Stokke, 1997).

The situation of lesbian women in the United States today reveals both gains and continuing conflicts. In 1994, the National Association of Social Workers declared lesbians to be an oppressed minority (Tully, 1995); at the same time, lesbian and gay organizations have received recognition and have achieved political power (Lacayo, 1998). The secrecy surrounding a gay identity seems to be giving way to greater openness; probably more gays and lesbians have identified themselves as such publicly today than ever before in this country (Lacayo, 1998). Yet open discrimination, homophobia, and often physical violence and other forms of harassment directed against the gay population persist as well (Tully, 1995).

Some political and religious groups are dedicated to promoting discrimination against the gay population, such as the Christian right, a strong faction of the Republican party. "Gary Bauer, head of the Family Research Council, and his mentor James Dobson, the Christian broadcaster who heads Focus on the Family, with its 2.3 million-name mailing list, have made opposition to gay rights a defining issue" (Lacayo, 1998, p. 36).

Although some protection of gay employment is afforded in federal employment (although not in the military) and in some municipalities, it is not universal. In 1996, the U.S. Senate "rejected a ban on job discrimination against gays and lesbians by a single vote," and at the same time barred "federal recognition of same-sex marriages" by an overwhelming majority (Hohler, 1996, p. A1). Many corporations and colleges provide benefits to the partners of lesbian and gay employees (Tully, 1995); in a court decision in 1998, homosexuals employed by the state of Oregon were granted benefits for their partners (Lewin, 1998c).

Legal issues, such as being at a disadvantage in custody disputes involving children from heterosexual marriages (discussed in Chapter 6), face lesbian women, and lesbian couples are not entitled to legal benefits of marriage, such as the right to inherit (from a partner) and tax benefits (Tully, 1995). Overt discrimination or more subtle lack of sensitivity to lesbian issues on the part of caregivers can be encountered when seeking psychotherapy and medical and social services.

Because many lesbians have had negative experiences with medical help, some stay away from doctors (Thompson, 1999b), which limits their ability to receive preventive interventions and early treatment for illness. Research findings reveal that "most lesbians avoid going to the doctor for routine checkups—especially gynecological exams—because of hostility from doctors, or because they are uncomfortable talking about issues that may reveal their sexual orientation" (Thompson, 1999b, p. A25). More health care centers providing services to lesbians have been developing.

Negative or ambivalent feelings of people toward lesbian life are also reflected in interpersonal relationships. Lesbians can experience overt rejection, but some prejudices are expressed in more subtle ways. Some lesbians have *internalized homophobia,* that is, they have internalized the negative feelings directed toward them by people in our culture, as other minority groups who face ongoing discrimination have done (Tully, 1995).

Gay Men

Male homosexuality is a term in disfavor by the gay movement, whose members have "adopted the slogan 'gay is good' and emphasized a newly found self-pride" (Berger and Kelly, 1995, p. 1064). Generally, men use the term *gay,* while women prefer to be called *lesbian* (Berger and Kelly, 1995).

Although often lifestyle differences exist between these groups, both gays and lesbians face many forms of discrimination. Gay men can also be members of ethnic and cultural groups, which may cause stress due to competing value systems and discrimination. Gay men who are Hispanic or black may find discrimination against them in both their own racial and ethnic communities as well as in the gay community (Adams Jr. and Kimmel, 1997; Berger and Kelly, 1995).

One of the major battles fought by the gay and lesbian communities has been with the psychiatric establishment, which classified homosexuality as a mental disorder until 1973; it was then accepted as one lifestyle and means of sexual expression among many, rather than a mental disorder (Kaplan et al., 1994).

Many psychoanalysts for more than ten years after this decision continued to describe "homosexuality as a 'perversion,' and analysts continued to speak of their ability to 'cure' the 'serious character disorders' of their gay patients" (in essence, to change them to heterosexuals) (Goode, 1998b, p. A19). Viewing homosexuality as an illness, the analytic societies refused to admit homosexual applicants to training institutes—a situation that has since changed.

Two years ago, Ralph Roughton, a faculty member of the Emory University Psychoanalytic Institute, wrote a letter to his colleagues announcing that he was gay; many people responded to his announcement with congratulatory messages (Goode, 1998b). Roughton, sixty-three, who had directed the analytic institute in the past and supervises other analysts, had been married for forty-one years and had been analyzed twice in an effort to change his sexual orientation, finding that his "perspective was the same as the whole analytic community, that this was something wrong with me that needed to be changed" (Goode, 1998b, p. A19).

Currently, nationwide between thirty-five and forty people undergoing psychoanalytic training and about fifteen psychoanalytic faculty are open about their gay and lesbian identities. However, one group of psychoanalysts, viewed as outside the mainstream by other analysts, started the National Association for Research and Therapy for Homosexuality. Headed by Charles Socarides, this organization emphasizes developing a heterosexual orientation in their homosexual patients (Goode, 1998b).

Many gay men have psychological issues related to conflicts and confusion about accepting their identities, as well as conflicts stemming from homophobia, which they may have internalized (Berger and Kelly, 1995). In addition, just like the general population, gay men as well as lesbians must cope with the general array of life issues, such as parenting problems and dealing with their own elderly parents. They may face the tendency of some therapists to reduce all of their problems to the matter of homosexuality rather than help them with other concerns.

Many gay men struggle with substance abuse (Berger and Kelly, 1995; Warn, 1997). Some clinicians working with this population assert that these men cannot work through substance abuse issues without working through their internalized homophobia as well (Warn, 1997). In fact, very often "other issues that typically emerge during treatment of gay men are impacted by homophobia: identity development and other life cycle issues, problems in socialization, body image, sexual behaviors, dysfunctional relational patterns, intimacy, and HIV/AIDS" (Warn, 1997, p. 389).

HIV/AIDS has had a major impact on the gay community and on the psychological well-being of its members. Although producing many devastating losses and much suffering, it has also involved many members of the community in political and public health education efforts (Berger and Kelly, 1995). HIV/AIDS is discussed at greater length in Chapter 12.

Transgenderism and Transsexualism

A gay male identifies himself as a man and a lesbian identifies herself as a woman; both feel sexual attraction to members of their own sex. A *bisexual* person is sexually attracted to members of both sexes but may or may not have sexual relations with people of both sexes (Zastrow and Kirst-Ashman, 1997). However, some people feel that they have been born the wrong sex; they feel deeply (and desperately) that they should have been the opposite sex, and many take measures to correct this situation. Jan Morris (1997), a writer who was born male, is now a woman after hormonal and surgical treatment. She recalls that at about three or perhaps four years of age she "realized that I had been born into the wrong body, and should really be a girl" (Morris, 1997, p. 11). Transsexualism, in Morris's (1997) view, is not a "sexual mode or preference. . . . not an act of sex at all," but a "passionate, lifelong, ineradicable conviction," of which "no true trans-sexual has ever been disabused" (p. 15). Consequently, until middle adulthood, a "sexual purpose dominated, distracted, and tormented my life: the tragic and irrational ambition, instinctively formulated but deliberately pursued, to escape . . . into womanhood" (Morris, 1997, pp. 16-17).

Transgender is the umbrella term used to encompass the spectrum of people who range from "cross-dressers (those who dress in clothes of the opposite sex) to transsexuals (those who surgically 'correct' their genitals to match their 'real' gender)" (Cloud, 1998, p. 48). The phenomenon of transgenderism is historically worldwide (Lesser, 1999). Some transgendered people have partially altered their sexual appearances with hormone treatments, electrolysis, clothing, or partial surgery. It is not known how many transgendered people there are in the United States, but more than 25,000 people have already had a sex-change procedure, and many more have signed up for it, with a very limited number of doctors in this country who do these operations (Cloud, 1998).

Harry Benjamin popularized the term *transsexual* in his book *The Transsexual Phenomenon,* which was published in 1966; the term subsequently received "medical-psychological status" (Lesser, 1999). Lesser cites the four criteria Benjamin ascribed to transsexuals: the first is "a lifelong gender dysphoria," (which is extreme misery with one's given gender); the second criteria involves "major disruption of identity development with resultant personal adjustment problems;" followed by seeking an actual sex change through treatment by means of hormone therapy and surgery; and, finally, engaging in cross-dressing (p. 182).

The request for sexual transformation surgery initially caused considerable controversy in the medical community, and a protocol, established by Benjamin, for medical intervention has been developed; compliance with its mandates is required before sexual surgery will be performed. These include: "a psychiatric evaluation, endocrinological screening, and a two-year, real life test in the preferred gender" (Lesser, 1999, p. 183).

Transsexuals have experienced prejudice and discrimination similar to that experienced by homosexuals, including hate crimes and murders, which have been increasing in incidence (Goldberg, 1999d). Transgenders have sometimes experienced discrimination by gays. The transsexual author and activist Riki Anne Wilchins, who considered herself lesbian, found that "gay and feminist groups long rejected her as not a 'real woman' and thus not a 'real lesbian'" (Goldberg, 1999d, p. A27), possibly on the grounds that she was not genetically female.

As the gay movement became mainstream, "it jettisoned transgenders as too off-putting" (Cloud, 1998, p. 48). Anger was expressed by transgenders against the Human Rights Campaign (the largest gay lobbying group in the country), which opposed including them in the Employment Nondiscrimination Act. However, greater rapport seems to be developing between these two groups, and the Human Rights Campaign facilitated a meeting between the Justice Department and transgender activists to discuss violence against transgenders (Cloud, 1998).

Transgenders have been building their own political power, and now have a lobbying group in Washington: Gender PAC. Lawyers have also been active with the Transgender Law Conference, and changes in laws in many states have helped transgenders, such as changing the sexual classification on their birth certificates, so that documents such as driver's licenses and passports "can reflect reality" (Cloud, 1998, p. 49). Some businesses have added nondiscriminatory clauses to protect their employment rights, and a number of cities (as well as the state of Minnesota) have protections in place against housing and employment discrimination.

STAGES OF ADULT DEVELOPMENT

Adult development is generally classified into three stages: early (from about ages twenty-two to forty); middle (ages forty to sixty); and late adulthood, (from age sixty to the end of life). Each life stage can bring its rewards and strains and presents opportunities for further psychological development.

How people change and develop is a complex conundrum, one of life's mysteries; it is one of the reasons novels, biographies, and case studies are so intriguing. Different theoretical schools continue to debate this subject.

A major controversy concerns the theory of *continuous development,* as opposed to the theory of *discontinuity.* Proponents of continuous development believe that childhood psychodynamics and behaviors remain throughout adulthood. Discontinuity advocates insist that longitudinal research studies demonstrate that discontinuity prevails during adulthood (Cohler and Galatzer-Levy, 1990); that is, people change, and personalities are not fixed in permanent patterns; life events (including unpredictable events) play a critical part in personality development (Cohler and Galatzer-Levy, 1990).

In favor of the discontinuous argument it has been shown that supportive relationships in adult life can serve as reparative experiences, enabling people to internalize the caring of others and grow further. Researchers have found that women who had been in orphanages as children would develop resilience as adults if they married supportive husbands (Vaillant, 1993). Vaillant (1993) adds that it is not just receiving support that is important in developing resilience, it is the capacity "to internalize those supports" (p. 332). Vivienne (discussed in the last chapter), who had the capacity to take in the support of others, such as her teacher, did not have the capacity to internalize this support, so these good feelings could not remain without his presence. The fact that Vivienne was unable to internalize support would argue in favor of the continuity theory; that is, her overwhelming feelings of low self-esteem, engendered in childhood, persisted and arrested, more positive developments.

The goodness-of-fit concept sheds light on adaptation and on the good adaptations people with various impairments in ego functioning may make in later life if they find the right niche. A person with limited cognitive skills, for example, can excel in a supportive work environment with concrete tasks to perform. A bright but overanxious student might function better, and thus gain self-esteem, in a small college rather than a large university.

People enter situations that may be regarded as dysfunctional but that nevertheless allow them to adapt. When people joined the Heaven's Gate cult, their psychological problems evidently meshed with the cult's philosophy and way of life (Chapter 5). People with poorly differentiated selves often enter marriages with others who also have poorly differentiated selves; if their "complementary" needs are met, their mutual adaptation may be served; when neither has sufficient ego cohesion to support the other, marital strife may ensue. Children are often triangulated into this union in the service of the couple's adaptation, but at their own developmental expense. We all have strengths and vulnerabilities, and our relationships and life experiences can foster either or both, depending on our capacities to adapt and to change, and the goodness-of-fit of the life circumstances in which we find ourselves.

Physician William Chester Minor (Winchester, 1998) was one of the major contributors to the making of the *Oxford English Dictionary* in the 1880s. Minor was a prolific and meticulous collector and annotator of words; his scholarship was outstanding. He was also a psychiatric patient at Broadmoor Hospital for the "criminally insane." Minor, who had murdered a man while in a delusional state, would do his careful dictionary work during the day; at night he was tormented by psychotic manifestations. He believed that "small boys . . . were put up in the rafters above his bed; they came down when he was fast asleep, chloroformed him, and then forced him to perform indecent acts" (Winchester, 1998, pp. 123-124).

Minor's success with the dictionary unfortunately did *not* ameliorate his condition; his condition actually deteriorated over the years. Minor had excellent cognitive and integrative capacities as well as good judgment with respect to his work. However, due to his mental illness (for which there was no treatment then), he was not capable of responding to developmental opportunities afforded by the life cycle, other than in an encapsulated intellectual realm. His early functioning was good; he had graduated from medical school and served as a doctor in the Civil War. His adult functioning was discontinuous (except for his intellectual powers) in relation to his earlier life. However, his paranoid schizophrenia, which developed in early adulthood, may have had its roots in his genetic makeup, while his childhood, adolescent, and adult wartime experiences shaped his core personality as well as the specific conflicts which were played out in his delusions; therefore, his life course was characterized by certain continuities.

A major criterion of mental health is the capacity to grow and to change. I would suggest that both continuities and discontinuities are present in a person's life, which become apparent when a person's life-cycle progressions and regressions, as well as underlying patterns of attachment and relationships, are examined. As we study any individual, we must do just that; individualize that unique person in terms of past history, including development of self-esteem, cohesion of self, ego functioning, defenses, coping mechanisms, and adaptation, in addition to significant themes in the person's life narrative. The biopsychosocial perspective is essential as individuals, with their biologically given attributes and deficits and their level of psychological development, interact with their environments (physical, cultural, political, and social). From an ecological perspective (Germain, 1991), both person and environment affect and change each other. The stages of adult development are presented in this chapter within this perspective.

Levinson's Life Course

Erikson (1963) received recognition as a leader in adding the perspective of adult development to child development studies. However, while underscoring the interaction of people and their environments, Erikson "leaves the mechanisms of development, as opposed to the content, essentially unexamined" (Stevens-Long, 1990, p. 138). Levinson and colleagues (1978) and Levinson and Levinson (1996), by contrast, were interested in the processes of adult development; they did not think that development took place the way our four-year-old (in Chapter 8) described it: "I used to be a little baby. Then I closed my eyes, and when I opened them up—all of a sudden I was a kid!"

Levinson (1986) discusses the life course, which describes the characteristics of a life in its "evolution from beginning to end" (p. 3). This evolution "involves stability and change, *continuity and discontinuity* [italics added], orderly progression as well as stasis, and chaotic flux" (Levinson, 1986, p. 3). Levinson and colleagues' (1978) original landmark study involved men; the second study (Levinson and Levinson, 1996) focused on the lives of women; "both genders go through the same periods of adult life structure development just as they go through the same periods of infancy and adolescence" (Levinson and Levinson, 1996, p. 36), but there are large differences in "life circumstances, in life course, in ways of going through each developmental period" (p. 36).

Each phase of the life cycle is an "era," which "has its own bio-psycho-social character" (Levinson and Levinson, 1996, p. 17). These eras overlap; "a new era begins as the previous one approaches its end. A *cross-era transition,* which generally lasts about five years, terminates the outgoing era and initiates the next" (p. 19). Levinson and Levinson's (1996) "key concept" is the "life structure: the underlying pattern or design of a person's life at a given time" (p. 22). They explain that "the primary components of a life structure are the person's *relationships* with various others in the external world" (Levinson and Levinson, 1996, p. 22). The life structure is not static but changes during life-cycle successions. Their research concern was with "how various aspects of self and world influence the formation of a life structure and shape its change over time" (Levinson et al., 1978, p. 42).

A life structure may have few or many components. The central components are those that have the greatest significance for the self and the life. They receive the greatest share of one's time and energy and they strongly influence the character of the other components. Only one or two components—rarely as many as three—occupy a central place in the structure. The *peripheral components* are easier to change or detach. (Levinson and Levinson, 1996, p. 23)

Levinson and Levinson (1996) also include people's concerns about what *does not* happen. What Schlossberg (1981) calls a "non-event," Levinson and Levinson (1996) refer to as "important *unfilled components*: a person urgently wants but doesn't have a meaningful occupation, a marriage, or a family; and this absent component plays a major part in the life structure" (p. 23). Family (including extended family) and occupation are usually major components of people's lives. "Underlying and permeating all relationships with the external world is the relationship to the self" (Levinson and Levinson, 1996, p. 24).

In addition to changes in the life structure over time, significant events in life also occur, such as a birth or an illness, which Levinson and colleagues (1978) refer to as "marker events," and they "are usually considered in terms of the adaptation they require" (p. 55).

Levinson (1986) predicts that the study of the life course will develop into an interdisciplinary field, because of the inseparability of people from their life situations and vice versa. He expresses concern that "each discipline has claimed as its special domain one aspect of life, such as personality, social role, or biological functioning, and has neglected the others"; he has observed that "the resulting fragmentation is so great that no discipline or viewpoint conveys the sense of an individual life and its temporal course" (p. 4).

Early Adulthood

The years from seventeen to twenty-two span the early adult transition, "a developmental period in which the era of childhood draws to a close and early adulthood gets under way" (Levinson and Levinson, 1996, p. 19). The early adulthood era itself begins at twenty-two and ends in the forties, during which life changes are made, and responsibilities assumed. Erikson (1963) refers to early adulthood as the stage of "intimacy versus isolation" and emphasizes the young adult's readiness for "intimacy, that is, the capacity to commit himself to concrete affiliations and partnerships and to develop the ethical strength to abide by such commitments, even though they may call for significant sacrifices and compromises" (p. 263). Intimacy has another significant dimension, which is permitting another to get physically and emotionally close to one's vulnerable self; this seems relevant in understanding the fears of intimacy that are so prevalent today, both in "normal" people and in people with actual psychopathology.

Erikson has been criticized for his exclusive emphasis on the intimacy of heterosexual relationships; however, the underlying principles he advocates also apply to many homosexual relationships, such as the emphasis on commitment and the integration of sexuality, trust, and mutuality within the relationship; the strong advocacy by many for recognition of homosexual marriages speaks to this point. Erikson's emphasis on procreation during this stage is also a priority of many gays and lesbians who become parents biologically or through adoption or fostering (discussed in Chapter 6).

Today, however, with the great diversity of lifestyles, people may not choose ongoing intimate relationships to have their needs met; many can have other types of rich relationships and lifestyles without feeling isolated. Levinson and Levinson (1996), when talking about the life structure, mention activities, books, and even locations with which people become involved. One might question whether a life that avoids exposure of the vulnerable self to another lacks something essential to complete fulfillment.

Erikson (1963) cites Freud who when asked "what he thought a normal person should be able to do well . . . was reported to have said 'Lieben und arbeiten' (to love and to work)" (p. 265). Erikson (1963) feels that "we cannot improve on the professor's formula" (p. 265). Levinson and colleagues (1978) also emphasize occupation, marriage, and family, "although there are significant variations in their relative weight and in the importance of other components" (p. 44). When Levinson and Levinson (1996) speak of the family, they include the extended family and observe that "the relationship to family is also interwoven with the relationship to ethnicity, race, occupation, cultural traditions" (p. 23).

Early adulthood is the era "of greatest energy and abundance and of greatest contradiction and stress" (Levinson, 1986, p. 5).

> Biologically, the 20's and 30's are the peak years of the life cycle. In social and psychological terms, early adulthood is the season for forming and pursuing youthful aspirations, establishing a niche in society, raising a family, and as the era ends, reaching a more "senior" position in the adult world. This can be a time of rich satisfaction in terms of love, sexuality, family life, occupational advancement, creativity, and realization of major life goals. But there can also be crushing stresses. (Levinson, 1986, p. 5)

Economic pressures and the need to make difficult choices are among the stresses faced by young adults; this is also a time when "we are most buffeted by our own passions and ambitions from within and by the demands of family, community and society from without" (Levinson, 1986, p. 5).

Systemic stresses may include lack of opportunities (such as high unemployment rates), discrimination, lack of adequate housing, economic problems, and living in violent neighborhoods. Family stresses encompass marital (and partner) conflict, sexual incompatibility, infertility, parent-child conflict, and problems with extended families. Divorce, a process that can be very painful and stressful, is a common occurrence.

Young adults may struggle with unresolved identity issues and attachment and self-esteem problems; they can become depressed and/or involved with substance abuse; this is also the period when schizophrenia tends to develop. Although men and women have the same rates of schizophrenia, men usually become schizophrenic at earlier ages (sometimes starting in adolescence) than women. Over 50 percent of male schizophrenic patients were hospitalized for schizophrenia before they were twenty-five. Most men develop this disorder between the ages of fifteen and twenty-five, while women generally develop schizophrenia between twenty-five and thirty-five (Kaplan et al., 1994).

Cognitive Development

Cognitive abilities continue to develop beyond the formal operations stage achieved in adolescence, although some adults never achieve the formal operations stage; as Piaget (1995b) noted, many adults remain "egocentric in their way of thinking" (p. 95). Michael Basseches postulated that *"dialectical thinking"* is a fifth (postformal) stage of cognitive development, beyond Piaget's formal operations, that develops in adulthood; it leads to a cognitive stance that acknowledges the role of conflict or contradiction in life (Stevens-Long, 1990, p. 131). The appreciation of *contradiction* and *paradox* is essential to the development of postformal or dialectical thought.

> Contradiction and paradox hold special interest. . . . Basseches believes that dialectical thought seeks contradictions among systems as a positive source for understanding change. Contradiction or paradox is not experienced as an unfortunate problem, but as an exciting opportunity for the emergence of a new idea. Basseches claims that the dialectical thinker understands how every effort to organize or systematize knowledge omits something—something that will eventually threaten the system with contradictions and create change. (Stevens-Long, 1990, p. 131)

Levinson (1986), reflecting a similar viewpoint, commented that "in studying the development of the life structure, we are not yet wise enough about life to say with precision that one life structure is developmentally higher, or more advanced, than another. We still know very little about the complexities and contradictions of the human life course" (p. 10).

Play in Adult Development

Colarusso (1993) reminds us to consider the role of play in adult development; it is as important in this phase as it was in childhood; as life becomes more complex, "play becomes an indirect approach to seeking an adaptive, defensive, skill-acquiring, and creative expression. It is a mode of coping with conflicts, demands, deprivation, loss, and developmental yearnings throughout the life cycle" (pp. 225-226). A close relationship exists between play and creativity; Noam (1996) views creativity "as an expression of the inner self taking the person into ever new, often surprising directions. . . . Wherever pursued, it always implies a deepening sense of awareness and curiosity, the most important counterforces to repetition and stagnation" (p. 152). Vaillant (1993) describes creativity as the "peculiarly human capacity for putting in the world what was not there before . . . [it] seems closely interwoven with the alchemy of the ego to bring order and meaning out of chaos and distress" (p. 2).

Play also involves the capacity to have fun—to be able to return, at least for a little while, to never-never land and enjoy it. This is related to the capacity for autonomous gratification (discussed in Chapter 2): being able to relax, to take pleasure in life, in one's body, and in one's sexuality, and in a variety of relationships to others. Being able to play (in action) and to enjoy playing (in feeling) add to one's pleasure in life; this can, for example, help a person adapt to retirement and feel entitled to enjoy it. In Chapter 13, the absence of the capacity to play and experience pleasure in schizophrenia and depression is discussed.

The ability to laugh with others and to laugh at oneself is another aspect of play. Humor, as Witkin (1999) points out, is generally missing in the social work literature, although it may be "making a comeback" (p. 101). Humor may "strengthen the immune system and act as a buffer against stress. Laughter . . . is a social lubricant" (Witkin, 1999, p. 101). Humor, with its healing functions, has been found to be effective with seriously sick children; for example, clowns are now part of some pediatric services. To a pediatrician who complained that clowns do not belong in intensive care units, one clown retorted: Neither do children!

Witkin (1999) cites Siporin, who states that laughter allows people to " 'have fun, to grow, to be free and human, to celebrate one's own life with the fellow members of one's community' " (p. 101). Humor is also a defense mechanism (Chapter 2) that can help people handle stress or conflict by draining the seriousness from situations and by providing an alternative and usually safe way of discharging tension, often with some element of hostility or aggression. "We all recognize that humor makes life so much easier . . . Freud suggested [humor] 'can be regarded as the highest of these defensive processes'" (Vaillant, 1993, p. 72).

Sexuality

That sexuality is an intrinsic part of adulthood states the obvious; sexuality is not compartmentalized within the person but is closely interrelated to the whole personality (Kaplan et al., 1994). Although sex outside of an extended relationship is not uncommon, many young adults seek marriage or long-term partnerships in which emotional and sexual intimacy are interrelated.

Sexual problems related to psychological, biological, or relationship difficulties frequently trouble young people; these factors are often interrelated. Although sex permeates our culture through movies, magazines, and television, personal communication about a couple's own sexual relationship is often lacking between partners. Sex can be a sensitive subject, tied up with taboos as well as deep feelings involving self-esteem and shame. "Performance anxiety" is not uncommonly a causal (sometimes *the* causal) factor in some sexual problems. Masters and Johnson in 1970, in their landmark study *Human Sexual Inadequacy,* described the problem of *"spectatoring"* (Scharff and Scharff, 1991, p. 28).

> In [spectatoring] a man stands outside himself looking on at his erectile difficulty, anxious lest his erection fail, thus precipitating its failure because of this anxiety. The concept of spectatoring is an important contribution to understanding the way anxiety about the situation contributes, as an independent factor with a life of its own, to sexual failure. (Scharff and Scharff, 1991, p. 28)

Certainly women, too, may be preoccupied with their sexual performance.

Physical and medical factors should be evaluated by a physician as part of understanding a client's (and a couple's) sexual difficulties. Substance abuse, for example, can affect sexual functioning in many ways, and serious "sexual dysfunction occurs within a month of significant substance intoxication or withdrawal" (Kaplan et al., 1994, p. 669). Physiological factors can be the primary contributor to dysfunction. Men may develop orgasmic disorders after genitourinary tract surgery; dysfunction "may also be associated with Parkinson's disease and other neurological disorders involving the lumbar or sacral sections of the spinal cord. . . . Prozac [is one of the drugs] implicated in retarded ejaculation" (Kaplan et al., 1994, p. 668).

Endocrine diseases such as hypothyroidism and diabetes mellitus can impair a woman's ability to experience orgasm, as well as drugs such as antihypertensive medications, central nervous system (CNS) stimulants, and tricyclic drugs (Kaplan et al., 1994); endometriosis can also affect sexual functioning. People with physical disabilities may experience a variety of sexual dysfunction. "A key issue is the absence of discussion about sex and disability" (Olkin, 1999, p. 226).

> Texts on sexuality barely acknowledge disability. . . . Conversely, it is startling how many books on disability do not discuss sexuality, or do so only cursorily. Much is still unknown about the interaction of disability and sexuality. [When discussed], the focus usually is on adults with acquired disabilities.
> However, ignoring persons with congenital disabilities reinforces the prevailing myth that such persons are asexual, as if early onset of a disability prevents healthy psychosexual development. Furthermore, information for two partners with disabilities is virtually nonexistent and quite scant for gay or lesbian relationships with disabilities. (Olkin, 1999, pp. 226-227)

Olkin (1999) refers to the journal *Sexuality and Disability* as the major contributor of professional writing on this subject and adds that "a sizable proportion of the literature is about the mechanics of sex . . . to the neglect of psychosocial and interpersonal factors" (p. 227).

Psychological and interpersonal factors, such as attachment difficulties, can be the primary cause of sexual conflict. Writer Anton Chekhov, for example, was sexually impotent only when relationships with women became emotionally significant and veered toward permanency (Rayfield, 1997). A history of childhood abuse—especially sexual abuse—can lead to adult sexual problems (Cruz and Essen, 1994).

> Some victims tend to act out sexually, which may contribute to compulsive sexual involvement, indiscriminate, numerous sexual partners, and/or sexual preoccupations; while at the other extreme, some patients might avoid sexual contact and manifest sexual difficulties such as sexual inhibition, arousal problems, low or nonexistent sexual desire, or fear of sex. Problems with achieving orgasms or erections, flashbacks, numbing or pain during sexual intercourse, or feelings of guilt, shame, or anxiety during sex are all too common with some survivors. (Cruz and Essen, 1994, p. 141)

Sexual dysfunction can cause depression; conversely, depression itself can be the root of sexual dysfunction. Depression affects both mood and body, with distressing mixed *mood-based* and *vegetative* symptoms, including lowered interest in sex as well as a decline in sexual functioning (Kaplan et al., 1994).

A major sexual difficulty is low sexual interest or *hypoactive sexual desire* (American Psychiatric Association, 1994; Kaplan et al., 1994; Scharff and Scharff, 1991). Determining the *baseline* of this disorder is important, as it can be a chronic problem or one of recent onset related to emotional distress, marital problems, and/or physical condition. "Decreased desire is one of the disorders that exists most frequently at the interface between sexual and marital difficulty" (Scharff and Scharff, 1991, p. 29).

At the end of Chapter 1, I presented the case of Mrs. Billings, who was hospitalized for depression. The couple's sexual problems were intertwined with Mrs. B.'s inner state, psychological conflicts, and anxieties, as well as her low self-esteem and poor self-image. Early relationship problems with her parents led to her anxiety about being a mother and fears of becoming pregnant. Communication problems between Mr. and Mrs. B. existed; they did not discuss their relationship, and their hurt feelings about sexual failure made it more difficult to address this problem (see case illustration in Chapter 1).

Gay, lesbian, bisexual, and transgender couples also develop sexual problems in their relationships, as varied as those presented by heterosexual couples. These problems also need to be assessed within a biopsychosocial framework.

Family Development

Varieties of family organizations were discussed in Chapter 6, and internal structural organization of family life and family problems, in Chapter 7. Family planning, becoming a parent, and separation-individuation issues are addressed in the following section.

Family planning. Many couples plan a family; some have children without planning. Not being able to have children when one plans to is usually an unanticipated event, which can cause great distress to a couple (the fertility crisis was discussed in Chapter 8).

Birth control is of concern to many; presently, the use of condoms is widely discussed as a precaution against contracting HIV and other sexually transmitted diseases. The birth control pill is also a very popular contraceptive, but many other varieties of birth control are available, the use of which is a matter of personal preference. Recent legislative and legal actions are being taken to mandate that insurance companies cover birth control costs for women (Goldberg, 1999; Lewin, 2000). Goldberg (1999) reported that "women between the ages of 15 and 44 spend 68 percent more on out-of-pocket health costs than do men, much of it on contraception"; in addition, although "93 percent of health maintenance organizations cover contraceptives, only about half of indemnity plans do so" (p. A15).

In July 2000, Planned Parenthood filed a class-action lawsuit in a Seattle court "charging that a company whose insurance plan covers most prescription drugs but excluded contraceptives is illegally discriminating against its female employees" (Lewin, 2000, p. A16).

Abortion has been a major political issue for many years and continues to be a key platform item in many elections, both on local and national levels.

Cultural attitudes vary toward birth control and the concept of family planning. But attitudes do change, and it is important not to make assumptions about an individual's interest in pursuing this subject. Major changes have occurred in Mexico, where families have tended to be large. The surge in population, which has "quintupled since 1940" with resultant problems in economics and employment, has led the government to establish a Population Council to curtail population increases; at the same time, government clinics were established to help couples with family planning (Dillon, 1999).This movement coincided with women's changing attitudes in Mexico toward birth control; "ignoring the Government and the Roman Catholic hierarchy, many women in the 1960's and early 1970's were buying contraceptives on the black market" (Dillon, 1995, p. A15). Consequently, the government's "family planning services began satisfying a repressed demand, and Mexican families began changing dramatically, almost overnight" (Dillon, 1999, p. A15).

Although many women in the United States welcome the right and ability to determine the size of their families, some prefer "to let nature take its course." Some women with deep unmet attachment needs may be motivated to become pregnant many times in succession because it protects them from "feeling empty."

In Chapter 2, we discussed Mrs. Kramer, an African-American woman who was pregnant and lived in a housing project with her husband and their ten children. Mrs. Kramer was responsive to the supportive services of a homemaker and to the intervention of a clinician who helped her feel better about herself and her future. Prior to the delivery of her eleventh child, the clinician asked Mrs. Kramer what she thought about the possibility of having her tubes tied when she gave birth. Mrs. Kramer reacted positively to this suggestion; when she came home with her new baby, she was not depressed that she had just had her last child, but jubilant. She had decided that eleven children were enough, and that life could be more enjoyable for her without further increasing the size of her family.

Some women, whose emotional needs are greater than their capacity to meet or regulate them, continue to have babies they are unable to mother; many of these children become wards of the child welfare system at some point.

Parenthood as a developmental phase. Becoming a parent can be a transforming psychological experience. Children have added a richness and pleasure to many lives, evoked a special love, and provided the opportunity to participate in a child's evolution from babyhood to adulthood.

At the same time, parents often undergo more subtle internal personality changes. Benedek (1970) refers to the parents' "emotional investment in the child [which] brings about *reciprocal intrapsychic processes in the parents* [italics added] which normally account for developmental changes in their personalities" (p. 124). Elson (1984) suggests that the "factors impinging upon the parent-child relationship are reciprocal and complex. The child influences the parent to nearly the same extent that the parent influences the child. This is the unique significance of the simultaneous ongoing process of the self experience in parents and children" (p. 302).

Ross (1984) discusses the changes in a father's identity as he assumes a "parental identity" (p. 382), which can lead to progressive or regressive changes in personality. (Ross utilizes the popular Piagetian concepts of assimilation and accommodation in his description.)

> They *assimilate* [italics added] images of their children and of themselves as parents with the available structures of their existing personality and in turn *accommodate* [italics added] to the repeated novelties occasioned by parenthood. In the face of these inner and outer demands, fathers may be thrust toward higher levels of identity organization. Or else they may capitulate, regress, or simply retreat from their newfound generational status. (Ross, 1984, p. 382)

Ross (1984) emphasizes how a father's psychological reactions can shift in relation to the changes in the child's developmental stages and their evolving interactions. The "subtle psychological changes within the adult resonate with the more visible upheavals in the child's momentous emotional growth. Thus, in order to comprehend the child's and father's relation to each other, one must glimpse at least the dialectical nature of their multifaceted, ongoing interaction" (Ross, 1984, p. 382). Ross's observations about fathers apply equally to mothers.

Parenthood affects the marital relationship, necessitating changes in the couple's lifestyle and relationship. No longer can a couple devote their primary attention to each other; the new child becomes the focus of concern. For many, parenthood is a joyful experience and can deepen the marital relationship. However, the adaptations required and the new demands on money, time, and occupational constraints can create strain, as can the requirement for emotional giving (when one or both parents possess limited emotional resources, a rivalry with the infant may develop, sometimes with disastrous consequences). Researchers studying marital relationships longitudinally have noted a general decline in marital satisfaction during parenthood; "generally the changes involved in rearing children and the accompanying stresses have been hypothesized as the reasons for that regression" (Mackey and O'Brien, 1999, p. 587). The stresses often involved in being a single parent can affect parent-child interactions and may complicate or thwart parental developmental progression.

Separation-individuation in young adulthood. The separation-individuation process continues throughout the life cycle (Mahler et al., 1975). Blos (1962) has observed adolescents going through a second individuation process, and Akhtar (1995) described a third individuation process occurring in people during the immigration experience (Chapter 5).

Colarusso's (1997) concept of a third individuation process relates to parenthood. He discusses the "continuous process of elaboration of self and differentiation from objects that occur in young adulthood, focusing in particular on involvements with children, spouse and parents" (pp. 77-78).

Separation-individuation dilemmas permeate young adulthood, whether or not one becomes a parent. Usually a progression evolves toward separation from parents, the development of greater autonomy, and achievement of a more integrated sense of identity. Many young adults and their parents successfully adapt to the changes in their relationship, although separation can be both an internal and interpersonal struggle. Subtle forms of separation-individuation conflicts include parents' attempts to control, be possessive, or become preoccupied with the lives of their adult children; young adults, in turn, may cling, often turning excessively to parents for emotional and financial support and advice.

Young adults' relationships to their parents are also colored by their choice of a spouse or partner. Although parental response may be positive, it is not unusual for tensions to develop in this arena, as in-laws can object or relate negatively to the partner or spouse on the basis of race, ethnicity, social class, sexual orientation, educational achievement, earning capacity, personality, their own internal conflicts, or changes this produces in their involvement with their children.

Cultural values shape one's adaptation to adulthood and parenthood. In Asian families, for example, as discussed earlier, a strong value is placed on interdependency within the family rather than independence (Wong and Mock, 1997). Education is often emphasized (especially for males), and parents may exert a strong influence on educational and career choices, discourage early dating, and oppose interracial relationships. However, Asian Americans "like all young adults . . . may begin to see young adulthood as a means to achieve physical and psychological distance from the family" (p. 197). Variations may occur in their response to separation-individuation and family loyalties.

Like most young adults, Asians experience a consolidation of their identity and values during this period. Some may question their own adherence to familial values. Some may stay closely allied to family values. . . . At the other extreme, some may not associate primarily with other Asians, unconsciously rejecting their family. Some Asians report having a "dual identity" defined by specific context. When they are at home, they are Asian ethnic identified . . . as per parental expectations. When they are away, this identity may be suppressed, and they may represent themselves as more Americanized. (Wong and Mock, 1997, p. 197)

Achieving parenthood may consolidate the young adult's sense of adulthood, and relationships with parents may enter a new phase, as the grandparents accept the adulthood of their offspring and share in the joy of a new child; it may be a time of "fence mending," as old conflicts fade in the midst of the excitement of participating in a new life. Parenthood can also be a time of renewed conflict, when the grandparents not only refuse to let go, but become more involved and controlling of their grandchildren and how they are raised (see Norris case in Chapter 7). If the grandparent becomes the primary caretaker of the child, the ground becomes fertile for an intensification of parental conflict; a complicated course of continued identity development and individuation may ensue for the adult child.

Development at Midlife

Midlife spans the ages from forty to sixty-five. Although physical capacities may gradually decline, most people are capable of leading an "energetic, personally satisfying and socially valuable life" (Levinson, 1986, p. 6). Erikson (1963) terms this the "generativity versus stagnation" phase; he views midlife as the "central" stage of development, because "generativity encompasses the evolutionary development which has made man the teaching and instituting as well as the learning animal" (p. 260). Generativity is "the concern in establishing and guiding the next generation" (Erikson, 1963, pp. 260-261); without the motivation and capacity to do this, Erikson observes, there is often a "pervading sense of stagnation and personal impoverishment" (p. 261).

During midlife people often reflect on their life and progress and may, as a result, become more mature, creative, responsible, and loving (Levinson, 1986). Kaplan and colleagues (1994) acknowledge the pressures and depressions which may develop but believe that midlife can be a positive time. Levinson (1986), crediting Erikson, also emphasizes generativity and the responsibility "for the development of the current generation of young adults" (p. 6), observing that many people "become 'senior members' in [their] own particular worlds, however grand or modest they may be" (p. 6). Levinson and colleagues (1978), however, see stagnation (which Erikson views in negative terms) as having positive attributes, commenting that "both generativity and its opposite pole, stagnation, are vital in a [person's] development" (Levinson et al., 1978, p. 30). The fight against stagnation is part of the developmental struggle, which leads to the recognition of vulnerability in the self, which "becomes a source of wisdom, empathy and compassion for others" (Levinson et al., 1978, p. 30).

Levinson and colleagues (1978) also comment that "unfortunately, middle adulthood is for many persons a time of progressive decline—of growing emptiness and loss of vitality" (p. 20). People can experience internal conflict and external pressure in midlife; sometimes an interaction of both occurs. Studies have indicated that people in midlife can experience "particular disharmony, lowered morale, increased concerns about health, and increased anxiety and depression" (Cohler and Galatzer-Levy, 1990, pp. 225-226). Cohler and Galatzer-Levy (1990) suggest that these anxieties "appear to account for first appearances of psychiatric illness in mid-life" (p. 226).

A person can be a leader at work, or recently laid off, can be surrounded by friends, family, and colleagues or have just ended a marriage (or partnership) with its multiple disrupted relationships with family, extended family, and social network; can be financially secure, or financially strapped by children starting college, paying for the care of elderly parents, or living at a poverty level; can feel overburdened by responsibilities with little time (or capacity) to play and experience pleasure. One can enjoy good health with minor ailments or face a debilitating or life-threatening illness. Unresolved inner stresses and conflicts and unresolved self-esteem issues may make a difference between a relatively benign versus a more disturbed midlife period.

Midlife traditionally is the time when children reaching adolescence leave home and parents face the empty nest syndrome; some parents would love to have an empty nest, as their children, now college graduates, choose to return home to live. People of midlife age often become grandparents and consider retiring; couples may turn toward each other as they contemplate enjoying their leisure years without the responsibility of children. Today, many women in their forties (and men in their forties and older) become parents of infants; grandparents may be assuming major (or full) responsibility for raising their grandchildren; people often chose to work into their seventies and beyond; and formerly married couples are now divorced and living alone or with blended families (or are going through successive divorces).

Although generativity concerns are important, midlife adults are often preoccupied with the generation *before* them—their own parents, who are aging and living longer. Parent caring can become a major task; people in midlife, known as the "sandwich generation," must deal with the needs of their parents as well as their children and grandchildren.

Physical Changes in Midlife

Midlife brings about major bodily changes and signs of incipient aging; these can become "a major, sometimes dominant, influence on mental life" (Colarusso, 1997, p. 80). Most people in midlife have good health and vitality; however, gradual declines and changes in the body can include having less physical energy, a decreasing level of metabolism (which can result in weight gain), the development of joint pains, changes in heart and kidney functioning, and problems with the gastrointestinal tract (Zastrow and Kirst-Ashman, 1997). Vision may decline, and hearing problems can develop. There tends to be a general increase in health problems such as diabetes, heart problems, and cancer.

Many people with health problems nevertheless continue to have high levels of functioning. Others find that disabilities dramatically alter their lives, their self-image, and relationships. Some people are responsive and supportive caretakers for their ill or disabled spouse or partner; other spouses or partners may feel overwhelmed by the new responsibilities and separations or divorces often ensue; the divorce rate is higher for couples in which a partner has a disability than for nondisabled couples.

Changes in bodily appearance and functioning, including the onset of menopause in women and changes in male sexual functioning (sometimes complicated by urinary and/or prostate problems), can affect psychological well-being, but the potential exists for positive adaptations (Colarusso, 1997). People often "mourn for the lost body of youth," and when they come to terms with the reality of their physical changes, this is "is experienced to a large degree as a separation-individuation phenomenon" (Colarusso, 1997, p. 81); if this is achieved, this can lead to attaining "new experiences and . . . developmental potentials" (p. 81).

Generally midlife adults remain sexually active; for some, sexual activity increases and/or becomes more pleasurable as child care responsibilities fade, and couples can be more attentive to each other. The onset of menopause can remove fears of pregnancy and add to the feeling of greater sexual freedom. People may also experience sexual dysfunction, in part physical and sometimes psychological or relational, or an interaction of these factors. The recent advent of Viagra has made available a medication to ameliorate male erectile disorders, and the large demand for it bears witness to the numbers of men with this problem. Recent advances have occurred in promoting Viagra and similar drugs for women with sexual problems related to impaired blood flow to the genitalia; this is often caused by menopausal changes, atherosclerosis, and diabetes (Mann, 1998).

Psychological Development in Midlife

Jung referred to the development of increased psychological *introversion* (a tendency to turn inward) in midlife. Neugarten has termed this "interiority" (Cohler and Galatzer-Levy, 1990, p. 225). There is "increasing preoccupation with the meaning of life" and a tendency to become aware of the passage of time and mortality. Colarusso (1997) has observed that people go through a fourth individuation phase, focusing on the dilemmas of attachment and loss, involving the "ironic awareness that one will die and be deprived of involvement with loved ones at the very time that a mature understanding of the importance of others for one's health, happiness, and security is at its peak" (p. 79). Colarusso (1997) observes that "at no other point in life is the potential for attachment—and loss—so great" (p. 79).

Grandparenthood in midlife is one factor promoting the fourth individuation phase (Colarusso, 1997). The grandparents' investment in and idealization of their grandchildren serves reparative developmental functions, including bonding and comforting, which can protect against anxieties about aging and dying. Becoming a grandparent may also raise anxiety about aging: "grandparenthood is often greeted with ambivalence, reflecting, in part, the struggle to accept a personal end" (Colarusso, 1998, p. 132).

Colarusso speaks of the grandchild granting "genetic immortality" to the grandparent; but genetic immortality cannot be a literal fact for those grandparents who have no genetic connection to their grandchildren. Regardless of genetics, continued emotional connection through their grandchildren's memories of them may promise a kind of immortality to many.

Some grandparents experience greater freedom to involve themselves with their grandchildren than they could with their own children, in part because they do not have the full responsibility for care. They may have also worked out their psychological conflicts over parenting with their own children and are free to see these new little people in their individuality, rather than as ghosts from the past.

Parent Caring

As the baby boomers reach their fifties, their parents are becoming older and "are moving into the ranks of what is often called 'the old-old,' where disability and thus the need for care become increasingly likely" (Toner, 1999, p. A1). For some midlife adults, parent caring can produce great stress—greater than the emotional upheavals of dealing with the empty nest syndrome (Neugarten, 1979).

It has been estimated by the National Alliance for Caregivers "that about 6.5 million people, nearly a fifth of the population 65 years and older, required assistance and about 22 million families—nearly 1 in 4—are providing some form of assistance to an older relative or friend" (Rimer, 1998a, p. A1). Caring for elderly relatives is costly to caregivers in actual financial expenditures for maintenance needs and services, loss of time spent at work, and missed opportunities for advancement. Almost three-fourths of participants in one survey reported that "elder care had affected their health" (Rimer, 1999, p. A8). Caring for elderly relatives with dementia can cause particular stress and bring on depressive symptoms in caregivers. "Their caregiving burden has long been recognized as a major public health concern" (Kennedy, 2000, p. 144).

Most elderly people live in the community, and their daughters or daughters-in-law usually care for them; more than half of these women are also employed, and approximately 40 percent have their own child care responsibilities (Kaplan et al., 1994). Joyce Rudock, a gerontologist, has observed that " 'elder care is to the 21st century what child care has been for the last few decades' " (Rimer, 1999, p. A8).

Clinicians must assess the degree of disability affecting an elderly client, the type of care needed, the availability of other caretakers and resources, the personalities of both the adult child and the parent, and the quality of their relationship to each other. The attitudes (and helpfulness) of children, spouses or partners, and siblings also affect the felt burden on the midlife caretaker. Although women are often primary caretakers, in many situations, men become caretakers to spouses, partners, or parents; it is not rare to find elderly men serving as caretakers for their wives.

Development in Late Life

Simone de Beauvoir once said in an interview that it is easier for people to contemplate their death than it is to contemplate their own old age. Most of us have fears and apprehensions about aging; perhaps this helps to explain why we may have difficulty dealing with this subject, and why we tend to stereotype the elderly (*ageism*); for in this process the old become *they,* and not *us.* Another difficulty in generalizing about the elderly and their problems is that we may forget that the elderly are a group of unique individuals; as unique in their later years as they were throughout the rest of their lives.

Gerontologists have classified the elderly, who are the fastest-growing age group in this country, into two groups: the young-old, ages sixty-five to seventy-four, and the old-old, ages seventy-five and older (Kaplan et al., 1994). A third group, sometimes referred to as the "frail elderly," who are past age eighty-five, has been added more recently. According to census data, "the 85-and-older population rose 274 percent from 1960 to 1994, and is the fastest growing group among those over 65" (Toner, 1999, p. A11).

As we search for some commonalities to help us understand this phase of adulthood, we are thwarted by extreme differences in the aging process itself. In early childhood, the differences among children in achieving developmental landmarks were slight; perhaps weeks or months. In adolescence, the range of variation was greater; it might take one thirteen-year-old boy two years to catch up to the growth spurts and maturational level of his same-age friend. For older adults, the range of variation can be measured in decades, and life trajectories can differ drastically. One can be youthful at eighty-five, physically healthy and intellectually vigorous; someone else can be old at sixty, totally incapacitated by a severe stroke.

In the elderly population, "only 5 percent require institutional care and only 10 percent require assistance in the community. Two-thirds of older adults report themselves in good to excellent health. Three-quarters report no more than minor if any limitations in activities of daily living" (Kennedy, 2000, pp. 4-5). The frail and the sick elderly, however, need a variety of medical, psychiatric, and social services, as well as assisted-living arrangements from relatives, community caretakers, assisted-living apartments, and nursing homes. The medical needs of the frail and sick elderly "have become enormous" (Kaplan et al., 1994, p. 65), and "the costs of their health needs, both personal and societal, pose substantial economic and policy challenges" (Kennedy, 2000, p. 1). "Dementia is the major cause of functional dependence in the elderly" (Kennedy, 2000, p. 5).

Mr. Hunter is at an age when some of his contemporaries are indeed "frail elderly," yet appears to be accomplishing the Eriksonian (1963) task of "developing integrity versus despair," being involved in living and maintaining attachments to others.

Mr. Hunter, a black, eighty-seven-year-old man living in a small town in Staten Island, was described to the writer, Joseph Mitchell (2000), as "one of those strong, self-contained old men you don't see much any more. He was a hard worker, and he retired only a few years ago, and he's fairly well-to do. He's a widower, and he lives by himself and does his own cooking" (pp. 6-7). When Mitchell phoned to arrange a meeting, Mr. Hunter told him that he was too busy that day for a visit. "An old lady I know is sick in bed, and I made her a lemon-meringue pie, and I'm going over and take it to her. Sit with her awhile. . . . You'll have to make it some other time" (Mitchell, 2000, p. 7).

When the visit does takes place, Mr. Hunter discusses his cooking and church activities with Mitchell as he frosts a three-layer cake:

> The preacher at our church is a part-time preacher. . . . Most Sundays, he and his wife take Sunday dinner with me, and I always try to have something nice for them. . . . A gospel chorus from down South is . . .

coming to my house for Sunday dinner. . . . Did you have your lunch?
(Mitchell, 2000, pp. 8-9)

Mr. Hunter appears to be in control of his own destiny and to have found
meaning in his religion, the social affiliations with his church, and involvement with caring for others. He takes pride in his accomplishments and his
mastery over his daily life. Mr. Hunter would fall within the high-functioning end of the spectrum of late adulthood.

The present population of elderly is "healthier, more active, and in better
financial condition than any previous cohort of persons age 65 or older"
(Kennedy, 2000, p. 5). However, many elderly people do have serious economic problems which impact on their quality of life and their health
(Kaplan et al., 1994). Elderly people living below the poverty level number
about 3.5 million; the lowest incomes are found in elders over age eighty-
five (Kaplan et al., 1994). Women live longer than men and "are twice as
likely as men to be poor. Black elderly women over 65 are five times more
likely to be poor than are white elderly women" (Kaplan et al., 1994, p. 72).

The number of older people of color is increasing; "the doubling and
even tripling in the numbers of elders of color is a significant part of the de-
mographic transformations taking place in the United States" (Sotomayor,
1997, p. 26). (Sotomayor includes many groups within her usage of people
of color, including African Americans, Latinos, Asians and Pacific Islanders, and Native Americans). She observed that they experience many socioeconomic problems, including having poor housing, tending to be more disabled, and being at greater risk because of their multiple living problems;
the economic status of elder Native Americans "is far worse than that of any
other elderly population of color" (Sotomayor, 1997, p. 31).

Biopsychosocial Concerns of Older Adults

People in late adulthood face multiple losses and depletion on many levels; but, like Mr. Hunter, many are actively involved in life and make plans
for the future. Colarusso (1998) reflects "that maintaining the ability to continue to be valued, valuable and relevant in a present dominated by younger
generations is a central developmental task of late adulthood" (p. 131).

Levinson and Levinson (1996) discuss the term *adolescing*, which connotes " 'moving toward adulthood' and suggests positive growth toward a
potential optimum" (p. 21); by contrast, "*senescing*, which means moving
toward old age . . . suggests negative growth and dissolution" (p. 22).Viewing
the life cycle from a child-development perspective will probably lead to
drawing a "rather bleak picture of adult development, since they [this per-
spective] tend[s] to ignore the often rich potentialities and achievements of
middle and late adulthood" (Levinson and Levinson, 1996, p. 21).

In late adulthood we are mostly senescing, but some vitally important adolescing may be done toward the end of the life cycle as we seek to give fuller meaning to our lives, to life and death as ultimate stages, and to the condition of being human. The approach of death itself may be the occasion of our growing to full adulthood. (Levinson and Levinson, 1996, p. 21)

Older adults have made major strides over the years in combating ageism, the stereotypical, prejudicial way of measuring older people in terms of their limitations, with an emphasis on their decline. Advances have been made, such as prohibitions against discriminating against the elderly in employment. Senior citizens are now a political presence felt at state and federal levels of government.

Work and Retirement

Some older adults eagerly anticipate retirement, with plans for activities including leisure pursuits, involvement with grandchildren, volunteer work, travel, or study. For others, forced retirement can produce turmoil and depression. An increasing number of older adults continue to be employed; the Age Discrimination in Employment Act, which ended the practice of mandated retirement at seventy, was passed by the U.S. Congress in 1967.

Many political figures and others prominent in their fields are themselves "young old" and "old old." In 1985, a man was killed by a New York City police car driven by an officer who was intoxicated (Lacayo, 1988).

[His widow] sued the city for $29 million, partly for the loss of her husband's future income. Because her husband was 71 at his death, the jury might have concluded that his income-producing years were mostly behind him. No problem. Her attorney was 86. . . . Octogenarian Harry Lipsig . . . perhaps the winningest liability lawyer in America. (Lacayo, 1988, p. 56)

Social Involvement

For some people, losing work means losing their social networks; the social life of elderly people is another important area of inquiry. Some older adults maintain large social networks; some prefer (and may always have preferred) a more solitary existence. Often people outlive their social networks and experience loneliness; as disabilities increase and mobility decreases, simply getting to where social activities take place can be difficult.

One elderly man, a former physician, living in a nursing home, outlived his wife and his colleagues with whom he had been actively involved. He had no children, and physical infirmity necessitated his move to a nursing home; one cousin, his only remaining relative, visited him regularly but was now moving to another state as her husband was retiring. The nursing home's social worker enabled him to feel less depressed and alone and to think of ways, even in these limited circumstances, in which he could feel more fulfilled and less isolated.

Adult children are often an important source of emotional comfort as well as helpful to their parents in their daily coping. Relationships with adult children are varied and can be complex; role reversal is not uncommon and is a frequent cause of conflict—now it is not the parent telling the teenager that he or she cannot have the car this Saturday—it is the adult child telling the parent that he or she should not be driving at all! In addition, prior chronic family dysfunction can complicate dealing with the parent's life changes. The new life crisis of aging, on the other hand, can present opportunities for families to work out past issues and reach a higher level of compatibility.

Relationships with grandchildren (and great-grandchildren) can be very meaningful to the elderly, through a sense of continuity and hope they will be remembered, enhanced by sharing family history and passing on mementos of their lives (Colarusso, 1998). The "feeling held" engendered by loving responses of the grandchild can be very soothing. However, if the grandparent is feeling depletion anxiety, grandchildren may be rejected because they "become but another painful reminder of the nearness of death" (Colarusso, 1998, p. 133).

When people reach late adulthood, their children and grandchildren may be so involved in their own lives that the elderly person becomes "increasingly aware of feelings of irrelevance or redundancy" (Colarusso, 1998, p. 134). Friends of the same age are very important to elderly people; if they are friends from the past, they can share memories and "confirm the importance and reality of a distant past" (Colarusso, 1998, p. 134). Newly made friends can also be an important source of support.

> Friends of the same age confirm and substantiate one's importance in the present. . . . They share a common position in the life cycle and similar relationships . . . serve as buffers against an increasingly short and precarious future. The end of life, in the presence of mental or physical illness, is less threatening when the developmental task is shared. (Colarusso, 1998, p. 134)

The "ethnic enclave" has been important for many elderly immigrants. In one study, a group of immigrants left their communities to move with their children and so were "uprooted again. . . . This group was unable to rejoin or locate an ethnic enclave in their new locale and within weeks to months developed depression and/or other mild organic symptoms" (Kao and Lam, 1997, p. 210).

Some elderly people have found new friends in retirement communities, assisted-living programs, foster homes for the elderly, and community programs, such as old-age centers. But many remain isolated. In San Francisco, for example, some elderly people have died alone; sometimes their bodies have not been discovered for weeks, "with no one to arrange their funerals, settle their estates or mourn their passing. So far this year, 275 people in the city have died this way, said city officials, compared with about 300 a year for the last decade" (Nieves, 2000, p. 9).

The beneficial effects of pets on children and adults in many settings have received increasing attention in the literature (Germain, 1991). When provided with pets, many older adults who had been living alone responded with improved mental states and a decrease in physical symptoms. "As companions, animals may assist in minimizing loneliness and may provide opportunities for tactile stimulation. In addition, touching a pet has been shown to affect the cardiovascular system. As nonjudgmental companions pets can provide informal emotional support" (Netting et al., 1987, p. 61).

Cognitive Development

Mental abilities do not inevitably decline in the elderly, and considerable variation exists. Dementias, which can be all encompassing, do develop in some people, while many have only minor problems with short-term memory. Conversely, some older adults can think in *more* complex ways, a continuation of the postformal mode of thinking developed in midlife.

Older adults often appreciate the complexities of a problem, including the interrelationships of motivation, logic, and irrationality. Therefore, they may no longer do well on tests of formal operations, because, finding the underlying assumptions unacceptable, they may "no longer see problems of pure logic as relevant or interesting" (Stevens-Long, 1990, p. 133).

> Edelstein and . . . Noam (1982) have described the intellectual behavior of older adults as a reunion of logic and affect. . . . the search for a socially adequate solution to problems rather than acceptance of the most "logical" solution. Wisdom . . . develops from an appreciation of the long-term consequences of action, and from the attempt to mediate between the demands of logic and emotion. The experience of re-

sponsibility in adult life is prerequisite to the development of wisdom. (Stevens-Long, 1990, p. 134)

Reminiscence

Reminiscence, recalling and talking about the past, is a common and normal process in late adulthood, which serves as adaptation but can lead to emotional problems if used excessively (Colarusso, 1998). Reminiscing can protect people from a painful present; it is a way of renewing memories and internalized ties to important people in their past; it aids self-esteem by helping people remember and feel good about past experiences and accomplishments; it can help people adapt to the idea of dying. Listening to family stories from the past can bring people closer together, as memories become shared knowledge. Colarusso (1998) emphasizes "that in no other phase of development does the focus on the past have such a positive impact on the adaptive functioning of the ego as occurs in late adulthood. With each reminiscence, the self is redefined and delineated in relationship to one's position in the life cycle" (p. 131).

Reminiscence has been used successfully in working with elderly Asian immigrants, as "it is helpful to encourage the client to talk about their birthplace or native land and skills they feel proud of" (Kao and Lam, 1997, p. 217). This creates "an emotional connection with clients [which] opens the way to engage them in treatment" (Kao and Lam, 1997, p. 217). This suggestion is applicable to elderly clients from many backgrounds.

A word of caution about the use of reminiscences: it should not be "pushed" on clients as a "helpful" therapeutic procedure, as some people may be made uncomfortable talking about the past; for some, the past is full of sadness and trauma. Although talking of these events can be healing for some, for others this can be distressing and retraumatizing. The basic social work principle of "starting where the client is" must be applied here.

Sexuality

One of the myths about the elderly is that they become asexual in feelings and behavior. This is far from the truth; overall, older people may have some decrease in the frequency of sexual activity and may experience biological problems complicating (or slowing down) their sexual response. But many remain both sexually interested and active. One problem for older heterosexual women is the relative absence of men, as women tend to outlive their male partners. "At age 80 there are four women for every man. Most women over age of 65 are widowed; most men are married" (Kennedy, 2000, p. 176).

Dating is of great interest to many in retirement communities; generally, men look for younger women, and although many women prefer younger men, they do not have the same choice (Rimer, 1998b). One eighty-five-year-old woman, who was rejected by many men after their first date with her because they wanted someone younger, commented: "Where do bald men with arthritic knees get off acting like this?" (Rimer, 1998b, p. A1). Many older men find that they are much sought after; this, however, "lasts only until they lose their driver's license . . . or lose their health" (Rimer, 1998b, p. A1). Many seniors have expressed anxieties about dating behavior.

Many people (including doctors) believed until recently that senior citizens were not at real risk for acquiring AIDS. However, this group, including many older heterosexual men and women, is "one of the fastest-growing HIV-infected populations in the U.S." (Drummond, 1999, p. 84H). South Florida (with a high concentration of retirees) has found that 14 percent of them are infected, in contrast to the national average of 10 percent among the elderly (Drummond, 1999, p. 84H). This includes some older people who had become infected with HIV earlier and were receiving successful treatment. HIV is transmitted in older adults primarily through sexual relationships, which occur often without the protection of condoms. "Physically fit single men, dubbed 'condominium Casanovas,' often flit from one woman to the next, sometimes passing along AIDS. Widowers often hire prostitutes" (Drummond, 1999, p. 84H).

Kennedy (2000) predicts an increase in AIDS in the elderly. One of the major concerns of this illness in the elderly is the development of the "AIDS-related dementia complex," which progresses more quickly in late adulthood (Kennedy, 2000, p. 176).

Many nursing homes have restrictive rules (or unspoken patterns of regulation) regarding the expression of a patient's sexual behavior (Kennedy, 2000; Zastrow and Kirst-Ashman,1997). Staff (and relatives of patients) sometimes must be educated "about the rights to privacy that competent, sexually consenting adults retain as residents of nursing homes" (Kennedy, 2000, p. 188). This attitude existed for years prior to the present concern with AIDS. Public health measures about safe sex in institutions might be easier to encourage if this were an open topic of discussion rather than a subject that is ignored. The same dilemma exists in high schools, where sex education is increasingly emphasizing abstinence.

Some patients with dementia may act out sexually, which must be handled appropriately and distinguished from normative sexual interests (Kennedy, 2000). If nursing homes have a problem with heterosexual sexuality, problems about accepting homosexual behavior within the nursing home may be compounded.

Research indicates that most elderly gay and lesbian people are well-adjusted; many have a large social network, are often part of a committed couple, and have an ability to cope with aging as they have coped with other problems, such as homophobia. Their basic concerns and problems are similar to those faced by heterosexual elders (Zastrow and Kirst-Ashman, 1997). Gay and lesbian elders tend to have specific concerns about legal matters, such as the rights of a partner to inherit, which may be opposed by the biological family, and they have institutional concerns, such as discrimination on the part of institutions or hospitals (Zastrow and Kirst-Ashman, 1997).

An interest in having special facilities built for homosexual elders has developed in response to fears of institutional discrimination (Bragg, 1999, p. A1). Many of the developers, who are also gay, are building retirement communities and assisted-care facilities "marketed specifically for homosexuals, places that will allow gays to grow old surrounded by other gays, where they do not have to live, and ultimately die, amid lingering condemnation" (Bragg, 1999, p. A1).

This might not be the preferred solution for everyone; some may lack funds to finance this type of private care. People from different cultural and ethnic groups might prefer other lifestyles or may feel discrimination from white gay and lesbian people based on their "other identities." African-American gay men, for example, may be uncomfortable living in institutions with white gay men; this may be related to preexisting tensions between some members of both groups (Adams Jr. and Kimmel, 1997).

Mental Health Problems of the Elderly

Although a close connection exists between physical health and mental health throughout the life cycle, this is especially true in the elderly population. "For both causality and course of illness, mental and physical health are inseparable in aged persons" (Kennedy, 2000, p. 2). Although physical illness, depression, and dementia increase with age, most seniors nevertheless "are neither demented nor seriously depressed. *Physically healthy seniors* [italics added] have the lowest rates of anxiety, depression, and substance abuse among the adult population" (Kennedy, 2000, p. 3).

The effects of prescription and nonprescription drugs often mimic symptoms of emotional disorders in the older population, due to such factors as incorrect dosage, changes in an older person's ability to absorb a drug, the patient's difficulty in following intake instructions, idiosyncratic sensitivity to the medication, and the effect of interacting medications—so-called polypharmacy—which might be prescribed by different physicians (Kaplan et al., 1994).

The many changes experienced by the elderly, including their own sense of physical and cognitive depletion, can place them at risk for mental illness (Kaplan et al., 1994). Another stressor can be the anticipation of their own death.

Being an immigrant can be stressful, and emotional problems have developed in both first- and second-generation elderly immigrants who have lost their network of friends and relatives on whom they have depended to deal with their new environments. "With the loss of these helpers, as a result of geographic moves or death, such individuals may experience such symptoms of emotional trouble as depression, hypochondria, insomnia, or even paranoia" (Kao and Lam, 1997, p. 208).

The emotional problems with which elderly people struggle can be exacerbations of chronic conditions, reactive difficulties in adapting to multiple losses and transitions, or a combination of these. According to Kaplan and colleagues (1994), the most common psychiatric problems in the elderly are depressive disorders, cognitive disorders, phobias, and alcohol use disorders, which are discussed next. The elderly also tend to suffer from sleep disorders, vertigo, somatoform disorders (physical symptoms which are psychologically based), and hypochondriasis (preoccupation with, and exaggeration of, physical complaints).

Most of the treatment for mental illness in older adults is not provided by psychiatrists but by primary care physicians; many doctors as well as other practitioners in the health field receive insufficient education in mental health problems of the elderly (Kennedy, 2000).

Depression. Approximately 30 percent of elderly patients seeing primary care physicians have depressive symptoms, and about half of this group have an actual depressive disorder (Kennedy, 2000). The elderly are organically reactive to depressive symptoms, which can worsen symptoms of their physical illness and impair their functional capacities (Kennedy, 2000). They also experience serious depression after bereavement more frequently than younger people do; however, depression in the elderly seems to be associated more with the development of physical illness and disability (Kennedy, 2000). It has been observed, for example, that over 50 percent of elderly people who have had strokes become depressed within a period of six months.

The suicide rate in the elderly is high, occurring in forty per 100,000 population (Kaplan et al., 1994); although depression is usually present, physical illness is often a major precipitating factor (Kennedy, 2000). Depression in the elderly is not always easy to diagnose; it often occurs in conjunction with physical problems, and some of its symptoms, such as memory loss and inability to concentrate, can be misdiagnosed as dementia (the reverse is equally true).

Cognitive disorders. Dementia (major significantly irreversible, global, and/or partial impairments of cognitive functioning) affects 4 million people in the United States at an estimated cost in direct services for physicians, hospitals, and caretaking agencies of $100 billion a year (Kennedy, 2000). The indirect costs, which are related to the expenses and lost wages of family members, is estimated to be another $100 billion. It is projected that the number of persons developing dementia will double during the next forty years (Kennedy, 2000).

Dementia, as a classification, covers a number of disorders, including dementia produced by AIDS, syphilis, vascular impairment, strokes, brain tumors, and chronic alcoholic intoxication. Patients with dementia experience a steady downhill loss of cognitive abilities, which seriously impair their overall psychosocial functioning (Kennedy, 2000). One of the most common and publicized forms of dementia is Alzheimer's disease (AD), "which develops gradually and at first almost imperceptibly, with symptoms that resemble ordinary memory lapses. Soon the lapses become more pervasive, and people with AD lose the ability to learn and remember anything new" ("Alzheimer's Disease—Part I," 1992).

> Sometimes slowly, sometimes rapidly, they descend from forgetfulness into confusion. They can no longer remember the names of friends and family members or find their way around in places that are not completely familiar. They begin to avoid social contacts, because they cannot follow the drift of a conversation. Cooking, driving, using tools, handling money, and even obeying simple instructions become overwhelmingly difficult. At this stage they can still function adequately using simple routines in a familiar environment, but they seem apathetic and withdrawn. ("Alzheimer's Disease—Part I," 1992, p. 2)

Patients may have difficulty controlling their impulses and emotions, and in their confusion "they dimly sense that they are losing everything, so they sometimes become suspicious and develop delusions, talking to imaginary persons or accusing family members of being impostors" ("Alzheimer's Disease—Part I," 1992, p. 2). In the last stages, they become totally disoriented and may not even know who they are, lose control of their bowel and bladder functions, have serious sleep problems, and often cannot take care of themselves in the most basic ways, such as dressing themselves or eating.

Deterioration proceeds, and patients are ultimately bedridden "and apparently oblivious" ("Alzheimer's Disease—Part I," 1992, p. 2); they die of "malnutrition, dehydration, infection, or heart failure. In nearly half of cases the immediate cause of death is pneumonia" (p. 2). The time between onset of the symptoms and death ranges from two to twenty years; it averages seven to ten years.

It is important to make an accurate differential diagnosis of this disease, and a neurological assessment is imperative, with the performance of neuropsychological and memory tests. Sometimes what appears to be Alzheimer's is not and may be drug intoxication, thyroid disorders, subdural hematoma, or other diseases that can often be treated. It is also important to differentiate AD from depression; complicating this diagnosis is the fact that depression is often present in Alzheimer's disease as well as coexisting with other dementias.

Families, who differ in their capacities to cope with this illness as well as with the required caretaking responsibilities, assume care for the majority of dementia patients; the toll on them is particularly high (Kennedy, 2000). Kennedy (2000) finds that some of the most difficult behaviors for families to cope with are incontinence, nighttime wandering, and assaultiveness. "Perhaps cruelest of all is the patient's loss of capacity to recognize the loved caregiver" (Kennedy, 2000, p. 74). Many families who attempt to take care of the relative at home feel guilty when this is no longer feasible.

> One client discussed with her student social worker her decision to place her husband, who had Alzheimer's disease, in a nursing home. She explained that her husband, formerly a gentle and loving man, had beat her, and how he often wandered away from the house, and she had to go in search of him. She had feared both for her own safety and his. It took her two years initially to make the decision that she could not take care of him at home. She said that, in retrospect, she should have placed her husband in a nursing home a year earlier than she did. Then, as if feeling guilty for saying that, she became tearful, and while showing the social worker a photo of her husband and herself before he became sick, she said he had expected her to take care of him when he got old, and that she had let him down. She said, "It's not fair, if it were any other illness, I could have cared for him—but not this one." Later in the session, she discussed how lonely she felt without her husband. "I miss him so much. I am nothing without him."

Anxiety Disorders. Anxiety disorders are found in the elderly, often (but not necessarily) in people who have had a history of problems with anxiety. Although the severity of symptoms may be milder than those in younger people, the actual impact on older people can be severe; the elderly may have more difficulty adapting to stress due to a weakened autonomic nervous system (Kaplan et al., 1994). Experiencing post-traumatic stress disorder also tends to produce more serious symptomatology in this population (Kaplan et al., 1994).

Substance Abuse

Many elderly people who are dependent on alcohol often have chronic drinking problems that have existed since they were young or midlife adults (Kaplan et al., 1994). They have serious medical problems (often liver disease) and tend to be unmarried, widowed, divorced, or never married; many are men in the homeless poor population. Kaplan and colleagues (1994) report that 20 percent of patients in nursing home are dependent on alcohol. They also report that alcohol and abuse of other substances are involved in 10 percent of mental health problems in the elderly; furthermore, the elderly have greater dependence on certain medications than is generally known, including hypnotics, anxiolytics (tranquilizers), and narcotics, as well as nonprescription drugs, and nicotine and caffeine.

Death

Human existence is time limited, and it is our human destiny to know that. It is also part of our human nature to rail against this fact, to seek fountains of youth and magic elixirs, to deny its inevitability, and to change the subject whenever possible. There is no one way to die, as there is no one way to live; nor is there just one way that people feel about this experience. Some people have deep religious beliefs, which may include strong beliefs in an afterlife. Some have made a peace with the end of life without the support of religion. Some are able to reconcile life conflicts with themselves, their close friends, and family, and face death with equanimity. Others do not.

Erikson (1963) talks about an older person facing aging and death with integrity. Colarusso (1998) reflects that if one has lived a fulfilled life, has reconciled the demands of the superego with the ego ideal, and has come to terms with "the inevitability of the death of all living things," then the person may have achieved "wisdom" (p. 136).

Older adults need an opportunity to discuss their fears, their wishes as to how they want to die, and whatever is on their mind that needs to be "settled." Some have many fears but do not want to talk about them, or at least not in the orderly way we might wish them to. In working with people who are dying or fearing death, it is important to listen and to understand both direct expressions of fears as well as metaphors or other indirect ways of expressing concerns.

Although many, if not all, mental health professionals and physicians (and social work students) feel anxious in dealing with death and dying because it stirs up their own personal fears as well as feelings of guilt and incompetence—because they not only are "surviving" but can't "solve this problem"—it is nonetheless important for you as social work students to realize that what you have to offer is a connection to the dying person (and their families) so that they are not alone—and not alone with their thoughts and their fears.

Systemic issues do not leave us even in the process of dying. Although we may ask people about how they might want to die, this often is irrelevant to what actually happens. Cloud (2000a), in reporting on this subject, asserts that "we should choose to die well. Too many of us don't" (p. 60). Citing a recent TIME/CNN poll, Cloud (2000a) observes that although seven out of ten Americans express a wish to die at home, three-fourths actually die in medical institutions; more than a third of terminally ill people are in intensive care units for a minimum of ten days. "Specialists say 95 percent of pain in terminally ill people can be mollified, but studies show that nearly half of Americans die in pain, surrounded and treated by strangers" (Cloud, 2000a, pp. 61-62). The need for hospice care and well-funded home care services exists; a recent dramatic decrease in federal funds for home health care has seriously affected needed services, "forcing many Medicare patients to spend more time in hospitals and nursing homes" (Pear, 2000, p. A1).

Death, of course, can occur at any stage in the life cycle; death and loss are discussed further in the next chapter.

Discussion

Biopsychosocial problems of the elderly exist on many levels, including the struggle to find appropriate opportunities for the young-old to have a sense of meaning in continuing work, volunteer activities, and leisure pursuits. Although some elderly people are economically comfortable or wealthy, many live in straitened circumstances and struggle to make ends meet. Lack of adequate housing, adequate food, and medical care present problems to them. The rural elderly, for example, many of whom are minorities, comprise about 30 percent of people over age sixty-five and live in a variety of locations and circumstances; many live alone, do not have transportation, and are isolated. Services are often not accessible to them (Germain, 1991).

As people age and many become disabled, physical, psychiatric, social, and economic problems become more critical. One major issue in the 2000 presidential race was inclusion of a prescription drug plan for the elderly under Medicare; this is a critical issue, as older people need more medication, which is usually expensive, and they often have difficulty paying for it with modest or low fixed incomes. Current debates also center on nursing homes (many of which provide inadequate care), lack of Medicare funds for assisted living at home (including hospice care for the dying), and lack of uniform standards of home health care. These topics are discussed further in Chapter 12.

CONCLUSION

Chapter 9, on latency children and adolescents, ended with Peter Pan's never-never land. Although some adults remain forever in Peter's realm, many do move ahead into the world of adults while hopefully retaining his spirit of play and humor. Attaining maturity, and with it the capacity to assume responsibilities, is the ultimate achievement of adulthood—perhaps never fully attained as we struggle with residues from earlier periods. The achievement of maturity also enables us to regulate our emotions—a task central in infancy but continuing in importance as our emotions, relationships, and life situations become more complex. Maturity ideally allows us to be at peace with ourselves; to appreciate our strengths and accept our vulnerabilities; to be able to meet our needs while being open to meeting the needs of others and putting those first when necessary, as when our children cry out to us in the middle of the night and we are tired. Maturity means the capacity to forgive ourselves for our past mistakes and to forgive others for theirs.

Gaining maturity affords us a greater perspective on life and our relationships. Life's struggles and pain can endow us with a sensitivity and compassion for others, including people who are different from us, and give a deeper appreciation of life and close relationships. As Colarusso (1997) reminds us, deeper connections to others produce feelings of poignancy as we realize the prospect of loss, especially as we move into later phases of adulthood.

Life is full of transitions and changes; the meanings we make of these, beyond the objective happenings themselves, are critical to how we react and adapt; it is important to understand "how people 'make sense' of the course of their lives, including problems in maintaining a coherent sense of self" (Cohler and Galatzer-Levy, 1990, p. 222). Levinson's concern with the life structure and its meanings to people at varying points in time carries a similar message (Levinson and Levinson, 1996).

The search for meaning, however, is a cognitive exercise (albeit with an affective connection) occurring at a conscious level; but our past history is always with us, even if not acknowledged, recognized, or remembered—even if avoided or hidden out of sight in the depths of our selves. If we asked Susan B.'s mother (in Chapter 8) about the meaning of her daughter to her and of her attachment to her daughter, she could answer this. But she did not seem to be aware of the meaning of the deep emotional impact on her of her own mother's early death and how this connected to her fears of being apart from Susan. In what has been described as anniversary suicides, people have committed suicide at the same age a parent was when that parent also committed suicide. Does the suicidal offspring always understand the meaning of this act?

As we turn to the next chapter on transitions, crises, and loss, the combined perspectives of looking at objective events, the cognitive meanings people make of these events, their affective reactions, and the conflicts and traumas these events evoke will further our deepest understanding. If indeed the wisdom of late adulthood enables people to integrate logic and emotion (Edelstein and Noam [1982] as cited by Stevens-Long, 1990), let us borrow this wisdom as we continue to explore and understand human development.

LEARNING EXERCISE

1. Interview an elderly person (not a relative or client) and discuss his or her views of life and social world. What values does he or she hold to be important, and what are some of the main factors that contribute to his or her present satisfaction and/or dissatisfaction with life? What are his or her views about the needs of the elderly population?

SUGGESTED READINGS

Articles

Cain, B. (1988). Divorce among elderly women: A growing social phenomenon. *Social Casework, 69,* 563-568.

Mackey, R. A. and O'Brien, B. A. (1999). Adaptation in lasting marriages. *Families in Society, 80,* 587-596.

McDermott, C. J. (1990). Empowering elderly nursing home residents: The resident's campaign rights. *Social Work, 35,* 155-157.

Books

Berman-Rossi, T. (1986). The fight against hopelessness and despair: Institutionalized aged. In A. Gitterman and L. Shulman (Eds.), *Mutual aid groups and the life cycle* (pp. 333-358). Itasca: F. E. Peacock Publishers, Inc.

Kennedy, G. J. (2000). *Geriatric mental health care: A treatment guide for health professionals.* New York: The Guilford Press.

Levinson, D. and Levinson, J. (1996). *The seasons of a woman's life.* New York: Knopf.

Nemiroff, R. and Colarusso, C. (1990). *New dimensions in adult development.* New York: Basic Books.

Scharff, D. and Scharff, J. (1991). *Object relations couple therapy.* Northvale: Jason Aronson Inc.

SECTION III:
SPECIAL ISSUES

Chapter 11

Life Transitions, Crises, and Loss

There is a sadness in coming to the end of anything in life. Man's instinct clings to the Life that will never end.

Lewis Carroll

We like to think that a permanency exists in our lives, a constancy that will remain; we will remain, our parents will, our homes will stay the same. But perhaps, as it has been said before, the only permanent aspect in our lives is the inevitability of change. Change begins from the moment of conception and continues during the steady, progressive evolution of the baby's embryonic state in utero. Birth brings with it the child's expulsion from the womb into the world, and a mother's experience of holding a real child that for so long had been part of her own body and who existed in her imagination. Otto Rank saw this expulsion from the womb as the birth trauma, the root of all separation anxiety.

Change can bring with it anticipation, excitement, anxiety, and new opportunities, but also often the loss of what has been. Watching their child walk across the stage to receive a high school diploma is one of life's most poignant moments for many parents; pride and love are intermingled with sadness and the realization that the child has begun the transition from adolescence into the beginnings of early adulthood, often accompanied by leaving home. "The pain of loss and suffering that so assuredly accompanies living is ever present at all stages of the life cycle" (Kramer, 1998, p. 211).

This chapter discusses the nature of life transitions and how people adapt to them; it also discusses crises people encounter in life and how they can produce breakdown but also have the potential of producing further growth. Losses are addressed from the perspective of those inevitable in transversing the life cycle as well as those experienced in painful life events, such as divorce.

Loss is frequently experienced in relation to positive life events; changes, even those most eagerly anticipated events—such as a child's going away to camp, or a couple moving into a new "dream" house—involve saying good-bye, even if temporarily for summer camp or more permanently if the couple has sold their old house. A promotion, eagerly awaited, means saying good-bye to one's old position and perhaps to one's colleagues. Loss can also mean relinquishing less tangible realities, such as aspects of one's self-image or of other meaningful possibilities, including the "road not taken" or hopes for other outcomes or reconciliations.

This chapter is concluded with a discussion of death, the ultimate loss, including death of people close to us as well as the anticipation of our own passing. Mourning and the expression of grief vary in individuals and in cultures. But acknowledging losses (be it death or other life losses) and grieving for them are considered essential for good mental health. Although the loss of a loved one or anticipating our own death can be frightening and extraordinarily painful, it also presents opportunities for working out conflictual relationships, renewing a sense of meaning of life, and enhancing closeness to others through feeling love and feeling that we are valued.

TRANSITIONS

People go through many transitions in life with major and minor consequences. Schlossberg (1981) has developed a useful model for the analysis of transitions and how people adapt to them. She includes three sets of factors: the first relates to the characteristics of the transition itself, such as whether it represents a loss or a gain; the second relates to the characteristics of the pretransition and posttransition environments, such as the presence of support systems; and the third relates to the characteristics of the individual, such as the person's psychosocial competence.

Schlossberg (1981) asserts that a transition has occurred if the event brings about new ways in which people think about themselves and the world, which then calls for a "corresponding change in one's behavior and relationships" (p. 5). She includes nonevents (which are events that have not occurred, such as not becoming pregnant) in her definition. This is a subject raised in the last chapter; it is what Levinson and Levinson (1996) refer to as "important *unfilled components* in the life structure (p. 23). When clients seek clinical services because they are upset, it is our inclination to ask: what happened? We might not think to ask: what did *not* happen?"

Characteristics of the Transition

Schlossberg (1981) describes the following seven specific attributes that characterize transitions.

Role Change: Gain or Loss

Transitions often involve changes in one's role. Becoming engaged might represent achieving a *role gain*. Losing a job, by contrast, might represent a *role loss*. Schlossberg (1981) observes that whether a negative or positive change occurs, "some degree of stress" is experienced by the person (p. 8).

Affect: Positive or Negative

People have feelings about going through a transition, which can be primarily positive (as in getting married) or primarily negative (as in bereavement). Schlossberg (1981) observes that ambivalence usually accompanies role changes; new parents, for example, typically have mixed emotions.

Source: Internal or External

People often have a choice in their life decisions; at other times, a determination is made for them by life circumstances or by other people. Some people may, for example, choose to go to medical school because that is their dream; others might feel they are left without a choice, because it is their parents' dream. The key element involved here is the perception of "control over one's own life" (Schlossberg, 1981, p. 9).

The concept of *locus of control* has received recent attention in the psychology of motivation. People who believe that they have no control over their lives are said to have an *external* locus of control. It is thought that people who have (and believe they have) a *internal* locus of control have better mental health; this has also been cited as an important indicator of resilience in children (Richman and Bowen, 1997). It should be noted that learned helplessness is also regarded as a feature of some types of personality disorders and that the stance of some individuals that their life circumstances are imposed on them from without may be a defensive posture against taking responsibility. Pinderhughes (1983) has popularized the concept of *empowerment* in social work, which she sees as "the treatment goal for all clients"; it is defined as "the ability and capacity to cope constructively with the forces that undermine and hinder coping, the achievement of some reasonable control over their destiny" (p. 333).

Timing: On Time or Off Time

In the life-cycle perspective, major life events occur at relatively predictable points in time. This can play an important part in how people react to life transitions. Schlossberg (1981) refers to Neugarten's (1979) concept of on-time and off-time events, and to the fact that many people compare themselves with others with regard to where they are in terms of life-cycle events. It is not uncommon, for example, to hear a childless young woman talk about her "biological clock running out," in terms of a hoped-for pregnancy, or a thirty-year-old worrying that she no clear career goals. Neugarten (1979) has claimed that timing has become less relevant because events in our diverse society today are now occurring at off times. Schlossberg contends that the timing of life events is still relevant. She feels people remain concerned about where they are in comparison to others of the same age.

Onset: Gradual or Sudden

Many of life's events are expected, gradual, or planned for, such as graduations, marriages, and the birth of a baby at the end of a pregnancy. Generally, it is easier to adapt to an event that one has anticipated and prepared for than to be surprised by a sudden event, such as a natural disaster, a heart attack, or, more positively, a promotion one had not anticipated (Schlossberg, 1981).

However, although life events of gradual onset enable people to prepare for them, it does not mean that they necessarily do so. People may deny an upcoming change and do nothing mentally or in reality to plan for the change. Paradoxically, some people may be better prepared for sudden changes, because they may have fantasized about them, even if they thought the event was unlikely to happen.

In Chapter 8, we discussed a four-year-old about to have back surgery who playacted the event with her grandfather. This helped her to anticipate what was going to happen to her and to cope with it. The technique of anticipatory guidance applied by clinical social workers can be helpful to clients facing a transition; children about to be placed in a foster home, for example, may feel less overwhelmed if they have a chance to process this, to anticipate the steps of what might happen, and to rehearse what they might do and feel in this new situation.

Duration: Permanent, Temporary, Uncertain

How long the transition will last affects one's adaptation to it; if the transition event is something positive, such as a promotion, one can feel good about it being permanent; if the event is undesirable, one will feel better to think that it will be over soon (Schlossberg, 1981). The lifestyle changes you have had to make to be a social work student and the academic and field placement expectations placed on you are more tolerable when you realize that schooling will not go on forever. It should be added that the idea of "permanency," even of a desirable event, such as the thought of being married to a person forever, can add to one's anxiety.

Schlossberg (1981) states that probably the greatest distress is connected to events which are uncertain in outcome. This would be especially true of negative events, such as illness. If someone has a serious illness, what can be expected? To be left with ambiguities rather than answers can be devastating. Social workers, among others, have been employees in agencies where it is known that some people will be laid off, but it is not known who or when or which services will be curtailed. The uncertainty can contribute greatly to anxiety and demoralization.

Degree of Stress

Although all transitions involve some stress, it is important to look specifically at the magnitude of stress involved for a person in the process of transition. Schlossberg (1981) refers to the well-known Social Readjustment Rating Scale devised by Holmes and Rahe in 1967. The premise of the Holmes-Rahe scale is that all change, whether negative or positive (even vacations and holidays), produces stress, and people who have gone through multiple changes in a short time are at greater risk for becoming sick. The scale ranks types of stress; the highest stress is associated with the death of a spouse; and the lowest stresses are events such as vacations. A person's general state of mental and physical health are also ranked. Schlossberg (1981) has some reservations about the Holmes-Rahe Scale, including the lack of attention to individual variation, since the subjective reactions people may have to a given stressor vary.

Schlossberg (1981) also places emphasis on the "balance between a person's deficits and resources at the time the event occurs" (pp. 9-10). By resources she refers to the person's general biopsychosocial state, including supportive relationships and capacity to cope. She observes that the ratio of strengths to deficits can vary over time.

Characteristics of Pretransition and Posttransition Environments

Schlossberg (1981) categorizes environmental influences affecting a person's adaptation to transitions as follows: interpersonal support systems, institutional supports, and physical setting.

Interpersonal Support System

In emphasizing the importance of supportive relationships in helping people adapt to transitions involving losses and stress, Schlossberg (1981) specifies three types of systems: intimate relationships, the family unit, and the network of friends. She emphasizes the ability to care for others as well as to receive and accept support oneself. This would relate to the concept of mutual aid groups discussed in Chapter 4.

Institutional Supports

Institutions refer to a wide variety of community organizations and their roles in providing services and emotional support (Schlossberg, 1981). Work organizations, for example, can be sources of stress and/or support for their employees. Societal rituals, such as weddings and graduations, provide needed support and validation to people. By contrast, no supportive rituals are offered to people going to court for a divorce.

Physical Setting

Schlossberg (1981) discusses the physical setting in a comprehensive way, including weather, neighborhoods, and living arrangements. In discussing personal space, she emphasizes the importance of "comfort, privacy, and aesthetics" (p. 12). (This topic was also addressed in Chapter 4.)

Characteristics of the Individual

Schlossberg (1981) discusses eight attributes of the individual contributing to adaptation to transitions, including:

- psychosocial competence
- sex (in the sense of gender and sex-role identification)
- age (and life stages)
- state of health
- race-ethnicity
- socioeconomic status
- value orientation and
- previous experience with a transition of a similar nature.

As these psychosocial characteristics are similar to those already discussed in this book, we will not detail them here.

CRISIS THEORY

The concept of crisis has been used in different ways by different authors; it is most often applied to external crises, often disasters, and usually unanticipated crises, such as witnessing (or being wounded in) a school shooting, facing the sudden death of a loved one, or losing one's home in a fire. Erikson (1963), among others, has discussed *developmental* or *maturational crises,* which accompany changes through the life cycle; Mahler and colleagues (1975) refer to the *rapprochement* crisis. Crisis, however, in a clinical sense is generally equated with overwhelming stress; people are said to be in a state of crisis if they are experiencing such extreme stress that their usual coping mechanisms are not adequate to facilitate adaptation.

The source of the stress can also be maturational, such as when a panic reaction ensues in the context of severe separation anxiety associated with the transition of leaving home for the first time. A crisis state can be experienced when going through an anticipated life event in an unanticipated manner, such as the premature birth of a child. A crisis state can be triggered by internal conflicts, such as those related to performance anxiety or sexual confusion. These can trigger states of anxiety and/or depression and precipitate a suicidal crisis.

Many clinicians agree that a state of crisis may be produced by both external and internal conditions. The classical writings on crisis theory address both; today, however, many place emphasis in practice only on the external systems elements of crisis management and on cognitive-behavioral adaptations, that is, helping the person with crises affecting social functioning by utilizing problem solving, finding appropriate resources, and enhancing coping mechanisms.

In discussing crisis intervention in the emergency room, Puryear (1984) states:

> The five main principles of emergency room crisis intervention are: setting limited goals, employing focused problem solving, expecting the individuals or family to take some action on their own behalf, providing support for that action, and building self-reliance and self-esteem. These principles are employed in six basic steps: establishing rapport, taking charge, assessing the patient or family's problems and assets, closing and follow-up. . . . Specific techniques, such as assigning tasks, active listening, positive reinforcement, reversing, and reframing are employed to help mobilize people in crisis. (p. 33)

Caplan's definition of a crisis as "an upset in a steady state" (Rapoport, 1970, p. 277) is frequently used. People generally manage to adapt to change and "maintain a state of equilibrium" (Rapoport, 1970, p. 276). However, through life-cycle changes, life transitions, and external and internal crises, people may experience "sudden discontinuities by which the homeostatic state is disturbed and which result in a state of disequilibrium," but they may nevertheless be able to cope with these sudden changes through "adequate adaptive or equilibrating mechanisms" (Rapoport, 1970,

p. 276). If not, they may enter a state of crisis, as their usual ways of solving problems are inadequate "to the task for a rapid reestablishment of equilibrium. The *hazardous events* [italics added], or stress factors that precipitate the crisis require a solution that is novel to the individual in relation to his previous life experience and usual and normal repertoire of problem-solving mechanisms" (Rapoport, 1970, p. 276).

The factors (or hazardous events) precipitating the crisis may be related not only to present life stresses but to past events and "may reactivate and trigger off unresolved or partially resolved unconscious conflicts" (Rapoport, 1970, p. 276). Although often overwhelming the person with strong emotions, the crisis can at the same time serve as a catalyst in fostering recall of old memories and feelings; this offers an opportunity not only to resolve the present crisis but to work through past conflictual material. "Thus the crisis with its mobilization of energy may operate as a 'second chance' in correcting earlier distortion and maladaptions" (Rapoport, 1970, p. 277).

Three basic types of events are hazardous for the homeostatic state: "a threat, a loss, or a challenge" (Rapoport, 1970, p. 277).

> A threat may be directed to instinctual needs or to an individual's sense of integrity or autonomy. A loss may be that of a person or an experience of acute deprivation. A challenge may be to survival, growth, mastery, or self-expression. Each of these states has a major characteristic affect. Threat carries with it high anxiety. Loss is experienced with affect of depression or mourning. Challenge is accompanied by some anxiety but carries with it an important ingredient of hope, release of energy for problem-solving, and expectation of mastery. (Rapoport, 1970, p. 277)

Rapoport (1970) highlights the major goals and techniques of crisis intervention. Since time is of the essence, clients should be seen as soon as possible; long delays on waiting lists will adversely affect this group. Crisis work does not lend itself to a lengthy diagnostic process; "diagnosis and treatment go hand in hand" (Rapoport, 1970, p. 288); immediate help is essential while the state of crisis is ongoing and before it resolves into a "new state of equilibrium [which] may be the same as or worse or better than that achieved before the crisis" (p. 277). Individuals and families may become more resistant to clinical intervention once the crisis has passed; in the midst of a crisis, they are more amenable to reorganization (psychologically) individually and as a family. "A little help, rationally directed and purposefully focused at a strategic time, is more effective than more extensive help given at a period of less emotional accessibility" (Rapoport, 1970, p. 287). Although time limits are set (usually not more than six weeks, and often less), a flexible use of time is recommended; that is, people might need to be seen several times a week or for longer periods than one hour.

A primary task of the clinician is to lower the client's anxiety; one effective way to do this is for the clinician to share his or her thoughts with the client about what the problem is and what the "operating dynamics" are in a way that "enables the client to get a manageable cognitive grasp of the situation" (Rapoport, 1970, p. 288). This understanding is very important as cognitive confusion often exists and the person is "bewildered and literally does not know how to grasp and understand what has been happening to him, how to evaluate reality, or how to anticipate, formulate, and evaluate the possible outcome of the crisis" (Rapoport, 1970, p. 281).

It is important to convey a sense of hope to the client; this involves having a "quality of intensity and investment in the client" (Rapoport, 1970, p. 289). Clinicians "should communicate actively both concern and authenticity," and at the same time utilize their "authority based on expertness and competence" (Rapoport, 1970, p. 300). Giving direction and advice, while at the same time helping the client develop a sense of autonomy and mastery as soon as possible, are often very effective when clients are overwhelmed. The establishment of a contract with the client is emphasized, as this helps establish time boundaries, structure, and goals with the client's full participation.

Some variation exists in how crisis intervention ends; time limits are considered important, and clients are helped to anticipate future stress and think about how they might cope with this. In some models of crisis intervention, the client is given the choice of continuing in more conventional therapy (usually with another clinician) or is offered the option of returning in the future.

Many writers stress the importance of knowing the precipitating problem leading to the crisis. Rapoport (1970) has observed that sometimes the cognitive mastery that the client gains from understanding and realistically perceiving the precipitating stress can be so therapeutically helpful that the client needs no additional clinical help. Some writers have emphasized that the precipitating factor might have stirred underlying psychological pain, which in itself needs to be explored. Hoffman and Remmel (1975) are cautious about accepting the precipitating event at face value as the main focus; they talk about the *precipitant*, which is "the thought or feeling aroused by the precipitating event. . . . It is the pain connected with the earlier unresolved conflict, and it is precisely this experience that impels the client to pick up the telephone to call for help" (p. 260).

Hoffman and Remmel (1975) are referring primarily to the traditional clinical model of clients seeking help with internal psychological distress, even if precipitated by an external event, such as a wife calling for help because her husband left her. Although this experience of being rejected and abandoned will be upsetting to most wives, the precipitant might be the pain arising from past and previously unexplored losses and/or rejections.

Crisis intervention, however, is often applied to situations in which clients do not pick up the phone and call for help but in which they are offered help, as in extreme, externally produced crises such as fires and school shootings. Complex and subtle distinctions must be considered here; some crises, such as those produced by external disasters, are so overwhelming that most people will be in a state of shock and disequilibrium after experiencing them. However, even in these crises, people still bring with them a past history of attachment and loss that will eventuate in differentiated and individual ways of responding both to the crisis and to offers of help.

The degree to which the emotional meaning of the crisis and the conflicts underlying the crisis are addressed also relate to the theoretical orientation of the clinician and helping agency. Smith (1976) has observed that two divergent approaches are taken to crisis treatment: "Jacobsen, Strickler and Morley (1968) refer to them as the generic and individual approaches to crisis intervention" (p. 167). Clinicians using the *generic* model analyze specific hazardous events (such as going through the divorce process), then develop specific treatment protocols related to the stresses this crisis produces and the tasks needed to resolve it. In the *individual* approach, no tasks are predetermined, but the focus is "on the problem-solving activities that each individual must accomplish in resolving the crisis. . . . Psychological tasks are used to resolve the crisis but these tasks differ from one client to another" (Smith, 1976, p. 167).

The following case illustrates an individual approach; this is followed by a discussion of a generic approach to crisis intervention.

Case Illustration of the Individual Approach to Crisis Intervention

Aguilera and Messick (1974) discuss the case of Mr. Z., which illustrates an effective use of crisis intervention techniques. Mr. Z., forty-three, president of a large corporation, was married and had three children. He apparently was in a state of equilibrium until the day he collapsed at work with a heart attack and was immediately hospitalized. He had been in good health and had no history of cardiac problems. However, his father and one brother died at about his age and his only living brother was seriously incapacitated, all due to heart problems. Mr. Z. had taken good care of his health and diet and exercised vigorously; he was "determined to avoid dying young or becoming an invalid like his brother" (Aguilera and Messick, 1974, p. 100).

Mr. Z. was an "exceedingly difficult patient," who was anxious, slept poorly, denied being worried about his physical problem, and demanded constant explanations of everything. His heart attack was judged to be mild with a good prognosis. His doctor felt he was not coping well with his illness and referred him for crisis intervention.

> In the first session the therapist observed Mr. Z.'s overt and covert signs of anxiety and depression and determined, through discussion with him his *perception* of what hospitalization meant to him, his usual *patterns of coping* with stress, and available *situational supports* [all italics added]. (Aguilera and Messick, 1974, p. 102)

This approach is generally used in crisis work: assessing how the client perceives the problem, the client's usual ways of coping, and using available situational (or environmental) supports, which, in this case, involved talking with Mr. Z.'s wife and doctor. The crisis therapist felt that the primary problem was Mr. Z.'s fear that he would either die or become an invalid; she also felt that his wife needed emotional support to be able to support her husband in this situation. Understanding the source of Mr. Z.'s anxiety and observing his poor coping in the hospital, the crisis therapist recommended that he be removed from intensive care to a private room, and be allowed half-hour periods of phone calls three times a day so that he could continue to be involved with his business.

When this was accomplished, Mr. Z. relaxed considerably and adapted to the hospital regimen. He shared with the clinician his feelings about the past losses of his father and brother and his anxieties about his own future. The following excerpt illustrates how an interview focused on concerns in the here and now becomes a critical tool in crisis intervention.

> Through discussion and verbal feedback, it was possible to get Mr. Z. to view his illness and the changes it would make in his life in a realistic perspective. No, he was *not* an invalid. Yes, he would be able to work and live a normal life. No, he would not have to give up sailing, just have someone else do most of the crewing. Yes, he would be able to resume his activities but would continue them at a more leisurely pace. . . . Gradually he became more accepting as he began to realize the impending myocardial infarction was a warning he should heed and that with proper care and some diminishing of his usual hectic pace he could continue to live a productive and useful life. (Aguilera and Messick, 1974, p. 104)

In addition to providing emotional support to his wife, the clinician discussed with her some needed changes in his lifestyle, but Mrs. Z. was also helped to understand that her husband was not fragile and *could* cope, thus relieving some of the burden on Mrs. Z. "The children and Mrs. Z. were encouraged to continue in their daily activities so that Mr. Z. would not feel that his being at home was disrupting to their lives" (Aguilera and Messick, 1974, p. 105). Anticipation of future events, such as Mr. Z. returning home, were discussed; this is typical in crisis intervention. Six sessions took place, which were contracted in advance; emphasis was on his strength and autonomy—all features of crisis work.

Mr. Z. and his wife were helped to adapt, and their anxiety was greatly reduced. Mr. Z. could "intellectually understand his reasons for his denial and dependence/independence conflicts" and could accept the possibility that his illness could recur: " 'At least now I've learned to relax and roll with the punches' " (Aguilera and Messick, 1974, p. 105).

Mr. Z. was in a crisis: he was overwhelmed with anxiety; his basic equilibrium was disturbed, as was his family's equilibrium. Mr. Z. was fortunate to be referred to a clinician; many people with sudden life-threatening illnesses or medical conditions which will drastically alter their way of life are not afforded this opportunity. Mr. Z. received important psychological help; his losses and his fears about his own mortality and disability were able to surface as he faced his own worst nightmare and coped with it.

Analyzing the Z. case in terms of Schlossberg's (1981) classification of transitions:

1. We observe a role change, as Mr. Z. temporarily lost his role as executive and took on the role of patient.
2. His affect was negative, as his anxiety level was high and he was depressed.
3. The source was external, as he had no control over this event (even though it occurred internally, within his body).
4. The question of whether this was on time or off time is debatable (he was in the prime of life, and not "old enough" to be disabled this way, although it is not uncommon for people to have heart attacks at his age; it was, however, an on-time event in terms of his family history).
5. The onset was sudden (extremely so), although at some level he may have been anticipating this could happen.
6. The duration of this transition was permanent, in that it was clear that he was vulnerable to heart problems, and some damage had been done.
7. It was also temporary, as the critical point of the illness had passed, and he could resume his previous level of functioning, with some limitations.
8. It was also uncertain because the condition could recur.
9. The degree of stress he experienced was very high, although this improved with intervention.

In looking at the pretransition and posttransition environments, we observe that he was able to control his employment status, and he had a good interpersonal family support system. However, due to this stress, his wife was "caving in," and, without the intervention, she might not have been able to deal with his demanding and anxiety-provoking behaviors; her inability to support him appropriately might have led to further maladaption and to disequilibrium in the marital situation. The couple's sexual relationship and how Mr. Z.'s heart problem might affect this, realistically and subjectively, was one factor not discussed in this case. Olkin (1999) has observed that there is often an "absence of discussion about sex and disability" (p. 226).

Mr. Z.'s immediate physical setting, the cardiac intensive care unit, was not advantageous for him emotionally, adding to his distress. An environmental modification was made, as the clinician recommended that he be moved to a private room; the change improved his mental state.

In terms of his individual characteristics, we can say that Mr. Z. had a high level of psychosocial competence, that he was identified with his male role, that he was in Levinson and Levinson's (1996) transition-building life stage of young adulthood going into middle adulthood, that his state of health had been good, and that he made a good recovery (with a good prognosis) from his cardiac problem. Mr. Z. had a high socioeconomic status, his value orientation seemed dominated by work and success. He had no previous experience with a transition like this before, but he faced a similar situation with his father and his two brothers and probably with himself in fantasy. His success in mastering this event, entailing as it did his being in a temporarily dependent state, would probably enable him to cope better if he were to fall ill again, although he might benefit from additional support in that event.

Absent Mr. Z.'s high level of psychosocial competence, not every person going through this experience would have adapted so well in such a short period of time. Someone, for example, with a fragile ego, a latent psychotic fear of annihilation, or a panic disorder might have seriously decompensated during such a medical crisis and been in need of more extensive help; a marriage on the verge of dissolution may also have produced different consequences.

Illustration of the Generic Model of Crisis Intervention

Clinicians using the generic model analyze specific hazardous events and develop specific treatment protocols related to the stresses these crises produce and the tasks needed to resolve them. One well-known generic model involves working with mothers who have given birth to premature babies (Kaplan and Mason, 1965). The authors have analyzed the stresses that mothers go through in such an event, including: having an unanticipated delivery; experiencing anxiety about whether the baby will live and, if so, be normal; returning home without the baby (who usually needs to remain at the hospital); and adapting to the baby's return home.

Kaplan and Mason (1965) found that the mother must complete four psychological tasks which are necessary for her adaptation and for the development of a positive relationship with her child. When the baby is delivered, the mother's first task is "preparation for a possible loss of the child" (p. 124); next she must come to terms with "her maternal failure to deliver a normal full-term baby" (p. 124). (This statement refers to the mother's self-criticism, not the authors' judgment of the mother.) As she grapples with these tasks, "anticipatory grief and depression" occur simultaneously (p. 124). The third step, after the baby has been in the hospital for several weeks, is "the resumption of the process of relating to the baby" (p. 124); finally, she learns in what ways a premature baby is different due to "its special needs and growth patterns" (p. 125).

As they are structured and specific, the protocols that have proliferated for specific tasks related to crisis types have often been carried out by paraprofessionals. Protocols can also sensitize clinicians to clients' possible reactions in a specific crisis. In addition, knowing that many people have similar feelings in similar situations, the clinician can validate a client's feelings about the crisis.

Analyzing hazardous events has led to the development of prevention programs, such as *primary prevention* programs set up before an anticipated crisis might occur. Working with patients and families prior to admission to hospitals or nursing homes, for example, can help them anticipate problems and their own adaptations and prepare them to work on these specific issues.

News reports of community disasters often mention that crisis teams are being sent to help people deal with their feelings and changed life circumstances. This form of *secondary prevention* can help people express their feelings, gain support, and hopefully prevent emotional decompensation.

However, when generic crisis intervention deals only with tasks inherent in a specific hazardous event, the specific meaning of the crisis to the individual and psychological conflicts that may be precipitated by this event are often left unexplored; in addition, variations in individual adaptations are not acknowledged, even though they may be highly significant. Recognition of such variations (for example, the presence of severe psychopathology or characterological patterns) requires some effort at differential diagnosis.

Woods and Hollis (1990) discuss a case in which a supportive policewoman, using a generic model, was providing crisis intervention for a woman who had been raped. The policewoman, who had learned in her training that the expression of anger was an essential piece of the rape protocol, pressured the woman to talk about her anger; but the woman, unbeknownst to the helper, was experiencing flashbacks and was still too frightened even to feel her anger. Woods and Hollis (1990) express concern about generic models that are designed and utilized in a rigid way; in addition, they express concern about inadequacy of training for many of the people carrying out this work.

Discussion

Crisis intervention is widely practiced today. From the systems perspective, it is one of the short-term models in particular favor with managed care companies. Generally, it is time limited, focused on a primary (that is, immediate and apparent) problem, and aims to help clients restore their previous level of functioning and equilibrium. Crisis intervention has been used very effectively in many situations, as we saw with the case of Mr. Z. However, a number of serious problems with this approach are encountered: (1) the ways in which a crisis may mask underlying psychological issues can be overlooked; (2) it may be applied blindly to people for whom crisis is a way of life; and (3) it may be seen as a cure-all substitute for needed ongoing support and psychotherapy.

Psychological Issues in Crisis Intervention

As originally envisaged, crisis intervention has the potential not only to return people to their baseline level of functioning but to help them reach higher levels of personality organization by working on key issues while the person is open to change. However, the views of different clinicians as to how this happens, or even if this should happen, reveal inconsistencies. In fact, some lack of clarity exists in this regard in Rapoport's (1970) classical article on crisis intervention. On the one hand, Rapoport asserts that crisis intervention has a strong focus on the here and now and relies heavily on problem-solving approaches. However, without describing the mechanisms involved, she also comments that crisis intervention can produce important personality changes and help resolve old conflicts, also the view of Woods and Hollis (1990).

Hoffman and Remmel (1975), as noted earlier, do not accept the premise of simply applying specific tasks to help clients solve their presenting problems; they are concerned with discovering the underlying precipitant, which is what actually motivates the call for help. Golan (1980) expresses concern that if clinicians look with a narrow focus only at the problem to be solved, they may "miss entirely the clues that other, more lasting disruptions are taking place concurrently" in the client's life (p. 547). Golan (1980) discusses transitional issues in a person's life that might be "obscured by the acute aspects of the immediate situation" (p. 543).

Crisis As a Way of Life

Although crisis is generally seen as a disturbance in a steady state, for some people living in crisis is a "quasi-steady" state; crisis work has sometimes been misapplied when working with this population (Rapoport, 1970). Some of these people have borderline personalities or character disorders; Reiner and Kaufman (1959) have described people with these underlying tendencies to be impulsive and to act out, creating chaos for themselves and others in their world; their crisis orientation is a way of protecting themselves from feeling their underlying depression. "Persons with character disorders are constantly threatened by the anxiety stemming from an unresolved depression. Much of their activity is designed to ward off the anxiety" (Reiner and Kaufman, 1959, p. 7).

> These impulse-ridden people appear to be in a perpetual state of crisis. It is not so much that they enjoy the uncertainty and chaos, as that they must have "something happening" in order to feel alive. . . . One must relate to these clients in the midst of their crises, or not at all. A further difficulty is that these acting-out persons—in spite of the intensity of their emotions—cannot enter into a discussion of their feelings and behavior. Their way of communicating is through action. (Reiner and Kaufman, 1959, p. 8)

Because of the intensity of the feelings of these clients, their manipulativeness, and their tendency to enmesh the clinician in their chaos, it is not unusual for the latter to be drawn into this maelstrom. Beginning social work students are especially vulnerable as they attempt to "fix" the problem and restore peace. It is also not uncommon to see this anxiety and chaos transmitted to the agency itself, as staff become involved in an atmosphere of crisis.

People with character disorders and borderline personalities need long-term, supportive treatment, and traditional crisis-oriented work is not the treatment of choice, although in certain situations emergency help is essential (Rapoport, 1970; Woods and Hollis, 1990).

Crisis Intervention As Insufficient Treatment

Time limits for crisis treatment are strictly adhered to; usually six weeks is the maximum time allowed. Some clients need more time to work out their crisis-related problems, and these time constraints can result in pressuring clients who need a slower pace and more time to integrate the traumatic events they have experienced (Woods and Hollis, 1990). Caplan (1976), the father of crisis theory, has questioned his original recommendation for six weeks of therapy following bereavement. He has observed that although people can mobilize useful resources during the initial crisis, this state is "usually followed by a prolonged period of adjustment during the adaptation to a radically new pattern of life . . . the issues involved . . . demanded that [one] continue supportive contact (Caplan, 1976, p. xv). Applegate and Bonovitz (1995) express concern about underlying developmental issues being left untouched in brief treatment; patients' "core psychosocial issues [remain] unseen and untreated. They remain frozen in failure" (p. 10).

Crisis intervention serves many useful purposes and can help restore functioning when it has been derailed; it can also be beneficial as part of ongoing therapy when a client becomes immobilized. It was suggested in Chapter 2 that when executive functioning and cognitive functioning falter, it is important to restore these functions, and methodologies developed through the application of crisis theory can be very helpful in this process. Crisis therapy is frequently valuable when it is the treatment of choice; it is problematic today because often no choice is given. Instead, it is mandated by managed care and its providers because it appears to be efficient, "neat," and inexpensive.

LOSS AND GRIEF

Loss, in a normative way, accompanies us throughout the life cycle, as we separate from our parents, change jobs, watch our children become adults and move away, face the death of people we know, and contemplate our own ending. Throughout this book other losses have been discussed, present in experiences such as giving up a baby for adoption, being placed in a foster home, becoming an immigrant, and learning one is infertile. During the divorce process, parents mourn the ending of a marital relationship, and children witness the end of their family as they knew it and may grieve for the parent now absent from their home; these children may experience additional losses, such as the familiarity of the family home and leaving their old school, neighborhood, and friends (Davies, 1999). Disability and illness present many losses, including: depletion of energy, sensory deprivation (resulting from loss of hearing and sight), loss of a sense of body integrity (as in amputations or mastectomies), and loss of ability to communicate (as in aphasia produced by strokes). These *primary* losses can lead to *secondary* losses related to an inability to take care of oneself, the dissolution of a marriage or partnership, and the loss of a social network, which can, in turn, produce lowered self-esteem, reactive depression, and anxiety states.

Parents of children with disabilities, chronic illness, and psychiatric illness also experience the loss of the child "that might have been," and some writers have discussed the perpetual mourning such parents experience.

Gombosi (1998), a psychoanalyst who is also the father of an autistic child, discussed the "trauma" of this discovery when his son was two and the sense of "dislocation" that he has observed in parents of autistic children, "accompanied by intense feelings, including sadness, rage, fright, and intense attachment to the child" (p. 262). He feels that parents can adapt to having an autistic child, but "I think most successful parents of autistic children have a profound sense of the tragic in their lives" (Gombosi, 1998, p. 263).

FACING DEATH

It is painful to think of those we are close to dying; it is especially painful to think of ourselves dying; perhaps this is why most of us tend to deny that this will happen. Noam (1996) cites Woody Allen as saying: " 'I do not want to gain immortality through my work, I want to gain it through not dying!' " (p. 155). Dying means saying good-bye to all that we know and all whom we know. It also faces us with the existential dilemma of not being. Colarusso (1998) cites the psychoanalyst Martin Grotjohn as he contemplates his own death:

> "I did not do badly in the almost 80 years of my life. I even learned how to live a little from the people who did not know and came to me to learn. But now I am stuck again. I am not ready to die, not ready to say good-bye to this life. I am not ready to say good-bye to myself. That seems to be the worst: to say good-bye to myself" (Grotjohn, 1985, p. 297). (Colarusso, 1998, pp. 127-128)

Because it is so difficult a subject for us to face, we tend to assume no one wants to talk about it, least of all a person who is facing death. But terminally ill patients usually want to talk about dying; the frequent problem is no one wants to listen. Dempsey (1971) talks about the inaccessibility of doctors and other helping professionals when it comes to listening. A patient is quoted by Dempsey as saying: "It's hard to carry on a conversation with Dr. X. when he comes in the room with a stethoscope in his ears and puts a thermometer in my mouth." It was observed, in one large hospital in Chicago thirty years ago, that while the professional staff was certain patients were too emotionally vulnerable to talk about their impending deaths, the patients were able to find one group of staff members who would listen: the cleaning women, usually conversing with them in the middle of the night.

One of the most distinguished pioneers in the field of death and dying is Elisabeth Kübler-Ross (1969), who stressed the importance of bringing this subject out into the open and talking freely about it with patients and their loved ones. Death has always been with us; however, changes have occurred in the way we respond to death now from the way people responded in the past. Paradoxically, as Kübler-Ross herself emphasizes, it is a fact that we generally handled this event better in the past than we seem able to do now, despite (or perhaps because of) all the advances in our modern medicine. In fact, these very advances may have complicated the whole process of dying.

People generally died at home in the past, with family and friends around them. The family physician probably knew the patient most of his or her life and was part of the social network of the family. Today, people tend to die in hospitals, attached to the best machines modern medicine has discovered. Kübler-Ross (1969) asks: "Is this approach our own way to cope with and repress the anxieties that a terminally or critically ill patient evokes in us?" (p. 9).

Through her experience in talking to dying patients, Kübler-Ross developed a typology of five stages of coping mechanisms with which these patients deal with their terminal illness, which are: denial and isolation, anger, bargaining, depression, and acceptance.

Stages of Coping with Death

First Stage: Denial and Isolation

Initially when told about the seriousness of their illness, most patients react with denial that this is happening; " 'No, not me, it cannot be true' " (Kübler-Ross, 1969, p. 38). Patients will gradually give up their denial, but how and when (its timing) they do this varies considerably.

Second Stage: Anger

Once people no longer deny the problem, feelings of "anger, rage, envy, and resentment" tend to dominate their feelings; the question now is: " 'Why me?' " (Kübler-Ross, 1969, p. 50); this stage can be difficult for family and staff to deal with; "this anger is displaced in all directions and projected onto the environment at times almost at random" (p. 50). Doctors and especially nurses are frequently criticized; families are "received with little cheerfulness and anticipation" (Kübler-Ross, 1969, p. 51); families generally react "with grief and tears, guilt or shame, or avoid future visits, which only increases the patient's discomfort and anger" (p. 51).

Third Stage: Bargaining

In bargaining, the patient, who has gone through the first two stages, now makes some compromise or bargain to receive an extension of time, or some special privilege. Many of these bargains are made privately with God and often are kept a secret. Sometimes the patient will make special requests to the staff. "The bargaining is really an attempt to postpone; it has to include a prize offered for 'good behavior,' it also sets a self-imposed 'deadline' (e.g. [attending] the son's wedding), and it includes an implicit promise that the patient will not ask for more if this one postponement is granted" (Kübler-Ross, 1969, p. 84).

One woman wanted very much to leave the hospital for her son's wedding. The hospital took special measures to ensure that this could happen. "She had made all sorts of promises if she could only live long enough to attend this marriage" (Kübler-Ross, 1969, p. 83). She looked very happy when she left the hospital. "I will never forget the moment when she returned to the hospital. She looked tired and somewhat exhausted and—before I could say hello—said, 'now don't forget I have another son!'" (p. 83).

Fourth Stage: Depression

As terminally ill patients weaken or undergo more surgery or treatments, they no longer deny their illness, and their anger is usually superseded by deep feelings of loss. This loss can be on many levels, such as bodily depletion or disfigurement, finances (in part related to medical costs), employment, and ability to care for their children. Kübler-Ross (1969) distinguishes the ensuing *preparatory depression* from a *reactive depression:* a preparatory depression "does not occur as a result of a past loss, but is taking into account impending losses" (p. 86). Kübler-Ross (1969) emphasizes the point that "the patient is in the process of losing everything and everybody he loves"; he will not really be helped by reassurance but if "allowed to express his sorrow he will find a final acceptance much easier" (p. 87). It is not necessary even to talk; "It is much more a feeling that can be mutually expressed and is often done better with a touch of a hand, a stroking of the hair, or just a silent sitting together" (Kübler-Ross, 1969, p. 87).

Fifth Stage: Acceptance

If the patient has successfully gone through the first four stages, he will reach the final stage of acceptance. Kübler-Ross (1969) observes that "this is not a happy stage" and in fact "is almost void of feelings" (p. 113). During this final phase, "It is as if the pain had gone, [and] the struggle is over," and the patient has gained some "peace and acceptance" (Kübler-Ross, 1969, p. 113). The patient may lose interest in the outside world, and this may be an especially difficult time for the family. This is a time that "we may together listen to the song of a bird from the outside," and the presence of others may be reassuring to know "that he is not left alone when he is no longer talking" (Kübler-Ross, 1969, p. 113).

Hope

Although each stage has its own tasks, Kübler-Ross (1969) talks about hope, "the one thing that usually persists through all these stages" (p. 138). She notes that "no matter what we call it, we found that all our patients maintained a little bit of it and were nourished by it especially in difficult times" (p. 139).

THE MOURNING PROCESS

Bereavement places a person in a vulnerable state; their physical and mental health can be negatively impacted (Kramer, 1998). The importance of grief and mourning have been emphasized in the literature; "loss and the incapacity to mourn appropriately is one core aspect of most types of psychopathology, not only depression" (Noam, 1996, p. 167). Although mourning is discussed most frequently in relation to death, it is also necessary to grieve other important losses in life.

Normal Grief

People are often in a state of shock when faced with the immediacy of a loss; it is often an encompassing feeling that affects both the person's mind and body. People feel sad, cry frequently, and may feel that they are losing control of themselves or that they are "going crazy;" this is related to the intensity of the feelings, being flooded by emotions when they are unanticipated (or sometimes being numb and unable to feel). The person is usually preoccupied with the memory of the person lost and may have difficulty concentrating on other things. Sleep is often disturbed and frequent dreams of the one who died may trouble the bereaved. There can be disturbances in eating, and weight loss (or weight gain) can occur; physical symptoms such as headaches may be present.

The person's preoccupation with the deceased may be expressed by wearing the deceased's clothing, touching his or her possessions, talking about him or her to others, and sometimes sensing the deceased's presence or having a visual illusion of him or her. These experiences are considered within the range of normal reactions (and sometimes people need to be reassured about their "normalcy"). In one study of widows and widowers in Wales, it was found that hallucinations of their deceased spouses were very common; most of the people interviewed felt that the presence of the hallucinations "helped" them (Rees, 1975, p. 70).

Linda Valli (a client discussed in Chapter 2) reported the following experience after her aunt died.

> At her aunt's funeral when she was a child, she saw her aunt in the coffin, which was a very upsetting experience for her. Shortly after this, she "saw" her Aunt sitting in a chair in the living room. . . . "She was sitting there—smiling!"

This "hallucination" was viewed as an "encapsulated" incident, occurring at the time of a death and its associated trauma for her.

Lindemann (1965), a pioneer in the field of bereavement (following his study of survivors of the Coconut Grove fire in Boston), has observed that if grief work is successfully accomplished, a person will achieve "emancipation from the bondage to the deceased, readjustment to the environment in which the deceased is missing, and the formation of new relationships" (pp. 10-11).

Bereavement rituals, found in all cultures, are often beneficial to mourners, although one can go through the rituals outwardly without mourning internally, and although support and the sharing of feelings with others is often very important to people, coming to terms with the loss is basically a personal process. "Beneath the surface of consciousness remains a core of deep sorrow that the bereaved person has to work through alone. Profound sorrow is silent" (Szalita, 1974, p. 673).

People vary in how and when they mourn; for many, after a loss, major life readjustments must take place, which (as noted in the previous discussion on crisis work) often take a long time; many people need support during this period as well.

Experiencing Grief

It is difficult to face loss, both in terms of the reality of the lost object itself and of feeling the intense feelings that usually accompany this loss. Erich Lindemann (1965) observed that "many patients try to avoid both the intense distress connected with the grief experience and the necessary expression of emotion" (p. 11). The intense pain of loss was expressed eloquently by George Foy (1999), who wrote about the death of his infant son in an intensive care unit when he was one month old. Foy, who is a professional writer, did not know if he would be able to write this story; he was so overcome with emotion that it seemed writing about it might prove impossible.

Foy was intensely involved with his son, Olivier, during his month of life. When Olivier died, Foy and his wife arranged a private burial; his preparations for the funeral helped sustain him, maintaining his feeling of connection with his son. The night before Olivier was to be cremated, Foy was unable to sleep; he realized that after the cremation, the loss would be final, and that it would be impossible for him to do "anything more to take care of him. And then you will know, finally and absolutely, that you have lost [Olivier]" (Foy, 1999, p. 51). But the worst part is the "beast," which is "quite simply, missing him, knowing he will not be with you ever again except in the makeshift and unworthy stories you tell" (Foy, 1999, p. 51).

Pathological Grief

The inability to mourn can produce a number of physical and psychological symptoms. People can experience pathological forms of grief, including depression, suicidal thoughts, substance abuse, and/or acting-out behaviors. People may develop somatic symptoms similar to those of the deceased person. "A woman whose late husband had suffered for years from Parkinson disease developed a Parkinson-like tremor, gait, and masklike face" (Szalita, 1974, p. 674).

People who have strongly ambivalent feelings toward the person who has died generally have more difficulty mourning that person and are more prone to pathological grief, which is often accompanied by intense (and usually irrational) feelings of guilt.

Children and Loss

Children react to grief and loss in terms of their general developmental and cognitive stages, as well as their individual psychological makeup. A three-year-old boy was faced with the sudden death of his mother after a school shooting and continually asked his father where his mother was. His father tells him that his "mom's stomach was hurt," or "Mom went to sleep," or "You know where Jesus lives, don't you? Mama went to see Jesus."

> But [the boy] continues to look under the bed for his mommy. "Mom's in heaven," [father] tries to explain.
>
> "She'll fall out," [the boy] says, "When is she going to come home?"
>
> [The boy] talks to his rocking horse, whom the family named Cactus. "Cactus, my mom can't come home."
>
> And then at night, [the boy] tells his father, "I want to go to heaven too." (Labi, 1998, p. 37)

In this dialogue, we see the boy's deep distress over feelings of loss and abandonment and his age-appropriate lack of understanding permanency; he thinks concretely and attempts to master the situation by explaining it to his toy horse. But he returns again to the wish that mother reappear; his primary concern is reconnecting to his mother.

Children suffer after parental loss and need considerable support, a chance to mourn their parents, and retain some connection and memories of them. They respond best if supportive caretakers to whom they are already attached (if possible) are available, or if not, people who have the capacity and motivation to reach out and attach to them.

Loss of Parents with AIDS

AIDS has taken the life of many adults and "left tens of thousands of children with dead or dying parents" (Aronson, 1996, p. 422). Although loss of a parent is always painful, children struggling with the trauma of parental AIDS and loss face multiple social problems and internal conflicts. For children experiencing parental loss to go through the mourning process successfully, "caring, supportive figures are crucial . . . [and] provide a 'holding environment'" (Aronson, 1996, p. 423). Many of these children do *not* have a supportive, holding environment; they have had "significant gaps in their care as they are shifted to various relatives during [parental] hospitalizations" (p. 424). The ways the children and their parents "cope with such breaks in their connectedness can be critical to a more adaptive grief process" (Aronson, 1996, p. 424).

One of the successful outcomes of mourning is the development of a positive identification with the lost object. Complicating this process for some children are a combination of their own ambivalent feelings toward the dead parent as well as criticisms about this parent from current caretakers.

In one case, a therapist worked with two sisters, Caitlin, twelve, and Mary, eight (Aronson, 1996). Prior to their mother's death, the girls were neglected by her and experienced abuse at the hands of her boyfriends. Caitlin and Mary were lying and stealing, and their grandmother threatened to put them in a foster home. The grandmother had a long-standing conflictual history with the girls' mother. The therapist attempted to help the sisters with their identification issues about their mother.

> During the course of treatment, the girls decided, on their own, to make two lists entitled "Ways to remember our mother" and "Ways *not* to remember our mother." Ways to remember mother included talking, crying, looking at pictures, and eliciting stories from their grandmother about the mother. Ways not to remember her included stealing, lying, cursing, playing hooky, not listening to adults, using drugs—all behaviors that they had heard attributed to their mother. Over time, the girls came to realize their pathological identification with their dead mother and began to develop identifications that were more positive, often based on stories told by their grandmother. (Incidentally, it took much work to help the grandmother understand the

importance of relating stories that cast the mother in a positive light.) (Aronson, 1996, p. 426)

In another situation, Melissa, twelve, a Hispanic girl whose mother died of AIDS, told her therapist that she would make a point to walk by the cemetery where her mother was buried every day on her way home from school (Aronson, 1996). Melissa lived with an aunt and was "forbidden" to discuss her mother's death in her aunt's home. She spoke of her great distress at not being able to "ameliorate her mother's condition. . . . Melissa also described tearfully but helplessly pleading with her mother not to shoot up. She began to weep openly over the loss of her mother and the profound changes that had occurred in her life as a result" (Aronson, 1996, p. 429). Melissa and her therapist discussed her loss and also how she missed sharing her progress with her mother. The therapist (in a variation of anticipatory work) discussed with Melissa how she might miss her mother in the future.

> We began to discuss what it would be like at the time of her prom and graduation, events that she would be unable to share with her mother. With help, Melissa acknowledged that through each stage of her life— graduation, marriage, and childbearing—she would be thinking of her mother and would need to reevaluate the loss in light of both her own development and her mother's wishes and aspirations for her. (Aronson, 1996, p. 429)

Other specific problems tend to complicate the mourning process and subsequent adaptation for this group of children. The person who becomes the caretaker for a child following parental death plays a very important role in that child's life; "the caretaker should ideally be a substitute object already known to the child, to whom the child may transfer attachment" (Aronson, 1996, p. 429). This can be problematic for these children, many of whom have come from broken homes and have lived with various relatives and in foster homes.

It is also important that the child be allowed to express grief; this is not always permitted, "especially if the dead parent was an IV drug user or a homosexual—issues that the family . . . may not wish to have verbalized" (Aronson, 1996, p. 430).

It is not uncommon for children to identify with a parent and with the parent's illness. Adolescent girls whose mothers have breast cancer are discussed in the next chapter; they are fearful that they will acquire this illness. A similar process occurs in children whose parents have AIDS.

There is fear and social stigmatization associated with AIDS. Some of the children whose parents have this disease have suffered social ostracism; some have been expelled from school (Aronson, 1996). Many children experience shame, and it is one of the therapeutic goals to "help to diminish [this] shame. . . . Several of the children I work with describe slinking around the school corridors, trying not to draw attention to themselves. By instilling in them the belief that they are not alone, one can help these children find solace and some relief from shame" (Aronson, 1996, p. 433). AIDS is discussed further in Chapter 12.

Although these issues are characteristic of the problems surrounding AIDS, they are also relevant for many other children whose parents suffer from other protracted and disruptive illnesses in comparable circumstances. The approaches to intervention just described may also be applicable to them.

Factors Complicating the Mourning Process

Grief can be difficult for people to express for many reasons, such as having conflictual feelings about the person who died or abandoned them. People may also not be able to express grief about situations which do not receive social approval. This has been termed "'disenfranchised grief'" (MacGregor, 1994, p. 164), which is encountered when people have been disenfranchised by society from the normal grieving process because their loss is not "'openly acknowledged, publicly mourned, or socially supported'" (p. 164).

Disenfranchised grief can exist when one partner in a "secret" lesbian or gay relationship has died, and the grieving partner has no one with whom to share this pain. In Chapter 9, I discussed latency-age children having difficulty sharing trauma-related grief (related to a friend being murdered) because they often felt shame and humiliation about the events. Children whose parents have AIDS experience disenfranchised grief. MacGregor (1994) suggests parents of children with a serious mental illness experience disenfranchised grief because the mental illness is stigmatized and the parents feel a lack of support in expressing their loss.

In some situations, bereavement ceremonies and rituals themselves have become disenfranchised. Families of psychiatric patients who have died in institutions often receive no assistance with bereavement when the patient has died, and peers in the institution as well as staff members close to the patient may not have any opportunities within the institution for memorial services or other alternative ways to share their sadness (Fauri and Grimes, 1994).

In the past, many Native Americans have been denied opportunities to formalize their burial rituals (Chapter 1). The Lakotas not only suffered massacres and other traumas of loss, but for many years were denied their ritual mourning ceremonies by the U.S. government (Brave Heart, 1998). "For American Indians, historical unresolved grief involves the profound, unsettled bereavement that results from generations of devastating losses which have been disqualified (Doka, 1989) by prohibiting indigenous ceremonies and by the large society's denial of the magnitude of its genocidal policies" (Brave Heart, 1998, p. 288).

Mourning Past Losses

Past losses that have never been resolved are often discovered during the course of clinical work, and therapy offers a second opportunity to help clients work through these losses. Such losses can be related to an actual death or other life events, including separations relating to divorce or abandonment. Adoptive children, even those adopted from infancy, often have active fantasies about their "lost" birth parents (Chapter 6).

Sometimes clients see no value in exploring these losses. "For reasons, then, of death or remoteness, these figures seem totally unavailable, and frequently clients consider them insignificant or unimportant in their lives" (Hartman and Laird, 1983, p. 249). However, when clients are ready to look at these losses and their effects on their present life, this may be the "turning point in the client's family work, the most effective strategy for change" (Hartman and Laird, 1983, p. 249).

Earlier in this chapter, we mentioned Linda Valli, who had some visual hallucinations after her aunt's death. Linda's mother died when she was thirteen; she felt her mother was angry with her before she died, and Linda assumed that she herself was bad and at fault. She never fully grieved for her mother, but experienced anxiety, a poor self-image, and inner constriction instead.

> Linda's mother died of a cerebral hemorrhage when Linda was thirteen. With feelings of sadness, Linda described how, from the time she was twelve, she worried about her mother's health and had fears of her death, as her mother's health declined and her headaches increased. Father, from her description, was a distant figure who had little involvement with the family. Although there was "probably" an early positive relationship with her mother, Linda could not clearly remember this, and felt her brother was preferred. There was significant marital discord, and Linda's mother appeared to have been depressed, but it seemed as though she was not as chronically unhappy as she was during her last year. Linda cried as she talked about going to church and lighting a candle for her mother and saying a prayer for her to live.

During the course of her therapy, Linda's phobic symptoms cleared up, her self-esteem improved, and her tendency to internalize her negative and angry feelings decreased markedly. Reconnecting to her feelings and memories about her mother, and looking at their relationship, her mother's death, and her reactions to it from a different perspective were among the critical issues addressed in helping Linda integrate a stronger self-image.

Pill and Zabin (1997) offered time-limited, twelve-week group therapy sessions to women whose mothers had died when they were children, observing that they had a chronic and deep sense of isolation stemming from their early feelings of loss. The authors felt that the group method was effective in helping them process this experience, as it provided both emotional support and validation for their feelings and a decreased sense of isolation. Because they did not have mothers, they often felt they were different from other children and felt embarrassed and stigmatized. Their grief was compounded by "not being allowed to talk about their mothers," and if they had the rare opportunity of meeting someone else who had this experience, "they felt an immediate bond" (Pill and Zabin, 1997, p. 187).

Difficulties in separation, transitions, endings, and feelings of inadequacy were among other common themes Pill and Zabin (1997) found, as well as difficulty acquiring social skills; as other children seldom came to visit, "social skills were not reinforced" (p. 189). Because of their sense of unworthiness, they often were not comfortable having their needs met by others; many assumed a caretaking role in relation to others instead. Linda Valli, at age thirteen, had also assumed a caretaking role when, after her mother's death, she felt responsible for her ten-year-old sister; she "felt sorry for her." Linda "feels heartbroken now to see the unhappiness in her sister's current life."

Many of the women in the group felt fear and insecurity, "could not trust that others would remain available for them," and lived with frequent "fears of abandonment and rejection" (Pill and Zabin, 1997, p. 190). Guilt, which is frequently found in children experiencing parental bereavement, was often expressed. The group experience also helped the women mourn and share their grief. Many of the women made psychological efforts to connect with their mothers, both through internal processing and sometimes by discussing their mothers with others who knew them. Some of the group members also had poor pre-existing relationships with their mothers, involving various forms of rejection or maltreatment; the group experience gave them an opportunity to work through some of these feelings.

Individual and group therapeutic experiences offer people the opportunity to work through past losses. Although loss may not be the focus of treatment, another way this issue may surface is in the process of termination of therapy.

Termination of Therapy

Termination of therapy often brings with it ambivalent feelings for the client, including positive feelings of accomplishment and achievement (assuming the therapy was successful), fear of being "on one's own," as well as feelings of loss. Termination is usually a difficult experience for social work students to face, as they must deal with a multitude of feelings themselves, including their sadness in saying good-bye to clients and their discomfort in hearing the client's feelings of loss and anger directed at them. It is usually most agonizing for students to bear their feelings of guilt upon termination; this is especially so when the termination is based on the student's ending a placement because of the academic calendar rather than a planned ending based on the client's needs and accomplishments.

The ending of therapy, with its focus on separation, can catalyze a client's past experience with separation and loss; this can bring up past losses that were never resolved, which the client now has the opportunity to resolve or at least begin to recognize. A child, for example, who was abandoned by a parent and is now being "abandoned" by a student-clinician may share his or her conviction that the clinician is leaving him or her because the child was "bad"; this can provide much "grist for the mill" and lead to the opportunity to correct the distorted self-image as well as the irrational guilt.

Many people who have endured losses in the past did not have the opportunity to say good-bye or discuss the relationship and its meaning to them at the time. A good termination can enable people to experience saying good-bye, which can leave them feeling that they will be missed, that they and the clinician have a meaningful relationship, and that they are valued. Fleeing from or avoiding saying good-bye forecloses this opportunity.

CONCLUSION

Transitions, crises, changes, and losses are inevitable parts of the life cycle; a person's experience with these events must always be examined within the biopsychosocial framework. People react differently to different crises and may also respond in different ways to the same type of crises at another point in their lives. Life events always have both an objective reality as well as a subjective meaning to people.

Major losses are deeply felt by most people, but some people with a history of past early losses may be especially vulnerable. People suffering from schizophrenia are also particularly vulnerable to loss and may seriously decompensate during such times. For some people, like Vivienne, a loss may represent not only the loss of a loved person but the loss of a selfobject, after which the person is left not only bereaved but devastated, "empty," and without direction.

One point that stands out in most writings on this subject is the importance of not isolating people who have losses or impending losses, and the need to engage them in discussion at a level of which they are capable and motivated for. Another critical point is the realization of how painful feelings of loss can be and how people, including clinicians, often try to avoid them. We have to be ready to listen and to come to terms with our own pain.

A final point is that people may need help in dealing with the loss experiences which underlie many presenting problems. For example, applying cognitive-behavioral approaches exclusively to a couple with marital problems, each married for the second time, may overlook the fact that neither partner has resolved the ambivalent feelings toward the first spouse, which is coloring present interactions with each other.

A major arena in which loss is evident is in the medical field, when people are confronted with serious illnesses and disabilities that can create havoc in every aspect of their lives. We turn our attention to this in the next chapter.

LEARNING EXERCISE

1. In your small group, discuss your cases in terms of the various losses the clients experienced, how these were handled, and the overall impact these losses have had on the clients' lives.

SUGGESTED READINGS

Articles

Omin, R. (1989). To die in treatment: An opportunity for growth, consolidation and healing. *Clinical Social Work Journal, 17,* 325-336.
Siebold, C. (1991). Termination: When the therapist leaves. *Clinical Social Work Journal, 19,* 191-204.
Zambelli, G. and Clark, E. (1994). Parentally bereaved children: Problems in school adjustment and implications for the school social worker. *School Social Work Journal, 19*(Fall), 1-15.

Books

Davids, J. (1993). The reaction of an early latency boy to the sudden death of his baby brother. In A. J. Solnit, P. B. Neubauer, S. Abrams, and A. S. Dowling (Eds.), *The psychoanalytic study of the child, Vol. 48* (pp. 277-292). New Haven: Yale University Press.
Kübler-Ross, E. (1969). *On death and dying.* New York: The Macmillan Company.
Vastola, J., Nierenberg, A., and Graham, E. H. (1986). The lost and found group: Group work with bereaved children. In A. Gitterman and L. Shulman (Eds.), *Mutual aid groups and the life cycle* (pp. 75- 90). Itasca, IL: F. E. Peacock Publishers, Inc.

Chapter 12

Illness and Disability

Minor surgery is that which is performed on someone else.

Aphorism

INTRODUCTION

The social worker was asked by the chief pediatrician to talk to a new patient, Mary, twelve, who had undergone unsuccessful eye surgery several days ago; the prognosis is poor, and it is expected that Mary's eyesight will deteriorate, eventuating in blindness. The family and the doctors had been optimistic about this surgery; no one had expected such a poor outcome. The doctors did not know Mary or her family personally as she had come to the hospital from an outlying rural area; they felt it would be helpful for the social worker to talk with Mary and her family and to share her impressions and recommendations with the doctors before they met the family. The biopsychosocial assessment of Mary and her family is discussed in the next section.

This chapter focuses on the impact of illness and disability on individuals and families at various points in the life cycle. Space does not permit a full discussion of the range of disorders that seriously affect people's health and functioning. What is emphasized in each vignette chosen is the specific medical disorder itself with its physical ramifications as well as its interaction with the biopsychosocial factors in the patient's life.

Although controversy continues to exist about the interactions of the body and the mind, my point of view is that a very close interrelationship exists in both directions. As we shall shortly see, Mary is facing impending blindness, not psychological in etiology, but physical pain and emotional suffering are present. Paul Norris, five, discussed in Chapter 7, had problems with recurrent vomiting for which no physical basis was found; the etiology was psychological, and Paul was somatizing his anxiety. People subject to multiple transitions and high degrees of stress are susceptible to illness (Chapter 11); for example, due to the multiple stresses involved, caretakers of patients with dementia are at high risk for both depression and physical illness (Kennedy, 2000). The interactions of physical health and illness and psychosocial influences are expanded upon later in this chapter.

One of the paradoxical situations that we face today is the ability of medicine to prolong life, in the process often increasing the number of people who live with disabilities, sometimes of a chronic nature. In Chapter 10, we saw the dramatic increase in the numbers of people who live past age eighty-five but who are more subject to chronic illness and infirmities. In addressing this paradox, Robert L. Kane, a gerontologist at the University of Minnesota, commented that " 'we are spending megabucks to understand the genome, but . . . we still don't have a basic system of care that responds to chronic disease. . . . We can't come up with a health care system that really responds to what people need'" (Rimer, 1998c, p. A20).

Advances in reproductive technology (Chapter 8) have resulted in many babies being born prematurely. Many of these babies develop serious chronic disabilities. In addition, children who would have died at early ages in the past now survive but live with illnesses such as cystic fibrosis, spina bifida, and congenital heart disease. "Chronic disease and its effect on children and families has replaced acute illness as the most serious issue in pediatric medicine" (Boice, 1998, p. 927).

Medical science has made tremendous advances in promoting good sanitation, developing antibiotics and effective vaccines, and in eliminating many but not all infectious diseases. However, doctors sometimes lose in the war against viruses. One of the most overwhelming defeats has been in the fight against HIV (human immunodeficiency virus), the agent responsible for the development of AIDS. Although progress has been made in recent years, the gains have been primarily in "containing" the disease and prolonging life rather than in finding a cure. AIDS now affects many men, women, and children in this country and throughout the world, producing untold misery and causing particular devastation in some countries, particularly in Africa and Asia. AIDS is further discussed later in this chapter.

Relevant systemic factors are considered throughout this presentation, and the chapter concludes with a discussion of such complex issues as the impact of economics on medical services, managed care, the crisis in nursing home care, and the cutback of funds for home and hospice care. In addition, the social worker's function itself in many settings has been reduced from active psychosocial intervention to a primary focus on discharge planning, often performed in a brief, perfunctory manner with a focus on concrete services.

On a more positive note, the tremendous advances in legal protections and services for people with disabilities are recognized; the Rehabilitation Act of 1973 and the Americans with Disabilities Act (ADA) of 1990 have been lauded as landmark legislation. According to Orlin (1995), "During the past 20 years the United States has experienced a public policy revolution affecting people with disabilities" (p. 233).

THE BIOPSYCHOSOCIAL PERSPECTIVE IN CLINICAL WORK WITH PEOPLE WITH ILLNESS AND DISABILITY

This case discussion of Mary, who had an unsuccessful eye operation, is now presented at some length to illustrate the biopsychosocial approach to people with medical problems; this is followed by a presentation of case vignettes illustrating illness and disability through the life cycle.

Case Illustration of Impending Blindness

The social worker went to Mary's room and found her alone. She was a pretty, slightly overweight, Mexican-American girl who seemed quiet and solemn but friendly, and she related positively to the social worker. She did not complain, indicated she felt no pain, and appeared to be stoic, but one sensed an underlying anxiety concerning her eyes and her hospitalization. Later that day, the social worker met with Mary's parents. The mother spoke Spanish with little English while the father had greater command of English; they were accompanied by their young daughter-in-law who spoke English well and acted as an interpreter. They were warm and friendly people, but at the moment all were anxious and very concerned about Mary's well-being. They presented the following information about their family and current life.

> Mary's father, thirty-six, and mother, thirty-seven, have been married seventeen years and have six children, Claudia, fifteen, Mary, twelve, Vincent, eleven, Joan, seven, and Jo, two and a half. The oldest child, Jim, eighteen, has been married for eight months and lives with his wife in the family home. (It was Jim's wife who participated in the interview with Mary's parents.) The family lives on a ranch with other Mexican-American families in a rural area in a southwestern state. Mr. F. is employed as a laborer, and Mrs. F. is a homemaker. The family is active in the Catholic church.

As the medical problem was the major focus of concern, the social worker asked the family about Mary's eye condition and Mary's feelings about this problem. In talking with people about their physical illness, information related to the onset of the problem, the patient's (and family's) understanding of the condition, and attitudes toward it are critical.

When Mary was four, physically healthy and developing well, a younger sister poked her in the eye, and she has had trouble seeing since then. Currently, the tentative diagnosis is acute glaucoma as a result of associated iris bombe, right eye. The operation several days ago was a peripheral iridectomy on the right eye. Parents reported that Mary had anxiety about this hospitalization and was afraid she might lose both eyes. Father has no hospitalization insurance and has made arrangements to pay the bill on a monthly basis. "We want to do what is best for her . . . if she gets her eyesight back, it's OK."

Another important point of inquiry is the degree of functional incapacity the medical condition might cause. According to the ADA, disability refers to "a physical or mental impairment that substantially limits one or more of the major life activities of such individuals" (Orlin, 1995, pp. 234-235). Mary's major life activity at twelve would be attending school. Closely related to this would be her social life and peer relationships; the social worker also inquires about how this aspect of her life is affected by her eye problem. To understand the degree of present and future impairment, it is essential to obtain a baseline of Mary's academic and social functioning, within the context of her family, social, and cultural domains.

The children attend school near the ranch, and the family has positive feelings about this facility. "It's a small school—you can learn more." Although Mary is twelve, she remains in the second grade, as her eye problem has led to lack of progress in reading. No facilities are available for children with visual disabilities in this school, and no referrals have been made to other resources (which are very sparse in the county). Theresa, Mary's sister-in-law, reports that Mary gets tired in school and says her head hurts. But Theresa notes that if she is not in school, she is OK. "I guess reading affects her eyes." Theresa feels that her eyes are holding her back. Sometimes in the mornings, Mary will ask her sister-in-law to write her a note to tell the teacher that "when she gets tired of reading she doesn't have to read anymore, can put her head down."

Theresa describes Mary as being very quiet, shy, and "quick to cry." However, she is usually more cheerful and outgoing than she seems in the hospital. She "likes to joke around, likes to dance." But sometimes she feels sick, then she wants to go to bed and rest. When she is in bed, she does not seem to want to talk to anyone. Theresa reports that Mary has frequent headaches (sometimes as many as three a week, other times she has none); Theresa attributes this behavior to her eye problem.

Mary has a serious functional incapacity in terms of her impaired school functioning. A number of pieces to this puzzle are missing; it is not clear why Mary cannot read. Does she have a learning disability interacting with her visual problem? We do not know the cause of her headaches (pressure from the glaucoma; eye strain; a secondary physical problem, and/or depression). Signs suggest that Mary may be depressed, such as crying easily, frequently needing to go to bed (stating she is in pain), and not wanting to talk to anyone at these times. It is possible that depression could be causing the headaches; it is also possible that she might feel depressed because she has so many headaches or that she just wants to be alone because she is in so much pain.

On a systems level, it is of serious concern that Mary continues to remain in the second grade (which may also be very depressing for her) and that these questions have not been explored. Ideally, an intensive, comprehensive medical/psychiatric, educational, and psychological evaluation should be done, but this was not routine in the rural area in which Mary lived. A public health nurse is involved with the family, but, other than making recommendations, her role is not clear.

> There has been some discussion, according to the family, with the public health nurse about sending Mary to the school for the blind in a city ninety miles away. Theresa says that Mary "is little and afraid to go." Mary's parents state that she cries when this is discussed and does not want to go there; they have not decided what to do, but the whole family seems reluctant to go along with this possible change.

The nurse is apparently attempting to make what to her seemed like a helpful suggestion but runs counter to the family's core way of life. It is quite possible that not only is Mary scared about losing her eyesight, but she is probably terrified about being separated from her family and living in an institution. Although some discussion has taken place about "solutions," it does not seem that the family or public health nurse are "attuned" to Mary's inner anxieties, and it is probable that this has not been openly discussed. When Mary goes to bed and does not want to talk to anyone, it suggests she may be suffering in silence.

It does not seem that any interventions have been made by the school to offer special education or provide Mary with special materials and consultation so that she can read and her education can continue. It is possible that prejudice toward Mexican Americans is involved in this situation; we would hypothesize that if a middle-class Caucasian child had the same presenting problems, more active intervention on her behalf would have occurred, and her educational status would have received considerable attention.

The social worker also explored Mary's family life and relationships.

> Family relationships appear to be warm and supportive, and no family problems were reported. Theresa states that the parents are very understanding to the children, "never hit them, always explain." The children get along well, and all enjoy playing with the baby. The children "watch out for Mary" when they play with her because of her eye problem.
>
> No psychiatric problems were reported in the family, nor serious health problems. The parents came from large families and had little schooling, chopping cotton at an early age. Mother's pregnancy with Mary was uneventful, and Mary's developmental landmarks were within the normal range.

Mary's family life seems stable and supportive; the family appears sensitive to Mary's vulnerability in terms of her eye problems. The social worker inquires about Mary's social environment and social relationships.

> The atmosphere on the ranch is very congenial, and the neighbors are cooperative and helpful. The children play together, and Mary has many friends, although it is not clear if she has any close friends (or chumships). Mary was described as a quiet girl who does not "like to run around much." Theresa, who grew up on the ranch and has known Mary a long time, reported that "the children make fun of her being chubby."

Mary lives in an environment in which people are friendly; she is part of this world, yet she experiences some "discrimination" as she is teased about her chubbiness. It is possible that her playmates sense her visual problems and are frightened and uncomfortable about this, so they displace it by teasing her about her weight, a "safer" subject. If she does become blind and is different in this way, how will this affect her friendships? Paradoxically, can this social group, while being of the same ethnicity and class and being supportive on one level, also be rejecting because she is different—and will become more different as her eyesight deteriorates? And if Mary, age twelve, remains at the second-grade level (with seven-year-olds), might this not set her further apart socially?

Discussion

Mary cried when she was admitted to the hospital for surgery. She was afraid she would lose both her eyes; therefore, she must know (and feel apprehensive) about her eye problems. It was the social worker's impression that Mary needed a supportive, ongoing relationship so that she could share her deep fears about becoming blind and her fears about being sent away. The family would probably be responsive to support and seemed open to talking about their concerns about her eyesight as well as future plans. Theresa should be included in the family work; she would be an asset in terms of her positive relationship to the family and her sensitivity to Mary's feelings.

Developmental stage. Developmentally, Mary is entering adolescence, marked by increases in growth, the development of sexuality, emotional turbulence, working out separation from the family, and planning for a future. She is at an age in which self-consciousness about appearance is considerable (and she is already being teased about her "chubbiness"), as is the need to be accepted by peers. Adolescents often share secrets with each other and feel best understood by a close circle of friends. Will Mary find no one with whom to share her special anxieties and physical similarities?

Blindness. Barbara Ceconi, the social work student cited in Chapter 1, who lost her eyesight suddenly while in college, commented that "the feelings I experienced during this time were akin to those of grieving the loss of a significant friend or family member. I was mourning the loss of my eyesight" (Ceconi and Urdang, 1994, p. 181). Becoming blind is an overwhelming event for anyone at any age. Krauz (1980) worked with legally blind veterans from diverse religious, ethnic, and racial backgrounds and found that although these differences existed, blindness was experienced by all as a major trauma. Krauz (1980) cites the Reverend Thomas Carroll who stated that blindness is not only a injury to the eyes; it is a "destructive blow to the self image . . . a blow almost to [one's] being itself" (p. 37).

Many people do adapt to blindness, as Barbara Ceconi did, and can lead rich and productive lives. After receiving training in adapting to the limitations imposed by lack of vision (such as mobility training and the use of modern technological devices), many blind people go to school, work, have families, and enjoy leisure activities and a social life (Asch, 1995). Although Asch acknowledges that upsetting emotions often accompany knowledge of impending blindness, she emphasizes the importance of people receiving information about the resources that are available to help them adapt to daily life. Although acknowledging that some individual visually impaired people and families may need psychological help, Asch (1995) stresses the point that blindness itself does not cause major personality disruptions.

Certainly, having knowledge of and access to appropriate resources is imperative; not every person facing blindness or any other major disability is in need of intensive psychotherapy. Having good educational resources in place for Mary's visual impairment so that she can learn to read and advance past the second grade would certainly be helpful for Mary. Mary probably does not need intensive psychotherapy; however, she needs sensitive psychosocial help as does her family. They are in a crisis; they are facing a great loss, and they will need to make major adaptations, on multiple levels, in their lives.

Krauz (1980), in discussing her work with legally blind veterans, makes the strong point that many of the veterans, although having access to rehabilitation services, would not use them; some had been blind for several years without applying for assistance. She attributes this phenomenon to the fact that the men were strongly defended against accepting their blindness; this denial kept them from accepting rehabilitation services; it also kept them from mourning their loss and, as a result, many were lonely and depressed. Krauz cautions against confronting denial too rapidly and emphasizes the need for first developing a supportive relationship with the patient. (This is an important example of why knowledge of defenses and how to utilize them needs to be a critical part of social work knowledge.) Denial is a defense frequently found in patients with serious disabilities; "a person with a severe handicap often denies it on a conscious as well as an unconscious level" (Szalita, 1974, p. 679).

Cultural perspective. Mary and her family are Mexican American and live in a small ethnic community. From a socioeconomic perspective, the family is in the lower class. The family was not known long enough to assess the impact of cultural influences in depth; however, some information about Mexican-American families is offered tentatively, in terms of possible applicability to this family. Family solidarity and the incorporation of the kinship family model is important; the pattern of interdependence with extended family groups has been referred to as " 'familism' " (Falicov, 1982, p. 138). We do not know about extended family members; however, Theresa, Mary's new sister-in-law, lives with the family, which is also a common pattern.

The family is protective toward its members and expects loyalty from them. We see evidence of the family's tendency to protect Mary and to watch out for her blindness. Value is placed on being honest and on maintenance of *"dignidad* (dignity) . . . Individuals pride themselves as being *pobre pero honesto* (poor but honest)" (Falicov, 1982, p. 138). Mr. Fernandez demonstrated dignity in shouldering the burden of the hospital bills.

"Autonomy and individual achievement are not particularly emphasized" (Falicov, 1982, p. 138), which may be why Mary's parents do not seem to be upset that she is in the second grade; a middle-class Caucasian family would probably be very upset about this situation and actively advocate for change. (Although many Mexican-American families today are actively engaged in advocacy for better education.) However, "Mexican parents are less pressured . . . to achieve developmental goals or to correct minor deviances from the norm" (Falicov, 1982, p. 141). Although the parents say that they like Mary's school because it is small and children can learn more (and this may indeed be true for the other children), they also may be comfortable with the school because it is part of their community.

It is understandable both from the point of view of family dynamics and cultural expectations why the family would be upset about Mary being sent to a state institution ninety miles away; most families probably would be distressed. However, the family seemed very open, and the social worker had the impression that they might be willing to go along with some modification in Mary's schooling or use of local resources if this were feasible. It also would be culturally compatible to continue the involvement with sister-in-law Theresa, in terms of the involvement of extended family members.

Although autonomy and achievement are not always emphasized in this cultural group, it would be especially important (at an appropriate time) to highlight the necessity that Mary develop these characteristics both to counteract the potential intrinsic dependence blindness can produce and to prepare her for appropriate employment; the combination of inadequate education, disability, and minority status can create special problems for employment and earning capacity. "Hispanics with disabilities have the highest proportion of unemployment" (Olkin, 1999, p. 21). The social worker felt that the parents were accessible to further work, and her efforts in this regard might be aided by the fact that in Mexican-American families "from early on the therapist is respected as an authority on human relations" (Falicov, 1982, p. 147).

Physical Illness and Disability in the Life Cycle

In this section, physical illness and disability are discussed from both a biopsychosocial and a developmental perspective, emphasizing the role life phase issues play in adaptation.

Childhood Health Problems

Today, the major health problems facing young children in this country are related to disabilities, although acute illnesses can produce familial stress and can lead to further medical complications. Disability in very young children has not been uniformly defined; classifications are based on an assessment of the child's functional capacities. It is not uncommon to see children with multiple disabilities, such as retardation, severe orthopedic problems, and hearing impairments. However, in terms of this book's organization, mental retardation and autism are discussed under mental health problems (as they are classified in the DSM-IV), in Chapter 13, with the understanding that they often overlap with physical problems.

More premature children are born today, and many more survive at very low birth weights than in the past. For approximately the past twenty years, doctors have been able to save very premature infants, and major break-throughs in neonatology have greatly improved their chances of survival during the past ten years; many of these children have early problems such as central nervous system immaturity, which can impede the development of self-regulatory patterns (Chapter 8).

A recent study, which followed a group of premature children, found that although many had developed without difficulties in their early years, problems with academic work and behavior were observed in later school years (Stolberg, 2000). It was also observed that in this group of "150 teenagers who weighed 2 pounds or less at birth, nearly one-third had significant physical disorders, including cerebral palsy, blindness and deafness"; in addition, "even those children with minor physical problems scored significantly lower on achievement tests than those in the control group" (Stolberg, 2000, p. A20).

In addition to disabilities secondary to low birth weights, some disabilities are genetic and others can develop in utero, for example, due to maternal illness, such as German measles or substance abuse. Developmental, neurological, and psychological problems can also be caused by child maltreatment. It is not uncommon to find an interaction of these factors; for instance, a child born with fetal alcohol syndrome might also be subjected to parental maltreatment. In fact, "although the findings are not consistent, many studies report higher rates of abuse for children with disabilities" (Olkin, 1999, p. 232).

Poverty, which is associated with a number of risk factors, such as a lack of adequate care during pregnancy, is a major risk factor for the development of disabilities and developmental delays in children (Zipper and Simeonsson, 1997). Poor housing, financial pressures, and other stresses may make it more difficult for caretakers to meet their children's physical and emotional needs (Zipper and Simeonsson, 1997).

The advent of an extremely premature baby presents one of the most difficult dilemmas facing parents, obstetricians, and pediatricians. Not only is care extremely costly (up to $2,000 a day) but achieving the infant's survival is often only the beginning of a very difficult path. The recent study on the sequelae of extreme prematurity (previously discussed) adds to the controversy about the ethical issues involved in this situation (Stolberg, 2000).

For very young children with disabilities, early intervention programs are critical, as discussed in Chapter 8. When children with disabilities are older, multiple systemic factors impinge on their adaptation, including the severity of the disability itself, the child's coping abilities, relationship to caretakers (as well as caretaker's attitude toward the disability), educational and rehabilitative resources available to the family (and their ability to use those services), adequacy of educational opportunities, and the child's acceptance by peers and others.

Clinical social workers have an important role to play in helping parents deal with the often overwhelming emotional and physical demands of raising a disabled child. A comprehensive biopsychosocial approach is needed, focusing both on psychological and relationship factors as well as on the systems issues involved in obtaining needed resources.

Of course, while this section has focused on disabilities, children can also experience other illnesses. Paul Norris, five (Chapter 7), had required hospitalizations for vomiting, which was understood to represent somatization and which responded for a time to mother-child therapy. Some children have life-threatening illnesses (or accidents); they and their parents often respond positively to supportive interventions. Children facing death often want to talk about it; with support they can feel less anxiety and more "held," and the terror of being "abandoned" can diminish.

Adolescents and Illness

Adolescence, accompanied by its own inner turbulence, can be an especially difficult time to cope with illness. As peer relationships are so important, social acceptance can be critical for those who feel "different." If the illness is terminal or if the prognosis is uncertain, anxiety can be overwhelming. Disabled adolescents' sexual concerns may not be addressed, and if they have a genetic disease, their concerns about transmission to their own offspring may go unheard (Boice, 1998). The following illustrates some of these issues.

Susan, seventeen, is a bright, very short, pretty adolescent who has spina bifida, a chronic congenital condition. This is due to an embryological failure of the two sides of the vertebral column to close; the presence and severity of the symptoms depend on the degree to which the spinal cord is involved (in many instances, seen as an incidental finding on X rays, the spinal cord is not involved, and the person has no symptoms). Unfortunately, Susan had serious impairments, including lack of mobility and minimal bowel and bladder control.

> Susan propelled herself in a wheelchair. She related very well to the social worker and was open in talking about herself. She had a sense of humor and appeared good natured and easygoing, but her frequent eye tics seemed one indication of an underlying tension.
>
> Because of her difficulties with bowel and bladder control, she wore diapers and was changed by her mother. Susan attended high school, where she excelled academically and was going to graduate in four months. In many respects, Susan functioned very well and had friends and extracurricular activities in school. But Susan's adolescent

issues were greatly intensified by her physical condition and parental attitudes toward it.

No plans had as yet been worked out for Susan after her upcoming graduation; her mother appeared to be denying this event, saying, "it is still far off." Susan and her mother disagreed regarding social activities; Susan wanted to have some freedom—to be permitted to go places by herself. She wanted to attend her senior prom, but her parents would not permit this. Susan stated: "Some day, I will be on my own . . . my parents do not prepare me for it." In talking about her physical problems affecting her life, Susan stated: "I guess that's four-fifths of my problem."

Susan has many strengths: she is a high-functioning teenager who relates well and is actively engaged in a full high school life. She does not appear to be "stigmatized" nor isolated, and talks of having many friends. Susan's adolescent problems center around separation-individuation problems in relation to her parents, compounded by restrictions imposed by her illness, such as the reality of her mother changing her diapers.

A clinical social worker could offer individual supportive help to Susan regarding family issues and future planning; she could discuss their attitudes toward her illness and her future with Susan's parents. Although physical illness is certainly complicating normal development, Susan's parents, in addition, may have trouble facing separation from Susan. The utilization of appropriate rehabilitative and higher educational resources in the community, as well as possible resistance to using them, could be explored. Susan might benefit from the services of a part-time attendant who could help with diaper changes and other bodily needs as a step in the "weaning-away" from mother. This may be a complex and difficult process requiring insight into the dynamics and developmental issues involved.

Diabetes in adolescents is another illness that can complicate the adolescent's psychological adjustment, as well as increase the normative parent-child conflict of this stage. Although the severity of diabetes can vary, some patients, such as those with insulin-dependent diabetes mellitus (IDDM) (Schwartz et al., 1989), need regular doses of insulin to keep their illness under control.

Diabetes can have severe long-term consequences and can lead to blindness and heart and kidney problems; short-term problems, such as fainting and comas, can occur if the balance between sugar intake and insulin is not appropriately adjusted as a result of mismanagement, intercurrent illness, stress, etc. Although good adaptation and resilience is often shown by many diabetic teenagers, the delicately balanced demands of insulin management, diet, and control can provide fertile ground for the acting out of preexisting as well as newly developing parent-child conflicts (Schwartz et al., 1989).

It is not uncommon to find a lack of compliance among adolescents in managing their own treatment regimes. "The secretive and self-destructive manner in which some adolescents manipulate their diabetes is the cause of much concern in both therapy and research" (Seiffge-Krenke, 1997, p. 342). In one study, mothers were often found to be overinvolved with their children's care and often assumed more responsibility for monitoring the diabetes than the adolescent assumed; this often reflects separation-individuation problems. However, Seiffge-Krenke (1997) observed that over time most of the adolescents in the study progressed toward independence and assumed responsibility for their own care. A case presentation in that paper highlighted the exacerbation of a basically pathological case of mother-daughter enmeshment by the problems of the daughter's diabetes and its management.

In the Seiffge-Krenke study, all the mothers of adolescents with diabetes were found to feel stressed; a process similar to the "chronic sorrow" experienced by mothers of children with disabilities (Chapter 11) was identified here as " 'chronic worries' " (Seiffge-Krenke, 1997, p. 353). Seiffge-Krenke suggests that the suffering experienced by these mothers, which often involved their identification with their child's suffering, was similar to the suffering of parents experiencing other traumas, such as kidnappings, endured by their children.

Serious illness and disabilities with which adolescents live can have profound psychological consequences for them as well as for their families; comprehensive clinical social work services should be available to this population.

Health Problems in Middle Adulthood

During middle adulthood people are often involved in building their careers, developing a family life, and extending their friendships; illness and disability can cause a major disruption in their basic functioning, relationships, and plans. Two cases are discussed here; one is of a fifty-year-old man who underwent a leg amputation; the second case is of a midlife woman who is living with multiple sclerosis.

A man with a leg amputation. Mr. J., fifty, an unmarried man, was a foreman in a plastics factory, lived with his father, and was in excellent health until a recent industrial accident necessitated the amputation of one leg below the knee. Mr. J. became depressed, so his physician asked the social worker to see him, as Mr. J. felt hopeless about his condition. His medical prognosis was good; he would eventually be fitted with a prosthesis, and if some modifications were made in his job, he should be able to return to work.

Mr. J. is a stocky man of medium height, who appeared indifferent to the social worker when she came to his hospital room to see him. His affect was flat; he was fairly unresponsive and conveyed the impression that he could manage on his own and did not need any help. The social worker understood his discomfort with her but did not accept his statement that he did not need help at face value. She brought out into the open his reluctance to talk to her and expressed her interest in getting to know him, talking about how his accident had affected his life and how she could assist in making plans for when he left the hospital. Mr. J. accepted this with reservations and gradually began to talk more about his work.

Over several meetings, he talked of his anxieties about managing, not being as much of a man anymore, and his discomfort about other people staring at him; they would just think about his leg and would not be at ease with him. He also could not stand the idea of being helpless. Mr. J. cried as he talked about how he always managed to cope and how he helps his elderly father who lives with him. "Now I am the invalid . . . the cripple."

During the course of their work together, Mr. J.'s depression lifted, and he made plans to be fitted with a prosthesis, to move ahead with his life, and to return to work. Although Mr. J.'s disability is not life threatening nor disabling in a major way, and he can resume his major roles and responsibilities in life, nevertheless the loss of his leg was traumatic to him at a deeper level. Any major change in the body image (such as disfigurements from burns or mastectomies) can affect feelings about body integrity, self-image, and identity. It is a loss that must be grieved, as any major loss must be grieved. The feelings of loss must be validated by others who may be too quick to reassure: Oh, it's all right—you can manage without it!

A woman with multiple sclerosis. Mrs. Brown, forty-one, requested therapy because she has multiple sclerosis, has been having troubling accepting this, and is feeling depressed. Although midlife is often the time for a woman to expand her horizons, as her children are growing up, in this situation Mrs. Brown's horizons are becoming more limited. Even though her husband has been supportive to her, her two daughters, sixteen and eighteen, are finding it difficult to accept her condition, and family tensions have increased; she thinks family counseling might be helpful.

Multiple sclerosis is an inexorably progressive, degenerative disease of the white matter of the central nervous system (CNS), with lesions that are characteristically scattered over time and in different parts of the CNS; it progresses by acute episodes with local symptoms that typically partially but never completely disappear. After each episode residual damage is left, which cumulatively debilitates the individual and ultimately leads to death.

Symptoms can include poor coordination, difficulty in walking, visual impairment, and speech difficulties.

> Mr. and Mrs. Brown came together for the first appointment. Mrs. Brown, a neatly dressed woman, has pleasant features, which became more noticeable as her mood lifted. Her gait is uneven and unsteady, but she can walk by herself. She is a bright woman, somewhat reserved, who has a baseline of high-functioning and good family relationships. Mr. M., forty-three, presents a distinguished appearance, is intelligent, reserved, and quite concerned about his wife. He seems very stable and is well functioning.
>
> Mrs. Brown has had symptoms of her illness for three or four years but did not know her diagnosis until one year ago. Her major symptoms are lack of coordination and dizziness; at times, her eyesight is affected; the words start to blur after she reads one or two pages. She walks erratically, and her right side has been affected. She has not been able to write for the past two years, although she can do some printing with her left hand, and she is not able to sew. She has had trouble with her bladder (another typical symptom), but this has subsided. The illness fluctuates; sometimes she is in a state of remission. Although she does not have a "real bad case," she was also told that she would never be any better. "It was like the friendly undertaker!"

Mrs. Brown, who had been a very active woman, has become functionally impaired; she continues to do some housework and some cooking, but her ability to do this is erratic, depending on the course of her symptoms. She had a "good day" yesterday, when she attended her oldest daughter's graduation from high school. She defines a "good day" as one in which she does not feel too dizzy. Mrs. Brown, who has a good work history, has also been a committed homemaker, and her inability to carry out responsibilities as in the past upsets her. In addition, she has delegated some of her responsibilities to her daughters, which has caused "some tremendous battles." The girls are also ashamed of their mother's condition.

> Joan, the oldest girl who is about to enter college, is a "tremendous girl"—has friends and many activities but "goofs off at home" and will not help out. Hilda, sixteen, is "a bear for work" but is upset about Mrs. B.'s being different; "other mothers are normal." One day, Hilda was shopping with her mother when Mrs. B collapsed in the parking lot. "She was very embarrassed." Sometimes, when walking down the street, her oldest daughter will walk behind Mrs. B.

The second session was a family meeting; when they arrived, Joan stated she did not want to be there and she did not want to talk but nevertheless became involved in the discussion. The family's baseline relationships were very warm; this was apparent beneath the tensions that were present. At one point, all three women were crying and explained: "We're a very emotional family." Mr. and Mrs. B. also expressed warm feelings for each other, and Mrs. Brown stated, "he's my best ally." Family therapy enabled the family to share their feelings about Mrs. Brown's illness and the consequent changes in their lives. It also gave them an opportunity to examine their interactions, which had become dysfunctional under the changed circumstances.

> Mrs. Brown said that one of the most difficult things for her is to be in a situation in which she needs to ask for help; she spoke of feeling guilty; this then led into a discussion of how her guilt about this produces guilt in the girls. Joan stated: "She expects us to read her mind!" Mrs. Brown responded: "I do feel guilty; no question about that—I feel guilty about being sick!" She also spoke about being angry— "my life is being turned upside down." When the clinician commented that she must wonder why this was happening to her, she commented that she frequently did wonder that.

The Browns terminated treatment after seven sessions. Mrs. Brown found she was feeling much better and was less depressed. She felt that family relationships had improved and that "things were out in the open and aired." In this case, the mother was the primary patient, but her illness affected her husband as well as her children, who were going through adolescence with their own needs to separate and their self-consciousness about being different in any way. They also feared losing their mother.

Children and adolescents are affected by any major illness of their parents and need an opportunity to talk about this. In discussing the impact of breast cancer on women, Spira and Kenemore (2000) observed that teenage daughters are particularly affected by this occurrence and were often noted "to be more withdrawn, fearful, hostile, or rejecting" (p. 187). Their concerns included: fear of their mother dying; and if the cancer were in remission, fear that it could recur; fear that they might get the illness; fear of their own sexuality (which might also lead to this illness); and concerns about changing roles in the family.

Spira and Kenemore (2000) emphasized the importance of open communication between mothers and their daughters about their disease; improved communication can, as was observed in the Brown case, lead to less anxiety and closer relationships. The more this openness develops, "the easier it may be for the adolescent girls to have their own reactions and thus facilitate the tasks of separation and reconnection" (Spira and Kenemore, 2000,

p. 190). I would add that adolescent sons may also be quite devastated by maternal cancer and may find it more difficult to talk about than daughters; it can be assumed erroneously that they are adapting well and do not need help.

Illness in Late Adulthood

Mrs. Gibson, a black woman, lived by herself in a rural area of a small city. Although only fifty-three, she is approaching late adulthood; she seems closer to the elderly in her life problems because of her ill health and its effect on her lifestyle. She also faces the social problems of elderly black women living alone in poverty. She has no children; her second husband from whom she had been divorced had remarried and subsequently died a few years ago. Mrs. Gibson was diagnosed with lupus erythematosus and pulmonary insufficiency secondary to it.

Lupus is an inflammatory disorder of the body's connective tissues, which are the structural, supportive tissues of all organs. The disorder is believed to be the body's immune reaction against its own tissues, but its cause is unknown. Because connective tissue is universally present throughout the body, many organ systems are typically involved, and the symptoms therefore vary considerably. Recurrent inflammation of the outer lining of the lungs may occur.

The social worker described meeting Mrs. Gibson.

> Mrs. Gibson has pleasant features, wears glasses, and was neatly dressed. She is intelligent and related well. She is a quiet, reserved person who is very concerned about her illness and feels pressured by her financial situation. Although generally composed, she began crying as she talked about herself; underlying depression and anxiety were present.

As the social worker talked with Mrs. Gibson about her living situation, a picture of poverty and hardship emerged.

> Mrs. Gibson receives a small social security allotment for disability. Although her mortgage payments on her home and her utilities are minimal, she is left with fifty dollars a month, after she paid for her medicine. She finds that often she does not have enough left for food. Sometimes at the store, her sisters let her add her groceries on to their bills. She would like to work, but she feels that she is "undependable" due to her health. Some days she feels well; other days, she does not. On Wednesdays, she "helps out" one sister and receives a few dollars for this. She sometimes helps another sister clean her house on Satur-

days—earns another few dollars; both jobs are "difficult" for her. "I get so short of breath."

Until several months ago, Mrs. Gibson had been receiving her medicine from a local private charity; they stopped doing this without giving her a reason. She did not apply for public assistance; when she applied two years ago, she was told she would not be eligible for disability unless she was bed-ridden or confined to a wheelchair. She also felt that the man who spoke to her on the phone was angry with her, so she never pursued this further.

Mrs. Gibson was very worried about her health: "I try not to think about my condition." In addition to her lupus, she also needs new glasses and a new lower dental plate, as "this one is too big—it hangs out."

For the last two months, she had been hearing a noise in her head [this is a lupus-related symptom]. "I hear it day and night—sometimes it stops, but for the most part it is continuous." Occasionally, it is ex-tremely loud—"seems like firecrackers." She can drown out this noise with a radio or by sitting close to a loud, ticking clock. She is bothered by this noise at night and usually does not sleep well; sometimes she is "so deaf" she cannot hear anything, and sometimes one side of her face "feels dead."

She finds she eats fairly well, but "sometimes I don't want it—I eat a lot of things I don't want—I can't always afford milk and stuff I like."

Mrs. Gibson has had to cut back on her activities; she cannot walk very much and tends to get dizzy if she does. She has trouble making her bed and sweeping: "I get out of wind." Recently, she used parts of two days to mop her floor; it would have been a strain to do it all at once. She has had to stop her enjoyable activity of sewing on her sew-ing machine; it makes her head feel worse.

Mrs. Gibson was never a "sickly person"; lupus began eight years ago. Sometimes the lupus flares up, and she has to go to the hospital; she "never knows" when this will happen. Sometimes she is hospital-ized for four to five days; other times it lasts for two weeks.

Mrs. Gibson, although living alone, is socially involved with her sisters, her niece, and her church; while these involvements are sustaining in many ways, the social worker had the impression that Mrs. G. could not fully en-joy them due to her physical state and her anxieties in relation to her illness.

Although people do come by to see her, she reports that "I stay gone most of the time—I just leave—I can't bear to look at the house." She spends a lot of her time at a sister's home (who lives close by) but mostly "just sits there." Her sister has six children, and her sister's thirteen-year-old daughter comes over to Mrs. Gibson's house to sleep at night. When she does not come, Mrs. Gibson spends the night with her sister. She is afraid to sleep alone in case she gets sick.

Mrs. Gibson is active in a Methodist church. She attends church services on Sundays and goes to the Ladies Circle every Tuesday night and a prayer meeting on Wednesday evenings. She finds she usually feels "pretty good" when she first gets there, but sometimes feels "sick" as the evening proceeds.

Mrs. Gibson is aware of and openly discussed her anxiety; the social worker felt Mrs. Gibson was afraid she might die but that this could not be directly addressed at this point. Her feeling "sick" in church could be related (at least in part) to mental associations to religious subjects such as eternity, funerals, and death.

Mrs. Gibson stated that her nerves are "real bad." She tends to worry, and is "bothered if the least little something happens—if a friend dies, it stays in my mind—makes me sick." She could not be specific as to how this affected her—"You can't hardly explain—it is just something you can't explain."

She finds that now "when the phone rings, it scares me so bad." She feels that "sometimes it seems like people call me up more to tell me things." The other night, for example, she received a phone call from her niece who lives in another state. She called to tell Mrs. Gibson that she just learned she has diabetes. At first, Mrs. Gibson discussed this as though it were an indication of her niece's hostility, then she stated that she had "practically raised" her niece; "maybe she wanted me to know."

Mrs. Gibson had what appears to have been an anxiety or panic attack seventeen years ago. She described it as a "nervous attack—I don't know what my problem was—everything just scared me." She was instructed to stay in bed for two weeks—"not answer the phone—do nothing." Mrs. Gibson, prone to feeling anxiety, has reacted to her present illness, with its overwhelming physical symptoms, with anxiety as well as depression.

Mrs. Gibson's case brings out the diverse issues uncovered by a comprehensive biopsychosocial assessment of a person with a serious illness. From a biological perspective, a consultation with Mrs. Gibson's physician is needed to understand more about the course of her illness, prognosis, and recommendations of what would be realistic for her in terms of her daily functioning. The degree to which depression and anxiety are affecting her physical symptoms also needs to be evaluated; conversely, is the lupus itself causing any specific biologically based emotional changes? Mrs. Gibson might benefit from an occupational therapy evaluation, to explore activities in which she might engage within the confines of her physical limitations. Mrs. Gibson might benefit from part-time homemaker services, but this did not exist in her locale.

From a social perspective, Mrs. Gibson's desperate financial situation was a major concern. The social worker encouraged Mrs. Gibson to reapply to the welfare department, informing them that she had already qualified as disabled under social security. Mrs. Gibson called the social worker back later to say that she had done this. When the welfare worker questioned if she was really disabled, Mrs. Gibson informed her about her social security disability; she reported that the worker then "smiled" and proceeded to fill out her application.

Mrs. Gibson was also experiencing considerable psychological distress because of her anxieties about her illness; it was thought that she would be very responsive to an ongoing supportive social work relationship, considering her positive response to the social worker and her readiness to talk about herself. Mrs. Gibson had many social supports in her life; from a cultural perspective, the involvement with extended families and church often found in the African-American culture were present. However, her anxieties and suspiciousness of the motivations of others (in terms of their response to her illness) may keep her from fully internalizing these supports; at times, she withdraws from people who seem to be reaching out to her.

When dealing with service providers, Mrs. Gibson, who is reserved and stoic, can easily fall between the cracks and thus fail to obtain necessary services. Concrete needs are critical, but so is her emotional state. Mrs. Gibson did not seek out the social worker but responded readily when approached. The medical social worker is in a crucial position to reach out to patients in the hospital; it is indeed tragic to think that the Mrs. Gibsons of today would be neglected as social workers disappear from medical settings and, when present, are often permitted to offer only brief concrete services.

THE BODY-MIND INTERACTION

The controversy surrounding mind-body dualism—that is, that mind and body are separate entities and operate independently of each other, has never abated over the centuries. Oliver Sacks (1990) observes that this dispute partly arises from our "almost irresistible desire to see ourselves as being somehow above nature, above the body" (p. 44). He advocates an integrated approach and notes that it is important to realize "how individual persons grow and become, and their growing and becoming are correlated with their physical bodies. Dualistic approaches prevent us from developing such a concept" (Sacks, 1990, p. 47). The new field of "psychoneuroimmunology (PNI) [which] poses a systemic model that assumes ongoing reciprocal influence among psychological and physiological processes" provides a basis for an integrated approach (Wood et al., 1989, p. 400).

As early as 1949, Alexander asserted that " 'every bodily process is directly or indirectly influenced by psychological stimuli because the whole organism constitutes a unit with all of its parts interconnected' " (Wood et al., 1989, p. 400). Wood and colleagues (1989) note that it has taken forty years for the nonpsychiatric medical community to accept this idea. They credit PNI research, which showed the linkage between psychological and somatic systems.

Today, paradoxically, the psychiatric community is itself divided on the subject of the effect of psychological forces on the body as well as on mental health. Some psychiatrists place strong emphasis on genetic and biological factors exerting primary influence on all psychiatric problems, and some view psychodynamic thinking as "unscientific."

Infant research has led to observations of psychosomatic interrelatedness; young children react physically to emotional factors in their lives (Mrazek, 2000). Many years ago, the early work of Bowlby and Spitz (Karen, 1990) demonstrated the serious effects of maternal deprivation on young children, resulting in failure to thrive—sometimes even leading to death.

Chapter 8 discussed the close relationship between neurobiology and emotional relatedness, affect, and the regulation of affect (Shapiro and Applegate, 2000). Chapter 10 noted the strong relationship between physical and psychological problems in the elderly (Kennedy, 2000). Trauma in children and adults may be followed by a post-traumatic stress disorder, which often includes a "physiological reactivity" to stimuli eliciting associations to the traumatic events, as well as "difficulty falling or staying asleep" (American Psychiatric Association, 1994, p. 428). Depression is marked by both psychological and physical distress, including fatigue and lack of energy, sleep problems, significant weight loss or weight gain, physical pain such as headaches, and sexual dysfunction (American Psychiatric Association, 1994).

Sleep problems illustrate the integrality and interaction of mind and body within the context of social and systemic factors.

Sleep Problems

Sleep is a basic biological need; it "is as powerful as the drive to eat or breathe" ("Sleep Disorders—Part I," 1994, p. 1). In *Macbeth,* distraught in the aftermath of the murder of the king, to which she has vehemently urged her husband, Lady Macbeth is utterly incapable of sleep. Shakespeare describes what she has lost: "Sleep that knits up the ravell'd sleeve of care/The death of each day's life, sore labour's bath/Balm of hurt minds, great nature's second course/Chief nourisher in life's feast."

Many Americans struggle with sleep problems related to an inability to fall asleep (insomnia) as well as difficulty staying awake as a result of insomnia and/or other contributory factors. Sleep disturbances are especially prominent in the elderly population (Kennedy, 2000). The United States, a "chronically sleep-deprived" country, "long ago exchanged the effortless biological cycle of sleeping and waking for the tyranny of electric lights, job-plus-kids living, graveyard shifts and packages that absolutely, positively have to be there overnight" (Goode, 1998a, p. D1).

In extreme sleep deprivation, when people have been kept awake for a week, "they become irritable, disoriented, and uncoordinated; they have difficulty in concentrating and may develop hallucinations and delusions" ("Sleep Disorders—Part I," 1994, pp. 1-2); in less extreme situations, disturbances in sleeping can "affect physical as well as mental health" (p. 2). Psychiatric conditions themselves, such as anxiety disorders, substance abuse, and especially depression, can cause sleep disorders. Sleep deprivation often leads to accidents, which are not uncommonly fatal. In a national study presented to Congress, it was observed that people working on shifts and young men driving long distances at night "were the most vulnerable to fatigue-related automobile accidents" ("Sleep-Depriving," 1999, p. A22). Over 1,500 deaths and 40,000 injuries each year are related to driving accidents, attributed "at least in part . . . [to] fatigue" ("Sleep-Depriving," 1999, p. A22). It has also been reported that "two-thirds of workplace accidents . . . are caused by human error, many of them the result of a failure of alertness" (Goode, 1998a, p. D1).

Eating Disorders

Although eating disorders are generally classified under psychiatric disorders, they are included in this section because of their close interrelationships with psychological issues (such as body image, overvaluation of thinness, its associations with identity difficulties, and anxiety) and its clear and critical relationship to the body (disrupting major physiological processes to such a degree that serious illness or death may result).

In anorexia nervosa, the person (most typically female, although this disorder has been found to occur in men) is intensely preoccupied with being thin and usually has a distorted body image, insisting that they are overweight, even when in reality they appear skeletal. From the physiological point of view, it is reminiscent of the failure-to-thrive infant problem, in which the infant does not eat (related to lack of adequate nurturing and subsequent anaclitic depression), which leads to growth failure and possibly death.

By contrast with the infant's situation, avoidance of eating by teens and adults, even when related to emotional difficulties, is very much under conscious control (in fact, the theme of control is one of its central and defining characteristics). Yet anorexics persist in not eating, despite the serious consequences. Paradoxically, people with anorexia may be quite preoccupied with food, often collecting recipe books and cooking for others. "They may cut food into tiny pieces, weigh it, hoard it, or pocket it and throw it away" ("Eating—Part I," 1992, p. 1). Denial is a major defense; they do not think that they have a problem and are highly resistant to intervention; hospitalization is often required. Physical symptoms in women include:

> Symptoms of starvation: dry skin, brittle nails and hair, constipation, anemia, loss of bone, swollen joints. The level of female hormones falls drastically, and sexual development may be delayed or arrested in very young women. Body temperature, heart rate, and blood pressure sometimes become dangerously low; potassium may be lost, with the resulting danger of cardiac failure. ("Eating—Part I," 1992, p. 1)

Bulimia nervosa occurs more frequently than anorexia; it involves episodes of binge eating usually followed by self-induced vomiting or use of laxatives. Referring to the DSM-IV definition, it is noted that "bulimia implies two or more episodes of binge eating (rapid consumption of a large amount of food) each week for at least three months" ("Eating—Part I," 1992, p. 1). Cases are encountered in which both anorexia and bulimia may occur simultaneously or at different times. People with this disorder may go on severe diets or eat normally between binges; they may also exercise compulsively. Although not considered as life threatening as anorexia, nevertheless serious physical consequences can occur:

> It can cause stomach aches, nausea, bloating, fatigue, weakness, sore muscles . . . erosion of dental enamel by acidic vomit, and scars on the hand from pushing fingers down the throat. Probably the most serious physical dangers are dehydration, loss of potassium, and rupture of the esophagus. ("Eating—Part I," 1992, p. 1)

Somatization

Somatization is another connecting link between psychological problems and the production of physical symptoms. This defense mechanism, discussed in Chapter 2, was described as a conversion of psychological tensions and conflict into somatic (physical) problems and complaints. Lipowski (1988) defines somatization as a "tendency to experience and communicate somatic distress and symptoms unaccounted for by pathological findings, to attribute them to physical illness, and to seek medical help for them" (p. 1359). So it is not uncommon for people to appear in the general practitioner's office with presenting symptoms of physical distress, which are masking and at the same time reflecting and expressing psychological distress. In many cultures, such as the Chinese, asking for help with physical problems is more acceptable than reporting psychological distress. This is not untrue of our own culture.

It has been observed that people with post-traumatic stress disorders or dissociative disorders often initially exhibit only somatic symptoms. It was noted in Chapter 5 in the discussion of group work with traumatized Cambodian women that their anxieties appeared most often as physical symptoms (Nicholson and Kay, 1999).

Research conducted on the etiological factors involved in the development of somatization has lent support to the idea that early childhood influences play a major role, and that if children observe illness and pain in their family, they may be vulnerable to developing somatizing traits (Lipowski, 1988). These observations would apply to the Paul Norris case discussed in Chapter 7.

People with panic disorders usually have such considerable anxiety about their physical health that some researchers "suggest that hypochondriasis is its essential feature" (Lipowski, 1988, pp. 1363-1364). Somatizing patients have been known to provoke feelings of antipathy in their doctors, who can become very frustrated when people insist that they are sick, demand medical care, often complain about their treatment, "and are inclined to doctor-shop" (Lipowski, 1988, p. 1361).

Although many patients present with the somatizing syndrome described by Lipowski, not all people with somatization symptoms have similar behaviors, nor are the origins necessarily similar; somatic symptoms expressed in people victimized by trauma, for example, may be specific to the trauma experience. Somatization has occasionally been observed in adolescent girls whose mothers had breast cancer; in one case the daughter developed migraines, and in another a daughter reported breast pain (Spira and Kenemore, 2000).

It is equally important to be aware of the opposite situation. A person may present with complaints of a psychological disorder which may in actuality be masking an underlying physical disease. A person presenting with symptoms of anxiety, for example, could be suffering from hyperthyroidism. Psychotic symptoms can be caused by acute intermittent porphyria, believed to have been the cause of the "madness" of King George III. The excessive secretion of adrenal steroids in Cushing's disease can cause depression; patients who take steroids for various medical conditions may also experience depression. A patient presenting with mood changes, hallucinations, and unprovoked aggressive behaviors may have temporal lobe seizures; the inattention seen in a person with petit mal seizures can be confused with attention deficit disorder. It is always sound practice to ask patients seeking clinical intervention to have a medical evaluation as part of the assessment process.

AIDS

During the past twenty years, an epidemic of AIDS (acquired immune deficiency syndrome) has swept through the United States, causing death, disability, and severe hardships for many adults and children. Initially, medical science was totally powerless against this newly arrived disease, and many patients suffered prolonged illnesses, culminating in death, often at very early ages. General prejudice toward those initially stricken by the disease, believed to be mainly homosexual men, was a major reason for the lag in funding for medical research. The death of the secretly gay popular actor Rock Hudson, who "came out" during his final struggle with AIDS, was a turning point for more positive attention to this disease.

HIV is transmitted primarily sexually and through intravenous drug use by the sharing of contaminated needles. HIV spread to many drug users, men and women, who also acquired this disease through heterosexual or homosexual involvement with infected partners. Children have also been victims; many are born with HIV, which has been transmitted to them by their infected mothers. It has also been contracted through the medical use of contaminated blood for blood transfusions.

AIDS is caused by the "human immunodeficiency virus (HIV), which is transmitted only through blood, semen, vaginal fluid, and possibly other body fluids" ("AIDS—Part 1," 1994, p. 1). HIV can be transmitted to a baby through the mother's placenta or by drinking the mother's breast milk (Steiner, 1995). The virus invades the body cells, in which it may lie dormant for approximately eight to ten years, and then "multiplies by undermining the immune system, the body's main defense against biological invaders" ("AIDS—Part I," 1994, p. 2).

> Like many viruses, HIV often causes a brief flu-like illness in the first few weeks after infection. The symptoms—fever, rash, muscle aches, and swollen lymph glands—represent the body's defenses at work as killer T cells multiply and destroy infected cells. Recovery is quick, and the antibodies created to lie in wait for further invaders can be detected within six weeks to a year. But some infected T cells survive, and the virus continues to deplete the immune system, causing the symptoms formerly known as AIDS-related complex (ARC), which

include fatigue, night sweats, and weight loss. ("AIDS—Part I," 1994, p. 2)

Ultimately, the body is no longer able to fight against these continued infections, and other diseases invade the body; "the most common infectious disease among people with HIV is pneumocystis carinii pneumonia, which is caused by a microorganism that normally inhabits the lungs" ("AIDS—Part 1," 1994, p. 2). In the past, once AIDS developed, death would occur in about eighteen months.

In the past few years, medical breakthroughs, although not curative, have been able to prolong the lifespan of AIDS patients and decrease their suffering. It is important that these new medications be started as early as possible; therefore early detection of AIDS is considered imperative. It is even more critical that HIV infection be prevented; many public health education measures, such as emphasis on safe sex and clean needles for intravenous drug use, have been promoted, although not with uniform success.

Paradoxically, while advances in AIDS treatment have alleviated much suffering, the sense of urgency and crisis has also been reduced, and "some gay men have grown disturbingly complacent about safe sex in recent years"; this phenomenon has been observed more in younger gay men (Sack, 1999, p. A8). Drug use has added to this problem. And although attention has focused on intravenous drug use, danger also exists in the use of recreational drugs such as ecstasy, which can lower inhibitions and add to feelings of complacency (Sack, 1999).

A new alarming trend is the dramatic increase in AIDS cases in black and Hispanic populations. The numbers of white gay men with AIDS has been declining, while the percentages of gay black and Hispanic men with AIDS is increasing (Altman, 2000). The overall death rate for AIDS has declined, but for black people age twenty-five to forty-four, AIDS is the main cause of death (Stolberg, 1998). The Haitian population has been particularly devastated by this epidemic (Boice, 1998).

The stigma associated with homosexuality in the black and Hispanic communities is very strong, which makes it more difficult for gay people to identify themselves as such; this (in addition to the stigma against drugs) keeps many people in these groups from seeking medical services for AIDS. In addition, many black and Hispanic organizations are reluctant to address this problem publicly.

David Satcher, the surgeon general, commented that the black church, which was part of his early life, is not accepting of homosexuality. "A real problem has been getting ministers that are even willing to talk about it in their pulpits" (Stolberg, 1998, p. A1). Representative Louis Stokes, Chairman of the Congressional Black Caucus's health committee, requested that the spread of AIDS among black people be declared a national public health emergency. " 'But,' he said, 'this is one [issue] that black leadership has shied away from' " (Stolberg, 1998, p. A12).

AIDS is an increasing problem among minority women, who acquire this disease more from sexual activity than through intravenous drug use; the latter was more prevalent in the past (Stolberg, 1998). Many of these women are not aware that they are at risk for AIDS and often find out through blood tests done during prenatal checkups that they have contracted the HIV virus (Stolberg, 1998). Because AIDS can be transmitted to infants during the mother's delivery and through her breast milk, provided the mother's condition is known, modern medical techniques can often reduce these dangers. Many children are born with HIV infections, and many are orphaned by AIDS (Chapter 11). Helping mothers face the prospect of dying, thus in effect abandoning their children, and the need to arrange custody are all very important but extraordinarily difficult issues for the mother, her family, and the social worker to face.

One study, by the Centers for Disease Control and Prevention (CDC), on women who entered the federal Jobs Corps program from 1990 to 1996, found that "young black women were much more likely to be infected with the AIDS virus than others" in this program. Although the study was "not representative of all young people," nevertheless it demonstrated "the extent of AIDS among the economically and educationally disadvantaged." It also revealed that the infection rate was higher in women between the ages of sixteen to eighteen than it was in men, and CDC referred to their findings as "alarming" ("HIV Infection," 1998). In another study, conducted by Kristen Mertz, it was found that high rates of venereal disease were prevalent in women prisoners (Altman, 1999a). In addition to venereal disease being a serious problem per se, it also predisposes women to AIDS infections.

Lesbian women tend to acquire AIDS through intravenous drug use; some women become infected through sexual contact with other women; and some may have had previous sexual contact with men, and may currently be bisexual (Friedman, 1997). Friedman asserts that lesbian women have been excluded from much of the research on AIDS.

Minority teenagers are especially at risk, as they fail to recognize the seriousness of the disease; in addition, "public health campaigns to promote safe sex have not been directed at the communities that need them the most, advocates said" (Steinhauer, 1999b, p. A14). Many homeless teens and teenage prostitutes are also at risk for AIDS (Chapter 9).

In one innovative program in New York City, teenagers provide AIDS prevention education to their peers ("Teen-agers Learn," 1999). Dante Notice, seventeen, involved in an AIDS committee at his high school in the Bronx, observed that many of his peers were sexually active but were indifferent to learning about AIDS. He advocates the advantages of peer-to-peer communication in educating teens about AIDS. " 'I can put it in words they can understand in a way that adults can't do,' he said. 'I can break it down for them in a street kind of way'" ("Teen-agers Learn," 1999, p. 29).

AIDS is also an increasing problem in the elderly population, which was addressed in Chapter 10.

AIDS is highly prevalent in the prison population and is "five times that of the general population"; 29 percent of deaths (involving 907 individuals) in the state prison population in 1996 were attributed to AIDS (Altman, 1999a, p. A14). HIV was transmitted to most of these men through pre-prison intravenous drug use; a greater number of men than those infected with HIV contracted other sexually transmitted diseases, such as syphilis (Altman, 1999a). Although some prisons diagnose and treat HIV/AIDS, the numbers of inmates treated and the quality of their care remains variable and inconsistent. Theodore Hammet, who conducted this comprehensive study, observed that "the new findings highlight not only inadequacies in prison health care but also in preventing transmission of infections after the prisoners are released" (Altman, 1999a, p. A14).

AIDS is an international crisis; more than 50 million people are infected with HIV throughout the world, and it is increasing most rapidly in Africa, India, China, and the Caribbean (Kahn and Kifner, 2000). The epidemic is especially severe in sub-Saharan Africa; in some countries, 25 percent of the people have the HIV virus "and will probably die within 10 years" (Daley, 1998a). One of the major complications in combating the problem in Africa is the very strong stigma attached to this disease (Altman, 1999c; Daley 1998a). People feel shame about the disease and often suffer discrimination when others find out about it, such as losing employment and experiencing social ostracism in their communities. This deters people from seeking diagnostic and treatment services or taking preventive measures; for example, some mothers who know they are HIV positive will continue to breast feed for fear of being noticed if they switch to a bottle containing a formula. It has been suggested that the strong emotional reactions to this disease are related to "two subjects that are highly taboo in many parts of Africa: sex and death" (Daley, 1998a, p. A12).

One of the consequences of the AIDS epidemic is the large number of orphaned children; a United Nations report indicated that, since 1981, "more than 11 million children have been orphaned by AIDS . . . and the number is expected to rise to 13 million by the end of 2000"; 95 percent of these children live in African countries south of the Sahara Desert (Altman, 1999c, p. A10).

The country with the highest percent of orphans is Zambia. Although many of these children are being taken care of by extended families, this system, in a country in which poverty is endemic, is breaking down as families are overburdened by this responsibility. "Many children are being squeezed out. In 1991 Lusaka had 35,000 children living on the street; today there are more than 90,000" (Daley, 1998b, p. A12). AIDS orphans are at high risk for malnutrition and various forms of child maltreatment; they also "face the stigma and discrimination that often shadow the disease" (Altman, 1999c, p. A10).

In the United States, debates continue about legal protections and sanctions related to the transmission of HIV. On one side, civil libertarians are concerned with protecting the privacy of individuals with the disease; others want laws that permit notification of partners of AIDS patients, and some demand exists for legal sanctions against those who knowingly transmit this disease to others. Currently it is considered a criminal offense in twenty-nine states to "transmit or expose others knowingly to H.I.V.," and a number of other states are considering similar legislation (Richardson, 1998, p. A1). According to data available, this figure has changed little as of mid-2001. Several cases that have received considerable media attention have fueled this trend toward punitive action.

In one such case, a twenty-one-year-old member of a street gang in Brooklyn, with a history of eight arrests and three convictions, allegedly knew he was HIV positive when, living in Jamestown, in Chautauqua County, New York, he had sexual relations with a number of women from ages thirteen to twenty-two over a period of time (Bellafante, 1997). He allegedly did not practice "safe sex" nor tell his partners that he had HIV; according to health officials, he was "the source of a near epidemic of HIV in the county of 141,000 and has caused the greatest public health crisis the area has ever faced" (Bellafante, 1997, p. 58). It has been established that 110 people in the county were infected by him directly or indirectly (through sexual involvement with people with whom he had sex). He was subsequently sent to prison in New York City on drug charges and stated that he had had sexual relations with fifty to seventy-five women in the New York area during the past year. He will be charged with "first-degree assault in the cases of those who contracted HIV from him" by prosecutors in Chautauqua (Bellafante, 1997, p. 58).

AIDS has spawned many complex biological, social, and psychological problems; it is not surprising that legal and ethical issues about controlling it are so complex. General agreement now exists between health official and advocates for AIDS patients "that early testing and tracking can do a great deal to slow the epidemic, although how the reporting of H.I.V. cases should be conducted remains a contentious issue" (Richardson, 1998, p. A25).

Unfortunately, prison has often become the "treatment of choice" for such problems as drug use and mental illness in adolescents, while therapeutic and rehabilitative measures are seriously lacking. The escalation of AIDS in disenfranchised populations requires creative and constructive outreach programs, offered within the social context of the lives of the people affected and the myriad interacting social problems they face.

Clinical Considerations in Working with AIDS Patients

Working with patients with AIDS follows the basic biopsychosocial framework of the medical social work approach, discussed in this chapter. Martin and Henry-Feeney (1994) cite NASW's statement on AIDS, which supports the conviction that the psychosocial aspects of AIDS "are similar to those of other life threatening, catastrophic illnesses: social isolation, discrimination, anxiety, depression, concern about body image, financial problems, feelings of loss of control, and a confrontation with one's own immortality" (p. 339).

As in work with patients with any disease, it is important to understand the nature of the disease process itself, the progression of this disease in the individual patient, and the patient's prognosis; collaboration with the patient's medical providers and an understanding of the patient's functional capacities are also critical. Patients may need considerable help with daily management activities and home health nursing care. Many AIDS clinics offer multiple services to their clients; AIDS support groups are beneficial to many people.

Death may be an imminent concern; helping clients talk about their fears of death, their impending multiple losses, and, for parents of young children, their wishes for their children's future caretaking is critical. Clinical work with partners and family members can prove a great source of support to them as well as to the patient through these painful times.

Some people with AIDS find that their life span has been extended through major medical advances such as the development of new protease inhibitors. Paradoxically, this new promise for life introduces a dilemma for patients who were planning for death. "Now a community that had become so accustomed to death is grappling with the implications of this new lease on life. There is elation of course. But not far behind is an unexpected ambiguity, anxiety, even dread" (Carton, 1996, p. A1). Any transition is difficult; the unanticipated transition from facing death to facing the complexities of living, including facing the fact that one has no money left and must find a job, can create its own stress.

Many disabling conditions are stigmatizing; AIDS carries with it a very strong social stigma, due, in large measure, to its associations with homosexuality and drugs; it also produces fear of possible contagion (and sometimes panic) in many people. From a cultural perspective, many black and Hispanic communities have negative attitudes toward AIDS, and clients from these groups may need special help confronting this.

Many young, poor minority people (a large at-risk population for AIDS) may have complex psychosocial problems in their lives; some may be "throwaway" or homeless, and may be engaged in multiple at-risk behaviors; AIDS (and AIDS prevention) needs to be worked with in the context of each individual's life situation.

One is always faced with confidentiality issues with clients; this dilemma can be exacerbated with AIDS patients, and clinicians may find themselves struggling with the ethical dilemma of dealing with a client's refusal to tell a partner about the presence of AIDS.

SYSTEMS ISSUES

Medical care today is an extraordinarily complex issue. As a science, medicine has made incredible progress; constant advances are achieved in many realms, including heart surgery, cancer treatments, the use of human organs as transplants, reproductive technologies, and neonatal care for extremely premature infants. Decoding the human genome promises future advances in fighting disease and promoting health and longevity. In many ways, our technical advances outrun our ethical and legal judgments concerning the use or misuse of these advances. This includes the dilemma of keeping patients alive, many times against their will, in questionable states of health, pain, and severe disability.

Economic Problems

Many medical advances, including open heart surgery and organ transplants, require huge expenditures of money; prescription medications are also a major factor in the rising costs of medicine. Economic issues are at the root of many of the conflicts and political debates on the financing of medicine. Long-term hospitalizations and/or prolonged intensive care for chronic conditions can bankrupt the average family. Health insurance is usually the most important part of a benefits package to employees; strikes have occurred to protest the lack or inadequacy of medical insurance. HMOs and the overriding concept of managed care have been one of the "solutions" to this crisis of providing affordable medical care.

Whether these solutions have created new problems, especially in the human services fields at all levels including professional education, remains a pressing question.

The American Association of Health Plans reports that managed care today covers 61 percent of the population (Kilborn, 1998). Managed care emphasizes health preventive measures and reducing unnecessary medical procedures; many doctors and patients have expressed dissatisfaction with this system because of its concerns with cost effectiveness rather than the quality of medical care. Doctors who in the past were free to make independent medical judgments based on their clinical experience now must have them seconded by bureaucrats. They often see more patients in less time, leaving little if any time to get to know them in a more rounded way and to establish the vital doctor-patient relationship with them. Many doctors have left the profession or have found alternative ways to practice (Gorman, 1999).

Although complaints continue about managed care, many Americans have no insurance coverage at all. In 1998, an increase of 833,300 people without medical insurance occurred, bringing the total uninsured to 44.3 million, although this was a year with the lowest unemployment rates in thirty years and with increased family incomes (Pear, 1999a). Three major reasons for this problem include: (1) some employers ask their workers to pay a higher share of insurance costs, which many are not able to manage; (2) new jobs often exist in small businesses which do not provide coverage; and (3) many people who have left the welfare rolls no longer have Medicaid or any other coverage (Pear, 1999a).

In stark contrast to many prosperous countries, 11.1 million children in this country are without health insurance (Pear, 1999a). Although Congress allotted funds for children's health care in 1997, many states did not actively recruit eligible children; less than 20 percent of the allotted money has been used (Pear, 1999b). Studies have revealed that many very poor elderly people are not receiving Medicare "safety net" supplements (Kilborn, 1999a, p. A7). Although they are entitled to these benefits (after a means test), many have not applied. This lack of enrollment is thought to be due to "conflicts between Federal and state agencies as well as a dearth of program leadership and coordination, labyrinthine red tape and demeaning application procedures" (Kilborn, 1999a, p. A7).

Hispanics are the largest ethnic group to be uninsured (Pear, 1999a); a third of Hispanic Americans do not have health coverage (Kilborn, 1999b).

Organ Transplants

Organ transplants have stirred considerable controversy; initially a rare, experimental procedure, organ transplantation has become commonplace today, and it is not surprising that this still relatively new procedure has raised many legal, systemic, and ethical issues. One recent controversy receiving much publicity relates to both the scarcity of available organs for transplants and questions about distribution. It is estimated that 62,000 people in this country are on waiting lists for a heart, lung, liver, or pancreas; "last year alone, 4,000 people died waiting" (Stolberg, 1999, p. A25). Congress has debated the question of changing the distribution of organs so that uniform standards can be established for sending organs outside the geographical area where the organ was donated to meet the most urgent patient needs. On November 16, 2000, the United Network for Organ Sharing (UNOS) adopted a new organ-allocation system for liver transplants (the

Mayo End-Stage Liver Disease Model [MELD]) based on disease severity rather than exclusively on the region where the organ was donated; this new system has not ended the debate (Bonfield, 2000).

In what has been considered a "revolutionary" procedure, live donors (often relatives of patients) have donated a portion of their liver; this procedure, performed less than 100 times (on adults) in this country, is seen as a possible solution to the shortage problem (Grady, 1999a). It had been determined that the "right lobe could be removed safely for adults"; nevertheless, doctors have expressed concern about donors who may feel pressured to agree and "may be taking too much of a risk" (Grady, 1999a, p. A12). Other transplant procedures have occurred using live donors, such as kidney and bone marrow transplants.

In one well-publicized case, a seventeen-year-old girl with leukemia was expected to die unless she had a bone marrow transplant; when no donors were found after an extensive search, the parents decided to have another child, in the hope that the baby's bone marrow would be compatible with that of the ailing sister (Morrow, 1991). The mother, forty-three, became pregnant and delivered a healthy baby girl who was judged to be a compatible donor.

When the baby was fourteen months old, the procedure (which is considered harmless for donors) took place, and the older daughter received the transplant. Although this family was seen as a warm, nurturing family who welcomed the baby in her own right, many ethical dilemmas were stirred up. "Is it morally acceptable for parents to conceive a child in order to obtain an organ or tissue to save the life of another one of their children?" (Morrow, 1991, p. 54). It has been demonstrated that tissue from an aborted fetus may be beneficial to patients with Parkinson's disease and Alzheimer's disease. A similar ethical concern has been voiced that some women might "conceive [and then abort] just to provide material for relatives in need" (Morrow, 1991, p. 56).

Recent advances have also occurred in transplanting nonvital organs to people, such as hands and knees, also raising ethical issues. "With rare exceptions, transplant recipients must, for the rest of their lives, take powerful anti-rejection drugs, whose side effects include increased risks of infection . . . cancer and other conditions. Who should decide if the risk is worth the reward?" (Altman, 1999b, p. 1). Additional questions, such as who would have the responsibility for paying for these transplants and whether people would be willing to make orthopedic donations for conditions that are not essential for life, have also been asked. The impact on the future relationships of live donors to recipients, when they are known and especially when they are in the same family, is another dilemma.

It is generally agreed that donors should give consent to have their organs transplanted (usually after death, and sometimes during life) and that organs not be sold. Chinese officials have been accused of selling the vital organs of executed prisoners to wealthy people in other countries (Gorman, 1998a). Whether the prisoners ever gave consent for this and whether the crimes for which people can be executed were expanded to increase the supply of organs have been questioned.

A controversial bill was introduced in Missouri that would allow prisoners on death row to donate either a kidney or bone marrow in exchange for a sentence reduced to life imprisonment with no parole. "Although doctors have attacked the bill on moral grounds, arguing that a choice between death or transplantation is never free, defense attorneys have called it 'fascinating'" (Gorman, 1998a, p. 76).

Nursing Home Care

Nursing homes have come under increasing scrutiny as many provide inadequate services to their residents, who are often helpless to protest. In California, where an intensive investigation was undertaken, it was alleged that "in 1993 alone, more than 3,000 people died as a result of unacceptable care" ("Toward Nursing," 1999, p. A26). Former President Clinton, in 2000, requested additional money for strengthening regulatory inspections. Barbara Hengstebeck, the executive director of the Coalition to Protect America's Elders, asserted that "until states are given the resources to beef up nursing home staff with qualified personnel, little or nothing can be done to protect the elderly in abusive, neglectful situations" (Beaucar, 2000, p. 15).

The lack of psychiatric care in nursing homes for those in need has been challenged; it has been estimated that "less than 1 percent of elderly nursing home residents who might benefit from psychiatric intervention receive it" (Kennedy, 2000, p. 262). In addition to patients with emotional problems complicating aging, such as those with depression or anxiety, many nursing homes now care for psychiatric patients who have been deinstitutionalized from state hospitals (Borson et al., 1987). "Considerable evidence indicates that psychiatric problems are frequently undiagnosed or misdiagnosed and that opportunities for effective intervention may be obscured by diagnostic bias toward 'incurable' conditions" (Borson et al., 1987, p. 1413).

Patients in nursing homes are extremely diverse in culture, ethnicity, education, lifestyle, and personality. One unfortunate tendency in nursing home life is to ignore the individuality of patients, infantilizing them and placing priority on their adaptation to institutional needs. Nursing home practices "can exacerbate loneliness, boredom and depression rooted in an environment where residents have lost control over basic physical and social aspects of their lives" (Levenson, 1998, p. 3). Special problems include lack of food choice (especially important to ethnic minorities), lack of choice about roommates, daily schedules, and activities, and failure to respect end-of-life choices. It has been recommended by the multidisciplinary group Pioneers in Nursing Home Culture Change that residents should be provided with "companionship, opportunities to help others, variety and spontaneity," and that residents should be surrounded by "other living things, including children, plants and animals" (Levenson, 1998, p. 3).

Home Health Care

Although it is generally believed that people do better living at home than in institutions when care is needed, a recent dramatic decrease in federal funds for home health care has occurred, resulting in the dependency on hospitals and nursing homes (Pear, 2000). As a consequence, home health care agencies have received less money and can provide services only to more serious cases involving those seniors who are so infirm that they cannot leave their homes at all. These figures do not "show how many people simply go without treatment after losing home care benefits, or how many such patients have died. But health care providers and lawyers for the elderly say they have evidence people are going uncared for" (Pear, 2000, p. A1).

Health care agencies avoid working with seriously ill patients, because these patients require more care (and more expenditures of money), exceeding Medicare limits. Many long-term patients are excluded from services, such as stroke patients who need extensive rehabilitation (Pear, 2000). Decreased Medicare funding of hospice services has also led to diminished use of hospice care. Hospice programs enable terminally ill people to die at home or in hospital-related hospice services, in an environment emphasizing comfort and pain alleviation (Cloud, 2000a).

Although many alternatives exist for older people, such as assisted living residences, the most popular choice is to remain at home. Conover (1997), writing three years before the current Medicare crisis, noted that seven million Americans were receiving a variety of home-care services which kept them from being institutionalized. One level of home care is provided by homemakers who help with cooking and housework but provide no medical or physical care, such as bathing. Many people can manage with assistance of this nature. Others, needing more care, require the services of a licensed home health aide.

The demand for home health aides is growing at a very rapid pace, and it has been predicted that from 1994 to 2005 there will be a 119 percent increase in these positions (Conover, 1997). Some health care agencies have been accused of fraudulent billing. Selection and ongoing supervision of workers remain problems; neglect and abuse have been observed in some situations. Older adults with paid caretakers can be "vulnerable in the same way as babies left with nannies"; now, however, "there is a new kind of nanny—and a caretaking relationship fraught with guilt, resentment and love that we are very likely to be wrestling with for years to come" (Conover, 1997, pp. 126-127).

CONCLUSION

Illness and disability are normative parts of the life course; however, as advances in medicine have been made and life has been prolonged, we see more people living with disabilities across the life cycle. Paradoxically and sadly, as medicine has made more magnificent scientific and technological advances, the humanistic qualities that were present in the family doctor of the past are often lacking; patients, viewed as organ systems, are shunted from specialist to specialist.

The present crisis in managed care has only intensified this trend away from humanistic medicine. Efficiency, productivity, and enormous amounts of paperwork take precedence over sitting and talking with, and getting to know, patients. Medical social work, with its expertise and experience, is vanishing in many sectors, replaced by solution-oriented and task-focused discharge planning and referral.

On a systemic basis, problems relating to health care (and paying for it) are tremendous and complex, a subject of national discourse. Almost every medical advance brings in its wake new moral and ethical dilemmas.

One major advance has been that the voices of the ill and disabled are now being heard, legislation is being passed in their behalf, and employment practices are changing in their favor. We read of Special Olympics and wheelchair entrants in marathon races. The front page of *The New York Times* reported that Brooke Ellison would be the first quadriplegic to graduate from Harvard, and quoted her as saying: " 'I've always felt that whatever circumstances I confront, it's just a question of continuing to live and not letting what I can't do define what I can' " (Steinberg, 2000, p. A1). Brooke and her mother, Jean Ellison, have written a book, *Miracles Happen: One Mother, One Daughter, One Journey,* recounting their experiences, which is set to be released in early 2002.

In working with people who are physically ill, the support and caring that we as clinical social workers can offer are part of the healing process. The body and mind are a unit, each affecting the other.

LEARNING EXERCISE

1. *Case Presentation:* Ask for student volunteers to present cases in which issues of illness and disability exist. Discussion can include:

type of illness, effect on functioning, attitudes toward illness and receiving care, available supports, adaptation and strengths, and special problems.

SUGGESTED READINGS

Articles

Lawrence, S. A. and Zittel, K. M. (2000). Heart transplantation: A behavioral perspective. *Journal of Human Behavior in the Social Environment, 3*(2), 61-79.

Spira, M. and Kenemore, E. (2000). Adolescent daughters of mothers with breast cancer: Impact and implications. *Clinical Social Work Journal, 28,* 183-195.

Books

Bloch, J. and Margolis, J. (1986). Feelings of shame: Siblings of handicapped children. In A. Gitterman and L. Shulman (Eds.), *Mutual aid groups and the life cycle* (pp. 91-108). Itasca, IL: F. E. Peacock Publishers, Inc.

Fadiman, J. (1997). *The spirit catches you and you fall down: A Hmong child, her American doctors and the collision of two cultures.* New York: Farrar, Straus and Giroux.

Friedman, E. (1997). The impact of AIDS on the lives of women. In S. L. A. Straussner and E. Zelvin (Eds.), *Gender and addictions: Men and women in treatment* (pp. 197-221). Northvale: Jason Aronson Inc.

Olkin, R. (1999). *What psychotherapists should know about disability.* New York: The Guilford Press.

Chapter 13

Mental Health Problems

. . . Mrs. Tickit, finding no balsam for a wounded mind . . . suffered greatly from low spirits . . .

Charles Dickens
"Little Dorritt"

Most people have experienced mental health problems in their lives, ranging from minor bouts of anxiety and depression and psychosomatic distress to more severe problems, such as major depressions or panic disorders. We have seen throughout this book how mental health problems are intertwined with social problems, often in a vicious circle. For example, depressed mothers, living in socially adverse conditions, are often unable to respond to their babies, who then fail to thrive or are otherwise neglected, and a spiral of state intervention, further deterioration, and increased depression may then ensue. It becomes difficult to tell where social adversity begins and individual illness leaves off or vice versa.

Schizophrenia, which usually develops in early adulthood, affects large numbers of people in this country. It is often a factor in homelessness and in family malfunction, which in turn may lead to foster placement for children. Substance abuse pervades our culture, often resulting in family problems, loss of employment, and illness. Pathological gambling, although not a physical addiction, can dominate a person's life, causing considerable personal distress, financial hardships, and family breakdown.

Social workers often work with people with borderline personalities who tend to be impulsive, anxious, manipulative, have serious interpersonal problems, and are often in a state of crisis. People also suffer from a range of anxiety disorders; post-traumatic stress disorder (PTSD) is a common consequence of physical abuse, sexual abuse, and torture and other atrocities frequently experienced by refugees.

People with mental retardation and serious developmental disorders, such as autism, also can have difficulties with social functioning and family relationships that can be compounded by psychiatric illness.

This chapter, although not dealing with many important mental health problems, focuses on the major issues just discussed because of their significance in social work practice. The combination of deinstitutionalization and managed care has led to a serious shortage of adequate mental health services, which is also addressed in this chapter.

Positive advances in educational services and supports also have been provided to patients and to families, and greater recognition of civil, political, and employment rights of this population has occurred. In many instances, families and sometimes patients have been involved in strong advocacy pursuits; this is discussed later in the chapter.

SCHIZOPHRENIA

Schizophrenia, present throughout recorded history, has been viewed over time through different perspectives and different cultural lenses. People suffering from this disease have been treated in varying ways, ranging "from kindness, and soothing medications, to restraints, cruelty, and even putting the unfortunate sufferer to death" (Karon and VandenBos, 1996, p. 7). Schizophrenia remains a mystery to us; although we know more about the brain chemistry involved and how to reduce its severe symptomatology, no cure exists as such. For many, it is a lifelong, chronic disease with remissions and decompensations. Although a number of people with this illness make good recoveries and attain a high level of functioning, many others face a tragic life of missed opportunities.

Because considerable variability is found in symptoms, etiology, and the course of the disease, many clinicians view it as "not one, but a group of clinical entities" (MacKinnon and Michels, 1971, p. 230). MacKinnon and Michels (1971) observe that "one patient may present with extreme social withdrawal, retreating to bed for weeks at a time, another with episodes of depersonalization and feelings of being controlled by external forces, and still a third has marked anorexia with severe weight loss" (p. 230).

Schizophrenia touches every aspect of a person's life. It most frequently occurs in late adolescence or early adulthood. People with schizophrenia often are aware that they are different, which may add to their difficulty in fully participating in life. Mr. S., who is thirty-five, had his first schizophrenic breakdown as an adolescent; he talked about how he had been a "loser," and about being "weird" and "different from everyone. . . . He was always "afraid of everyone and everything." They often miss the on-time events of adult development. When Mr. S. first became ill, he "wanted to come to the hospital," because he hoped people could make him well; he "wanted to go to college, have a job, and have a girlfriend." Now in adulthood, none of his hopes have been fulfilled.

Schizophrenia is a "disorder that affects the total personality in all aspects of its functioning: emotion, volition, outward behavior, and most particularly, the thinking process. While not all patients show the same range or magnitude of disturbances, and even the same patient's symptoms will vary in time, the hallmark of this disorder is that it permeates every aspect of the individual's functioning" (Bemporad, and Pinsker, 1974, p. 524).

Arieti (1974) made the point that meaning and logic lie beneath schizophrenic thought processes which, on the surface, can appear totally meaningless and illogical (Chapter 2). Karon and VanderBos (1996) described a patient who was considered " 'confused' because he drank from his own urinal"; another patient, who was paranoid, shed light on this action by commenting: " 'If you only drink your own urine and only eat your own feces, you will never die' " (p. 54). Since fear of annihilation and death is so common in schizophrenia, this "defense against death" becomes understandable.

Mark Vonnegut (1975) wrote an autobiography in which he discussed his severe schizophrenic break which occurred after graduation from college (Chapter 2). At one point, he picked up a quantity of tobacco tins in a store and walked out with them without even thinking of paying. His friend Simon questioned his need for this large quantity of tobacco. Mark's act had its own logic; it was very important to have a continual supply of cigarettes, although not for the usual reasons most people have for smoking.

> Smoking was an important reminder of who I was. It was my clock. Cigarettes seemed to keep time. They had a continuity with the real world that I seemed to be losing. As long as I smoked cigarettes I was alive. As far as I knew, dead people didn't smoke cigarettes. (Vonnegut, 1975, p. 102)

Karon and VanderBos (1996) cite Lidz (1973), who described schizophrenic thought as having an " 'egocentric overinclusiveness,' " meaning that a person has "the feeling that things which logically are not related to the self *are* related to the self, or that things which realistically one cannot influence are being influenced by one's actions" (p. 54). In addition, sometimes "the patient regresses under stress and uses modes of thought that were more typical of an earlier period in life, or were dreamlike" (Karon and VanderBos, 1996, p. 55). Karon and VanderBos (1996) also note Rudolf Ekstein's (1971) observation that "while there is no general schizophrenic language, each patient has a meaningful personal language which the therapist must learn" (p. 55).

It is ironic that the DSM-IV (American Psychiatric Association, 1994) does not include thought disorders at all, which most clinicians (past and present, including Kaplan et al., 1994) view as the core characteristic of schizophrenia; the American Psychiatric Association's (1994) preference was to list disordered speech, as this was observable, and "inferences about thought are based primarily on the individuals' speech," whereas there was an "inherent difficulty in developing an objective definition of 'thought disorder'" (p. 276).

Thought disorders are a composite of the actual content of the thoughts as well as the thought processes themselves; a person, for example, may lack coherence, logic, be unable to abstract, have loose associations, and sometimes use frequent puns (Kaplan et al., 1994). The listener often cannot "make heads or tails" of what the person has just said.

The following letter was addressed by a patient to one of the male physicians in the hospital where she was under treatment (Noyes, 1953). The content itself is bizarre, but it is also difficult to understand just what the patient is trying to communicate; illogic and incoherence predominate, and some puns and clang associations such as "plant" and "tant'" are present. This communication serves to distance the reader from the letter writer, rather than enhancing a rapport between them. Only the first paragraph of this letter is presented here.

> Dear Dr. _____ ,
>
> "My Plan," or as my mother used to call you, "the Little Plant," or else one little Plant for I was the other Plant, called "Tant." Will you please see that I am taken out of this hospital and returned to the equity court so I can prove to the court who I am and thereby help establish my identity to the world. Possibly you do not remember or care to remember that you married me May 21, 1882, while you were in England and that I made you by that marriage the Prince of Wales, as I was born Albert Edward, Prince of Wales, I am feminine absolutely, not a double person nor a hermaphrodite, so please know I am England's feminine king—the king who is a king.
>
> [Two paragraphs follow, and then the letter is signed.]
>
> Sincerely,
>
> "Tant"
>
> Queen of Scotland, Empress of the World, Empress of China, Empress of Russia, Queen of Denmark, Empress of India, Maharajahess of Durban, "Papal authority" as a Protestant. (Noyes, 1953, pp. 374-375)

This degree of thought disturbance is not present in all people with schizophrenia; some—especially patients with paranoid schizophrenia—may have thought processes that are more intact, and their thought disturbances may be limited to specific areas of dysfunction. In Chapter 10, for example, we discussed William Minor, who suffered from paranoid schizophrenia) and was a major contributor to the first *Oxford English Dictionary;* his cognitive abilities were excellent but unfortunately they did not protect him from the delusions which took over at night.

The ego functions (Chapter 2) of a schizophrenic person are extensively impaired to one degree or another; but it is important to assess them on an individual basis and track their variation over time. In addition to thought, a major disturbance exists in the patient's expression of emotions or affect: "the patient's subjective emotional experience may be diminished, flattened, or blunted. . . . He has difficulty expressing and communicating the emotional responses of which he is aware. This affective deficit not only leads to estrangement from others, but also to an inability to enjoy the solitude that results. The patient is a lonely, unhappy person. Anhedonia, or the absence of pleasure, characterizes his entire life, although it is rarely the presenting complaint" (MacKinnon and Michels, 1971, p. 231).

Executive functioning is typically markedly impaired; many people with schizophrenia are unable to work; often they cannot manage without the "auxiliary ego" of others. Hence the need for living with families, foster families, or in group homes (and sometimes hospitals). Frequently when the acute symptoms, such as hallucinations, disappear (or are controlled by drugs), "background or *residual symptoms* [italics added] remain" ("Families in the Treatment," 1989, p. 1).

> Schizophrenic patients are still likely to be apathetic, socially withdrawn, and emotionally unresponsive. Their gestures and movements are peculiar, their speech slow, hesitant, and repetitious. Often they . . . develop annoying or dangerous habits like wandering alone at night. . . . They have difficulty in managing money and remembering to take their drugs. They cannot concentrate, initiate activity, or even take much pleasure or interest in anything. Providing for their daily needs, holding a steady job, or maintaining even casual social relationships is often too much for them. ("Families in the Treatment," Part I, 1989, p. 1)

Their perceptions of outer reality are usually disturbed; the actions and activities of others are often misinterpreted, and often severe distortions of perception occur marked by "secondary symptoms such as hallucinations, illusions, delusions" (MacKinnon and Michels, 1971, p. 239). Inner perception, i.e., self-awareness and attunement to inner feelings, is markedly impaired, while at the same time a preoccupation with inner states exists; this is often a fragmented rather than an integrated process.

The capacity to relate is markedly impaired; "he has few friends and does not trust people. . . . He learns to protect himself by maintaining emotional distance, preferring his own autistic world to shared experiences in the world of others. . . . The mistrust, fear of closeness, ambivalence, and clinging dependency of the schizophrenic patient influence all of his human contacts" (MacKinnon and Michels, 1971, pp. 237-238).

The person with schizophrenia has a weakened sense of identity, ranging from a poor self-image to fragmented ego states, with fears of bodily disintegration and annihilation. Boundaries are often diffuse; in Chapter 2, we noted how Mark Vonnegut begged his friend to hypnotize him so that he could control Vonnegut; being under his friend's control, Vonnegut would know that he himself existed.

It is not uncommon to find that many chronically mentally ill patients also have serious problems with alcohol abuse, which can cause serious treatment complications, including regression and the possible need for hospitalization (Mulinski, 1989).

> Although symptoms of schizophrenia can be controlled with medication, these patients are often non-compliant with treatment. Acute intoxication can exacerbate psychotic symptoms. Alcohol abuse undermines psychosocial interventions and interferes with compliance with medication. (Mulinski, 1989, p. 339)

To schizophrenic patients, the world is often puzzling and very frightening; it loses its solidity as patients lose their sense of cohesiveness and identity. One woman felt she had been "ordered" by her ten-year-old daughter and her friends to buy materials so they could make valentines. As she "obeyed" and opened the door, she felt as though her arms and legs were becoming dismembered from her body, and an absolute panic set in; this psychotic state lasted for some time.

The person with a sense of total dissolution and fear of annihilation, living in a world that is also felt to be crumbling, needs to feel safe; structure and caring relationships that are warm but not intrusive are of primary importance. Herein lies much of the complexity involved in working with schizophrenic people; they need closeness but fear it, and relating to others is usually a major problem. They need structure and limit setting but often fight this, not wanting to be controlled by others. The hospitalization they may desperately need, because it provides a safe haven, may nevertheless terrify them, at least initially.

General agreement (although not unanimous) prevails on the benefits of medication; medication advances provided the first breakthrough in psychiatric treatment of schizophrenia and enabled the deinstitutionalization movement to begin. For the first time, a way was found to decrease psychotic thought processes and help people maintain better contact with reality as well as behavioral control.

Concerns have been expressed about the side effects of the continual use of antipsychotic medication. Many patients are resistant to taking these medications and often do not take them if they are without supervision; this problem is compounded by the lack of care and supervision that exists for many people with mental illness. Ethical and civil rights issues have also been involved in this problem; some people feel it is a violation of a patient's rights to mandate either medication or hospitalization; this is discussed further at the end of this section.

In the following instance, Mr. S., discussed previously, who was in a state psychiatric hospital, had been taken off all medications for two weeks as he was being prepared to take part in trials of a new antipsychotic drug. In the following session, he was being seen by a social work intern, who was hopeful that they could continue their constructive discussions about positive activities in which Mr. S. might be able to engage.

> Instead of talking about activities, he talked about death, decay, and the maggots that were eating his brain and body. He told me about people who were chasing him with clubs, who wanted to beat his brains out, and spoke about eating cats, and rotting in hell. I did not know how to handle this psychotic process, so I just allowed him to continue talking, as I listened anxiously.

Some guidelines are generally followed in working with schizophrenic patients. These are based on the nature of the illness. They include providing structure and limits; reality testing; development of skills in daily living; enhancing relationships; and enhancing self-esteem. Some theorists are primarily behaviorally oriented; others incorporate psychotherapy as part of the overall treatment.

Although about one-third of schizophrenic patients live with their families (while many are homeless), advances have been made in the provision of group homes for the mentally ill. Work with families, using such services as psychoeducational therapy for the families, as well as family therapy has also been emphasized.

Work with Schizophrenic Patients

The clinician can help patients anchor their anxieties and navigate the complexities of life, and they can provide a model for thinking, solving problems, and interacting with others. If patients can internalize these functions, they will achieve a higher level of integration. From a self psychology perspective, the therapist becomes an important selfobject for the patient. Semrad emphasized providing support through effective, empathic human responsiveness, which permits a withdrawn or confused schizophrenic person to make effective contact with another person (Adler, 1979). Winnicott's concept of the holding environment has been applied to case management with schizophrenic clients (Kanter, 1990), and was discussed in Chapter 3.

The Clinical Relationship

Because schizophrenic patients are generally uncomfortable with people, a clinician can find it difficult to establish relationships with them. "Sessions may be characterized by frequent silences which the worker must fill, monosyllabic answers to questions, awkwardness, apparent disinterest in proceeding with treatment, or highly inappropriate discussion" (Nelsen, 1983, pp. 337-338). Shifts can occur within one session from fairly rational discussion into psychotic deterioration. Mr. S., for example, after talking about some of his earlier experiences in a realistic way, changed the subject.

> Mr. S. began to complain about how bad he felt, and how it was because people at the hospital were taking gallons and gallons of his blood. He said that "blood is brain and brain is blood," and people are taking away his brain and making him crazy. He said that it was an "atomic insanity" that caused him to have to suffer for all of his life. He began to rock back and forth rather violently in his chair and shake his legs rapidly.

The student realized that Mr. S. was having trouble tolerating this long period of talking; when she suggested they discontinue now and talk more the following week, Mr. S. seemed very relieved "and his rocking and shaking decreased." (It understandably and undoubtedly relieved the social worker's anxiety as well.)

Although many schizophrenic patients have the ability to relate to the therapist and can accept the positive aspects of the holding environment, they can also become frightened by the closeness, and it is not uncommon to see some oscillation between closeness and retreat from it. In response to the social work student's expression of concern, the following dialogue occurred at the end of a session, which reflects Mr. S.'s confusion about what caring means and some boundary problems.

> He looked at me and smiled, asking, "Are you a member of my family or something?" I said that I wasn't a member of his family and won-

dered what made him ask me that question. He said that usually only family members would talk to him for this long. I again told him that I was not a family member, but his therapist. He thanked me and then left the room.

After several sessions in which Mr. S. was positive and cooperative in talking with the student, a session occurred in which he was avoidant and resistant.

He turned his head away from me and wouldn't look at me during the session; he responded with one-word answers. I said that it seemed like he didn't want to talk; I wondered if he had something on his mind that he wasn't saying. He said in an angry tone that he didn't have anything on his mind but that he didn't feel like talking to me.

I wondered if he were angry or disappointed with me, which he denied. I told him that it would be okay if he were mad at me, and that I'd like to talk about it if he were. He said that talking to me didn't do any good and that he was sick of it. When I suggested that he was disappointed about our work together, he said it didn't matter, that no one in the hospital helped him anyway; we all just made him worse. After a few minutes, he got up and said he didn't want to talk anymore, and he left. I told him that I would be in my office for the rest of this half hour, which was the time reserved for him, if he changed his mind and wanted to come back; but he didn't.

Later in the day, the student saw Mr. S. on the ward; he approached and asked: "You're coming back next week, aren't you?" She assured him that she was and confirmed their appointment. Their work together continued positively after this incident; however, at a later date, after some good progress, further deterioration occurred, which the student attributed to his fear of his own progress and anxiety about possibly leaving the hospital in the future. However important these issues are, this decompensation also occurred when the social work student returned from a vacation, a point which was not openly discussed; the loss (even temporary) of a therapist can produce decompensation in a patient.

Another important point in considering the therapeutic relationship is the reaction of the clinician; the intensity of the patient's feelings can arouse intense feelings in the clinician, and the "inevitable hopelessness, helplessness, and despair that these patients experience in therapy will inevitably be felt by the therapist" (Adler, 1979, p. 135). The use of intersubjectivity is very relevant in this work; tuning in to one's subjective reactions to the patient can often alert a clinician to the patient's unverbalized feeling state

(Adler, 1979). A clinician can also feel frustrated, disappointed, and unsuccessful, because of the slow rate of progress and frequent regressions.

The social work student is especially vulnerable to these feelings, as one often feels one's success as a clinician is measured by the improvement of the patient. Paradoxically, at the same time that students struggle with these feelings, it has often been observed that student therapists are very successful with chronic schizophrenic patients because of their genuineness, the intensity of their involvement, and their expectations for the patients' improvement, which may be novel to each patient's experience. In this excerpt, the student shares her feelings after one of Mr. S.'s regressive episodes.

> It was not until this session that I was able to admit how intensely I was being affected by Mr. S. and his psychosis and hopelessness. I thought it was "unprofessional" and even unkind to feel so miserable, frustrated, or hopeless during our sessions. It was difficult to acknowledge insecurities about my own competence and ability as a social worker. I felt like I had no idea what I was doing! I was sure that a "better social worker" would be able to help Mr. S. more than I. I was equating Mr. S.'s lack of progress with my failure as a social worker.

The Focus on Reality

The consensus in work with this population seems to be that a reality orientation is extremely important; the patient's preoccupations with the inner world needs to be directed outward, with an emphasis on enhancing coping capacities. The following discussion took place after Mr. S. complained about having a stomachache and feeling depressed and bored.

> I suggested that if we thought about why his stomach was bothering him or why he was so depressed and bored, maybe we could come up with ways to help him feel better. I asked if he would like to try, and he said "OK." I thought we could start by thinking about what kinds of things he had been doing lately and how he was spending his time. He said that today he drank seven cups of coffee (by 11:00!) and skipped breakfast. I asked him about other things he did with his time. Sometimes he smoked cigarettes or watched TV but usually he sat around. When asked about groups, he mentioned that he liked music and art. I inquired if he had had a chance to think about his "mental torture" while playing an instrument or drawing; he said "only sometimes." He hadn't been going to groups lately, because he "didn't feel well." When asked if he thought going back to the groups might help him feel better, he said he would go—especially to his music group, which he liked.

I also asked if he had seen the nurse about his stomach, and he told me that she wouldn't think anything was wrong. I wondered if there was anything that he could do to help make his stomach feel better. He thought and said that maybe he could eat breakfast and he might not be hungry. I agreed and said that I when I don't eat breakfast, sometimes my stomach hurts, too.

Mr. S. began attending more activities, and through a behavior modification design earned rewards, such as going to the canteen through his increased activities; following these advances, the student discussed with Mr. S. more about his feelings and disappointments related to "emotional issues and relationships." Schizophrenic patients are often responsive to this type of discussion, and as they learn to connect with their feelings and express them, they can experience relief, and their anxiety often decreases. Although some clinicians work with schizophrenic people only with a concrete, task-centered orientation, many patients have the capacity to develop self-awareness and to make some connections between their inner states and their behaviors.

Generally, it is important to have team collaboration as part of the therapeutic plan. Clinicians often work constructively with doctors, nurses, recreation therapists, etc. Working with families is also important; the student felt that Mr. S.'s positive relationship with his parents "served as a motivating factor for him to work on his programs."

Community Care

When state psychiatric hospitals began closing, community care, in the form of assisted-living arrangements such as group homes for the mentally ill, was seen as the ideal alternative. Many of these facilities have been very effective, providing structure, support, and guidance for their residents and encouraging their involvement in the community. Different levels of care and supervision exist depending upon the needs of the patients.

Some patients are involved in community day care programs or are enrolled in other rehabilitative projects. Support and self-help groups are also available in the community, which many people find helpful, and case management has often been provided. Case management with the chronically mentally ill is a major method of intervention in the community.

Case Management

The case manager plays a coordinating role, in particular in arranging therapeutic services. Case managers are often social workers who work with patients living either in their own apartments or with their families.

Visits by the manager may range from being occasional or as-needed to involving intensive daily supervision to ensure medication compliance and assistance with the basic requirements of daily functioning. Kanter (1990, 2000) emphasizes that provision of a holding environment is of major importance in case management; this raises case management to a level beyond the mere provision and coordination of concrete services, as it is often viewed.

Work with Families

About forty years ago, schizophrenia was generally thought to be have developed as the result of family factors, such as faulty communication. The term schizophrenogenic mother was often used to characterize mothers of these patients as sending mixed messages to them throughout their lives, which they could neither obey nor disobey, nor comment on, resulting in a state of total schizophrenic confusion. Therefore families often were ignored or "kept at a distance" when their children were hospitalized.

> Parents were seen as overprotective, or cold and indifferent, or it was said that they confused the child with mixed emotional messages. . . . The symptoms were said to be a response to "double binds," "pseudo-mutuality," and other destructive forms of communication. It was suggested that the family "needed" the schizophrenic disorder to maintain its own stability, or somehow created it to prevent the adolescent from maturing normally and leaving home. ("Families in the Treatment—Part I," 1989, p. 1)

This perspective on schizophrenia influenced mental health approaches and at times kept clinicians from looking outside this framework. Major breakthroughs in our understanding of schizophrenia have led to understanding its strong genetic and biochemical basis, and parents are no longer held to be the causative agents (although relationship factors can certainly contribute to exacerbations or precipitation of decompensations). At the same time that attitudes toward families were changing, many patients were returning home after deinstitutionalization. Now, families were becoming paramount in the treatment of their schizophrenic children, and professionals began to find ways of working with them. Rather than viewing the family primarily as the root of the problem, they were now viewed as reacting to and being affected by the chaotic world of their schizophrenic offspring. Families needed support; psychoeducational approaches were one way to help them with their schizophrenic children (Anderson, 1983). One major component of these programs related to understanding how schizophrenic people are vulnerable to stress, and finding ways to eliminate stress in their lives (Kopeikin et al., 1983).

Families need help understanding this complex illness and developing realistic expectations for what the patient can achieve; they need to help the patient deal with daily life, develop routines, and learn rules of behavior. The following is an example of this psychoeducational approach with families.

> People with schizophrenia must be approached calmly and patiently. They often prefer to be alone, and their privacy should be respected. . . . Both nagging criticism and overenthusiasm are bad. Requests and criticism should be expressed pleasantly, clearly, concisely, and specifically; for example, "you should help out more around the house" is bad, but "Please take out the garbage today" is good. Families are told that a patient's own requests, when they make simple sense, should be respected and not interpreted; if she prefers to eat alone in her room, she should be allowed to do so and her motives should not be questioned.
>
> Families are also taught to watch for signs of relapse: agitation, insomnia, loss of appetite, physical symptoms, a patient's growing conviction that people are laughing at her and talking about her. Parents are also given specific suggestions for coping with the patient's irrational fears and any threats of violence. ("Families in the Treatment—Part II," 1989, p. 2)

Another approach that many families find helpful is multiple family group meetings, or multiple family therapy ("Families in the Treatment, Part II," 1989; McFarlane, 1983). In this model, several families who have schizophrenic members meet together with several therapists (with or without the schizophrenic member, depending both on circumstances and the model used). It is often an excellent source of support for the families and tends to break down the isolation and guilt experienced by many of these families. It has been observed that "families often speak more candidly to one another than to therapists . . . and they begin to recognize in themselves what they have first seen in others" ("Families in the Treatment—Part II," 1989, pp. 2-3). McFarlane (1983) has noted:

> It readily enlists family participation and cooperation, reduces feelings of blame, and then provides several avenues for significant alteration in family interaction, all the while providing an opportunity for relatives to share their pain, guilt, and perplexity and to develop a critically needed social support system. (p. 170)

Some parents of schizophrenic adult children need supportive services, which they often do not receive, such as respite care to provide temporary relief to take care of their own needs. Many parents are becoming elderly themselves and, no longer able to meet the needs of their children, are concerned about their children's lack of preparation for the future. Even when family life is proceeding comfortably, does that mean that the patient is receiving optimal care, or that efforts are being directed toward community residences and employment?

The majority of families favor "group homes, foster homes, and halfway houses that provide a decent physical environment along with some counseling and supervision; the schizophrenic patients themselves often agree" ("Families in the Treatment—Part II," 1989, p. 3). It has been pointed out that "having learned that the family is not the main problem in schizophrenia, we must not act as though it is the main solution" ("Families in the Treatment—Part II," 1989, p. 3).

Family work with schizophrenic patients tends to focus on their parents; siblings are "an especially ignored component" of this work. Although some may become caretakers, their needs have been neither explored nor met (Riebschleger, 1991). In one study, siblings were noted to experience grief and loss, and to experience mixed feelings, including "anger, guilt, fear, shame, and sorrow. . . . They felt drawn to help the ill family member and at the same time were repulsed by their brother or sister's bizarre behavior" (Riebschleger, 1991, p. 3). Sometimes they observed themselves " 'feeling crazy' " when their ill siblings condition deteriorated (Riebschleger, 1991, p. 99). Recommendations for assistance included the siblings' need for support and education and their wish to be involved in the treatment team. Some support groups for siblings currently exist in the National Alliance for the Mentally Ill (NAMI).

One of the most active self-help groups parents have developed is the National Alliance for the Mentally Ill, whose membership grew to about 200,000 families in 1999 (Winerip, 1999b). This group is supportive, educational, and political, producing publications about schizophrenia and lobbying for legislation. It has been observed that participants are generally from the middle class; "ways must be found to include the poor as well" ("Families in the Treatment—Part I," 1989).

Community Groups for the Mentally Ill

One approach offering support to people with mental health problems is the clubhouse model; Fountain House, established with funding from the National Institute of Mental Health in 1976, was the model for this program; currently over 180 clubhouses are operating nationally, and about twenty-five new facilities are developed annually (Jackson et al., 1996). The clubhouse model is viewed as being different from the traditional day-treatment program (medical) model, which is held to be infantilizing and demeaning by its detractors. Dorothy Purnell, a former clubhouse member, working to earn an associate degree in human services, commented that when she was in day-treatment programs she "learned to be dependent. . . . I created ashtrays and clay animals that were stored on a shelf and eventually discarded . . . . I felt that I, too, deserved to be thrown away" (Jackson et al., 1996, p. 176).

The clubhouse model, in contrast, is a competency-based program that offers its members a sense of community and has egalitarian relationships between staff and members, who manage the clubhouses together. The major focus is on the clients' "participation . . . [and] empowerment, building on . . . strengths, and maximizing client self-determination" (Jackson et al., 1996, p. 177). Although members are helped to secure clinical treatment elsewhere, and most take medication, they are viewed positively, their contributions are encouraged and appreciated, and they are helped to develop their potentialities and abilities.

The Current Crisis in Care

Although some people with schizophrenia receive very good services and manage to function well, an overwhelming problem exists with the current lack of care and the general indifference to this situation. In Chapter 4, we discussed the problems created by deinstitutionalization, and how the promised alternatives for hospital care, such as group homes, did not materialize, or when they did, the resources were insufficient to meet the needs of this population. In addition, some patients continued to need the intensive structure and care provided in a hospital setting or might have a need for this service in the future course of their illness. Finally, managed care, with its dictates about limited hospitalizations and treatments, curtailed many mental health services, including the ability of general hospitals to maintain psychiatric patients for relatively long periods in their facilities.

The utilization of privatization in the mental health field is becoming more commonplace, whereby the care of mentally ill patients is contracted to private vendors, with the goal of monetary savings for the state. Dumont (1996) observed the disastrous results when this happened in Massachusetts, accompanied by the "destruction of community mental health capacities and inpatient care" (p. 293); he observed the resulting "increased rates of violence, homelessness, and imprisonment of psychiatric patients along with the deprofessionalization and demoralization of clinicians" (p. 293).

In 1999, in New York City, a tragic case receiving much publicity involved the murder of a young woman who was pushed to her death under a subway train by a twenty-nine-year-old schizophrenic patient who did not know her. Especially disturbing about this situation was the fact that this man knew that he was mentally ill, that he was desperately seeking help for himself, but it was not available. He pleaded for help with many mental health professionals, some of whom attempted to find alternative placements for him; when this failed, as there was no continuity of care, he drifted. It was also well known that he had assaulted thirteen people prior to this murder. Michael Winerip (1999b) reported his story because, he stated, this young patient and what happened to him typifies many of the present dilemmas facing other mentally ill patients who are receiving no care or inadequate care at best.

The man concerned had been hospitalized thirteen times; each time, he had signed himself in voluntarily. However, the difficulties started after his discharges. The social workers working with him knew that he should not be living alone, but they could not place him. The alternative care plans they looked into included long-term care at state hospitals, supervised group homes, or utilizing the services of an intensive case manager, who could make daily home visits. When in 1997 he himself "requested long-term hospitalization," he was referred instead to an emergency room and released after spending one night there (Winerip, 1999b, p. 44).

The following year, after a stay with a psychiatric service at a private hospital for a month, the staff documented three violent acts he had committed and recommended placement at the state hospital, which "agreed in principle" to admit him, but there was no room (Winerip, 1999b, p. 44). His last hospitalization, in a private facility, lasted for three weeks, and he was discharged although the hospital psychiatrist noted that he was "disorganized, thought disordered, and delusional" (Winerip, 1999b, p. 45). He was given enough medication for a week and referred to a psychotherapy center, which sees people for office appointments only and makes no home visits. Because he missed so many appointments, he received a form letter asking him to phone the clinic; if he did not, services for him would be terminated.

Winerip (1999b) cites a national study done in 1998, which reports that less than half of those suffering from schizophrenia "receive adequate care"; it has also been estimated that states spend "a third less" now on treating the mentally ill than they did in the 1950s (pp. 45-46).

Conflicts Between Empowerment and Beneficence

Many advances today promote the rights of the mentally ill, including legislation prohibiting employment discrimination against this group. Also, although patients with mental illness have the legal right to vote, many do not exercise this right; recently advances have been made in promoting their voting activity. The Mental Health Voter Empowerment Project "locates potential voters—whether in hospitals, at advocacy events, in housing projects, clinics or support groups—registering them, educating them about mental health issues and making sure they get to the polls on Election day 2000" (Goode, 1999c, p. A1).

Kruger (2000) emphasizes the importance of empowerment for the psychiatrically disabled and discusses his agency, the Mental Patients' Association (MPA), which works with present and former psychiatric patients; it began as a self-help group about thirty years ago. Their guiding principle is being "antipsychiatric, antisocial-control, and prohuman rights and mutual self-help" (Kruger, 2000, p. 430). Not only was it important to "destigmatize mental illness," but also to help others see it "as an integral part of the continuum of human life"; to improve the public image of psychiatric patients to enhance their own self-worth; and to engender the respect of others (Kruger, 2000, p. 430).

Self-determination and "having a voice" about one's life are important components of empowerment for patients, Kruger (2000) argues, and services should be available to people with psychiatric disabilities as they are to people with physical disabilities, "real world alternatives to forced hospitalization being one" (p. 435). Kruger (2000) recommends that research not focus on the "deficits" of this population, such as lack of motivation and poor social skills. The patient should be seen "in a context of oppression" and should learn more about "consciousness raising" (p. 436). Kruger expresses concern that people with psychiatric problems tend to internalize the negative attitudes of society toward them and asserts that we should not accept the idea that professionals be empowered to judge or determine the ideology or lifestyles of others. Professionals should not have a superior status; an equality should exist between those giving and those receiving help (Kruger, 2000).

The empowerment of oppressed patients model stands in opposition to the model advocating the need for protective intervention when necessary (Murdach, 1996). There are some clinicians in the empowerment camp who, while acknowledging the value of medication (when appropriate and "not used to punish patients"), nevertheless oppose forcing people to take medication if they refuse (Bentley, 1993, p. 102). Bentley (1993) asserts that "social workers must stand with the right of patients to refuse medication" (p. 104). In several well-publicized cases, involuntary commitment has been opposed by some civil rights groups. However, in opposition to this viewpoint, Satel (1999), a psychiatrist, asserts that "critics refuse to acknowledge . . . that about half of all schizophrenics have no insight into their own condition and no understanding of why they need medication. As for free will, the freedom to be psychotic is no freedom at all" (p. A31).

Murdach (1996) acknowledges the dilemma social workers confront when faced with curtailing client autonomy, because of the value they place on client self-determination. However, she is concerned about protecting clients when necessary, such as from their suicidal or other self-destructive impulses. She advocates a differential use of beneficence or "benevolent intervention," which depends "on the degree of rational impairment or decisional incapacity demonstrated by the client and the amount of risk or danger present in the situation if the client is left unprotected" (Murdach, 1996, p. 27). In essence, she argues, it is important to protect the client's decision making as much as possible, but some protection, ranging from mild to extreme, may be indicated depending on the degree of endangerment to the client.

DEPRESSION

Depression is classified as a mood disorder when symptoms become severe, yet depressed or sad moods also accompany us through the life cycle, especially during periods of loss or other crises. However, such depressed feelings are generally temporary and do not develop into full-blown clinical depression. When a depressive disorder develops, "every facet of life— emotional, cognitive, physiological, behavioral, and social—may be affected" (MacKinnon and Michels, 1971, p. 174).

Generally, a person with clinical depression has a lowered mood, little energy and fatigues easily, lacks motivation, does not experience joy or pleasure, and cannot look forward to future events; in fact, the depressed person often feels that no future exists, and suicidal thoughts and/or intentions may be present. Self-esteem is low, and hopelessness, helplessness, and feelings of guilt are usually present. Although thought processes are not distorted as they are in schizophrenia (unless a psychotic depression is present), thinking tends to be slowed down, and people may have difficulty concentrating and are often preoccupied with themselves and their troubles. There develops a "sense of isolation from people and things, the sense of a dull, dead world" (Nemiah, 1961, p. 149). Anger (not always obvious) is intermingled with depression; in extreme situations, homicidal wishes and acts may coexist with depression. Most of the time, the anger is not felt as such by the person (as this might be too threatening) but may be internalized and directed against the self.

Physical symptoms include disturbances in appetite, which can be diminished (accompanied by weight loss) or considerably increased, leading to overeating and weight gain (which in turn can add to depressive feelings). Headaches can occur; abdominal distress, especially relating to constipation, is common. There may be a preoccupation with being or becoming ill, which can eventuate in hypochondriasis. Many depressed patients may appear at the doctor's office with physical complaints that often are treated as such, while the underlying depression goes undiagnosed.

Mrs. Billings, who was discussed in Chapters 1 and 10, was admitted to an inpatient psychiatric facility for treatment of depression. She was tired, felt tearful, and stated that her symptoms were increasing. She complained of dizziness and shortness of breath and had gained forty pounds in the past three years, adding greatly to her self-consciousness. She had one previous psychiatric hospitalization for a suicide attempt and depression. She has very low self-esteem, strong feelings of guilt, and is very self-conscious. "It is hard for me to make friends. . . . I am uncomfortable with people."

Depression refers "both to a symptom and to a group of illnesses that have certain features in common" (MacKinnon and Michels, 1971, p. 174). Depression can range from a mild depression reactive to a life crisis (in which the person remains functional) to experiencing such an encompassing, immobilized state that hospitalization becomes essential. When depression become so severe that the patient appears almost catatonic, says little, and is preoccupied with very morbid and distorted thoughts, a *psychotic depression* may be present. Some people, on the other hand, can have a psychotic depression with agitated features; such a patient is usually restless and gives an "overall impression of intense anxiety" (MacKinnon and Michels, 1971, p. 180).

Some people have mood swings, from depression to elated moods, accompanied by extreme hyperactivity; they are said to be *cyclothymic*. In more extreme cases, bipolar disorder is present, in which manic phases may produce erratic, irrational behaviors, including impulsive acting out, such as excessive buying sprees (which the patient usually cannot afford), hypersexuality, and aggression. Mania in adolescents is often overlooked. Their symptoms can be attributed to an antisocial personality disorder or schizophrenia.; they may present with psychosis or substance abuse (Kaplan et al., 1994).

Some types of depression are thought to be primarily genetic, and often these depressions are severe, tend to respond to medication, and do not necessarily have clear precipitating events; biological factors are considered the primary etiology in bipolar illness. Lithium (for those who do not develop adverse physical side effects) has brought about remarkable control of the symptoms. Antidepressants have been used to treat many types of depression, often with good results. Debate continues about whether medication is effective or necessary for all depressive states, and whether psychotherapy (of various schools) is just as effective or more effective with more lasting results; some advocate both measures.

Seasonal affective disorder (SAD) has been recognized since the 1980s; this is "a major (serious) depression that recurs each year at the same time, starting in fall or winter and ending in spring" ("Seasonal Affective," 1993).

Treatment usually involves either antidepressant medication and/or the use of bright lights for several hours a day. Less severe forms are also known.

Depression very often does not exist alone but coexists with at least one other disorder. It is frequently found with borderline states, substance abuse, schizophrenia, anxiety disorders, including post-traumatic stress disorders, and somatization disorders. Depression is often not diagnosed in schizophrenia; it can be overlooked as the client's flat affect is attributed to schizophrenia rather than depression (Kaplan et al., 1994).

Some people who are depressed attempt to medicate their depression with alcohol; this can also have negative consequences as alcohol can aggravate depressive states. William Styron (1990), the novelist, has very vividly described his own bout with depression, which began when he suddenly stopped his ongoing use of alcohol. He, however, attributes his underlying depression to genetics as well as his inability to mourn the death of his mother when he was thirteen (Chapter 1).

It was initially thought that depressive disorders could not exist in children because their superegos were not sufficiently mature to experience the guilt and conflict associated with depressive guilt. Now it is recognized that a depressive state, with its listlessness, anhedonia, unresponsiveness, and failure to thrive, can occur even in infants; depressive symptomatology is also seen in young children who have been abandoned, maltreated, or have attachment disorders. Often the mothers of these children have been found to be depressed.

A high incidence of depression is found in adolescents. In Chapter 9, we observed that their depressions can often be masked by various at-risk and acting-out behaviors; this is often true in adults as well. Reiner and Kaufman's (1959) hypothesis, discussed in Chapter 11 (in reference to people in crisis), suggested that a depressive nucleus related to early deficits in nurturing underlies the acting-out behavior of the character disorder. Acting-out behaviors may blunt the pain of depressive feelings.

In the early editions of the *Diagnostic and Statistical Manual of Mental Disorders,* such as the DSM-I and DSM-II, depressions were apparently "classified among the personality disorders and neuroses." In a major change in 1980, the DSM-III "designated chronic depression as 'dysthmic disorder' and classified it as an affective or mood disorder, along with major depression and bipolar disorder" ("Is Lifelong," 1991, p. 8). Debate continues about whether depression is primarily a mood disorder or a characterological state in some people.

Normal Grief and Depression

Normal grief and depression share some features; sadness, loss of pleasure, and withdrawal from usual activities can occur in both. The bereaved person tends to be preoccupied with the loss, and it may take some time, ranging from weeks to months, before the person resumes former activities and develops new relationships (MacKinnon and Michels, 1971). Clear distinctions, however, are present; "the grief stricken individual does not suffer from a diminution of self-esteem. He is not irrationally guilty, and it is easy for the interviewer to empathize with his feelings" (MacKinnon and Michels, 1971, p. 181). Although the bereaved person may "feel that his world has come to an end . . . he knows that he will recover and cope" (p. 181).

Loss is most often the precipitating factor leading to depression. As noted in Chapter 11, it is not only loss that is critical, but it is the unresolved grief for this loss which can produce depression even years later. In addition, being bereft on an individual who fulfilled a deep psychological need can eventuate in feelings of emptiness, fragmentation, and sometimes suicidal despair. We saw this happen to Vivienne (discussed in Chapter 9) when her teacher (her selfobject) moved away. This experience "struck at the core of Vivienne's psychological vulnerability" (Mack and Hickler, 1981, p. 101).

Biopsychosocial Approach to Depression

Approaches to treating depression are diverse; some emphasize only medication while others recommend medication combined with psychotherapy. Cognitive therapy is considered by many to be one of the most helpful treatments for depression (Kaplan et al., 1994). Beck (1976) (Chapter 3) has identified a "depressive triad" of thoughts: "a negative conception of the self, a negative interpretation of life experiences, and a nihilistic view of the future" (Beck, 1976, p. 84). Utilizing this framework, patients are helped to reconceptualize their basic life assumptions.

Behavioral, behavioral-cognitive approaches, and interpersonal therapy, which focuses on impaired social relationships, are frequently applied to depression. Group therapy is sometimes the primary treatment or is an adjunct to other forms of therapy.

A biopsychosocial approach is the most comprehensive way to look at depression, and differential intervention plans are developed, depending on the motivation, capacities, and degree of impairment within the context of a person's life and problems. In many instances, a psychodynamic approach can be helpful to clients in overcoming their depression as well as enhancing their overall happiness and functioning.

In Chapter 7, we discussed Nora in relation to the issue of family enmeshment; she was chronically depressed and had experienced trauma and deprivation in her early life. Nora's behavior was also self-defeating in many ways, and entanglements with her family, followed by disappointments related to their uncaring attitudes toward her, would lead to the onset of her depressive symptomatology. A supportive relationship with her was the basis for enhancing self-esteem, and she gradually got in touch with her underlying sadness, loss, and feelings of being unloved; she became more reflective about her unmet needs, her behaviors, and their consequences. Although changing cognitive constructions of herself were part of the process, these were related to her specific life situation and were not changed in a formulaic manner.

Suicide

The U.S. Surgeon General, David Satcher, has called suicide "a significant public health problem" ("Surgeon General," 1999, p. A15); in 1997, there were more deaths (30,000) resulting from suicides than from homicides (19,000); it is the "eighth leading cause of death in the United States" (p. A15). Many more "unsuccessful" suicide attempts require emergency room care (about 500,000), often with serious physical and psychological consequences. More than 60 percent of suicides have been committed with handguns (Armstrong, 1998).

People who commit suicide are usually depressed; as we saw in Chapter 9, depression is present in most adolescent suicides. About half of schizophrenic patients, usually younger ones (in the early years of their illness), have made suicide attempts, of which 10 to 15 percent eventuate in death (Kaplan et al., 1994). Borderline personalities make frequent suicide threats and attempts, sometimes resulting in death. Many elderly people who commit suicide have serious physical problems (Chapter 10); suicide in children and adolescents is frequently associated with child maltreatment or intense and prolonged rejection.

Psychosocial factors have been associated with suicide; gay and lesbian adolescents, for example, have a higher suicide rate than do their peers (Chapter 9). Suicide among black teenagers has increased; this had been "quite rare, [but] has sharply increased over the last two decades, a troubling rise that might reflect the strain some black families feel in making the transition to middle-class life" (Belluck, 1998a, p. A1).

Police suicides have been increasing, usually by means of a handgun and often associated with serious alcohol use. John Violanti, a police suicide expert, observed that police today are "one and one half times more likely to commit suicide than their predecessors only a decade ago" (Armstrong, 1998, p. A8). This problem has been attributed to a number of factors: increased stress related to confronting more violence and criminals who are more dangerous; being under greater public scrutiny while receiving less public respect; and dealing with the many different levels of responsibility and involvement encountered in community policing. In addition, organizational problems within police departments are thought to play a role, including: "the perception of unfair promotional systems and arbitrary disciplinary procedures, the rigid requirements of a military-like hierarchy, midnight shifts, and long hours" (Armstrong, 1998, p. A8).

Cultural and societal attitudes toward suicide also play a role in suicidal behavior. In Ireland, the dramatic increase of suicides in young men, while related to changing social factors, is also related to the Catholic church's changing attitude toward suicide, which has become more "benign," so that suicide is "no longer vehemently condemned from the pulpit" (Clarity, 1999, p. 9). In Japan, by contrast, suicide "has little of the stigma it carries in Western societies; in literature, history and even today, suicides are often portrayed as noble, a matter of conscience or an honorable form of protest" (Strom, 1999, p. A8). In Japan, which in the past had very low suicide rates, the rate of suicide among men is reaching a record high (a rate higher than found in the United States). In China, where the suicide rates of women in rural areas is soaring and is five times the rate for women in other parts of the world, suicide is also not stigmatized, and sometimes it is recognized as an honorable act (Rosenthal, 1999).

In Ireland, while depression and alcoholism are considered important underlying factors, societal changes are also suspected as contributory, including difficulties men have in adapting to the "changing roles of men and women in what remains a male-dominated society" (Clarity, 1999, p. 9). In Japan, the serious economic recession, with its lower wages and accompanying numbers of layoffs, has led both to unemployment and job insecurities. It is considered very humiliating to be without work in Japan, and the shame and fear of condemnation by others for this disgraceful act is very strong (Strom, 1999). Chapter 4 discussed *karojisatsu,* which is the phenomenon of suicide being precipitated by extreme overwork, also a frequent phenomenon today in Japan, related to measures taken by employers to deal with the recession (Japan, 1999).

In China, the suicide rate among women is "the puzzling plague of rural China" (Rosenthal, 1999, p. 1). Despite theories advanced about this problem, no conclusive answers have been found; traditionally, suicide was usually committed by urban men. One consistent finding is that the means of suicide by rural women is the ingestion of pesticides; steps have been taken in some areas to restrict the most dangerous of these pesticides.

Some theories relate to socioeconomic changes in rural China. In one large study, suicides were observed to be "minidramas," in which immediate stress or an argument with a family member led to this sudden, impulsive act, using the easily available pesticide; mental illness, depression, and alcohol consumption, factors usually associated with suicide, were not observed. Some experts attribute this phenomenon to the basic low self-esteem in which Chinese women (and their society) hold themselves. In rural China, "customs and language reinforce women's feelings of worthlessness and helplessness. . . . Men control family assets, and women do not even eat dinner with them" (Rosenthal, 1999, p. 12). The key question in crisis intervention remains unanswered here: "But why now?"

Suicide Prevention

In Chapter 9, several points raised about the prevention of adolescent suicide are relevant here. These include listening for signs of hopelessness, despair, and depression as well as understanding serious at-risk behaviors in which the person might be engaged. Oblique communications are often overlooked because the lay public has not learned how (or been educated) to pick up on, interpret, and be comfortable responding to them. It is important to ask directly about suicide. Important issues to clarify are the intent, the means, and the purpose the suicide act will serve. Underlying mental health problems need to be clarified, and the person's judgment and impulse control are important factors to consider. If the person seems to be at serious risk, it is important to seek immediate psychiatric consultation and to consider the possibility of hospitalization.

Internalized anger is usually a significant component of depressive states and is often a motivator of suicidal behavior. It is not uncommon for the suicidal person to wish to punish the survivors: "they'll be sorry when I'm gone." Homicidal acts are sometimes carried out by depressed people; periodic newspaper accounts report people who have murdered their spouses, family, co-workers, and sometimes people they do not know, and then killed themselves.

Suicide Survivors

People who are survivors of those who have committed suicide often suffer a great deal related to the actual loss, the stigma associated with this, and guilt. "Survivor-victims of a suicide are often emotionally and psychologically disrupted to such an extent that immediate supportive intervention should be initiated" (Welu, 1975, p. 144). It has been observed that many families of police officers who have committed suicide have received no support of a financial (often no or few financial benefits) or of an interpersonal nature. Many have felt the burden of stigmatization as well as social isolation. The widow of a police officer who killed himself is treated in a dramatically different way from the widow of a police officer who died in service as a hero (Armstrong, 1998).

BORDERLINE PERSONALITIES

People with borderline personalities tend to live in a world of inner chaos, deep insecurity, and unstable moods; they have deep fears of being abandoned and an unstable sense of identity. Their inner world is often displaced (and acted out) onto the external world, arousing turmoil, confusion, and anxiety in others.

The term borderline personality was officially adopted as a diagnosis by the American Psychiatric Association in 1980; until then, people with this diagnosis were classified with various other disorders ("Borderline," 1994). Having officially recognized this group, the mental health field has taken a great deal of interest in these patients. Writings appeared and workshops were given; many of these workshops focused on transference and countertransference difficulties in working with borderline patients. Clinicians continue to struggle with the turbulence created in the wake of encounters with people with borderline personalities; the question of whether this is a discrete diagnosis or an overused diagnosis overlapping other categories remains unanswered.

> The symptoms of the . . . borderline personality . . . [are] instability in mood, thinking, behavior, personal relations, and self-image. Although people . . . with this disorder cannot bear to be alone and constantly demand attention, they are often difficult to work and live with. They plague friends, family, and lovers with unreasonable demands, provocative behavior, tantrums, hypochondriacal complaints, and suicide threats. They are chronically angry, quick to take offense, and easily depressed. They are susceptible to drug and alcohol abuse and other self-destructive impulsive behavior. They repeatedly follow idealization of another person with contemptuous rejection, and their intense attachments alternate with equally sudden breakups. ("Borderline," 1994, p. 1)

In the past, people with these symptoms tended to be classified as pseudoneurotic, narcissistic, infantile, paranoid, impulse-ridden, sociopathic, and "as-if" personalities, among others (Freed, 1980). People with depressive, cyclothymic personalities and bipolar disorders continue to present problems for the diagnostician attempting to differentiate these syndromes from the borderline personality disorder. More than half of borderline patients have had periods of depression and have a relatively high rate of depressive illness in their families. However, differences exist between them and people with mood disorders. "Their moods are much more susceptible to change in response to external events, and their depressions are often qualitatively different, with less guilt, appetite loss, and lethargy, but more loneliness, emptiness, and boredom" ("Borderline," 1994, p. 2).

Although borderline patients have mood instability and often display impulsive acting-out behaviors, their mood instability does not reach the heights of frenzied, uncontrolled behavior often displayed by the person with a bipolar disorder. The borderline personality is prone to psychotic decompensation when under stress, but these episodes are seen as brief and sporadic and tend to disappear when the stress dissipates.

Two of the major defense mechanisms of the borderline personality are projective identification and splitting. Projective identification (described in Chapter 2) is related to the defense of projection but extended to the point in which not only does the individual disavow a feeling by projecting it onto someone else, but this is done in such a way that the other person reacts with the same kind of behavior or attitudes being disavowed by the person utilizing this defense. A patient, for example, who is feeling angry will project this anger onto another person then through a psychological maneuver will say something to antagonize this other person, who will react in an angry way, which reinforces the borderline person's belief that, indeed, this person was angry.

In Chapter 2, we gave a variant of this mechanism in the example of Mrs. Bosworth, a child welfare client who was overwhelmed in caring for her young son. She asked the child welfare worker, Ms. Schmidt, to place him in a foster home, but when the worker tried to do this, Mrs. Bosworth verbally attacked the worker and then complained to the worker's supervisor. Mrs. Bosworth was disavowing her own angry feelings toward her son and her wish to be rid of him. She involved Ms. Schmidt in acting out this wish for her, and then attacked her for this hostile act, so she could be the innocent victim of this "outrage."

Clinicians are frequently subject to client's projective identifications in the treatment situation, and this adds to the complexity of treatment. Many borderline patients have the capacity to "tune in" to the unconscious feelings of others, and it is not uncommon for them to pick up on a therapist's vulnerability. If, for example, the therapist may have doubts about being adequate as a therapist, the patient will probably aim the provocation in this direction, so that the therapist will react in a personally defensive rather than in a clinically objective manner. Using an intersubjective approach, if clinicians tunes into the feelings stirred up in them by these clients, they can use them as a tool in therapy, rather than being controlled by them.

Splitting is frequently utilized as a defense by borderline clients; this occurs because they are not able to tolerate ambivalent feelings or mixed emotions, including negative as well as positive feelings toward a given event. Clients may also engage in splitting in relation to their self-concepts; "extreme repetitive oscillation between contradictory self concepts" is another manifestation of the mechanism of splitting (Kernberg, 1984, p. 16). In Chapter 3, in the discussion of the separation-individuation theory of Mahler and colleagues (1975), splitting was referred to as occurring because of a failure in the achievement of the final stage of object constancy. Also in that section, an example was given of splitting occurring in an institutional setting, in which a young male patient managed to pit the "good" staff (those he favored) against the "bad" staff (those whom he appeared to disfavor) causing institutional havoc and dissension.

Theoretical approaches to treating the borderline personality vary; a spectrum of function and dysfunction exists in people within this category, as well as varying degrees of motivation for treatment. Many of the writings address patients in outpatient or inpatient treatment settings, in which their symptomatology (whether acknowledged or denied) is the basis for their care. However, many social workers encounter people with borderline personalities in settings in which their mental health is not the focus of their concern, such as medical or child welfare settings. Mrs. Bosworth, in the previous example, was a client in a nontreatment setting. It is important for clinicians to be aware of the underlying diagnostic problems and find intervention strategies that can maximize support for the client and minimize the likelihood of the clinician being "swept away" by the client's overwhelming personality and manipulations.

It is generally agreed that one major aspect in treatment is the recognition of the defenses of splitting and projective identification, and utilizing one's subjectivity to understand how they are played out in therapy; appropriate clients can then be helped to see how they often get into complicated interpersonal situations by inappropriate use of these mechanisms.

People with borderline personalities frequently lack the capacity to self-soothe and often find themselves in turbulent emotional states that they cannot control. Adler (1985) sees helping the patient develop the capacity to self-soothe as a major goal of psychotherapy. Kernberg (1984) makes the point that in supportive psychotherapy with a borderline client, a major difference exists "between giving a patient advice on how to handle his life and helping him understand how certain 'automatic' ways of functioning are detrimental to his interests" (p. 156).

> The therapist's function is to acquaint the patient with the primitive defenses and their effects upon his evaluation of reality and decision-making processes. In contrast to efforts to override pathological character traits and primitive defenses by advice regarding more "normal" behavior, the therapist attempts to acquaint the patient with the conscious and preconscious aspects of his intrapsychic difficulties and to help him use such knowledge, which the patient potentially has and is actively avoiding. (Kernberg, 1984, p. 156).

In the following situation, a social work student was working with G., a woman with a borderline personality structure; she was aware of G. using the defenses of splitting and projective identification and brought this pattern and its negative social consequences to her attention. G. had been at a new job for two weeks and reported to her social work intern that she had alienated almost all her co-workers because she had stood up for one woman whom she thought was being mistreated.

> G. seems to experience authority figures as all bad, while she projects her feeling of being abused onto, and then identifies with, those whom she perceives as being mistreated. These people to her are all good. She devalues all the others who are not assisting the victim, thus preserving the goodness of herself and the victim. We discussed this situation in terms of G. looking at people and things in general as either all good or all bad, and black or white with nothing in between, and of her being oversensitive to some people because her feelings have been hurt. G. associated this with her expecting too much and of wanting the world to be perfect—wanting everyone to meet each other's needs. She then said that she was looking for the impossible and needed to work on being able to accept people's shortcomings.

People with borderline personalities often have intense needs for relationships but are often unable to maintain them because they fear engulfment (a primitive sense of danger of merging with the other person, possibly based on an equally primitive wish for this); they lack skills in forming relationships and in understanding the relationship binds in which they frequently find themselves.

> A young male patient . . . had allowed a friend who was "down and out" to share his apartment until he was able to "get it together again." After a few days the "friend" had taken money from his wallet, had damaged furniture with burning cigarette butts, and had seduced the patient's girlfriend. The patient was hurt and angry, but had no awareness of the type of interpersonal information he would need to process to make more accurate predictions about others' behaviors. Rather, he was driven by the need to hold on to the relationship. (Marziali and Munroe-Blum, 1994, p. 55)

People with borderline personalities are often helped by learning how to cope with the here and now, to develop a more cohesive sense of self and better self-image, to learn how to exercise good judgment, to "size up situations" appropriately, and to establish more stable relationships. Group treatment is often effective with this population; sometimes it is used as the sole treatment, sometimes as an adjunct to individual therapy. Group therapy has the potential advantage of diluting the relationship to the therapist (which can become very intense and tumultuous in individual treatment), fostering improved interpersonal skills, helping find constructive solutions to difficult reality situations, and learning to recognize emotions and their connection to behaviors. Marziali and Munroe-Blum (1994) were positive about the results of their group intervention with this population; in particular, they felt that group members learned to get in touch with their angry feelings and how to handle anger and confrontations with one another in a constructive manner.

Working with borderline patients is often one of the most difficult tasks for students; they are frequently caught in an emotional maelstrom and can feel confused and totally inept; Briggs (1979) addresses many of the problems posed by borderline personalities. "Trainees customarily personalize responses from borderlines; since these responses are often hostile, the therapist may take them as affronts" (p. 138). Setting limits with a borderline person is also an important key to successful work; this is "one of the hardest tasks for trainees" (Briggs, 1979, p. 144). This includes distinguishing between acceptance of clients and their feelings and limitless tolerance of their verbal abuse or other manipulations. She notes that with experience trainees "will appreciate the fact that early limit-setting, especially with homicidal or suicidal borderlines, will help to reduce their own anxieties" (Briggs, 1979, p. 136).

ANXIETY DISORDERS

Like depressed feelings, anxiety is experienced universally. Anxiety is an unpleasant affect, characterized by uneasiness, fear, worry, and physical and emotional distress. Sometimes it is relatively mild or temporary, as when one might worry about taking a test; however, for some, overwhelming anxiety can be precipitated by taking a test. Universal situations probably exist in which anxiety escalates into panic for most people, such as sitting on an airplane that suddenly develops serious mechanical problems midair. A patient, being told that he or she has cancer, can become highly anxious. The rule of thumb is that anxiety does not have a cause in reality but that fear does, although a mixture can certainly be seen in emergency situations, for instance.

Kafka's novels portray very vividly a state of constant anxiety and dread, and the potential of terror striking from anywhere. Such dread was experienced by a woman, about to take her first plane trip across the Atlantic Ocean, who woke her husband up in the middle of the night before her flight. "Have you ever thought about how big the ocean is?" she asked him. In her mind, she saw herself in a little plane with dim lights flying into the vast darkness into the middle of nowhere where no one would see it, and she would be lost; this would be an example of *existential anxiety*.

One characteristic of an anxiety state is "an apprehensive self-absorption which interferes with an effective and advantageous solution of reality problems" (Campbell, 1989, p. 48). Some people live in a constant state of anxiety and apprehension (a generalized anxiety disorder); for others, anxiety at times escalates into intense, overwhelming attacks of panic (panic disorders); for some, anxiety is displaced onto various external objects, such as a fear of dogs or elevators (phobic reactions); some people's anxiety is channeled into symptoms such as obsessions (continual preoccupation with certain subjects or thoughts), or into the development of routinized habits, the completion of which must be obeyed or the person will experience extreme discomfort, as in constant hand washing (compulsions). People who have been through traumas in early life (such as experiencing sexual abuse) or in later life (such as being a refugee fleeing from the horrors or war and torture) can develop serious symptoms of anxiety (post-traumatic stress disorder).

Sometimes anxiety is felt directly and/or channeled in bodily symptoms, as in various somatization disorders. It is not uncommon for anxiety and depression to coexist; anxiety and panic attacks are often part of the symptom picture of the borderline personality. Some people with severe anxiety may try to relieve it through excessive smoking or through the use of substances such as alcohol. One of the most common anxiety disorders, and often one of the most disabling, is the panic disorder.

Panic Disorders

Panic disorder usually begins before a person is thirty and frequently begins before the age of twenty; it is unusual for panic disorders to begin past the age of sixty-five ("Panic Disorder—Part I," 1990, p. 1).

> For five minutes to a half hour, the victim feels unbearable dread, a sense of unreality, and intense physical symptoms—choking sensations, labored breathing, a leaping, pounding heart, chest pain, dizziness, nausea, sweating, hot and cold flashes, numbness or tingling in the hands and feet, blurred vision. Victims fear that they will faint, lose control of themselves, go mad, or die. *Panic attacks* [italics added] constitute *panic disorder* [italics added] when many of these symptoms occur together repeatedly in a short period of time—say, once a week or more for a month—or when they create a persistent disabling fear of the next attack. ("Panic Disorder—Part I," 1990, pp. 1-2).

Panic attacks tend to continue to develop once the initial disorder starts; one of the most difficult effects is the anticipation of future attacks or "anticipatory anxiety," which can be "more serious than the panic attacks themselves" ("Panic Disorder—Part I," p. 2). People then become more avoidant of situations that they fear might produce another panic attack. Agoraphobia is a subset of the panic disorders but also can occur by itself, without being accompanied by a panic disorder. Agorophobia involves the avoidance of situations that trigger anxiety, usually public places. Its root is *agora,* which is the Greek word for marketplace. Marks (1987) noted that "this avoidance leads many agoraphobic people to become completely housebound" (Marks, 1987, p. 1161).

One client expressed her fear of driving; sometimes she is afraid to go to the mall (the modern "marketplace"). This client, who somatizes, discussed her symptoms in a somatic context; she has stated that she is "afraid that I might faint in the car on the way," rather than "I am afraid of crowds," but the end result is avoidance. Lipowski (1988) stated that several factors have been noted to account for somatization in anxiety disorders, which include "enhanced awareness and selective attention to bodily sensations and danger-related information generally, increased sympathetic nervous system arousal, and a negative bias in appraising one's health" (p. 1364). In Chapter 12 it was noted that people with panic disorders usually have such considerable anxiety about their physical health that some researchers "suggest that hypochondriasis is its essential feature" (Lipowski, 1988, pp. 1363-1364).

Some people with agoraphobia develop drinking problems, and "the rate of attempted suicide is about 20 percent—at least as high as it is in major depression" ("Panic Disorders—Part I," 1990, p. 2). Depression and agoraphobia are also closely linked; "a third to a half of people with repeated panic attacks develop major depression, and patients with major depression have a greatly increased risk of panic disorder" (p. 2).

The etiology of this problem is controversial; some attribute causation primarily to biological factors, others to psychological causes with varying perspectives related to psychodynamic, self psychology, cognitive, and learning theories. An editorial in the *American Journal of Psychiatry* noted: "The extraordinary amount of research on the panic disorders in the past several years has most recently focused on their biological features. . . . This explosion is all the more striking in that it occurs with respect to conditions that until recently were considered by many to be the least likely to have important biological aspects" (Ballenger, 1986, p. 516).

Opinions on treatment differ; medications (especially antidepressant drugs) are frequently used effectively (although they often do not prevent relapses); behavioral and cognitive interventions are popular ("Panic Disorders—Part II," 1990). As people with panic disorders usually do not know when an attack will strike, they live in anxious anticipation. Many are helped to "concentrate on their internal sensations first; for example, they can be taught to cut off panic at an early stage through muscle relaxation, meditation, self-hypnosis, and especially exercises in slow, calm, rhythmic breathing" ("Panic Disorders—Part II," 1990, p. 3). Bandura (1976) discusses a treatment model for agoraphobic patients, who are phobic about the world outside of their home, in which the therapist participates in activities with the patient (Chapter 3).

Cognitive therapy aims to help people deal with those faulty patterns or habits of thought that are related to exacerbating anxiety, such as the tendency to "catastrophize," which Beck (1976) describes as "a common characteristic of anxious patients, [that] illustrates anticipation of extreme adverse outcomes" (p. 93). They are helped to control this tendency and to alter their ways of thinking about events and, for example, "to distract themselves with substitute activities, concentrate on neutral details [for example, think about the design of a bridge, rather than that it could collapse], or give themselves reassuring suggestions" ("Panic Disorders—Part II," 1990, p. 3).

Beck (1976) also discusses the internal stressor, in which "the stress . . . is generated internally and consists of such psychological phenomena as the demands the person places on himself, his repetitive fears, and self-reproaches"; Beck points out that this mechanism can be detected by tapping into the "internal communication system" (1976, pp. 196-197).

Learning to tolerate and contain anxious feelings is an important part of most therapeutic approaches to panic disorders; however, the familiar dilemma of whether merely to eradicate symptoms or to understand underlying psychosocial problems presents itself. A woman might be experiencing panic attacks because she is unable to tolerate the impending death of her mother; events in one's current life can reactivate past traumatic events producing panic.

Chambless and Goldstein (1981) discuss the sense of entrapment that can develop when a person wishes to leave (even preconsciously) a partner that he or she is attached to, usually a spouse, and is emotionally unable to flee, leading to the development of agoraphobia (Chambless and Goldstein, 1981). Chambless and Goldstein (1981) also observe that often " 'inexplicable' panic attacks that agoraphobics experience happen after some unpleasant interpersonal interaction in which the agoraphobic feels ill treated or trapped by his inability to be appropriately assertive" (p. 126). Another interpretation is that the panic effectively targets a particular person in the patient's life who must accompany the person to allay his or her fears; this permits dependency on the targeted person.

Mahoney (2000) discusses panic disorder from the self psychology perspective and sees it resulting from "early selfobject failures" which "lead to diminished capacity to regulate anxiety and self-soothe later in life. Severe recurrent anxiety states during development may be later organized as a loss of sense of self . . . or may result in withdrawal or avoidance" (p. 205). Because panic attacks can be so disabling, people need direct help in overcoming them and managing in their lives; at the same time, many people may be capable of and motivated for looking beneath the surface reality of their panic.

Post-Traumatic Stress Disorder

Post-traumatic stress disorder (PTSD) was officially recognized in the 1980s. It was discovered in large numbers of veterans from the Vietnam War; for many years it went undiagnosed and untreated. It has been estimated that 30 percent of Vietnam vets have experienced this syndrome (Kaplan et al., 1994). Following is a description of a veteran who was seen ten years after his war experiences in Vietnam ("Post-traumatic Stress—Part I," 1991):

> During his year in the army his platoon was repeatedly ambushed, and in one of those ambushes his closest friend was killed while he stood a few feet away. He himself hit a boy Vietcong fighter with a rifle butt and killed him. He admits that his mind keeps returning to these events, and he still has nightmares about them, but he insists that he does not want to talk about any of that. He is constantly anxious and agitated, and he jumps at the sound of . . . [a] backfiring automobile. He becomes enraged at anything he regards as a mistake . . . by a person in authority, . . . he feels constantly bored and depressed and is "only going through the motions" at work and at home. He hardly talks to his family and has alienated most of his friends. He often carries a gun, and in moments of sudden anger he strikes his wife or starts fights with strangers over trivial annoyances. ("Post-traumatic Stress—Part I," 1991, p. 1)

Since PTSD has received recognition, additional study and research on this subject have been carried out, and other previously undiagnosed conditions have become better understood, including the psychiatric sequelae of severe trauma experienced by children (through maltreatment and witnessing violence); women, through rape and battering; adults who were abused as children; survivors of concentration camps and other war and torture situations; as well as catastrophic environmental events, such as hurricanes, tornadoes, and fires. Several researchers have questioned whether borderline symptomatology (found mostly in women) resulted from early experiences of childhood abuse.

The onset of the symptoms of this disorder can be almost immediate or delayed by years. People with PTSD experience symptoms such as nightmares, flashbacks, and intrusive memories of the trauma. It is not uncommon for events or people to trigger memories or associations; this may seem to come out of the blue, or may be related to the specific trauma. In the case just presented, the veteran would become agitated at the backfire of a car because of its association with gunfire. Greg, discussed next, who was being seen by a clinical social worker, experienced an "unprovoked" attack of anxiety.

> Greg, a teenager with developmental disabilities who exhibited some bizarre behaviors and often lived in a world of fantasy, was taken to an amusement park and allowed to drive one of the automated cars, which he wanted to do very much. However, after an enthusiastic start, he panicked and said that he never wanted to go back to this park again. Greg, who lived in a foster home, had a very traumatic child-hood; his father was murdered in a car, and although the teenager was not present at the murder, he believes he was, and that the father's body was hurled into the backseat where he was sitting. Although this boy was not capable of verbalizing this connection, it is quite probable that this is what produced his panic attack. Although he had been a passenger in cars many times without this reaction, it is possible that driving a car for the first time may have elicited association to (and identification with) his father, who was a taxi driver.

If Greg indeed does avoid this park and other amusement rides in the future, this might be considered "a conditioned response that resembles a phobia"; it is very common for people to "over-react to anything associated with the traumatic event" ("Post-traumatic Stress—Part I," 1991, p. 3); people have other ways of avoiding these traumatic memories; "they often succumb to a kind of emotional anesthesia. Under its influence, most of their feelings seem not quite real to them, everyone is a stranger, and activities that were formerly important no longer matter" (p. 2). It is not uncommon for people with PTSD to experience dissociation (discussed in Chapter 2); in dissociation the person's sense of identity or consciousness is disrupted.

A third set of symptoms relates to the development of *hypersensitivity;* "they are edgy, irritable . . . sleep poorly and find it difficult to concentrate. Some are tense with barely stifled rage and occasionally lose control in violent outbursts" ("Post-traumatic Stress—Part I," 1991, I, p. 2). Children tend to present a different symptom picture and do not have "flashbacks, emotional numbing, and amnesia." Rather, they present with "separation anxiety, school phobias, a fear of strangers, and recurrent nightmares. They also have headaches, stomach aches, and other physical symptoms" ("Post-traumatic Stress—Part II," 1991, p. 1).

Generally, therapy aims to help the patient remember and confront the traumatic event and see its connection to his or her feelings and symptoms. This can present many difficulties, including the patient's resistance to looking at this as well as the danger of retraumatization as the patient gets in touch with the trauma. Some behavior therapists use systematic desensitization (and implosive therapy, or purposeful massive flooding with images of the trauma under controlled and protected conditions) ("Post-traumatic Stress—Part II," 1991). Group therapy is often effective with PTSD patients as they can share experiences with others, learn how others have managed their feelings, develop new relationships, and lessen the burden of stigma (Berzoff, 1996a).

Not all people experiencing trauma develop PTSD; research is attempting to learn more about vulnerabilities and resilience in relation to this syndrome. Some opposition exists to doing this; "people with PTSD and their advocates have charged psychiatry with stigmatizing victims by belittling the significance of traumatic events. They fear that attention to individual vulnerability will encourage the belief that they are responsible for their own troubles" ("Post-traumatic Stress—Part I," 1991, p. 3).

In one study of rape victims, early experiences were found to be decisive in reactions to this experience; those women who coped well in the aftermath of this crisis came from backgrounds where they developed positive feelings about themselves and had "positive attachments to primary caregivers"; those women who had more difficulty coping had "negative self-schemas which reflect disrupted attachments with significant others or other childhood traumas such as sexual abuse [which] result in mistrust of others and uncertainty about one's power to ensure safety" (Regehr et al., 1999, pp. 181-182). Kaplan and colleagues (1994) affirm this point, suggesting that additional factors make people more vulnerable to developing PTSD, including a biological vulnerability to psychiatric disorders, characterological problems such as a borderline or antisocial personality, and recent alcohol abuse.

Two additional points were stressed by Kaplan and colleagues (1994). The first relates to the importance of assessing the stressor from the participant's subjective reaction rather than assessing the stressor itself. Second, they discuss whether adequate supports are present for the person after the trauma. Herman (1997) observed that during World War II soldiers were protected against feeling terror by the support they felt from their units and leaders; this is in sharp contrast to the loss of cohesion often experienced in combat by soldiers in Vietnam, intensified by the negative feelings they experienced from their countrymen when they returned home because they had fought an unpopular war. The adulation experienced by the returning World War II hero was lacking.

One of the reasons clinicians may have difficulty in working with PTSD is that they may experience great anxiety and other disturbances through being immersed in the client's world; vicarious traumatization is the term applied to this process. It has been noted, for example, that in working with victims of rape, clinicians may "experience a heightened sense of vulnerability and an enhanced awareness of the fragility of life or feelings of helplessness, depression, or despair" (Fox and Carey, 1999, p. 190). Child welfare workers have also experienced vicarious traumatization in their work with victims of various forms of trauma and maltreatment (see Chapter 6). Supportive supervision and staff support groups are often helpful to clinicians working with this population.

THE ADDICTIONS

Substance abuse is a major problem today and affects people of all ages starting with young adolescent and some preteens, and not excluding the elderly. The Substance Abuse and Mental Health Services Administration (SAMHSA) stated that the United States lost $276 billion in 1995 due to substance abuse (O'Neill, 1999). These figures were broken down to include: $34 billion for paying related health care expenses; $94 billion due to lost salaries because of illness; and $51 billion due to salaries lost related to criminal activities. Substance abuse is also highly correlated with physical and mental illness (O'Neill, 1999). "People with co-existing substance abuse and mental health problems are more likely to be severely impaired, require hospitalization, and need professional services" (O'Neill, 1999, p. 3).

Many problems related to substance abuse have been discussed throughout this book, including its negative effect on family relationships, parenting, and its relationship to child abuse (Chapter 7); its harmful effect on the developing fetuses of pregnant women (Chapter 8); its relationship to suicide, depression, and acting-out behaviors in adolescents (Chapter 9); and its prevalence in the homeless population (Chapter 4). Its relationship to mental health problems has been discussed in this chapter and will be expanded further in this section. Pathological gambling, although not a physical addiction, does produce a physical "high" in many people and has the same hold over them, as gambling becomes a primary motivator in life, responsibilities fade, and people often descend into spiraling economic ruin; this subject is discussed later in this section.

Alcohol Abuse

The consumption of alcohol is the predominant form of substance abuse (two-thirds); the remaining one-third of abusers use other substances (Kaplan et al., 1994). Alcohol abuse can have a serious effect on a person's health but is often not recognized by physicians when it is in its early stages ("In Study," 2000).

The roots of alcoholism are multicausal; they may include cultural factors (such as the attitude toward alcohol), familial, and psychological factors. More attention has recently been paid to the possibility of a biological predisposition toward alcoholism; this remains an unsettled question. Many people in our culture drink and usually can keep their alcohol consumption under control; those who may occasionally drink too much at a party are not necessarily dependent on regular drinking; alcohol dependence is "characterized by lack of control" (Mulinski, 1989, p. 334). As drinking increases, so do problems in the client's general functioning and social relationships. In addition, people who abuse alcohol typically utilize "rationalization and denial to hide their loss of control from themselves and from those around them" (Mulinski, 1989, p. 334).

One of the major problems in working with persons dependent on alcohol is their resistance to treatment; often their physical and psychological dependence is so great that they will deny the need for help and minimize their amount of drinking as well as its ensuing complications. Therefore, a major problem is to motivate people with substance abuse and involve them in treatment; sometimes this can be accomplished through caring confrontations from family members; sometimes it takes leverage from external sources of control to accomplish this, such as being mandated to alcohol treatment by a court. In some successful employee assistance programs, the aim of reaching workers while they are still capable of employment and using the leverage of dismissal from work if they do not comply with treatment has often been effective.

Alcohol has serious effects on the body and on brain chemistry, and withdrawal from serious alcohol usage must be medically monitored. Research points to the need for people with alcohol problems to abstain from drinking, although some clinicians argue in favor of occasional controlled social drinking (Kaplan et al., 1994; Wallace, 1992). It is important that treatment be focused on the drinking itself, in terms of the patient's need to drink, ways to control this, and finding alternate lifestyles and/or other interests when drinking stops. Some people have centered their life around drinking companions and have nothing with which to fill up their time and space when they attain sobriety.

For some patients, in need of structure and support, halfway houses can be helpful. Alcoholics Anonymous has been found very beneficial to people with drinking problems; it is often used an adjunct to other forms of treatment. Work with patients who abuse alcohol also needs to be culturally sensitive; due to the multiple stresses faced by Southeast Asian people, the abuse of alcohol, as well as other substances has been an important problem (Amodeo et al., 1996). Gay men tend to have a high rate of drinking problems, often associated with internalized homophobia, which also must be addressed in treatment (Warn, 1997).

Alcoholism is considered a chronic disease; people usually need some type of ongoing help even after drinking initially stops. Opinions differ as to whether to focus exclusively on alcohol-related issues or to involve the person in psychotherapy related to other life issues as well. One criticism of the work with substance-abusing mothers is that it is often focused only on treating the substance abuse without offering comprehensive services dealing with poverty, lack of education, past maltreatment, and difficult interpersonal relationships as well as mothering capacities and skills (Dore, 1999).

The problem of dual diagnosis (that is, substance abuse coexisting with other psychiatric disorders) in clients who abuse alcohol has been addressed with increasing frequency (Mulinski, 1989; O'Hare, 1995). Associations have been found with disorders including schizophrenia, depression, antisocial personality, borderline personality disorder, and anxiety. In the past, programs existed only for substance abusers or only for people with psychiatric disorders; today some progress has been made in the development of integrated programs, although, as in all substance abuse treatment programs, the need for services is far greater than the supply.

Drug Abuse

Drug abuse is a major problem in this country; in addition to the primary problems caused by this disorder, such as its serious psychological and physical effects on the user, secondary effects include its impact on employment and family relationships. An important additional secondary effect is the fact that drugs are illegal and most are very expensive. Many people have turned to crime and various illegal activities, including prostitution, to support their habits. In addition, a number of people who abuse drugs have been sent to prison (in alarming numbers, leading to the escalation of our prison population) where they generally receive punishment rather than treatment (Chapter 4).

Drug abuse has been difficult to treat, in part because of the variation of symptoms in individuals, even those taking the same drug. It has also been found that most people who abuse drugs usually do not abuse only one substance but several, in addition to frequent use of cigarettes. "Most heroin addicts have been, are, or will be alcoholic, and most people who start to smoke marijuana do not stop drinking alcohol" ("Drug Abuse—Part II," 1989, p. 3). Some people continually change drugs, and some will use drugs in combination with other drugs to "control each other's side effects" (the combination of a stimulant with a sedative or opioid is especially popular).

Unfortunately, space does not allow a description of the side effects of the many specific drugs on its users; following is a brief synopsis of some of the deleterious effects of drugs.

> Some acute physical effects are the impairment of reaction time and motor coordination by alcohol, diazepam, or marijuana; death from respiratory depression after an overdose of heroin or a combination of sedatives; cerebrovascular strokes caused by high doses of amphet-

amine or cocaine in people with high blood pressure or damaged arteries. Acute psychological dangers include . . . anxiety or paranoid reactions to marijuana; "bad trips" from hallucinogenic drug use; irritability, agitated paranoia, and unpredictable rage under the influence of stimulants; alcohol and cocaine hangovers; drowsiness caused by benzodiazepine or opiates. ("Drug Abuse—Part I," 1989, p. 1)

Although treatment of substance abusers has to take the complex physical reactions of a given person to a specific drug into account, the general principles of working with people with alcohol dependence, previously discussed, are similar ("Drug Abuse—Part II," 1989). People with drug abuse problems also frequently have coexisting psychiatric disorders that also need to be diagnosed and treated.

Compulsive Gambling

Gambling is an activity that many people engage in for enjoyment; church-sponsored bingo games, for example, are a popular social activity; occasional visits to a gambling casino or participating in gambling activities on a cruise ship are common. However, gambling becomes a way of life for some people, and then something which controls their lives; at that point, it can be said to become an addiction. Today, the increased availability of gambling opportunities, including state-run lotteries, gaming on Indian reservations, and real gambling on the Internet have increased the gambling activities of many people; in some cases, this has led to serious personal crises.

In a study by the National Gambling Impact Study Commission, it was found that over 5 million people in this country are "pathological or problem gamblers, and another 15 million are at risk of falling into the same morass" (Brody, 1999, p. D7). In the past, almost all gambling was attributed to men; now "nearly a third are women and a growing number are teen-agers" (p. D7). People are gambling over $500 billion a year, "an amount which has doubled in a decade" (p. D7).

Blume (1992) has described compulsive gambling as an addiction without drugs and provides the following succinct observations.

> Pathological gamblers make excuses for their losses or even deny them. A large loss of the kind any gambler should expect is an intolerable injury to their self-esteem, and they stake more and more to recoup. Losses increase erratically; the gambler's mood follows his luck, with ups and downs that can be compared to the alternating depression and hypomania of bipolar disorder. The gambler's family life and work situation deteriorate as debt grows and personal possessions, savings, and legitimate loan sources are exhausted. Lying, em-

bezzlement, and forgery are rationalized. Eventually the gambler may ask for a "bailout," a large loan or gift to pay off debts, usually in return for a promise to give up gambling. Like detoxification without rehabilitation for a heroin addict, the bailout merely enables the addiction to renew itself and continue. (Blume, 1992, p. 4)

Gamblers often fall prey to loan sharks as well.

A number of similarities have been found between pathological gambling and substance abuse; in fact, both are often found to coexist. Other diagnoses found in compulsive gamblers include: depression, bipolar disorder, schizoaffective disorder, and panic disorders (Robinson, 1997). Few treatment facilities exist for people with this problem; some private practitioners work with this group, and Gamblers Anonymous, similar to Alcoholics Anonymous, has often been effective (Robinson, 1997).

DEVELOPMENTAL DISABILITIES

In a biography of novelist Jane Austen, Nokes (1997) describes the large Austen household as always struggling economically but vibrant, lively, and warmly involved with each other. However, one member of this household, George (born in 1766), the second oldest son, did not seem to be developing normally. As a baby, George was "often subject to alarming fits," but the family was reassured that this often happened to young children (Nokes, 1997, p. 38). However, George "did not thrive. Already four years old, he struggled to form a syllable and was still subject to strange fits" (Nokes, 1997, p. 39); but when he reached the age of six, "the malady could no longer be disguised, nor the resolution longer delayed" (p. 43).

> Madness, or mental infirmity . . . was a sickness which afflicted not only the sufferer but also those . . . compelled to be the daily witnesses of its melancholy effects. For the sake of the other children it was agreed that little George should be sent away. . . . The Cullums [a family who provided this type of care] . . . had proved themselves quite equal to such a task. Cassandra [George's mother] made no protest . . . and the boy [was] removed into safe-keeping with . . . [this family]. There were to be no visits, no letters, . . . or family records beyond what was necessary for the maintenance of the poor child's life. It would be almost as if the boy had never existed. (Nokes, 1997, p. 43)

When George was sent to his new home, the family resolution of no contact was maintained. The Austens paid for George's care, and, later on, George's older brother visited to pay the fees "but did not linger for conversation" (Nokes, 1997, p. 522). As an adult, when Jane Austen tried to converse by the use of sign language with a man who was deaf and mute, she remembered conversing this way with George when he was a child. It was strange for her to "think of poor George," who was now past forty, and with whom she had not had contact during all this time. "But where nothing could be amended it was useless to repine, and she quickly dismissed all conscious thoughts of her idiot brother from her mind, as they had all been taught to do as children" (Nokes, 1997, p. 347). When George died, he was buried about twenty miles away from Jane Austen's tomb.

> George was laid to rest in an unnamed grave in the churchyard. . . . In death, as in life, he was to be forgotten, his remains unmarked by any stone. Only George Cullum [his caretaker] was in attendance at George Austen's death. It was he who noted for the death certificate that George Austen was "a gentleman." (Nokes, 1997, p. 526)

More than 200 years later, in an editorial in *Social Work,* Witkin (1998) expressed concern that today many people with mental retardation are also forgotten, and he referred to them as the "invisible" population. He observes that they do not usually "participate in the mainstream of community life," and that "when they do appear in public, we avoid them or develop 'special' programs for them, rendering them invisible once again" (Witkin, 1998, p. 293); it is also his impression that social workers "have shown little interest in this group" (p. 293). A stigma is often attached to the classification of retardation, and those with this diagnosis are often sensitive to this, have low self-esteem, and have internalized negative images of themselves.

Although George Austen was unfortunate in being isolated from his family (probably in part due to their shame about his condition), he nevertheless did receive good care (especially for the times he lived in); certainly he received far more humane treatment and respect than many mentally retarded people who came later. George Austen lived in what we would today call a specialized foster home for the retarded. During the past century and until the 1960s, many people with retardation lived in large state institutions, often with poor physical conditions and dehumanizing (at its worst) or infantilizing (at its best) treatment. Since retardation is a chronic disorder, little in the way of education or rehabilitation was provided; people had no preparation for living outside the institutions. Sometimes people who were not retarded were "dumped" into these settings because their behavior might have been difficult or serious family problems existed, or they were deaf (which was not diagnosed) or had other medical disorders, and no in-depth or ongoing evaluations were done.

Today, many people with retardation have been deinstitutionalized; federal legislation, including the Americans with Disabilities Act, is in force;

special educational services are federally mandated; special residences and group homes exist; vocational services and day programs are available. However, many programs do not have sufficient resources to adequately meet this population's needs.

For example, about 100,000 mentally retarded adults in the United States are on long waiting lists for homes and day care programs (funded by Medicaid) ("Suit Seeks," 1999). Some of the parents still caring for their adult children are in their sixties and seventies (this problem also exists for many parents of schizophrenic children). A lawsuit was initiated in Massachusetts in March 1999, demanding that the state provide appropriate services, which had been lagging. One plaintiff, a sixty-one-year-old woman, reported waiting "a decade for a residential program for her 41-year-old daughter . . . who is retarded, deaf and legally blind" ("Suit Seeks," 1999, p. 23); this woman had "been told repeatedly that her daughter was ineligible because she was not considered a 'crisis' case with nowhere else to turn" (p. 26).

Assessment of Mental Retardation

A person is considered mentally retarded only if this condition has started before the age of eighteen. Mental retardation can range from mild to moderate, severe, and profound. Functional assessment is an important part of the diagnosis, and the capacities of people to take care of their own hygiene, their daily living needs, work, or maintain themselves in the community are factors that are evaluated.

The specific cause of mental retardation in many people is not known. However, clear-cut causes of retardation can be determined in a number of patients, which include: genetic disorders (such as Down's syndrome), illness of the mother during pregnancy (such as German measles and AIDS), prematurity, substance abuse of the mother (fetal alcohol syndrome), complications of pregnancy (toxemia), and complications during delivery which can deprive the baby's brain of oxygen (anoxia) (Kaplan et al., 1994).

A child can acquire retardation after birth through illness (such as viral encephalitis), accidents, or child abuse, which cause traumatic brain injuries. Poor environmental conditions and various types of maternal deprivation and child maltreatment can cause what appears to be retardation; however, good early intervention programs often can reverse these conditions. Sometimes children who are not retarded have been diagnosed as such because of undiagnosed deafness and/or blindness. Mental retardation can coexist with psychopathology such as schizophrenia or mood disorders. Children with *pervasive developmental disorders* (such as autism) tend to have a high rate of serious cognitive impairments.

Clinical Issues

It is important to keep in mind that people who are cognitively limited also have the same human problems other people do and also progress through the life cycle. They are subject to a variety of psychosocial stressors and have family relationships that cover the spectrum from warm and supportive to abusive. Their psychosocial difficulties must be evaluated from a life-cycle perspective, in terms of the developmental changes, progressions and normal regressions, expectations, and stresses of their age.

Early diagnosis of developmental disabilities is important to enable early intervention efforts; this is critical in promoting optimal development for the disabled child as well as providing needed support and educational guidance for the caretakers.

Children with developmental disabilities are at greater risk for being abused than "normal" children (Olkin, 1999); this factor should be kept in mind when evaluating families. A special therapeutic problem exists for children who have been abused and need therapeutic intervention but may not have the verbal skills to engage in conventional therapy; special techniques have been evolving to work with this problem, although services in this area are scarce.

School-age children should receive special educational services to meet their needs; advances in special education programs have made a major difference in educating these children. As relationships with peers are so important at this age, cognitively impaired children are vulnerable to the hurtful insults (such as "retard"), prejudices, and discrimination that other children direct at them. One of the most pejorative terms anyone can use is calling someone a "retard!" Many retarded children and adults have problems with self-esteem, can feel different from others, and, as Witkin (1998) reminds us, remain outside the mainstream.

A variety of approaches, including support from school-based programs and families, can help counter these responses. Some children may benefit from individual clinical work; some may do well in groups in which the group support can help validate their need to feel worthwhile.

Teenagers in general go through a turbulent time; self-esteem issues of normal adolescence are intensified for retarded teens by their awareness of being different; this must be addressed. Struggles between dependence and independence surge; it can be difficult to find the right balance between granting the autonomy teens want and maintaining the protective controls they may need. Involvement of often overprotected and overcontrolled retarded youngsters in settings that foster independence and autonomy in as many spheres as is reasonable should be encouraged.

Separation-individuation issues must be worked out on many levels; some face the option of moving away from home into group homes, and this can also be a conflictual issue for them as well as their parents. Some, like George Austen, were sent away for varying periods of time in their childhood and may have reactive separation and loss issues resulting from these experiences.

Teenagers experience sexual changes and feelings and are often eager for help with sex education and their conflicting feelings about entering into sexual activity; this focus is often lacking with the cognitively impaired population. Some older teenagers and young adults may benefit from support and guidance about entering committed relationships, choosing career opportunities, making a life, and choosing a lifestyle which, depending on their needs and inclinations, might range from living with parents, independent living, to group (or foster) homes. As noted earlier, options for group homes are seriously limited; while living with parents can be a benign experience, it can also be conflictual and may serve to thwart independent strivings.

People in middle adulthood may have families of their own with successful family lives, or they may have family struggles, as many of their nondisabled peers do. Many in middle adulthood who have lived with their families all their lives might be facing separation for the first time, as their parents age and can no longer care for them.

Older retarded adults carry with them the diversity of health and lifestyle problems that many nondisabled elderly would have. Some people can continue in independent living; many find themselves in nursing homes. Generally, retarded people (especially those with severe or profound retardation) tend to die at an earlier age due to other physical problems (Kaplan et al., 1994).

Many clinicians believe that people with cognitive limitations are not amenable to psychotherapy; if help is provided to them, it follows a behavioral model (which usually permeates most of the settings in which they live and work). However, some clinicians have experienced successful therapeutic encounters with retarded people, who often respond positively to supportive relationships and want to talk and think about their lives, their fears, and getting along with others. Their low self-esteem can be improved, and they can experience (for some, it may be a unique experience) not being outside of the mainstream of human discourse and finding that someone is interested in what they think and what they feel.

Mikkelsen (1994) believes that people who are mentally retarded "experience the full range of human emotions, and in some situations their cognitive limitations may actually heighten the intensity of their feelings" (p. 8). He has observed:

> Many mentally retarded people who are not living with their families will have experienced repeated losses. Institutional staff members and

counselors to whom they have felt close will have gone away. They will have left friends behind on moving to new residences. A previous psychotherapist may have broken off treatment before it was completed. This accumulation of losses and the fear of further losses can make retarded people hesitant to begin a new therapeutic relationship. A therapist who is not aware of these issues may wrongly regard the resulting reticence as an effect of limited cognitive capacity. (Mikkelsen, 1994, p. 8)

Work with Families

It is an unanswered question as to why George Austen was socially isolated from his family throughout his lifetime. Was it a combination of the family's shame, anger, and overt rejection? Nokes (1997) refers to an episode in Jane Austen's novel, *Persuasion.* The Musgrove family had a very difficult son who was both "stupid" and "unmanageable," and who was "sent to sea," as he "deserved" this. The family rarely heard about him, and he was "scarcely at all regretted" (Nokes, 1997, p. 524). The implication here is that the motivation was overt rejection based on utter frustration and anger with this impossible son; by inference, this may be what the Austen family felt toward George.

However, Jane Austen's recollection as an adult of using sign language with George when he was a child is quite striking. Sign language is not easy to acquire; it takes some motivation and time to learn. This suggests the possibility that some involvement and investment was made in communicating with George. The brief, early descriptions of the parents' reactions to George and his medical problems sound caring. Therefore, another hypothesis is that the parents may have experienced deep grief and sadness at losing their second-born son; these feelings may have been "sealed off," so that they could deal with this act of exclusion, which was against their basic nature; if George could remain "sealed off," so could their feelings.

Having a developmentally disabled child produces many complex, conflictual feelings in parents; grief (followed by "chronic sorrow") (Chapter 11) combined frequently with guilt, anger, and resentment; many feel dazed and overwhelmed when hearing this news; some may seal off their feelings and choose to remain emotionally distant from the child rather than experience their devastating disappointment and sense of personal failure.

Families frequently overcome their distress, become supportive and positively invested in their children, and involve themselves in rehabilitative efforts on their children's behalf; many join support groups, take political action, and become active in organizations such as the National Association for Retarded Citizens. Many advances have been made in the field of developmental disabilities; and with good educational and rehabilitative efforts, many children can make good advances functionally, even if the disability itself cannot be reversed. Social workers can "instill in parents realistically positive expectations toward their children"; in addition, they can help parents learn "more effective skills" for both coping with their children's special problems and aiding in their growth (Proctor, 1983, p. 515). As typical in many early child intervention programs (Chapter 8), parents are seen as collaborators with the helping professionals.

Every family's subjective reactions, while having certain common features, are different, and every family is unique. The baseline biopsychosocial functioning of a family must be understood in the context of their social world and culture, and their strengths and vulnerabilities must be evaluated in terms of their attitudes, relationship (and attachment behaviors) to the child, and potential to respond (and to act as collaborators) for rehabilitative services for their disabled child.

Socioeconomic, racial, and cultural factors are important considerations in working with children with developmental disabilities. Poverty has been cited as a factor putting families under greater stress, and children under these circumstances are generally at greater risk for developmental problems; being a member of a racial minority can also add to a family's stress. For families already stressed for these reasons, having a disabled child can aggravate dysfunction, and both the child and siblings can be affected by the additional tension (Phillips, 1999). Families can also have other problems, including family dissolution, alcoholism, mental illness, and child maltreatment; adding the extra difficulty of a disabled child may be overwhelming.

A child with developmental disabilities can produce multiple stresses in any family in terms of demands on time, problems in controlling behavior, and difficulty in socializing with others, sometimes due to the child's negative behaviors. Depending on the degree of disability, the realistic demands placed on the family, and the capacity of the family to cope, *respite care* is often very helpful; this can also be critical for many well-functioning families.

A variety of programs (usually group models) have been designed for siblings of disabled children who may feel shame, confusion, and uncertainty about how to relate to their disabled brothers or sisters. Phillips (1999) expressed specific concern about the impact of a disabled child on siblings in African-American families who lived in socioeconomically disadvantaged households. The pilot program that was developed was motivated by the frequent concern on the part of parents about devoting so much time and energy to the disabled child that they did not have "enough 'left over' for their other children"; they were worried about the impact on these siblings (Phillips, 1999, p. 571). This program, carried out with 180 siblings (half of whom were in a control group) ages nine to twelve, provided a group intervention that lasted for fifteen weeks and included "group discussion about developmental disabilities, recreational activities, and homework assistance" (Phillips, 1999, p. 572). The program was found to be effective, and, at the end, the children experienced less stress, felt more supported, and had "less depression and anxiety and higher self-esteem" (Phillips, 1999, p. 576).

Autism

Pervasive developmental disorders, which seriously affect language, socialization, and behavior, include several specific syndromes (such as Asperger's disorder and Rett's disorder); however, only autism will be discussed here.

The etiology of autism, with its pervasive, disabling effects on a child's developmental processes, is still not known, although all evidence points to biological factors as being prominent in its etiology. From a phenomenological point of view, the child's lack of emotional connectedness and attachment to other people is its defining characteristic. The term *autism* comes from the Greek word *autos,* which means self; in this context, it means the absence of interest in others and a self-absorption; the more extreme the autism, the less the awareness of and the greater the indifference to other people.

Autism can develop during different stages of infancy and early childhood, but it is classified as autism only if it arises by the age of three (American Psychiatric Association, 1994). Variations occur in its severity and symptomatology as well as the presence of other disabilities, such as retardation (very frequent), epilepsy, blindness, deafness, and various physical illnesses. Serious deficits in communication (American Psychiatric Association, 1994) include no verbal language; few words; *echolalia,* a "stereotyped and repetitive use of language" (p. 70); and "restricted repetitive and stereotyped patterns of behavior, interests, and activities" (p. 71).

In some ways, autism is a "wastebasket" classification, as many developmental abnormalities that share some of these features have been labeled autism. Although it is clear that an organic basis underlies this disorder (in the past it was thought to be caused by parental coldness and rejection), the existence of different etiologies may explain the inconsistent symptoms and the fact that autism appears at different points during the first three years of development. German measles in the mother, for example, may produce autism in a child, which is present at birth. Some abnormalities do not appear until the child is a year and a half or two years old, possibly related to factors such as a viral illness or metabolic disturbance.

It is my impression that one of the distinctive features of autism is the difficulty for the child to process and integrate thoughts and feelings; although they maybe capable of learning, they tend to remain at a concrete level of thinking; often considerable rigidity characterizes both their thinking and behaviors. Some children have serious behavior problems, such as tantrums, and appear to be out of control; in part, this can be related to (or intensified by) parental confusion and inconsistency about how to deal with their child.

One mother described her seven-year-old son, Christopher, diagnosed as autistic; one concern was his speech: "He just doesn't talk unless he wants something." Another mother was pleased about the decreased echolalia in her son's speech, which is described as the "pathological repetition by imitation of the speech of another" (Campbell, 1989, p. 232). Some children have no speech at all; sign language is frequently used to compensate for this.

Christopher was recently toilet trained, and his mother was pleased about this and the fact that now "he makes only occasional mistakes." Toilet training is often a major problem in this population and a frequent focus of intervention.

Christopher does not have any friends; "he is a loner," although he does respond to his older sister. (It is not uncommon to see this variation; children may show varying amounts of affection, such as wanting hugs or kissing parents or seeming to have a favorite person, although basically the interpersonal world does not seem to be a major interest.) Peter Gombosi, a psychoanalyst, has written about his own autistic son, Andrew (Chapter 11). In discussing the lack of attachment behaviors attributed to autistic children, he notes:

> But all is not as it seems. Any parent or teacher of an autistic child, or anyone who does not diagnose and "understand" from a distance, will tell you of moments of intense interchange that are never spoken of in descriptions of autism. The capacity for some kind of object relationship is not missing, but in most autistic children it is distorted and severely restricted and takes other shapes. (Gombosi, 1998, p. 256)

Christopher enjoys the rides in amusement parks; "the wilder it is the more he loves it." He also enjoys the swings at home (swinging and other self-stimulating behaviors are often favorite pastimes of autistic children). Gombosi (1998) observed that "most develop a repetitive, circular behavior called 'stimming' [self-stimulation], which seems to occupy their senses, while ignoring the world. . . . My son's roommate likes to spend his free time squishing mud between his fingers . . . [another] boy will put his hand in front of his face and wave it to and fro rapidly" (p. 256).

Christopher's mother reports that "his only interest is in eating; he is constantly eating—cereal, soup, a popsicle; he will have supper and then want something else." (Eating habits are often a major concern; some children will eat only a limited diet of three or four foods and are insistent about this;

one ten-year-old girl would eat only oatmeal.) When Christopher eats in the yard, "he has a bad habit of throwing dishes into the neighbor's yard after he's finished eating"; the neighbor is "accepting of this and returns the dishes." Christopher is not destructive, and she can keep fragile things in the house (many parents, on the other hand, find that their children are destructive, damage things, and are difficult to control). The only thing Christopher destroys is colored newspapers.

Christopher is very active and very nervous; his fingernails are "bitten down." It is not unusual to find some autistic children engaged in self-abusive behaviors. One mother described her five-and-a-half-year old son as self-abusive at home, where he pinches himself, claws at his face, and sometimes scratches at his brother's face. Recently, he has been scratching his own testicles.

Another mother, with a fourteen-year-old son, felt that his demands on her were high. "His demands are always directed toward me"; he will tell her, for example, "You make the chicken!" He is also concerned with sameness and rituals (another common trait): he does not like anyone to be missing and often asks the whereabouts of family members who are not at home.

Treatment Considerations

Early intervention is critical in working with autistic children and their families. It is generally accepted that behavior modification including positive reinforcement and social skills training is the treatment of choice (Groden and Baron, 1988), and many of these children respond well and can progress to higher levels of functioning and communication within the basic parameters of this chronic disorder. Aversive approaches are to be very strictly limited, reviewed, and monitored. Gombosi (1998) recognizes the importance of a behavioral approach and has commented that "for those of us raised in the psychodynamic tradition, it is both inspiring and humbling to see the improvements some autistic children can make within a strictly behavioral, intensive program, sometimes to the point where they attend school without an aide in a regular classroom" (p. 272). He also credits the "experts in the trenches," the teachers who work with these children; "how they continue so loyally, enthusiastically, and with such good cheer, with children who are not their own, in the face of the difficulties relating to these children, is a wonder to me" (Gombosi, 1998, p. 274).

Working with families of autistic children and coordinating efforts at home with educational approaches at school are very important. I would add that the same biopsychosocial perspective discussed in relation to working with families of retarded children applies to this population.

CONCLUSION

This chapter discussed those mental health problems that frequently affect the populations served by clinical social workers and are deeply intertwined with complex family and social problems. This book has attempted to go beneath surface symptomatology and to understand human struggles; the biopsychosocial approach is especially relevant for people who have mental health problems and for their families. Developing awareness of intersubjectivity is imperative for working effectively with complicated individual and relationship disturbances.

Disparities exist in the mental health fields today; on one hand, tremendous advances in research and knowledge are occurring and exciting pilot programs are in development; at the same time, many people go unserved, are seriously neglected, and needlessly suffer. Dorothea Dix and her pioneering efforts on behalf of the mentally ill 100 years ago remain, unfortunately, relevant for us today.

LEARNING EXERCISE

1. In your small groups, choose one of the mental health problems discussed in this chapter, and role-play a clinical interview with a patient with this disorder and/or the family of the patient.

SUGGESTED READINGS

Articles

Briggs, D. (1979). The trainee and the borderline client: Countertransference pitfalls. *Clinical Social Work Journal, 7,* 133-145.

Solomon, A. (1992). Clinical diagnosis among diverse populations: A multicultural perspective. *Families in Society: The Journal of Contemporary Human Services, 73,* 371-377.

Books

Gee, K. K. and Ishii, M. M. (1997). Assessment and treatment of schizophrenia among Asian Americans. In E. Lee (Ed.), *Working with Asian Americans: A guide for clinicians* (pp. 227-251). New York: The Guilford Press.

Gombosi, P. G. (1998). Parents of autistic children: Some thoughts about trauma, dislocation, and tragedy. In A. J. Solnit, P. B. Neubauer, S. Abrams, and A. S. Dowling (Eds.), *The Psychoanalytic Study of the Child, Vol. 53* (pp. 254-275). New Haven: Yale University Press.

Jamison, K. 1996. *An unquiet mind: A memoir of moods and madness.* New York: Vintage Books.

Straussner, S. L. A. and Zelvin, E. (Eds.) (1997). *Gender and addictions: Men and women in treatment.* Northvale: Jason Aronson Inc.

Styron, W. (1990). *Darkness visible: A memoir of madness.* New York: Random House.

SECTION IV:
INTEGRATION

Chapter 14

Conclusion

Perplexity is the beginning of knowledge.

Kahlil Gibran

The biopsychosocial framework as a perspective for understanding and working with people has been discussed throughout this book. This is not a new idea and is generally thought to be the basis for clinical social work. However, many social work texts today focus on generic social work principles, macro issues, task-centered treatment, and cognitive-behavioral approaches. Although these approaches have value, they do not provide the depth of understanding of individuals and families that psychodynamic approaches provide.

For many people, psychodynamic means an exclusive psychoanalytic framework; this tends to overfocus on instinct theory. The current revisions within the psychoanalytic world itself, including the additions of object relations theory and self psychology, are often excluded from discussion.

A major theme is that people have an inner world (whatever you choose to call it) which is alive, dynamic, often does not make sense, contradicts itself, fuels our emotional lives, and affects the way we relate to others and feel about ourselves.

The psychodynamic emphasis of this book has in no way excluded the cultural, social, and physical environments or ignored social policy issues. A close interrelationship exists among all these factors; it is regrettable that for years a schism has undermined social work, splitting these approaches rather than synthesizing them.

This book has emphasized the importance of human attachments from birth throughout the life cycle. The examination of this concept provides but one example of how inner and outer worlds are interwoven. Without developing adequate attachment to others, our development and maturation will be stunted and go awry. We have seen, for example, in the children in *The Drifters* (Chapter 8) how their inadequate nurturing affected not only their relationship capacities but all their ego functions and their achievement of self-esteem and a solid self-identity.

551

Child welfare problems have received special attention in this book, because so many children are adrift today with no place they can call home and no family that they can say is "my forever family." Many troubled families also struggle not only with vital external problems, such as poverty, poor housing, and lack of services, but also with their own unresolved attachment problems and other emotional conflicts. These families need services on multiple levels; to be most effective, a solid psychodynamic orientation can provide the clinician with an empathic understanding of their many needs, their frequent distrust of others, how to develop relationships with them, and how to listen.

Winnicott (Grolnick, 1990) has spoken of the paradoxes and riddles involved in working with patients, forging a partnership with the client, and working toward a path of mutual discovery. Sitting with their clients, students must have a solid foundation to achieve this. One such base is the understanding of a client's ego functioning. This clarifies the client's psychological needs and appropriate ways to respond. In Chapter 13, for example, we discussed schizophrenic patients and the impairments in all their ego functions. Supportive reality-based work was deemed necessary to help them repair and rebuild these functions.

It is important always to address a client's ego functioning, how this changes over time, and how to adapt our treatment accordingly. Bandler (1963) comments that "all psychological forms of therapy are 'ego-supportive.' None of them aims to weaken or to overthrow the ego" (p. 27). In deciding which theory to follow and which techniques to use, the analysis of ego functions is one very important determining factor. In concluding, the case of Linda Valli is presented to illustrate how ego functions were analyzed in one client and the value derived from that analysis. It is interesting to note the variations present; some functions were strong and others needed strengthening. This case also illustrates how a psychodynamic orientation in work with a client can add a depth of understanding, which can help facilitate emotional growth.

CASE ILLUSTRATION OF EGO FUNCTIONS

As we discuss this case, each ego function is examined separately, and the strengths and vulnerabilities of each function are assessed. The reader may recall that Linda Valli has been discussed several times in this book—in Chapter 2, related to the development of her strengths (including her determination or will), and in Chapter 11, in terms of the loss of her mother when she was thirteen and the visual hallucinatory experience of her aunt she experienced after the aunt's death. Linda was seen in weekly psychotherapy for seven months.

Linda Valli, twenty-seven, a woman of Italian ancestry, was four months pregnant when she applied to a mental health clinic because her fears and anxieties, a chronic problem for her, had increased in intensity over the past eight months. She was afraid to drive, afraid to be by herself, and afraid to travel too far from the immediate vicinity of her home. Not only had these fears produced restrictions in living, but she also became preoccupied with them, spending time sitting and obsessing about overcoming them, and then feeling self-punitive when she gave in to the fears. She reported a positive relationship with her husband and her two-year-old daughter. She stated that no problems in her life were causing distress—"Only what is going on inside of me." Linda is a very attractive woman who is intelligent, and although "shy" and inhibited, she related positively to the clinician.

Linda's capacity for outer perception was basically sound though not optimal; despite good reality testing, she did have occasional difficulties with outer perception under stress. The "hallucination" she reported (seeing her aunt after she had died) was not viewed as a serious sign of mental disorder; this "encapsulated" symptom occurred at a time of death and trauma for her. It is not uncommon for bereaved people to have visual and auditory hallucinations of deceased persons, especially shortly after their death.

Linda's mother died when she was a teenager, and sometimes she has a sensation of her mother's ghost (which is frightening to her), when she is home. She does not hear her voice or see her: "It's just a frightening thought—it doesn't go beyond that." This was also seen as an "encapsulated" occurrence, related to her conflictual feelings toward her mother.

During therapy, Linda experienced growth in her ego functions. She could see her relationship problems with her husband more clearly, and we can see an increase in the capacity for outer perception.

She describes her husband as sometimes having a "glass barrier" around him. She also stated that this is not new, but before coming to the clinic, it was like being in darkness . . . she said she became more aware of her husband as a person when she started becoming more aware of herself as a person.

Linda had some difficulty with her ability for inner perception, but her capacity for this was excellent; she developed this capacity further during treatment. Linda did not initially recognize many of her feelings, nor did she see a connection between her anxiety attacks and underlying conflict. Linda further developed a very good *observing ego*. Initially, she tended to suppress her feelings and to internalize emotions, particularly anger, taking it out on herself. In the following incident, we can see that Linda started her narrative with no understanding of what precipitated her upset but was quick to make a connection, indicating that the potential for observing an issue was present but needed development.

> Linda had had an upsetting episode during the week but could not see any reason for being upset. As she began describing some of the events leading up to this distress, the significance of the events, some of which were rather humorous, became apparent. By the end of the interview, Linda could look back and laugh over it.
>
> She had been waiting for an aunt to come to her home so that she could give her a permanent wave. The aunt (to be driven by an "undependable" sister-in-law) was scheduled to arrive in the morning but did not come until the afternoon. In addition to having to wait all morning, the afternoon is not the best time for Linda. She did not really want to do it in the first place but did not want to hurt her aunt. On top of this, Linda does not like giving permanents at home because they are messy, etc. While she was giving the permanent, she was worried throughout that she would mess up the aunt's hair.

At the end of treatment, Linda described the development of her observing ego, but in her own terms. "It's like being outside myself and looking at myself—not keeping all my thoughts and feelings in—after twenty years of keeping everything in!"

Cognitive functions were minimally impaired. She was intelligent, used good judgment, had the capacity to integrate and reflect, spoke coherently and logically, and had no thought disorder. At times, her cognitive abilities were clouded by her anxiety; as the anxiety diminished and she became more self-aware, her cognitive ability gained in strength. When she terminated, she spoke of not being "nutsy" anymore.

She engaged somewhat in magical thinking, especially in regard to her husband.

> She expects her husband "will be able to read my mind." If she wants his help, she will not tell him but expects that he will know and then resents it if he does not. She realizes, she stated, that it would be better to tell him first so that he will know.

There were major problems in Linda's management of needs and feelings. She had difficulty not only expressing angry feelings but also acknowledging to herself that she had them, as was apparent in the incident of giving her aunt a permanent without awareness of her feelings of resentment. Impulse control was not a problem; in fact, the opposite, the strong inhibition of impulses, was an issue for her. She had problems with autonomous gratification and became aware that it was difficult for her to give herself pleasure.

> Linda described baking a cake and feeling that she had to rush whenever she did this, even if she had two hours. She enjoys preparing supper, too, but when it is on the table, she finds she rushes through it. "I am at my worst after supper." I raised the issue of whether she allowed herself pleasure. Does she feel she is entitled to enjoy herself?

Linda acknowledged that allowing herself enjoyment was indeed problematic; however, her observing ego enabled her to see other examples of this, and her integrative capacity helped her put her insights into action and to change.

Linda's management of object relationships was not seriously impaired, although aspects of her relationships were problematic. Linda's strength in relationship capacity was evident in her development of the therapeutic relationship. Initially shy and presenting in a somewhat superficial manner, she soon became more relaxed and open, sharing more about herself in a progressive manner and was emotionally responsive to the therapist. She showed no fear of the therapeutic relationship, did not pull away from its developing closeness, nor did she attempt to use it inappropriately, which indicated the absence of boundary formation problems. Although shy, she nevertheless did have the capacity to relate and had had friendships throughout her life. She was preoccupied with her present anxieties, which diminished her social relationships, but nevertheless bonds were retained. She was emotionally responsive to her two-year-old daughter. The relationship with her husband was basically stable, although some communication problems existed. As Linda's sense of self-identity was enhanced and as her outer perceptive capacities increased, she saw the potential for building a closer relationship to her husband.

During the intake process, Linda's therapist had some concern about the extent of Linda's anxieties and the degree to which she might be incapacitated in her daily executive functioning. Of particular concern to the therapist was Linda's two-year-old daughter: was she receiving adequate care from her mother at the present time? She therefore asked Linda about an average day at home.

> Linda gets up in the morning, gets breakfast, does some housework . . . if she starts to think of going somewhere, she becomes preoccupied with this and might "waste a lot of time" just sitting and worrying about it. Sometimes she is OK, and if she goes out, for example, to visit her sister, she will develop a "big fear" about having to drive home. Although Linda is not doing "the million things she can be do-

ing," she feels she is responsive to her daughter's needs; she feeds her, comes if she calls, etc. She referred to her daughter with positive feeling as "a little angel—a peach." During the day, her daughter is in the house playing. "She is pretty independent."

Linda's executive functioning seemed adequate: she was able to care for her daughter, and fulfill her basic responsibilities. However, it was not optimal; she spent time unproductively preoccupied with her anxieties. During the course of therapy, as she became more comfortable with herself and as her anxiety level diminished, her executive functioning improved.

As work with Linda progressed, it became apparent that she had an excellent capacity for integration. Her therapist felt that this factor contributed greatly to her making so much progress in treatment in the relatively short time of seven months. Often the capacity for integration can be difficult to assess at the beginning of therapy. The therapist "cannot usually evaluate the capacity of the client to learn and to change except as a result of helping efforts that offer the opportunity for new learning and that motivate and support the individual in his efforts to learn" (Upham, 1973, p. 147).

> During the fourth session, Linda brought out the feeling that she tends to put herself down. She realized this during the week in regard to placemats. If there are four mats, and one is the odd one, she will always give herself the odd one. This week she went out and bought something she wanted, just for herself. She stated that it is always more natural for her to go out and shop for other people. In the sixth session, she commented: "Maybe I do take things out on myself . . . like anger—I am starting to think." She also talked about reading an article in a magazine about how people see you . . . that there are good things about you, too. She has also been thinking about this in relation to herself.

In this excerpt, we can see that Linda is actively involved in the treatment process and is integrating what is happening on many levels. Linda's reading an article, for example, on self-image and then applying it to herself, is an excellent example of integration at work. She commented: "I think of what we talk about during the week and I work things through in my own mind." Furthermore, her insight about giving to others and not to herself is immediately followed by a behavioral change, which is at a high level of integrative capacity. It is noteworthy that this behavioral change was not suggested by the clinician but was derived internally from her own insight and emotional growth.

Finally, in examining her sense of ego identity, we note a number of problems related to her sense of self and self-esteem. Early in treatment, she stated that she usually feels uncomfortable with other people: "I don't know who I am." During the early part of her marriage, she had difficulty being comfortable with the sexual relationship. "I didn't want it—I wished it weren't part of marriage and part of me." During treatment, she grew to feel considerably more positive about herself and having a firmer sense of who she was. "I'm as good as anyone else—I don't put myself down or make apologies and excuses for other people." As noted earlier, when talking about outer perception, Linda had commented that she became more aware of her husband as a person when she started becoming more aware of herself as a person.

In summation, in assessing Linda's ego functioning, we see an uneven, skewed picture in terms of strengths and weaknesses among the various ego functions. We observe a basically well-functioning person who is able to carry out her major roles (although at a reduced capacity), whose cognitive processes were essentially intact, whose outer perception was reality oriented, and who, although socially inhibited (and presently preoccupied), had a basic capacity to relate. Her integrative capacities were potentially very strong, as was her capacity to learn and grow, as evidenced by her rapid progress in therapy. She manifested more serious problems with inner perception, management of needs and feelings, and identity formation, which were a major focus of therapy. Therapy afforded Linda the opportunity for continued personality growth. Not only did her symptoms of anxiety disappear, but all her ego functions improved dramatically. It was anticipated that this freeing of her ego functions from a growth-inhibiting, "frozen" state will enable this maturational process to continue.

In examining the treatment, several factors contributed to its success. First, important factors resided in Linda herself, including her motivation, her will to get better, her ability to involve herself in treatment and in a therapeutic relationship, her capacity to develop further an "observing ego," and her capacity to integrate. A good deal of hidden health emerged beneath the presenting picture of pathology.

The treatment, based on a psychodynamic perspective, was founded on the development of a therapeutic relationship, which enabled the work of therapy to proceed, as Linda's development of trust enabled her to reveal painful aspects of herself and her past life. Furthermore, from an object relations perspective, the relationship itself was a key factor in treatment, providing a holding environment in which Linda could feel sustained and her feelings contained. She internalized aspects of the therapeutic relationship, including the therapist's positive regard for her, which helped build a stronger sense of identity and esteem. As Bandler (1963) comments, the therapeutic relationship "is not merely the medium in which restitution and growth take place; we, as the objects to whom the patient relates (like parents and educators, via identification), take our place in his personality and contribute to its consolidation and modification" (p. 44). In addition, from a self psychology perspective, the therapeutic relationship and the utilization of empathy helped develop a more cohesive sense of self.

From a psychoanalytic perspective, Linda was able to see how her past life and relationships (e.g., the physical decline and subsequent death of her mother when she was a young teenager; her mother's preference for her brother; her father's emotional removal from the family) affected her present feelings about herself. The major focus of work was in the here and now; however, in looking at some of her patterns of behavior, it was helpful to relate these to her past. In addition, on an affective level, Linda grieved for her parents and became aware of and accepting of her angry feelings, which she stopped internalizing. She was able to discuss her superego conflict about finding it difficult to give herself pleasure.

From an ego psychological perspective, attention was directed to Linda's ego functions, which matured during treatment. Her coping skills were also addressed and were enhanced. Linda, for example, was concerned that she "might go crazy" while in the hospital giving birth to her child. "The doctor won't know . . . he won't do anything—it will be so bad, I'll be off the wall!" Her therapist asked why she felt she had to wait until it gets very bad if she becomes upset—why can't she tell someone? Linda could feel more empowered when she realized she could have some control over this situation. Also, in terms of coping, Linda was assisted by anticipatory guidance, in thinking ahead to what plans she might make when she went to the hospital, etc. Vaillant (1993) cites Heinz Hartmannn's comments on anticipation. " 'The familiar function of anticipating the future, orienting our actions according to it and correctly relating means and ends to each other . . . is an ego function and, surely, an adaptation process of the highest significance' " (p. 71).

THE LIFE COURSE

In looking at the life cycle, it has been stressed that the life course is full of both continuities and discontinuities; that core feelings about the self and central experiences remain with us. I have suggested that good mental health involves the capacity to change and to adapt. Linda Valli had this capacity, which she was able to fulfill with therapeutic help. Some people seem frozen in their development and unable to change but may be responsive to supportive and environmental help to facilitate their social functioning.

The ecological concept of goodness-of-fit is very relevant to understanding the adaptation of people along the life course. Although Linda Valli had some problems in her relationship to her husband, it was basically a strong relationship, as was her relationship to her daughter. She also had a small circle of friends. Her internal changes enhanced all her relationships; it did not upset a precarious interpersonal balance.

Edgar Allan Poe (Silverman, 1991) experienced painful losses in his life; his later adaptations provide interesting insights into the concept of goodness-of-fit and the continuities and discontinuities in his life course.

Poe was born in 1809 in Boston to a mother who was a beautiful and very talented actress, and who had achieved a great deal of acclaim. His father had theatrical aspirations, but was unsuccessful at this vocation, and deserted his family.

Poe had one brother and a sister, and he and his mother apparently had a very warm relationship. His mother suddenly died when he was about 3. His sister became a foster child (whom he saw occasionally), while his brother went to live with his father's family and was absent from Poe's life. Poe was taken in, but less than fully accepted as their child, by a wealthy, childless family in Baltimore, and was never adopted. He had an ongoing difficult relationship with his foster father. He assumed the foster father's last name, Allan, as his own middle name, perhaps in lieu of it being his last name, as it would have been had he been adopted (Silverman, 1991).

Poe experienced early maternal loss at an age when it would have been cognitively difficult to understand and process it; he also lost his siblings and was taken in, but never officially adopted. Silverman (1991) suggests that the recurring theme in his fiction about people who are dead, but not dead, reflect his wish for his mother to regain life and for reunion with her. One can only speculate about what might have happened if Poe had been in a family with a better goodness-of-fit, if he had been helped to mourn his loss, if he had not also lost his siblings, and if his biological father had reappeared in his life.

One of the most interesting aspects concerning his adaptation occurred in his later life. When he was twenty-seven, he married his thirteen-year-old cousin Virginia and lived with her and her mother (his aunt). Apparently this was a very congenial arrangement for all; Virginia's mother also "mothered" him (Silverman, 1991). Although we might question this nontraditional arrangement, it provided a positive goodness-of-fit for Poe.

However, tragically, Virginia developed tuberculosis and died when she was only twenty-four. At this point, Poe was overwhelmed, did not resolve his grief constructively, and soon his life descended into chaos. He became involved in unstable relationships with several women at the same time, and his drinking increased; he died when he was forty. During his marriage, he had a relatively stable life; but he was not able tolerate the loss of his young wife and the breakdown of his living arrangements (Silverman, 1991). We can speculate that the loss of his young wife precipitated inner distress related to his unresolved past grief.

Poe worked many years as a writer and critic for newspapers and magazines, gaining fame only later in his life. He was always concerned about his finances (and never received any inheritance from his foster family, because he was not an adopted heir). He would sometimes drink to excess; his drinking seems to have increased when he had employment problems (newspapers were an unstable source of employment) (Silverman, 1991). Again, we can only speculate what might have happened if he had a secure economic and employment base and had received recognition at an earlier period in his life for his tremendous talent. We also wonder how much his losses and other life vicissitudes, as well as how he experienced these, fueled his style, his subject matter, and his creative genius in general.

CONCLUSION

This book is meant to serve as an introduction to the biopsychosocial approach to working with people; it is not expected that you will have fully cognitively mastered and integrated all the material presented in this text. Time, experience, more reading, and more learning will help foster this development and integration. The development of self-awareness and the concept of intersubjectivity have been discussed in many chapters. Tuning in to the feelings evoked in one by clients is an additional rich source of understanding and learning, and contributes to the development of the professional self.

It can be frustrating to work in a profession with so many ambiguities and uncertainties; it also presents an exciting opportunity, as challenges confront us and new discoveries are waiting to be made. One can develop optimally if one is not lulled into accepting formulas and neat solutions but searches for a deeper understanding of the human condition.

LEARNING EXERCISE

1. In your small groups, discuss your impressions about the biographies and autobiographies you have read. Share your impressions with each other about the life course of your subjects and look for similarities and/or differences in your impressions.

References

A brief history of Ballot Measure 58 (2001). Center for Health Statistics (and Vital Records), Oregon Health Division, Oregon Department of Human Services. Available online at <http://www.ohd.hr.state.or.us/chs/certif/58update.htm>.

Adams Jr., C. L. and Kimmel, D. C. (1997). Exploring the lives of older African American gay men. In B. Greene (Ed.), *Ethnic and cultural diversity among lesbians and gay men: Vol. 3. Psychological perspectives on lesbian and gay issues* (pp. 132-151). Thousand Oaks, CA: Sage Publications.

Adler, G. (1979). The psychotherapy of schizophrenia: Semrad's contributions to current psychoanalytic concepts. *Schizophrenia Bulletin, 5* (1), 130-137.

Adler, G. (1985). *Borderline psychopathology and its treatment.* New York: Jason Aronson Inc.

Adnopoz, J. (1996). Complicating the theory: The application of psychoanalytic concepts and understanding to family preservation. In A. J. Solnit, P. B. Neubauer, S. Abrams, and A. S. Dowling (Eds.), *The psychoanalytic study of the child, Vol. 51* (pp. 411-421). New Haven: Yale University Press.

Aguilera, D. and Messick, J. M. (1974). *Crisis intervention theory and methodology.* St. Louis: The C. V. Mosby Company.

AIDS and Mental Health—Part 1 (1994). *The Harvard Mental Health Letter, 10 (7),* pp. 1-4.

Akhtar, S. (1995). A third individuation: Immigration, identity and the psychoanalytic process. *Journal of the American Psychoanalytic Association, 43,* 1051-1084.

Akhtar, S. and Kramer, S. (Eds.) (1998). *The colors of childhood: Separation-individuation across cultural, racial, and ethnic differences.* Northvale: Jason Aronson Inc.

Al-Krenawi, A. (1999). Social workers practicing in their non-western home communities: Overcoming conflict between professional and cultural values. *Families in Society: The Journal of Contemporary Human Services, 80,* 488-495.

Alexander Jr., R. and Alexander, C. L. (1995). Criminal prosecution of child protection workers. *Social Work, 40,* 809-814.

Alpert, J. L. (1995). Introduction. In J. L. Alpert (Ed.), *Sexual abuse recalled: Treating trauma in the era of the recovered memory debate* (pp. xix-xxiv). Northvale, NJ: Jason Aronson Inc.

Alquijay, M. A. (1997). The relationships among self-esteem, acculturation, and lesbian identity formation in Latina lesbians. In B. Greene (Ed.), *Ethnic and cultural diversity among lesbians and gay men: Vol. 3. Psychological perspectives on lesbian and gay issues* (pp. 249-265). Thousand Oaks: Sage Publications.

Altman, L. K. (1999a). Much more AIDS in prisons than in general population. *The New York Times,* September 1, p. A14.

Altman, L. K. (1999b). New direction for transplants raises hopes and questions. *The New York Times*, May 2, pp. 1, 38.

Altman, L. K. (1999c). U.N. issues grim report on the 11 million children orphaned by AIDS. *The New York Times*, December 2, p. A10.

Altman, L. K. (2000). AIDS surges in black and Hispanic men. *The New York Times*, January 14, p. A13.

Alzheimer's Disease—Part I (1992). *The Harvard Mental Health Letter, 9* (2), pp. 1-4.

American Psychiatric Association (1994). *Diagnostic and statistical manual of mental disorders*, Fourth edition. Washington, DC: Author.

Amodeo, M., Robb, N., Peou, S., and Tran, H. (1996). Adapting mainstream substance-abuse interventions for Southeast Asian clients. *Families in Society: The Journal of Contemporary Human Services, 70*, 403-412.

Anderson, C. M. (1983). A psychoeducational program for families of patients with schizophrenia. In W. R. McFarlane (Ed.), *Family therapy in schizophrenia* (pp. 99-116). New York: The Guilford Press.

Angell, G. B., Kurz, B. J., and Gottfried, G. M. (1998). Suicide and North American Indians: A social constructivist perspective. *Journal of Multicultural Social Work, 6*, 1-25.

Angelou, M. (1997). *I know why the caged bird sings*. New York: Bantam Books.

Applegate, J. S. and Bonovitz, J. M. (1995). *The facilitating partnership: A Winnicottian approach for social workers and other helping professionals*. Northvale: Jason Aronson Inc.

Arieti, S. (1974). Schizophrenia: The psychodynamic mechanisms and the psychostructural forms. In S. Arieti (Ed.), *American handbook of psychiatry: Vol. 3*, Fourth edition (pp. 551-587). New York: Basic Books, Inc.

Arieti, S. and Bemporad, J. (1978). *Severe and mild depression: The psychotherapeutic approach*. New York: Basic Books, Inc.

Armstrong, D. (1998). Police suicides rely on tools of guns, alcohol. *The Boston Globe*, August 24, pp. A1, A8.

Aronson, S. (1996). The bereavement process in children of parents with AIDS. In A. J. Solnit, P. B. Neubauer, S. Abrams, and A. S. Dowling (Eds.), *The psychoanalytic study of the child, Vol. 51* (pp. 422-435). New Haven: Yale University Press.

Asch, A. (1995). Visual impairment and blindness. In R. L. Edwards and J. G. Hopps (Eds.), *Social work encyclopedia*, Nineteenth edition, Vol. 3 (pp. 2461-2468). Washington, DC: NASW Press.

Ashford, J. B., Lecroy, C. W., and Lortie, K. L. (1997). *Human behavior in the social environment: A multidimensional perspective*. Pacific Grove: Brooks/Cole Publishing Company.

Attneave, C. (1982). American Indians and Alaska native families: Emigrants in their own homeland. In M. McGoldrick, J. K. Pearce, and J. Giordano (Eds.), *Ethnicity and family therapy* (pp. 55-83). New York: The Guilford Press.

Austin, D. (1997). The institutional development of social work education: The first 100 years—and beyond. *Journal of Social Work Education, 33*, 599-612.

Ballenger, J. (1986). Editorial. *American Journal of Psychiatry, 143*, 516-518.

Bandler, B. (1963). The concept of ego-supportive psychotherapy. In H. J. Parad and R. R. Miller (Eds.), *Ego-oriented casework: Problems and perspectives. Pa-*

pers from the Smith College School for Social Work (pp. 27-44). New York: Family Service Association of America.

Bandler, L. S. (1967). Family functioning: A psychosocial perspective. In E. Pavenstedt (Ed.), *The drifters: Children of disorganized lower-class families* (pp. 225-253). Boston: Little, Brown and Company.

Bandura, A. (1976). Social learning perspective on behavior change. In A. Burton (Ed.), *What makes behavior change possible?* (pp. 34-57). New York: Bruner/ Mazel, Publishers.

Barnes, A. and Ephross, P. H. (1994). The impact of hate violence on victims: Emotional and behavioral responses to attacks. *Social Work, 39,* 247-251.

Barovick, H. (2000). Fear of a gay school. *Time, 153,* February 21, p. 52.

Barrie, J. M. (1904). "Peter Pan."

Barth, D. (1991). When the patient abuses food. In H. Jackson (Ed.), *Using self psychology in psychotherapy* (pp. 223-242). Northvale: Jason Aronson Inc.

Barth, R. P. (1994). Shared family care: Child protection and family preservation. *Social Work, 39,* 515-524.

Barton, B. R. and Marshall, A. S. (1986). Pivotal partings: Forced termination with a sexually abused boy. *Clinical Social Work Journal, 14,* 139-149.

Basch, M. F. (1988). *Understanding psychotherapy: The science behind the art.* New York: Basic Books, Inc.

Bass, D. (1995). Runaways and homeless youths. In R. L. Edwards and J. G. Hopps (Eds.), *Social work encyclopedia,* Nineteenth edition, Vol. 3 (pp. 2060-2067). Washington, DC: NASW Press.

Bastien, M. (1995). Haitian Americans. In R. L. Edwards and J. G. Hopps (Eds.), *Social work encyclopedia,* Nineteenth edition, Vol. 2 (pp. 1145-1155). Washington, DC: NASW Press.

Bauer likens ruling on gay couples to terrorism (1999). *The New York Times,* December 28, p. A22.

Bearak, B. (1998). Caste hate, and murder, outlast Indian reforms. *The New York Times,* September 19, p. A3.

Bearak, B. (1999). To talk like a New Yorker, sign up for Spanish lessons. *The New York Times,* October 18, pp. A1, A25.

Beardslee, W. R. and MacMillan, H. L. (1993). Preventive intervention with the children of depressed parents: A case study. In A. J. Solnit, P. B. Neubauer, S. Abrams, and A. S. Dowling (Eds.), *The psychoanalytic study of the child, Vol. 48* (pp. 249-276). New Haven: Yale University Press.

Beaucar, K. O. (1999a). Bills seek to extend safety net for foster teens. *NASW News, 44* (7), p. 7.

Beaucar, K. O. (1999b). Case overload compounds children's peril. *NASW News, 44* (5), p. 3.

Beaucar, K. O. (1999c). Grandparent caregivers face hurdles. *NASW News, 44* (10), p. 12.

Beaucar, K. O. (1999d). The violence has come home to roost. *NASW News, 44* (6), p. 3.

Beaucar, K. O. (2000). Elder abuse is a crisis, groups say. *NASW News, 45* (1), 15.

Beck, A. T. (1976). *Cognitive therapy and the emotional disorders.* New York: New American Library.

Becker, E. (2000). Child care in military is praised as a model. *The New York Times,* May 17, p. A17.

Begun, A. L. (1993). Human behavior and the social environment: The vulnerability, risk, and resilience model. *Journal of Social Work Education, 29,* 26-35.

Beinert, P. (1998). How the California G.O.P. got a Spanish lesson. *Time, 151,* May 18, p. 58.

Belenky, M. F., Clinchy, B. M., Goldberger, N. R., and Tarule, J. M. (1986). *Women's ways of knowing: The development of self, voice, and mind.* New York: Basic Books.

Bell, Currer [Brontë] (1853). *Villette.* New York: Harper and Brothers, Publishers.

Bell, C. (1986). Adoptive pregnancy: Legal and social work issues. *Child Welfare, 45,* 421-435.

Bellafante, G. (1997). Deadly seduction. *Time,* 150, November 10, p. 58.

Belluck, P. (1998a). Black youths' rate of suicide rising sharply. *The New York Times,* March 20, pp. A1, A16.

Belluck, P. (1998b). Razing the slums to rescue the residents. *The New York Times,* September 6, pp. 1, 26, 27.

Belluck, P. (1999). A white supremacist group seeks a new kind of recruit. *The New York Times,* July 7, pp. A1, A7.

Belluck, P. (2000). Indian schools, long failing, press for money and quality. *The New York Times,* May 18, p. A1, A22.

Bemporad, J. R. and Pinsker, H. (1974). Schizophrenia: The manifest symptomatology. In S. Arieti and E. B. Brody (Eds.), *American handbook of psychiatry,* Second edition. (Volume Three—Adult Clinical Psychiatry) (pp. 524-550). New York: Basic Books, Inc.

Benedek, T. (1970). The family as a psychological field. In E. J. Anthony and T. Benedek (Eds.), *Parenthood: Its psychology and psychopathology* (pp. 109-136). Boston: Little, Brown and Company.

Bentley, K. J. (1993). The right of psychiatric patients to refuse medication: Where should social workers stand? *Social Work, 38,* 101-106.

Berger, R. M. and Kelly, J. J. (1995). Gay men overview. In R. L. Edwards and J. G. Hopps (Eds.), *Social work encyclopedia,* Nineteenth edition, Vol. 2 (pp. 1064-1075). Washington, DC: NASW Press.

Berlin, R. and Davis, R. B. (1989). Children from alcoholic families: Vulnerability and resilience. In T. F. Dugan and R. Coles (Eds.), *The child in our times: Studies in the development of resiliency* (pp. 81-105). New York: Brunner/Mazel.

Berman-Rossi, T. (1986). The fight against hopelessness and despair: Institutionalized aged. In A. Gitterman and L. Shulman (Eds.), *Mutual aid groups and the life cycle* (pp. 333-358). Itasca, IL: F. E. Peacock Publishers, Inc.

Berzoff, J. (1996a). Anxiety and its manifestations. In J. Berzoff, L. M. Flanagan, and P. Hertz (Eds.), *Inside out and outside in: Psychodynamic clinical theory and practice in contemporary multicultural contexts* (pp. 397-427). Northvale: Jason Aronson Inc.

Berzoff, J. (1996b). Drive theory. In J. Berzoff, L. M. Flanagan, and P. Hertz (Eds.), *Inside out and outside in: Psychodynamic clinical theory and practice in contemporary multicultural contexts* (pp. 17-47). Northvale: Jason Aronson Inc.

Berzoff, J. (1996c). Psychodynamic theory and the psychology of women. In J. Berzoff, L. M. Flanagan, and P. Hertz (Eds.), *Inside out and outside in: Psychodynamic clinical theory and practice in contemporary multicultural contexts* (pp. 247-266). Northvale: Jason Aronson Inc.

Berzoff, J., Flanagan, L. M., and Hertz, P. (1996). Inside out and outside in. In J. Berzoff, L. M. Flanagan, and P. Hertz (Eds.), *Inside out and outside in: Psychodynamic clinical theory and practice in contemporary multicultural contexts* (pp. 1-16). Northvale: Jason Aronson Inc.

Bill extends foster care aid (1999). *The Morning Sun,* Pittsburg, Kansas. Available online at <http://www.morningsun.net/stories/121599/usw_1215990028.shtml>.

Bloche, M. G. and Eisenberg, C. (1993). The psychological effects of state-sanctioned terror. *The Harvard Mental Health Letter, 10* (5), pp. 4-6.

Bloch, J. and Margolis, J. (1986). Feelings of shame: Siblings of handicapped children. In A. Gitterman and L. Shulman (Eds.), *Mutual aid groups and the life cycle* (pp. 91-108). Itasca, IL: F. E. Peacock Publishers, Inc.

Blos, P. (1962). *On adolescence: A psychoanalytic interpretation.* New York: The Free Press.

Blume, S. B. (1992). Compulsive gambling: Addiction without drugs. *The Harvard Mental Health Letter, 8* (8), pp. 4-5.

Boice, M. M. (1998). Chronic illness in adolescence. *Adolescence, 33,* 927-939.

Bonfield, T. (2000). Level of sickness will matter more. *The Cincinnati Enquirer.* November 24. Available online at <http://enquirer.com/editions/2000/11/24/loc_the_wait_for_organs.html>.

Borderline Personality—Part I (1994). *The Harvard Mental Health Letter, 10* (11), 1-4.

Borson, S., Liptzin, B., Nininger, J., and Rabins, P. (1987). Psychiatry and the nursing home. *American Journal of Psychiatry, 144,* 1412-1418.

Boszormenyi-Nagy, I. and Spark, G. (1973). *Invisible loyalties.* New York: Harper and Row.

Bowen, M. (1985). *Family therapy in clinical practice.* New York: Jason Aronson Inc.

Bowlby, J. (1969). *Attachment and loss: Vol. 1.* New York: Basic Books, Inc.

Bowlby, J. (1988). Developmental psychiatry comes of age. *American Journal of Psychiatry, 145,* 28-37.

Braga, W. (1989). Youth suicide risk assessment: Process and model. In B. Garfinkel and G. Northrup (Eds.), *Adolescent suicide: Recognition, treatment and prevention* (pp. 1-21). Binghamton, New York: The Haworth Press.

Bragg, R. (1999). Fearing isolation in old age, gay generation seeks haven. *The New York Times,* October 21, pp. A1, A16.

Brave Heart, M. H. (1998). The return to the sacred path: Healing the historical trauma and historical unresolved grief response among the Lakota through a psychoeducational group intervention. *Smith College Studies in Social Work, 68,* 287-305.

Brave Heart, M. Y. H. (1999). *Oyate Ptayela:* Rebuilding the Lakota Nation through addressing historical trauma among Lakota parents. *Journal of Human Behavior in the Social Environment, 2,* 109-126.

Brenner, C. (1974). *An elementary textbook of psychoanalysis,* Revised edition. Garden City: Anchor Press/Doubleday.

Bretheron, I. (1996). Internal working models of attachment relationships as related to resilient coping. In G. G. Noam and K. W. Fischer (Eds.), *Development and vulnerability in close relationships* (pp. 3-23). Mahwah, NJ: Lawrence Erlbaum Associates.

Brickel, C. M. (1986). Pet-facilitated therapies: A review of the literature and clinical implementation considerations. *Clinical Gerontologist, 5,* 309-332.

Briggs, D. (1979). The trainee and the borderline client: Countertransference pitfalls. *Clinical Social Work Journal, 7,* 133-145.

Brightman, B. (1984-1985). Narcissistic issues in the training experience of the psychotherapist. *International Journal of Psychoanalytic Psychotherapy, 10,* 293-317.

Brody, J. E. (1998). Children of depressed parents at risk. *The New York Times,* March 3, C7.

Brody, J. E. (1999). Compulsive gambling: The overlooked addiction. *The New York Times.* May 4, D7.

Bronner, E. (1999). In a revolution of rules, campuses go full circle. *The New York Times,* March 3, pp. A1, A15.

Brooke, J. (1999). Diary of a high school gunman reveals a plan to kill hundreds. *The New York Times,* April 27, pp. A1, A20.

Brooks, D., Barth, R. P., Bussiere, A., and Patterson, G. (1999). Adoption and race: Implementing the Multiethnic Placement Act and the Interethnic Adoption Provisions. *Social Work, 44,* 167-178.

Brown, D. (1972). *Bury my heart at Wounded Knee.* New York: Bantam Books.

Brown, E. M. (1998). The transmission of trauma through caretaking patterns of behavior in holocaust families: Re-enactments in a facilitated long-term second-generation group. *Smith College Studies in Social Work, 68,* 267-285.

Brown, M. (1986). Maintenance and generalization issues in skills training with chronic schizophrenics. In J. P. Curran and P. M. Monti (Eds.), *Social skills training: A practical handbook for assessment and treatment* (pp. 90-116). Washington Square, New York: New York University Press.

Bruni, F. (1997). A cult's 2-decade odyssey of regimentation. *The New York Times,* March 29, pp. 1, 8, 9.

Burman, S. and Allen-Meares, P. (1994). Neglected victims of murder: Children's witness to parental homicide. *Social Work, 39,* 28-34.

Burnette, D. (1999). Custodial grandparents in Latino families: Patterns of service use and predictors of unmet needs. *Social Work, 44,* 22-34.

Butterfield, F. (1998). Prisons replace hospitals for the nation's mentally ill. *The New York Times,* March 5, pp. A1, A26.

Butterfield, F. (1999a). As inmate population grows, so does a focus on children. *The New York Times,* April 7, pp. A1, A18.

Butterfield, F. (1999b). Indians are crime victims at rate above U.S. average. *The New York Times,* February 15, p. A12.

Butterfield, F. (1999c). Prisons brim with mentally ill, study finds. *The New York Times,* July 12, p. A10.

Butterfield, F. (2000). Racial disparities seen as pervasive in juvenile justice. *The New York Times*, April 26, pp. A1, A18.

Buxbaum, E. and Sodergren, S. S. (1977). A disturbance of elimination and motor development. In R. S. Eissler, A. Freud, M. Kris, P. B. Neubauer, and A. J. Solnit (Eds.), *The psychoanalytic study of the child, Vol. 32* (pp. 195-214). New Haven: Yale University Press.

Cain, B. (1988). Divorce among elderly women: A growing social phenomenon. *Social Casework, 69*, 563-568.

Campbell, R. J. (1989). *Psychiatric dictionary*, Sixth edition. New York: Oxford University Press.

Canino, I. A. and Spurlock, J. (2000). *Culturally diverse children and adolescents: Assessment, diagnosis and treatment*, Second edition. New York: The Guilford Press.

Caplan, G. (1976). Foreword. In H. J. Parad (Ed.), *Emergency and disaster management* (pp. xxiii-xxv). Bowie: The Charles Press Publishers, Inc.

Caplan, L. (1990). *An open adoption*. New York: Farrar, Straus, and Giroux.

Carlson, B. and Maciol, K. (1997). Domestic violence: Gay men and lesbians. In R. L. Edwards (Ed.), *Social work encyclopedia supplement*, Nineteenth edition (pp. 101-111). Washington, DC: NASW Press.

Carlson, M. (1997). Home alone. *Time, 150*, November 10, p. 30.

Caro, R. (1983). *The years of Lyndon Johnson: The path to power*. New York: Vintage Books.

Carton, B. (1996). Life after death: New AIDS drug brings hope to Provincetown, but unexpected woes. *The Wall Street Journal*, October 3, pp. A1, A6.

Carvajal, D. (1999). Slavery's truths (and tales) come flocking home. *The New York Times*, March 28, Section 4, p. 5.

Catalano, S. (1990). *Children's dreams in clinical practice*. New York: Plenum Press.

Ceconi, B. and Urdang, E. (1994). Sight or insight? Child therapy with a blind clinician. *Clinical Social Work Journal, 22*, 179-192.

Cermak, P. and Molidor, C. (1996). Male victims of child sexual abuse. *Child and Adolescent Social Work Journal, 5*, 385-400.

Chambless, D. and Goldstein, A. (1981). Clinical treatment of agoraphobia. In M. Mavissakalian and D. Barlow (Eds.), *Phobia: Psychological and pharmacological treatment*. New York: The Guilford Press.

Chan, C. S. (1997). Don't ask, don't tell, don't know: The formation of a homosexual identity and sexual expression among Asian American lesbians. In B. Greene (Ed.), *Ethnic and cultural diversity among lesbians and gay men: Vol. 3. Psychological perspectives on lesbian and gay issues* (pp. 240-248). Thousand Oaks: Sage Publications.

Chapman, C., Dorner, P., Silber, K., and Winterberg, T. S. (1986). Meeting the needs of the adoption triangle through open adoption: The birthmother. *Child and Adolescent Social Work, 3*, 203-213.

Chapman, C., Dorner, P., Silber, K., and Winterberg, T. S. (1987a). Meeting the needs of the adoption triangle through open adoption: The adoptee. *Child and Adolescent Social Work, 4*, 78-91.

Chapman, C., Dorner, P., Silber, K., and Winterberg, T. S. (1987b). Meeting the needs of the adoption triangle through open adoption: The adoptive parent. *Child and Adolescent Social Work, 4* (1), 3-13.

Chaskin, R. J., Joseph, M. L., and Chipppenda-Dansokho, S. (1997). Implementing comprehensive community development: Possibilities and limitations. *Social Work, 42,* 435-444.

Chast, R. (1998). Theories of everything [cartoon]. *The New Yorker, 74,* p. 42.

Chenot, D. (1998). Mutual values: Self psychology, intersubjectivity, and social work. *Clinical Social Work Journal, 26,* 297-311.

Chess, S. (1989). Defying the voice of doom. In T. F. Dugan and R. Coles (Eds.), *The child in our times: Studies in the development of resiliency* (pp. 179-199). New York: Bruner Mazel.

Child Abuse—Part I (1993). *The Harvard Mental Health Letter, 9* (11), 1-3.

Child Abuse—Part II (1993). *The Harvard Mental Health Letter, 9* (12), 1-4.

Choi, N. G. and Snyder, L. (1999). Voices of homeless parents: The pain of homelessness and shelter life. *Journal of Human Behavior in the Social Environment, 2,* 55-77.

Clarity, J. F. (1999). Lost youth in Ireland: Suicide rate is climbing. *The New York Times,* March 14, p. 9.

Clines, F. X. (1999). Smithsonian making room for Indian museum. *The New York Times,* September 29, pp. A1, A18.

Cloud, J. (1997). Out, proud and very young. *Time, 150,* December 8, pp. 82-83.

Cloud, J. (1998). Trans across America. *Time, 151,* July 20, pp. 48-49.

Cloud, J. (1999). Tracking down mom. *Time, 152,* February 22, pp. 64-65.

Cloud, J. (2000a). A kinder, gentler death. *Time, 156,* September 18, pp. 60-67.

Cloud, J. (2000b). The lure. *Time, 155,* June 5, pp. 62-67.

Cohen, A. (1998). Widow and the wizard. *Time, 151,* May 18, pp. 72-74.

Cohen, C. S. and Phillips, M. H. (1997). Building community: Principles for social work practice in housing settings. *Social Work, 42,* 471-481.

Cohen, D. and Fears, D. (2001). Hispanics draw even with blacks in new census. *Washington Post,* March 7, p. A01. Available online at <http://www.washingtonpost.com/ac2/wpdyn?pagename=article&node=&contentId=A32121-2001Mar6>.

Cohen, L. J. and Slade, A. (2000). The psychology and psychopathology of pregnancy: Reorganization and transformation. In C. H. Zeanah Jr. (Ed.), *Handbook of infant mental health,* Second edition (pp. 20-36). New York: The Guilford Press.

Cohen, M. N. (1996). *Lewis Carroll: A biography.* New York: Vintage Books.

Cohler, B. J. (1987). Adversity, resilience, and the study of lives. In E. J. Anthony and B. J. Cohler (Eds.), *The invulnerable child* (pp. 363-424). New York: The Guilford Press.

Cohler, B. J. and Galatzer-Levy, R. M. (1990). Self, meaning, and morale across the second half of life. In R. Nemiroff and C. Calarusso (Eds.), *New Dimensions in Adult Development* (pp. 214-263). New York: Basic Books.

Cohler, B. J. and Zimmerman, P. (1997). Youth in residential care: From war nursery to the therapeutic milieu. In A. J. Solnit, P. B. Neubauer, S. Abrams, and A. S. Dowling (Eds.), *The psychoanalytic study of the child, Vol. 52* (pp. 359-385). New Haven: Yale University Press.

Colarusso, C. A. (1993). Play in adulthood: A developmental consideration. In A. J. Solnit, P. B. Neubauer, S. Abrams, and A. S. Dowling (Eds.), *The Psychoanalytic study of the child, Vol. 48* (pp. 225-245). New Haven: Yale University Press.

Colarusso, C. A. (1997). Separation-individuation processes in middle adulthood: The fourth individuation. In S. Akhtar and S. Kramer (Eds.), *The seasons of life: Separation-individuation perspectives* (pp. 73-94). Northvale: Jason Aronson Inc.

Colarusso, C. A. (1998). A developmental line of time sense: In late adulthood and throughout the life cycle. In A. J. Solnit, P. B. Neubauer, S. Abrams, and A. S. Dowling (Eds.), *The psychoanalytic study of the child, Vol. 53* (pp. 113-140). New Haven: Yale University Press.

Coleman, D. (1996). Transference: A key to psychoanalytic social work. In J. Edwards and J. Sanville (Eds.), *Fostering healing and growth: A psychoanalytic social work approach* (pp. 46-58). Northvale: Jason Aronson Inc.

Comas-Diaz, L. and Jacobsen, F. M. (1991). Ethnocultural transference and countertransference in the therapeutic dyad. *American Journal of Orthopsychiatry, 61,* 392-402.

Comparing race/ethnicity between the 2000 census and earlier censuses (2001). Texas State Data Center, Department of Rural Sociology, Texas A&M University. Available online at <http://census.tamu.edu/Data/Redistrict/PL94-171/re-report.php>.

Condon, J. T. (1986). Management of established pathological grief reaction after stillbirth. *American Journal of Psychiatry, 143,* 987-992.

Conover, T. (1997). The last best friends money can buy. *New York Times Magazine,* November 30, pp. 124-130, 132.

Conte, J. (1995). Child sexual abuse overview. In R. L. Edwards and J. G. Hopps (Eds.), *Social work encyclopedia,* Nineteenth edition, Vol. 1 (pp. 402-409). Washington, DC: NASW Press.

Cook, C. A. L., Selig, K. L., Wedge, B. J., and Gohn-Baube, E. A. (1999). Access barriers and the use of prenatal care by low-income, inner-city women. *Social Work, 44,* 129-139.

Courtney, M. E. and Barth, R. P. (1996). Pathways of older adolescents out of foster care: Implications for independent living services. *Social Work, 41,* 75-83.

Crawford, J. M. (1999). Co-parent adoptions by same-sex couples: From loophole to law. *Families in Society: The Journal of Contemporary Human Services, 80* (3), 271-278.

Crockenberg, S. and Leerkes, E. (2000). Infant social and emotional development in family context. In C. H. Zeanah Jr. (Ed.), *Handbook of infant mental health,* Second edition (pp. 60-90). New York: The Guilford Press.

Crohn, J. (1997). Asian intermarriage: Love versus tradition. In E. Lee (Ed.), *Working with Asian Americans: A guide for clinicians* (pp. 428-438). New York: The Guilford Press.

Cruz, F. G. and Essen, L. (1994). *Adult survivors of childhood emotional, physical, and sexual abuse: Dynamics and treatment.* Northvale: Jason Aronson Inc.

Cummings, E. M., Davies, P. T., and Campbell, S. B. (2000). *Developmental psychopathology and family process: Theory, research and clinical implications.* New York: The Guilford Press.

Curran, J. P. and Monti, P. M. (1986). Social skills training with schizophrenics. In J. P. Curran and P. M. Monti (Eds.), *Social skills training: A practical handbook for assessment and treatment* (pp. 1-4). Washington Square, New York: New York University Press.

Cushman, L. F., Kalmuss, D., and Namerow, P. B. (1993). Placing an infant for adoption: The experiences of young birthmothers. *Social Work, 38,* 264-272.

Daley, S. (1998a). AIDS is everywhere, but the Africans look away. *The New York Times,* December 4, pp. A1, A12.

Daley, S. (1998b). In Zambia, the abandoned generation. *The New York Times,* September 18, pp. A1, A12.

Dalsimer, K. (1982). Female adolescent development: A study of *The Diary of Anne Frank.* In A. J. Solnit, R. S. Eissler, A. Freud, and P. B. Neubauer (Eds.), *The psychoanalytic study of the child, Vol. 37* (pp. 487-522). New Haven: Yale University Press.

Dane, B. (2000). Child welfare workers: An innovative approach for interacting with secondary trauma. *Journal of Social Work Education, 36,* 27-38.

Davenport, J. A. and Davenport III, J. (1995). Rural social work overview. In R. L. Edwards and J. G. Hopps (Eds.), *Social work encyclopedia,* Nineteenth edition, Vol. 3 (pp. 2076-2085).Washington, DC: NASW Press.

Davids, J. (1993). The reaction of an early latency boy to the sudden death of his baby brother. In A. J. Solnit, P. B. Neubauer, S. Abrams, and A. S. Dowling (Eds.), *The psychoanalytic study of the child, Vol. 48* (pp. 277-292). New Haven: Yale University Press.

Davies, D. (1999). *Child development: A practitioner's guide.* New York: The Guilford Press.

Day, D. (2001). Health emergency: African American and Latina women and their children. AIDS orphans. Report from the Dogwood Center. HEALTH EMERGENCY 2001. The spread of drug-related AIDS and hepatitis C among African Americans and Latinos. Available online at <http://www.dogwoodcenter.org/2001/12women.html>.

Dean, C. (1998). After a struggle, women win a place "on the Ice." *The New York Times,* November 10, pp. D1, D4.

de Anda, D. (1995). Adolescence overview. In R. L. Edwards and J. G. Hopps (Eds.), *Social work encyclopedia,* Nineteenth edition, Vol. 1 (pp. 16-33). Washington, DC: NASW Press.

Dedman, B. (1999). Clinton faults Senate over Hispanic judicial nominees. *The New York Times,* October 10, p. 22.

Deitz, J. (1991). When the patient is depressed. In H. Jackson (Ed.), *Using self psychology in psychotherapy* (pp. 193-202). Northvale: Jason Aronson Inc.

Delgado, M. (1997). Role of Latina-owned beauty parlors in a Latino Community. *Social Work, 42,* 445-453.

Dempsey, D. (1971). Learning how to die. *New York Times Magazine,* November 14, pp. 58-60, 64-74, 81.

DeParle, J. (1999). Early sex abuse hinders many women on welfare. *The New York Times,* November 28, pp. 1, 20.

DiGiulio, J. F. (1987). Assuming the adoptive parent role. *Social Casework: The Journal of Contemporary Social Work, 68,* 561-566.

Dillon, S. (1999). Smaller families to bring big change in Mexico. *The New York Times,* June 8, pp. A1, A15.

Dissociation and dissociative disorders: Part I (1992). *The Harvard Mental Health Letter, 8,* March, pp. 1-4.

Dissociation and dissociative disorders: Part II (1992). *The Harvard Mental Health Letter, 8,* April, pp. 1-4.

Doctor with breast cancer rescued from South Pole (1999). Imaginis.com Breast Health News. Imaginis Corporation, Durham, North Carolina. Available online at <http://www.imaginis.com/breasthealth/news/news10.18.99.asp?mode=1>.

Dolnick, E. (1993). Deafness as culture. *The Atlantic Monthly, 272* (September 3), 37-53.

Donner, S. (1991). The treatment process. In H. Jackson (Ed.), *Using self psychology in psychotherapy.* Northvale: Jason Aronson Inc.

Dore, M. M. (1999). Emotionally and behaviorally disturbed children in the child welfare system: Points of preventive intervention. *Children and Youth Services Review, 21,* 7-29.

Dowdy, A. (1998). Housing for old, young to debut in Dorchester. *The Boston Globe,* September 10, p. B1, B8.

Drachman, D. (1995). Immigration statuses and their influence on service provision, access, and use. *Social Work, 40,* pp. 188-197.

Drug abuse and dependence—Part I (1989). *The Harvard Medical School Mental Health Letter, 6* (4), pp. 1-4.

Drug abuse and dependence—Part II (1989). *The Harvard Medical School Mental Health Letter, 6* (5), pp. 1-4.

Drummond, T. (1998a). Busted for possession. *Time, 152,* December 7, p. 50.

Drummond, T. (1998b). Touch early and often. *Time, 152,* July 27, p. 54.

Drummond, T. (1999). Never too old. *Time, 153,* June 7, p. 84H.

Dugan, T. F. (1989). Action and acting out: Variables in the development of resiliency in adolescence. In T. F. Dugan and R. Coles (Eds.), *The child in our times: Studies in the development of resiliency* (pp. 157-176). New York: Brunner/Mazel.

Dulmus, C. N. and Rapp-Paglicci, L. A. (2000). The prevention of mental disorders in children and adolescents: Future research and public-policy recommendations. *Families in Society: The Journal of Contemporary Human Services, 81,* 294-303.

Dulmus, C. N., Rapp-Paglicci, L. A., Sarafin, D. J., Wodarski, J. S., and Feit, M. D. (2000). Workfare programs: Issues and recommendations for self-sufficiency. *Journal of Human Behavior in the Social Environment, 3* (2), pp. 1-12.

Dumont, M. P. (1996). Privatization and mental health in Massachusetts. *Smith College Studies in Social Work, 66,* 293-303.

Dupper, D. R. and Poertner, J. (1997). Public schools and the revitalization of impoverished communities: School-linked, family resource centers. *Social Work, 42,* 415- 422.

Dworkin, S. H. (1997). Female, lesbian, and Jewish: Complex and invisible. In B. Greene (Ed.), *Ethnic and cultural diversity among lesbians and gay men: Vol. 3. Psychological perspectives on lesbian and gay issues* (pp. 63-87). Thousand Oaks: Sage Publications.

Eagle, M. N. (1987). The psychoanalytic and the cognitive unconscious. In R. Stern (Ed.), *Theories of the unconscious and the self* (pp. 155-188). Hillsdale: The Analytic Press.

Eamon, M. K. (1994). Institutionalizing children and adolescents in private psychiatric hospitals. *Social Work, 39,* 588-594.

Eating disorders—Part I (1992). *The Harvard Mental Health Letter, 9* (6), pp. 1-4.

Edelstein, W. (1996). The social construction of cognitive development. In G. G. Noam and K. W. Fischer (Eds.), *Development and vulnerability in close relationships* (pp. 91-112). Mahwah, NJ: Lawrence Erlbaum Associates.

Edelstein, W. and Noam, G. (1982). Regulatory structures of self and "post-formal" stages in adulthood. *Human Development, 25,* pp. 407-422.

Edlefsen, M. and Baird, M. (1994). Making it work: Preventive mental health care for disadvantaged preschoolers. *Social Work, 39,* pp. 566-573.

Edmundson, M. (1998). Book review of: *Open minded: Working out the logic of the soul* by Jonathan Lear. *The New York Times Book Review,* August 16, p. 10.

Edward, J. (1996). Listening, hearing, and understanding in psychoanalytically oriented treatment. In J. Edward and J. Sanville (Eds.), *Fostering healing and growth: A psychoanalytic social work approach* (pp. 23-45). Northvale: Jason Aronson Inc.

Edward, J., Ruskin, N., and Turrini, P. (1992). *Separation/individuation: Theory and application,* Second edition. New York: Bruner/Mazel Publishers.

Egan, T. (1999a). Hard time: Less crime, more criminals. *The New York Times,* March 7, Section 4, p. 1.

Egan, T. (1999b). Poor Indians on rich land fight a U.S. maze. *The New York Times,* March 9, pp. A1, A20.

Elkind, D. (1981). *Children and adolescents: Interpretive essays on Jean Piaget,* Third edition. New York: Oxford University Press.

Elliott, L. and Bourette, S. (1999). A father's stunning anger. *Toronto Globe and Mail,* August 24, pp. A1, A5.

Ellison, R. (1980). *Invisible man.* New York: Vintage Books.

Elson, M. (1984). Parenthood and the transformation of narcissism. In R. Cohen, B. Cohler, and S. Weissman (Eds.), *Parenthood: A psychodynamic perspective* (pp. 297-314). New York: The Guilford Press.

Erera, P. I. and Fredriksen, K. (1999). Lesbian stepfamilies: A unique family structure. *Families in Society: The Journal of Contemporary Human Services, 80,* 263-270.

Erikson, E. (1963). *Childhood and society.* New York: W. W. Norton and Company, Inc.

Espin, O. M. (1997). Crossing borders and boundaries: The life narratives of immigrant lesbians. In B. Greene (Ed.), *Ethnic and cultural diversity among lesbians and gay men: Vol. 3. Psychological perspectives on lesbian and gay issues* (pp. 191-215). Thousand Oaks: Sage Publications.

Ewalt, P. L. (1997). Editorial: The revitalization of impoverished communities. *Social Work, 42,* 413-414.

Ewalt, P. L. and Mokuau, N. (1995). Self-determination from a Pacific perspective. *Social Work, 40,* 168-175.

Fadiman, A. (1997). *The spirit catches you and you fall down: A Hmong child, her American doctors and the collision of two cultures.* New York: Farrar, Straus and Giroux.

Falco, K. L. (1991). *Psychotherapy with lesbian clients: Theory into practice.* New York: Brunner/Mazel.

Falicov, C. J. (1982). Mexican families. In M. McGoldrick, J. K. Pearce, and J. Giordano (Eds.), *Ethnicity and family therapy* (pp. 134-163). New York: The Guilford Press.

Falloon, R. H. and Liberman, R. P. (1983). Behavioral family interventions in the management of chronic schizophrenia. In W. R. McFarlane (Ed.), *Family therapy in schizophrenia* (pp. 117-137). New York: The Guilford Press.

Families in the treatment of schizophrenia—Part I (1989). *The Harvard Medical School Mental Health Letter, 5* (12), pp. 1-4.

Families in the treatment of schizophrenia—Part II (1989). *The Harvard Medical School Mental Health Letter, 6* (1), pp. 1-3.

Farley, J. (1990). Family developmental task assessment: A prerequisite to family treatment. *Clinical Social Work Journal, 18,* pp. 85-98.

Fauri, D. P. and Grimes, D. R. (1994). Bereavement services for families and peers of deceased residents of psychiatric institutions. *Social Work, 39,* 185-190.

Fedarko, K. (1997). How a few firemen created a safe haven for some Chicago kids. *Time, 150,* November 17, pp. 72-73.

Fein, E. (1998). Secrecy and stigma no longer clouding adoptions. *The New York Times,* October 25, pp. 1, 30-31.

Felsman, J. K. (1989). Risk and resiliency in childhood: The lives of street children. In T. F. Dugan and R. Coles (Eds.), *The child in our times: Studies in the development of resiliency,* (pp. 56-80). New York: Bruner/Mazel.

Fewer high school students having sex, poll says (1998). *The New York Times,* September 18, p. A18.

Field, T. (2000). Infant massage therapy. In C. H. Zeanah Jr. (Ed.), *Handbook of infant mental health,* Second edition (pp. 494-500). New York: The Guilford Press.

Firestone, D. (1999). Murder reveals double life of being gay in rural south. *The New York Times,* March 6, pp. A1, A9.

First, R. J., Rife, J. C., and Toomey, B. G. (1995). Homeless families. In R. L. Edwards and J. G. Hopps (Eds.), *Social work encyclopedia,* Nineteenth edition, Vol. 2 (pp. 1330-1337). Washington, DC: NASW Press.

Fischer, N. (1994). An interactional view of developmental pathogenesis, and therapeutic process: Complexity and hazards. In S. Kramer and S. Akhtar (Eds.), *Mahler and Kohut: Perspectives on development, psychopathology, and technique* (pp. 99-116). Northvale: Jason Aronson Inc.

Flanagan, L. M. (1996). Object relations theory. In J. Berzoff, L. M. Flanagan, and P. Hertz (Eds.), *Inside out and outside in: Psychodynamic clinical theory and practice in contemporary multicultural contexts* (pp. 127-171). Northvale: Jason Aronson Inc.

Fox, R. and Carey, L. A. (1999). Therapists' collusion with the resistance of rape survivors. *Clinical Social Work Journal, 27,* 185-201.

Foy, G. M. (1999). Burning Olivier: The brief life and private burial of an infant son. *Harper's Magazine, 299* (1790), pp. 39-54.

Fraiberg, S. (1968). *The magic years: Understanding and handling the problems of early childhood.* New York: Basic Books.

Fraiberg, S., Adelson, E., and Shapiro, V. (1975). Ghosts in the nursery: A psycho-analytic approach to the problem of impaired infant-mother relationships. *Journal of the American Academy of Child Psychiatry, 14,* 387-422.

Frank, M. G. (1996). A clinical view of the use of psychoanalytic theory in front-line practice. In J. Edward and J. Sanville (Eds.), *Fostering healing and growth: A psychoanalytic social work approach* (pp. 59-76). Northvale: Jason Aronson Inc.

Frankel, S. A. (1994). The exclusivity of the mother-child bond: Contributions from psychoanalytic and attachment theories and day-care research. In A. J. Solnit, P. B. Neubauer, S. Abrams, and A. S. Dowling (Eds.), *The psychoanalytic study of the child, Vol. 49* (pp. 86-106). New Haven: Yale University Press.

Fraser, M. W. (1997). The ecology of childhood: A multisystems perspective. In M. W. Fraser (Ed.), *Risk and resilience in childhood: An ecological perspective* (pp. 1-9). Washington: NASW Press.

Freed, A. O. (1980). The borderline personality. *Social Casework: The Journal of Contemporary Social Work, 61,* 548-558.

Freed, A. O. (1985). Linking developmental, family, and life cycle theories. *Smith College Studies in Social Work, 55,* 169-182.

Freeman, D. M. A. (1998). Emotional refueling in development, mythology, and cosmology: The Japanese separation-individuation experience. In S. Akhtar and S. Kramer (Eds.), *The colors of childhood: Separation-individuation across cultural, racial, and ethnic differences* (pp. 17-60). Northvale: Jason Aronson Inc.

Freeman, M. and Freund, W. (1998). Working with adopted clients. *Journal of Analytic Social Work, 5* (4), 25-37.

French, D. C. and Tyne, T. F. (1986). The identification and treatment of children with peer-relationship difficulties. In J. P. Curran and P. M. Monti (Eds.), *Social skills training: A practical handbook for assessment and treatment* (pp. 280-308). Washington Square, New York: New York University Press.

Freud, A. (1946). *The ego and mechanisms of defense.* New York: International Universities Press, Inc.

Freud, Sigmund (1959). A note on the unconscious in psychoanalysis (1912). In E. Jones (Ed.), *Sigmund Freud: Collected papers,* Volume 4 (pp. 22-29). New York: Basic Books.

Freud, Sophie (1999). The social construction of normality. *Families in Society, 80,* 333-339.

Friedman, E. G. (1997). The impact of AIDS on the lives of women. In S. L. A. Straussner and E. Zelvin (Eds.), *Gender and addictions: Men and women in treatment* (pp. 197-221). Northvale: Jason Aronson Inc.

Gaensbauer, T. J. (1994). Trauma in the preverbal period: Symptoms, memories, and developmental impact. In A. J. Solnit, P. B. Neubauer, S. Abrams, and A. S. Dowling (Eds.), *The psychoanalytic study of the child, Vol. 49* (pp. 122-149). New Haven: Yale University Press.

Galanter, M. (1982). Charismatic religious sects and psychiatry: An overview. *American Journal of Psychiatry, 139,* 1539-1548.

Garbarino, J. (1982). *Children and families in the social environment.* New York: Aldine Publishing Company.

Garbarino, J. and Kostelny, K. (1997). What children can tell us about living in a war zone. In J. Osofsky (Ed.), *Children in a violent society* (pp. 32-41). New York: The Guilford Press.

Gay, P. (1988). *Freud: A life for our time.* New York: W. W. Norton and Company.

Gee, K. K. and Ishii, M. M. (1997). Assessment and treatment of schizophrenia among Asian Americans. In E. Lee (Ed.), *Working with Asian Americans: A guide for clinicians* (pp. 227-251). New York: The Guilford Press.

Geller, J. (1996). Mental health services of the future: Managed care, unmanaged care, mismanaged care. *Smith College Studies in Social Work, 66,* 223-239.

Germain, C. (1991). *Human behavior in the social environment.* New York: Columbia University Press.

Germain, C. and Gitterman, A. (1980). *The life model of social work practice.* New York: Columbia University Press.

Gilkerson, L. and Stott, F. (2000). Parent-child relationships in early intervention with infants and toddlers with disabilities and their families. In C. H. Zeanah Jr. (Ed.), *Handbook of infant mental health,* Second edition (pp. 457-471). New York: The Guilford Press.

Gilligan, C. (1982). *In a different voice.* Cambridge: Harvard University Press.

Giovacchini, P. (1993). Absolute and not quite absolute dependence. In D. Goldman (Ed.), *In one's bones: The clinical genius of Winnicott* (pp. 241-256). Northvale: Jason Aronson Inc.

Giovannoni, J. M. (1995). Childhood. In R. L. Edwards and J. G. Hopps (Eds.), *Social work encyclopedia*, Nineteenth edition, Vol. 1 (pp. 433-441). Washington, DC: NASW Press.

Gitterman, A. and Miller, I. (1989). The influence of organization on clinical practice. *Clinical Social Work Journal, 17,* 151-164.

Glaberson, W. (1998). Case tries to win siblings a right to be together. *The New York Times,* December 29, pp. A1, A12.

Gleick, E. (1997). "The marker we've been waiting for." *Time, 150,* April 7, pp. 31-36.

Glodich, A. (1998). Traumatic exposure to violence: A comprehensive review of the child and adolescent literature. *Smith College Studies in Social Work, 68,* 321-345.

Golan, N. (1980). Using situational crises to ease transitions in the life cycle. *American Journal of Orthopsychiatry, 50,* 542-549.

Goldberg, C. (1999a). Crackdown on abusive spouses, surprisingly, nets many women. *The New York Times,* November 23, pp. A1, A14.

Goldberg, C. (1999b). Harvard is returning bones, and a Pueblo awaits its past. *The New York Times,* May 20, pp. A1, A18.

Goldberg, C. (1999c). Insurance for Viagra spurs coverage for birth control. *The New York Times*, July 30, pp. A1, A15.

Goldberg, C. (1999d). Spotlighting issues of gender, from pronouns to murder. *The New York Times*, June 11, p. A27.

Goldberg, C. (1999e). Vermont's high court extends full rights to same-sex couples. *The New York Times*, December 21, pp. A1, A23.

Goldberg, C. (2000). Court says a partner can veto an embryo implantation. *The New York Times*, April 4, p. A14.

Goldberg, J. E. (1999). A short-term approach to intervention with homeless mothers: A role for social work clinicians in homeless shelters. *Families in Society: The Journal of Contemporary Human Services, 80,* 161-168.

Goldberg, S. (1995). Introduction. In S. Goldberg, R. Muir, and J. Kerr (Eds.), *Attachment theory: Social, developmental, and clinical perspectives* (pp. 1-15). Hillsdale: The Analytic Press.

Golden, F. (1999a). Good eggs, bad eggs. *Time, 153,* January 11, pp. 56-59.

Golden, F. (1999b). Smoking gun for the young. *Time, 153,* April 19, p. 48.

Goldstein, H. (1990). The knowledge base of social work practice: Theory, wisdom, analogue, or art? *Families in Society: The Journal of Contemporary Human Services, 71,* 32-43.

Goldstein, H. (1999). Editorial notes: "Different" Families. *Families in Society: The Journal of Contemporary Human Services, 80,* 107-109.

Goldstein, J. and Goldstein, S. (1996). "Put yourself in the skin of the child," she said. In A. J. Solnit, P. B. Neubauer, S. Abrams, and A. S. Dowling (Eds.), *The psychoanalytic study of the child, Vol. 51* (pp. 46-55). New Haven: Yale University Press.

Gombosi, P. G. (1998). Parents of autistic children: Some thoughts about trauma, dislocation, and tragedy. In A. J. Solnit, P. B. Neubauer, S. Abrams, and A. S. Dowling (Eds.), *The psychoanalytic study of the child, Vol. 53* (pp. 254-275). New Haven: Yale University Press.

Goode, E. (1998a). New hope for the losers in the battle to stay awake. *The New York Times*, November 3, pp. D1, D8.

Goode, E. (1998b). On gay issue, psychoanalysis treats itself. *The New York Times*, December 12, A19, A29.

Goode, E. (1999a). Clash over when, and how, to toilet train. *The New York Times*, January 12, pp. A1, A17.

Goode, E. (1999b). Deeper truths sought in violence by youths. *The New York Times*, May 5, p. A24.

Goode, E. (1999c). Gentle drive to make voters of those with mental illness. *The New York Times*, October 13, pp. A1, A16.

Goode, E. (1999d). Return to the couch: A revival for analysis. *The New York Times*, January 12, pp. D1, D6.

Goode, E. (2000). Sharp rise found in psychiatric drugs for the very young. *The New York Times*, February 23, pp. A1, A13.

Goolishian, H. A. and Winderman, L. (1988). Constructivism, autopoiesis and problem determined systems. *The Irish Journal of Psychology, 9,* 130-143.

Gorman, C. (1998a). Body parts for sale. *Time, 151,* March 9, p. 76.

Gorman, C. (1998b). Girls on steroids. *Time, 152,* August 10b, p. 93.

Gorman, C. (1999). Bleak days for doctors. *Time, 153,* February 8, p. 53.

Gottlieb, N. (1995). Women overview. In R. L. Edwards and J. G. Hopps (Eds.), *Social work encyclopedia,* Nineteenth edition, Vol. 3 (pp. 2518-2528). Washington, DC: NASW Press.

Grady, D. (1999a). Live donors revolutionize liver care. *The New York Times,* August 2, pp. A1, A12.

Grady, D. (1999b). What's missing in childbirth these days? Often, the pain. *The New York Times,* October 13, pp. A1, A16.

Greenhouse, L. (2000a). Case on visitation rights hinges on defining family. *The New York Times,* January 4, p. A11.

Greenhouse, L. (2000b). Program of drug-testing pregnant women draws Supreme Court review. *The New York Times,* February 29, p. A12.

Groden, G. and Baron, M. G. (1988). *Autism: Strategies for change.* New York: Gardner Press.

Grolnick, S. (1990). *The work and play of Winnicott.* Northvale: Jason Aronson, Inc.

Gross, E. R. (1995). Deconstructing politically correct practice literature: The American Indian case. *Social Work, 40,* 207-213.

Grotjohn, M. (1985). Being sick and facing eighty. In R. A. Nemiroff and C. A. Colarusso (Eds.), *The race against time: Psychoanalysis and psychotherapy in the second half of life* (pp. 293-302). New York: Plenum.

Guterman, N. B. and Cameron, M. (1997). Assessing the impact of community violence on children and youths. *Social Work, 42,* 495-505.

Guterson, D. (1995). *Snow falling on cedars.* New York: Vintage Books.

Gutheil, I. A. (1992). Considering the physical environment: An essential component of good practice. *Social Work, 37,* 391-396.

Halbfinger, D. M. (1999). U.S. accuses 3 of smuggling Mexican babies. *The New York Times,* May 27, pp. A1, A25.

Hall, C. S. and Lindzey, G. (1979). *Theories of personality,* Third edition. New York: John Wiley and Sons.

Hall, S. S. (2000). The smart set. *New York Times Magazine,* June 4, pp. 52-57, 90-91,100.

Hamilton, N. G. (1990). *Self and others: Object relations theory in practice.* Northvale: Jason Aronson Inc.

Hanley, R. (1999). New Jersey court overturns ouster of gay Boy Scout. *The New York Times,* August 5, pp. A1, A21.

Hart, J. (1998). Young and on the run. *The Boston Globe,* February 2, pp. A1, B4.

Hartman, A. and Laird, J. (1983). *Family-centered social work practice.* New York: The Free Press.

Hartmann, H. (1958). *Ego psychology and the problem of adaptation.* New York: International Universities Press, Inc.

Harvey, A. R. (1995). The issue of skin color in psychotherapy with African Americans. *Families in Society: The Journal of Contemporary Human Services, 76,* 3-10.

Hegeman, E. (1995). Transferential issues in the psychoanalytic treatment of incest survivors. In J. L. Alpert (Ed.), *Sexual abuse recalled: Treating trauma in the era of the recovered memory debate* (pp. 185-213). Northvale: Jason Aronson Inc.

Helping poor students achieve more (1999). *The New York Times,* May 9, p. 24.

Henry, J. (1999). Permanency outcomes in legal guardianships of abused/neglected children. *Families in Society: The Journal of Contemporary Human Services, 80,* 561-568.

Herbert, T. (1993). *Dearest beloved: The Hawthornes and the making of the middle-class family.* Berkeley: University of California Press, Ltd.

Herman, J. L. (1997). *Trauma and recovery.* New York: Basic Books.

Herman, J. L. (1989). Wife-beating. *The Harvard Medical School Mental Health Letter, 5* (10), 4-6.

Hess, P. M., Folaron, G., and Jefferson, A. B. (1992). Effectiveness of family reunification services: An innovative evaluative model. *Social Work, 37,* 304-311.

High percentage of inmates say they were abused as children (1999). *The New York Times,* April 12, p. A19.

Hilts, P. (1999). Largest study yet rates effect of fertility drugs. *The New York Times,* January 21, p. A12.

HIV infection rates among poor young women are called 'alarming' (1998). *The Boston Globe,* August 28, p. A10.

Hoberman, H. (1989). Completed suicide in children and adolescents: A review. In B. Garfinkel and G. Northrup (Eds.), *Adolescent suicide: Recognition, treatment and prevention* (pp. 61-88). Binghamton, New York: The Haworth Press.

Hoffman, D. L. and Remmel, M. L. (1975). Uncovering the precipitant in crisis intervention. *Social Casework, 56,* 259-267.

Hoffman, L. (1981). *Foundations of family therapy: A conceptual framework for systems change.* New York: Basic Books, Inc.

Hogan, L. (1990). *Mean spirit.* New York: Ivy Books.

Hohler, B. (1996). Senate OK's bar on gay marriages. *The Boston Globe,* September 11, pp. A1, A10.

Hollingsworth, L. D. (1998). Promoting same-race adoption for children of color. *Social Work, 43,* 104-116.

Holloway, L. (1999). Seeing a link between depression and homelessness. *The New York Times,* February 7, p. 3.

Holloway, L. (2000). Turnover of teachers and pupils deepens trouble of poor schools. *The New York Times,* May 25, p. A29.

Holmes, J. (1995). "Something there is that doesn't love a wall": John Bowlby, attachment theory, and psychoanalysis. In S. Goldberg, R. Muir, and J. Kerr (Eds.), *Attachment theory: Social, developmental, and clinical perspectives* (pp. 19-43). Hillsdale: The Analytic Press.

Holmes, S. A. (1999). Black groups in Florida split over school voucher plan. *The New York Times,* May 30, p. 15.

Homeless deaths are rising in San Francisco (1998). *The New York Times,* December 21, p. A16.

Honig, R., Grace, M., Lindy, J., Newman, C., and Titchener, J. (1993). Portraits of survival: A twenty-year follow-up of the children of Buffalo Creek. In A. Solnit, P. Neubauer, S. Abrams, and A. Dowling (Eds.), *The psychoanalytic study of the child, Vol. 52* (pp. 327-355). New Haven: Yale University Press.

Hopps, J. G., Pinderhughes, E., and Shankar, R. (1995). *The power to care: Clinical practice effectiveness with overwhelmed clients.* New York: The Free Press.

Hornblower, M. (1998). No Habla Español. *Time, 151,* January 26, p. 63.

Horwitz, T. (1999). Untrue confessions: Is most of what we know about the rebel slave Nat Turner wrong? *The New Yorker,* December 13, pp. 80-89.

Huang, L. N. (1997). Asian American adolescents. In E. Lee (Ed.), *Working with Asian Americans: A guide for clinicians* (pp. 175-195). New York: The Guilford Press.

Hughes, D. A. (1998). *Building the bonds of attachment: Awakening love in deeply troubled children.* Northvale: Jason Aronson Inc.

Hungerford, A., Brownell, C. A., and Campbell, S. B. (2000). Child care in infancy: A transactional perspective. In C. H. Zeanah Jr. (Ed.), *Handbook of infant mental health,* Second edition (pp. 519-532). New York: The Guilford Press.

Hunter, J. and Schaecher, R. (1995). Gay and lesbian adolescents. In R. L. Edwards and J. G. Hopps (Eds.), *Social work encyclopedia,* Nineteenth edition, Vol. 2 (pp. 1055-1063). Washington, DC: NASW Press.

Huse, M. (1989). *A study of adult adoptees who request background information.* Unpublished doctoral dissertation: Simmons College School of Social Work, Boston, Mass.

In study, diagnoses miss alcohol abuse (2000). *The New York Times,* May 12, p. A16.

Increase in eating disorders in Fiji linked to arrival of U.S. TV (1999). *The New York Times,* May 20, p. A11.

Intercountry Adoption (1999). *Innocenti Digest 4.* Unicef. Available online at <http://www.cepadu.unipd.it/centro/perfez/11_corso/modulo_4/07_adozioni.pdf>.

Irizarry, C. and Appel, Y. (1986). Growing up: Work with preteens in the neighborhood. In A. Gitterman and L. Shulman (Eds.), *Mutual aid groups and the life cycle* (pp. 111-140). Itasca, IL: F. E. Peacock Publishers, Inc.

Isaacs, M. B., Montalvo, B., and Abelsohn, D. (2000). *Therapy of the difficult divorce: Managing crises, reorienting warring couples, working with the children, and expediting court processes.* Northvale: Jason Aronson Inc.

Isaacson, W. (1999). The biotech century. *Time, 152,* January 11, pp. 42-43.

Ivanoff, A. and Riedel, M. (1995). Suicide. In R. L. Edwards and J. G. Hopps (Eds.), *Social work encyclopedia,* Nineteenth edition, Vol. 3 (pp. 2358-2372). Washington, DC: NASW Press.

Jackson, A. (1999). The effects of nonresident father involvement on single black mothers and their young children. *Social Work, 44,* 156-166.

Jackson, H. (1991). Introduction: Putting self psychology to work. In H. Jackson (Ed.), *Using self psychology in psychotherapy* (pp. 1-12). Northvale: Jason Aronson Inc.

Jackson, L. C. and Greene, B. (2000). *Psychotherapy with African American women: Innovations in psychodynamic perspectives and practice.* New York: The Guilford Press.

Jackson, R. L., Purnell, D., Anderson, S. B., and Sheafor, B. W. (1996). The clubhouse model of community support for adults with mental illness: An emerging opportunity for social work education. *Journal of Social Work Education, 32,* 173-180.

Jacobson, N. S. (1986). Communication skills training for married couples. In J. P. Curran and P. M. Monti (Eds.), *Social skills training: A practical handbook for assessment and treatment* (pp. 224-252). Washington Square, New York: New York University Press.

Jamison, K. 1996. *An unquiet mind: A memoir of moods and madness.* New York: Vintage Books.

Japan ordered to pay for worker's suicide (1999). *Providence Sunday Journal,* March 14, p. A5.

Jarmon-Rohde, L., McFall, J., Kolar, P., and Strom, G. (1997). The changing context of social work practice: Implications and recommendations for social work educators. *Journal of Social Work Education, 33,* 29-46.

Jarrell, A. (2000). The face of teenage sex grows younger. *The New York Times,* April 2, Section 9, pp. 1, 8.

Javier, R. A. (1996). Psychodynamic treatment with the urban poor. In R. Pérez Foster, M. Moskowitz, and R. A. Javier (Eds.), *Reaching across boundaries of culture and class: Widening the scope of psychotherapy* (pp. 93-113). Northvale: Jason Aronson Inc.

Jenkins, P., Seydlitz, R., Osofsky, J. G., and Fick, A. C. (1997). Cops and kids: Issues for community policing. In J. Osofsky (Ed.), *Children in a violent society* (pp. 300-322). New York: The Guilford Press.

Jiménez-Vázquez, R. (1995). Hispanics: Cubans. In R. L. Edwards and J. G. Hopps (Eds.), *Social work encyclopedia,* Nineteenth edition, Vol. 2 (pp. 1223-1232). Washington, DC: NASW Press.

Johnson, A., Edwards, R., and Puwak, H. (1993). Foster care and adoption policy in Romania: Suggestions for international intervention. *Child Welfare, 72,* 489-506.

Johnson, G. (1997). Comets breed fear, fascination and web sites. *The New York Times,* March 28, p. A9.

Johnson, K., Bryant, D. D., Collins, D. A., Noe, T. D., Strader, T. N., and Berbaum, M. (1998). Preventing and reducing alcohol and other drug use among high-risk youths by increasing family resilience. *Social Work, 43,* 297-308.

Jones, M. J. (1986). Speaking the unspoken: Parents of sexually victimized children. In A. Gitterman and L. Shulman (Eds.), *Mutual aid groups and the life cycle* (pp. 211-227). Itasca, IL: F. E. Peacock Publishers, Inc.

Kadushin, A. (1974). *Child welfare services,* Second edition. New York: Macmillan Publishing Co.

Kahn, E. M. (1979). The parallel process in social work treatment and supervision. *Social Casework, 60,* 520-528.

Kahn, J. and Kifner, J. (2000). World trade officials pledging to step up effort against AIDS. *The New York Times,* April 18, pp. A1, A11.

Kanter, J. (1990). Community-based management of psychotic clients: The contributions of D. W. and Clare Winnicott. *Clinical Social Work Journal, 18,* 23-41.

Kanter, J. (2000). Beyond psychotherapy: Therapeutic relationships in community care. *Smith College Studies in Social Work, 70,* 397-426.

Kao, R. S.-K. and Lam, M. L. (1997). Asian American elderly. In E. Lee (Ed.), *Working with Asian Americans: A guide for clinicians* (pp. 208-223). New York: The Guilford Press.

Kaplan, D. M. and Mason, E. A. (1965). Maternal reactions to premature birth viewed as an acute emotional disorder. In H. Parad (Ed.), *Crisis intervention: Se-*

lected readings (pp. 118-128). New York: Family Service Association of America.

Kaplan, H. S. (1974). *The new sex therapy: Active treatment of sexual dysfunctions.* New York: Brunner/Mazel.

Kaplan, H., Sadock, B., and Grebb, J. (1994). *Synopsis of psychiatry: Behavioral sciences/clinical psychiatry.* Baltimore: Williams and Wilkins.

Kaplan, M. D. and Pruett, K. D. (2000). Divorce and custody: Developmental implications. In C. H. Zeanah Jr. (Ed.), *Handbook of infant mental health,* Second edition (pp. 533-547). New York: The Guilford Press.

Karen, R. (1990). Becoming attached. *The Atlantic Monthly, 265,* February, pp. 35-70.

Karon, B. P. and VandenBos, G. R. (1996). *Psychotherapy of schizophrenia: The treatment of choice.* Northvale: Jason Aronson Inc.

Kaufman, J. and Henrich, C. (2000). Exposure to violence and early childhood trauma. In C. H. Zeanah Jr. (Ed.), *Handbook of infant mental health,* Second edition (pp. 195-207). New York: The Guilford Press.

Kegan, R. (1982). *The evolving self.* Cambridge: Harvard University Press.

Kelley, T. (1998). To surf, perchance to dream. *The New York Times,* October 1, p. E1.

Kennedy, G. J. (2000). *Geriatric mental health care: A treatment guide for health professionals.* New York: The Guilford Press.

Kernberg, O. (1965). Notes on counter-transference. *Journal of American Psychoanalytic Association, 13,* 38-56.

Kernberg, O. F. (1984). *Severe personality disorders: Psychotherapeutic strategies.* New Haven: Yale University Press.

Kierkegaard, S. (1938). *Purity of heart* (1846). New York: Harper and Row.

Kilborn, P. T. (1998). Reality of the H.M.O. system doesn't live up to the dream. *The New York Times,* October 5, pp. A1, A16.

Kilborn, P. T. (1999a). Medicare safety nets fail to catch many of the poor. *The New York Times,* January 23, p. A7.

Kilborn, P. T. (1999b). Third of Hispanic Americans do without health coverage. *The New York Times,* April 9, pp. A1, A18.

Kilgore, C. (1988). Effect of early childhood sexual abuse on self and ego development. *Social Casework, 69,* 224-230.

Kim, R. (2001). Chinese lead Asian tally. *San Francisco Chronicle,* May 16. Available online at <http://www.sfgate.com/cgibin/article.cgi?file=/chronicle/archive/2001/05/16/MN101414.DTL>.

Kinzie, J. D., Leung, P. K., and Boehnlein, J. K. (1996). Treatment of depressive disorders in refugees. In E. Lee (Ed.), *Working with Asian Americans: A guide for clinicians* (pp. 265-274). New York: The Guilford Press.

Kirby, L. D. and Fraser, M. W. (1997). Risk and resilience in childhood. In M. W. Fraser (Ed.), *Risk and resilience in childhood: An ecological perspective* (pp. 10-33). Washington: NASW Press.

Kiselica, M. S. (1995). *Multicultural counseling with teenage fathers: A practical guide.* Thousand Oaks, CA: Sage Publications.

Kohut, H. (1971). *The analysis of the self: A systematic approach to the psychoanalytic treatment of narcissistic personality disorders. The psychoanalytic study of the child: Monograph no. 4.* New York: International Universities Press, Inc.

Kolata, G. (1998). Researchers report success in method to pick baby's sex. *The New York Times*, September 9, pp. A1, A20.

Kopeikin, H. S., Marshall, V., and Goldstein, M. J. (1983). Stages and impact of crisis-oriented family therapy in the aftercare of acute schizophrenia. In W. R. McFarlane (Ed.), *Family therapy in schizophrenia* (pp. 69-97). New York: The Guilford Press.

Koscis, J. H. (1991). Is lifelong depression a personality or mood disorder? *The Harvard Mental Health Letter, 8* (2), p. 8.

Kotler, J. (1999). Tribe fights planned adoption of twins. *Toronto Globe and Mail*, August 20, p. A11.

Kramer, B. (1998). Preparing social workers for the inevitable: A preliminary investigation of a course on grief, death, and loss. *Journal of Social Work Education, 34*, 211-227.

Kramer, S., Byerly, L., and Akhtar, S. (1997). Growing together, growing apart, growing up, and growing down. In S. Akhtar and S. Kramer (Eds.), *The seasons of life: Separation-individuation perspectives* (pp. 3-22). Northvale: Jason Aronson Inc.

Krauz, S. L. (1980). Group psychotherapy with legally blind patients. *Clinical Social Work Journal, 8*, 37-49.

Kressel, K. (1997). *The process of divorce: Helping couples negotiate settlements.* Northvale: Jason Aronson Inc.

Kreuger, L. (1997). The end of social work. *Journal of Social Work Education, 33*, 19-27.

Kruger, A. (2000). Empowerment in social work practice with the psychiatrically disabled: Model and method. *Smith College Studies in Social Work, 70*, 427-439.

Kübler-Ross, E. (1969). *On death and dying.* New York: The Macmillan Company.

Labi, N. (1998). The hunter and the choirboy. *Time, 151*, April 6, pp. 28-37.

Lacayo, R. (1988). The case of the little big man. *Time, 132*, July 18, p. 56.

Lacayo, R. (1997). The lure of the cult. *Time, 150*, April 7, pp. 45-46.

Lacayo, R. (1998). The new gay struggle. *Time, 152*, October 26, pp. 32-36.

Lacey, M. (1999). Teen-age birth rate in U.S. falls again. *The New York Times*, October 27, p. A14.

Landau, R. (1998). Secrecy, anonymity, and deception in donor insemination: A genetic, psycho-social and ethical critique. *Social Work in Health Care, 28*, 75-89.

Landers, S. (1992). Grandparents trying to raise kids' kids. Second-time-around families find aid. *NASW News*, March, p. 5.

LaSala, M. (1998). Coupled gay men, parents, and in-laws: Intergenerational disapproval and the need for a thick skin. *Families in Society, 79*, 585-593.

Lawrence, S. A. and Zittel, K. M. (2000). Heart transplantation: A behavioral perspective. *Journal of Human Behavior in the Social Environment, 3* (2), 61-79.

Lee, E. (Ed.) (1997). *Working with Asian Americans: A guide for clinicians.* New York: The Guilford Press.

Lee, F. R. (1998). New York to teach deaf in sign language, then in English. *The New York Times*, March 5, p. A28.

Lee, J. A. B. and Swenson, C. R. (1986). The concept of mutual aid. In A. Gitterman and L. Shulman (Eds.), *Mutual aid groups and the life cycle* (pp. 361-377). Itasca: F. E. Peacock Publishers, Inc.

Lee, M. and Greene, G. J. (1999). A social constructivist framework for integrating cross-cultural issues in teaching clinical social work. *Journal of Social Work Education, 35,* 21-37.

Lemonick, M. D. (1994). The killers all around. *Time, 144,* September 12, pp. 62-69.

Lemonick, M. D. (1995). Can the Galapagos survive? *Time, 149,* October 30, pp. 80-82.

Lemonick, M. D. (1997). "It's a Miracle." *Time, 151,* December 1, pp. 34-46.

Lemonick, M. D. (1999). Designer babies. *Time, 153,* January 11, pp. 64-66.

Lesser, J. G. (1999). When your son becomes your daughter: A mother's adjustment to a transgender child. *Families in Society: The Journal of Contemporary Human Services, 80,* 182-189.

Lester, B. M., Boukydis, C. F. Z., and Twomey, J. E. (2000). Maternal substance abuse and child outcome. In C. H. Zeanah Jr. (Ed.), *Handbook of infant mental health,* Second edition (pp. 161-175). New York: The Guilford Press.

Levenson, D. (1998). Nursing homes: More than just medical. *NASW News, 43* (2), p. 3.

Levin, J. D. (1991). *Treatment of alcoholism and other addictions: A self-psychology approach.* Northvale: Jason Aronson Inc.

Levine, I. M. (1982). Introduction. In M. McGoldrick, J. K. Pearce, and J. Giordano (Eds.), *Ethnicity and family therapy* (pp. xi-xii). New York: The Guilford Press.

Levine, J. A. (1993). Involving fathers in Head Start: A framework for public policy and program development. *Families in Society: The Journal of Contemporary Human Services, 74,* 4-19.

Levine, K. G. (1990). Time to mourn again. In A. N. Maluccio, R. Krieger, and B. A. Pine (Eds.), *Preparing adolescents for life after foster care: The central role of foster parents* (pp. 53-72). Washington, DC: Child Welfare League of America.

Levinson, D. (1986). A conception of adult development. *American Psychologist, 41* (1), 3-13.

Levinson, D., Darrow, C., Klein, E., Levinson, M., and McKee, B. (1978). *The season's of a man's life.* New York: Knopf.

Levinson, D. and Levinson, J. (1996). *The seasons of a woman's life.* New York: Knopf.

Levy, A. J. and Wall, J. C. (2000). Children who have witnessed community homicide: Incorporating risk and resilience in clinical work. *Families in Society: The Journal of Contemporary Human Services, 81,* 402-411.

Lewin, T. (1998a). American colleges begin to ask, where have all the men gone? *The New York Times,* December 6, pp. 1, 38.

Lewin, T. (1998b). New families redraw racial boundaries. *The New York Times,* October 27, pp. A1, A18-A19.

Lewin, T. (1998c). Oregon's gay workers given benefits for domestic partners. *The New York Times,* December 10, p. A16.

Lewin, T. (1998d). Two views of growing up when the faces don't match. *The New York Times,* October 27, p. A19.

Lewin, T. (1999). Arizona high school provides glimpse inside cliques' divisive webs. *The New York Times,* May 20, p. 26.

Lewin, T. (2000). Insurance should cover cost of contraceptives, suit says. *The New York Times,* July 20, p. A16.

Lichtenberg, P. (1995). Men overview. In R. L. Edwards and J. G. Hopps (Eds.), *Social work encyclopedia,* Nineteenth edition, Vol. 2 (pp. 1691-1697). Washington, DC: NASW Press.

Lieberman, A. F., Silverman, R., and Pawl, J. H. (2000). Infant-parent psychotherapy: Core concepts and current approaches. In C. H. Zeanah Jr. (Ed.), *Handbook of infant mental health,* Second edition (pp. 472-484). New York: The Guilford Press.

Lieberman, F. (1984). Singular and plural objects: Thoughts on object relations theory. *Child and Adolescent Social Work, 1,* 153-157.

Liederman, D. S. (1995). Child welfare overview. In R. L. Edwards and J. G. Hopps (Eds.), *Social work encyclopedia,* Nineteenth edition, Vol. 1 (pp. 424-433). Washington, DC: NASW Press.

Lindemann, E. (1965). Symptomatology and management of acute grief. In H. Parad (Ed.), *Crisis intervention: Selected readings* (pp. 7-21). New York: Family Service Association of America.

Lipowski, Z. (1988). Somatization: The concept and its clinical application. *American Journal of Psychiatry, 145,* 1358-1368.

Longres, J. F. (1995a). Hispanics overview. In R. L. Edwards and J. G. Hopps (Eds.), *Social work encyclopedia,* Nineteenth edition, Vol. 2 (pp. 1214-1222). Washington, DC: NASW Press.

Longres, J. F. (1995b). *Human behavior in the social environment.* Itasca, IL: F. E. Peacock Publishers, Inc.

Lopez, S. (1998). Hide and seek. *Time, 151,* May 11, p. 60.

Loppnow, D. (1985). Adolescents on their own. In J. Laird and A. Hartman (Eds.), *A handbook of child welfare context, knowledge, and practice* (pp. 514-531). New York: The Free Press.

Lott-Whitehead, L. and Tully, C. T. (1993). The family lives of lesbian mothers. *Smith College Studies in Social Work, 63,* 265-280.

Luey, H. S., Glass, L., and Elliott, H. (1995). Hard-of-hearing or deaf: Issues of ears, language, culture, and identity. *Social Work, 40,* 177-182.

Lyman, R. (1999). Bush's run casts a shadow on a Texas hate crimes bill. *The New York Times,* May 13, p. A1.

Lynch, V. J. (1991). Basic concepts. In H. Jackson (Ed.), *Using self psychology in psychotherapy* (pp. 15-25). Northvale: Jason Aronson Inc.

MacFarlane, K. and Waterman, J. with Conerly, S., Damon, L., Durfee, M., and Long, S. (1986). *Sexual abuse of young children.* New York: The Guilford Press.

MacGregor, P. (1994). Grief: The unrecognized parental response to mental illness in a child. *Social Work, 39,* 160-166.

Mack, J. E. and Hickler, H. (1981). *Vivienne: The life and suicide of an adolescent girl.* New York: A Mentor Book, New American Library.

Mackey, R. A. (1985). *Ego psychology and clinical practice.* New York: Gardner Press, Inc.

Mackey, R. A. and O'Brien, B. A. (1999). Adaptation in lasting marriages. *Families in Society, 80,* 587-596.

MacKinnon, R. A. and Michels, R. (1971). *The psychiatric interview in clinical practice.* Philadelphia: W. B. Saunders Company.

Mahler, M., Pine, F., and Bergman, A. (1975). *The psychological birth of the human infant.* New York: Basic Books, Inc.

Mahoney, D. M. (2000). Panic disorder and self states: Clinical and research illustrations. *Clinical Social Work Journal, 28,* 197-212.

Main, M. (1995). Recent studies in attachment: Overview, with selected implications for clinical work. In S. Goldberg, R. Muir, and J. Kerr (Eds.), *Attachment theory: Social, developmental, and clinical perspectives* (pp. 407-474). Hillsdale: The Analytic Press.

Maluccio, A. N. (1980). Promoting competence through life experiences. In C. B. Germain and A. Gitterman (Eds.), *The life model of social work practice* (pp. 282-302). New York: Columbia University Press.

Maluccio, A. N., Pine, B. A., and Warsh, R. (1996). Incorporating content on family reunification into the social work curriculum. *Journal of Social Work Education, 32,* 363-373.

Mann, A. (1998). Cross-gender sex pill. *Time, 151,* April 6, p. 62.

Marans, S. and Adelman, A. (1997). Experiencing violence in a developmental context. In J. Osofsky (Ed.), *Children in a violent society* (pp. 202-222). New York: The Guilford Press.

Marin, R. (2000). At-home fathers step out to find they are not alone. *The New York Times,* January 2, pp. 1, 18.

Markoff, J. (1997). To gullible, Net offers many traps. *The New York Times,* March 28, p. A12.

Marks, I. (1987). Behavioral aspects of panic disorder. *American Journal of Psychiatry, 144,* 1160-1165.

Marmor, J. (1971). Dynamic psychotherapy and behavior therapy: Are they irreconcilable? *Archives of General Psychiatry, 24,* 22-28.

Martin, M. L. and Henry-Feeney, J. (1994). Clinical services to persons with AIDS: The parallel nature of the client and worker process. *Clinical Social Work Journal, 17,* 337-349.

Marziali, E. and Munroe-Blum, H. (1994). *Interpersonal group psychotherapy for borderline personality disorder.* New York: Basic Books.

Masaki, B. and Wong, L. (1997). Domestic violence in the Asian community. In E. Lee (Ed.), *Working with Asian Americans: A guide for clinicians* (pp. 439-451). New York: The Guilford Press.

Mattei, L. (1996). Race and culture in psychodynamic theories. In J. Berzoff, L. M. Flanagan, and P. Hertz (Eds.), *Inside out and outside in: Psychodynamic clinical theory and practice in contemporary multicultural contexts* (pp. 221-245). Northvale: Jason Aronson Inc.

Mattei, M. de L. (1999). A Latina space: Ethnicity as an intersubjective third. *Smith College Studies in Social Work, 69,* 255-267.

Mattick, I. (1967a). Description of the children. In E. Pavenstedt (Ed.), *The drifters: Children of disorganized lower-class families* (pp. 53-84). Boston: Little, Brown and Company.

Mattick, I. (1967b). Nursery school adaptations and techniques. In E. Pavenstedt (Ed.), *The drifters: Children of disorganized lower-class families* (pp. 163-204). Boston: Little, Brown and Company.

McCourt, F. (1996). *Angela's ashes: A memoir of childhood.* London: HarperCollins Publishers.

McDermott, C. J. (1990). Empowering elderly nursing home residents. The resident's rights campaign. *Social Work, 35,* 155-157.

McFarlane, W. R. (1983). Multiple family therapy in schizophrenia. In W. R. McFarlane (Ed.), *Family therapy in schizophrenia* (pp. 141-172). New York: The Guilford Press.

McFeely, W. S. (1991). *Frederick Douglass.* New York: W. W. Norton and Co.

McGirk, T. (1998). The sword of Islam. *Time, 152,* September 28, pp. 56-57.

McGoldrick, M. (1982). Ethnicity and family therapy: An overview. In M. McGoldrick, J. K. Pearce, and J. Giordano (Eds.), *Ethnicity and family therapy* (pp. 3-30). New York: The Guilford Press.

McGoldrick, M., Pearce, J. K., and Giordano, J. (Eds.) (1982). *Ethnicity and family therapy.* New York: The Guilford Press.

McGrath, C. (1998). Introduction. Being 13: A special photography issue. *New York Times Magazine,* May 17, pp. 29-30.

McKim, J. (1996). Marital split creates embryo custody case. *The Boston Globe,* December 4, pp. A1, A20.

McRoy, R. G., Grotevant, H. D., and White, K. L. (1988). *Openness in adoption: New practices, new issues.* New York: Praeger.

Mehta, P. (1998). The emergence, conflicts, and integration of the bicultural self: Psychoanalysis of an adolescent daughter of South-Asian immigrant parents. In S. Akhtar and S. Kramer (Eds.), *The colors of childhood: Separation-individuation across cultural, racial, and ethnic differences* (pp. 129-168). Northvale: Jason Aronson Inc.

Mercer, S. O. and Perdue, J. D. (1993). Munchausen syndrome by proxy: Social work's role. *Social Work, 38,* 74-81.

Mikkelsen, E. (1994). Is psychotherapy useful for the mentally retarded? *The Harvard Mental Health Letter, 11* (2), 8.

Miles, C. (1998). Mothers and others: Bonding, separation-individuation, and resultant ego development in different African-American cultures. In S. Akhtar and S. Kramer (Eds.), *The colors of childhood: Separation-individuation across cultural, racial, and ethnic differences* (pp. 79-112). Northvale: Jason Aronson Inc.

Minuchin, S. (1974). *Families and family therapy.* Cambridge: Harvard University Press.

Mishne, J. M. (1982). The missing system in social work's application of systems theory. *Social Casework, 63,* 547-553.

Mitchell, J. (2000). Mr. Hunter's grave. In D. Remnick (Ed.), *Life Stories: Profiles from The New Yorker* (pp. 3-26). New York: Random House.

Mitchell, S. (1988). *Relational concepts in psychoanalysis.* Cambridge: Harvard University Press.

Mittler, P. (1992). Educating children with severe learning difficulties: Challenging vulnerability. In B. Tizard and V. Varma (Eds.), *Vulnerability and resilience in human development: A festschrift for Ann and Alan Clarke* (pp. 163-181). London: Jessica Kingsley Publishers.

Mood disorders in childhood and adolescence—Part I (1993). *The Harvard Mental Health Letter, 10* (5), pp. 1-4.

Morales, J. (1995). Gay men: Parenting. In R. L. Edwards and J. G. Hopps (Eds.) *Social work encyclopedia*, Nineteenth edition, Vol. 2 (pp. 1085-1095). Washington, DC: NASW Press.

Moran, J. R. (1999). Preventing alcohol use among urban American Indian youth: The seventh generation program. *Journal of Human Behavior in the Social Environment, 2,* 51-67.

Morehouse, E. (1989). Treating adolescent alcohol abusers. *Social Casework: The Journal of Contemporary Social Work, 70,* 355-363.

Morris, J. (1997). *Conundrum.* London: Penguin Books.

Morrison, T. (1977). *Song of Solomon.* New York: The Signet Press.

Morrison, T. (1999). *Paradise.* New York: Plume.

Morrow, D. F. (1993). Social work with gay and lesbian adolescents. *Social Work, 38,* 655-660.

Morrow, L. (1991). When one body can save another. *Time, 137,* June 17, pp. 54-58.

Morton, N. and Browne, K. D. (1998). Theory and observation of attachment and its relation to child maltreatment: A review. *Child Abuse and Neglect, 22,* 1093-1104.

Moultrup, D. (1981). Towards an integrated model of family therapy. *Clinical Social Work Journal, 9,* 111-125.

Mrazek, D. A. (2000). Somatic expression of disease. In C. H. Zeanah Jr. (Ed.), *Handbook of infant mental health,* Second edition (pp. 425-436). New York: The Guilford Press.

Mt. St. Helens darkens land, lives; social, economic shock waves felt (1980). *NASW News, 25,* July, pp. 1, 12.

Mulinski, P. (1989). Dual diagnosis in alcoholic clients: Clinical implications. *Social Casework: The Journal of Contemporary Social Work, 70,* 333-339.

Murdach, A. D. (1996). Beneficence re-examined: Protective intervention in mental health. *Social Work, 41,* 26-32.

Murphy, L., Pynoos, R. S., and James, C. B. (1997). The trauma/grief-focused group psychotherapy module of an elementary school-based violence prevention/intervention program. In J. Osofsky (Ed.), *Children in a violent society* (pp. 223-255). New York: The Guilford Press.

Nadelman, A. (1986). Sharing the hurt: Adolescents in a residential setting. In A. Gitterman and L. Shulman (Eds.), *Mutual aid groups and the life cycle* (pp. 141-160). Itasca, IL: F. E. Peacock Publishers, Inc.

Nakashima, E. (2001). Administration calls halt to gun buybacks. *Washington Post,* July 26, p. A23. Available online at <http://www.washingtonpost.com/ac2/wpdyn?pagename=article&node=&contentId=A50620-2001Jul25>.

Nasjleti, M. (1980). Suffering in silence: The male incest victim. *Child Welfare, 49,* 269-275.

National Adoption Information Clearinghouse. (1999). Washington, DC: NAIC. Available online at <http://www.calib.com/naic>.

Native American Legislative Update (2001). Friends Committee on National Legislation, Washington. Available online at <http://www.fcnl.org/act_nalu_curnt/
indian_504_01.htm>.

Nelsen, J. C. (1983). Treatment issues in schizophrenia (1975). In F. J. Turner (Ed.),
Differential diagnosis and treatment in social work, Third edition (pp. 337-346).
New York: The Free Press.

Nelson, J. C. (1974). Teaching content of early fieldwork conferences. *Social Casework, 55,* 147-153.

Nelson, K. E., Saunders, E. J., and Landsman, M. J. (1993). Chronic child neglect in
perspective. *Social Work, 38,* 661-671.

Nemiah, J. C. (1961). *Foundations of psychopathology.* New York: Oxford University Press.

Nemiroff, R. A. and Colarusso, C. A. (1990). *New dimensions in adult development.*
New York: Basic Books.

Netting, F. E., Wilson, C. C., and New, J. C. (1987). The human-animal bond: Implications for practice. *Social Work, 32,* 60-64.

Neugarten, B. L. (1979). Time, age, and the life cycle. *American Journal of Psychiatry, 136,* 887-894.

Newhill, C. (1995). Client violence toward social workers: A practice and policy
concern for the 1990's. *Social Work, 40,* 631-636.

Newton, M. (1995). *Adolescence: Guiding youth through the perilous ordeal.* New
York: W. W. Norton and Company.

Nicholson, B. L. and Kay, D. M. (1999). Group treatment of traumatized Cambodian women: A culture-specific approach. *Social Work, 44,* 470-479.

Nieves, E. (1998). Homelessness tests San Francisco's ideals. *The New York Times,*
November 13, pp. A1, A21.

Nieves, E. (1999). California calls off effort to carry out immigrant measure. *The
New York Times,* July 30, pp. A1, A15.

Nieves, E. (2000). In San Francisco, more live alone, and die alone, too. *The New
York Times,* June 25, p. 9.

Noam, G. G. (1996). Reconceptualizing maturity: The search for deeper meaning.
In G. G. Noam and K. W. Fischer (Eds.), *Development and vulnerability in close
relationships* (pp. 135-172). Mahwah, NJ: Lawrence Erlbaum Associates.

Noam, G. G. and Fischer, K. W. (1996). Introduction: The foundational role of relationships in human development. In G. G. Noam and K. W. Fischer (Eds.), *Development and vulnerability in close relationships* (pp. ix-xx). Mahwah, NJ:
Lawrence Erlbaum Associates.

Noble, H. B. (1999). Study backs a drug for hyperactive children. *The New York
Times,* December 15, p. A16.

Nokes, D. (1997). *Jane Austen: A life.* Berkeley: University of California Press.

Nowinski, J. (1990). *Substance abuse in adolescents and young adults.* New York:
W. W. Norton and Company.

Noyes, A. (1953). *Modern clinical psychiatry,* Fourth edition. Philadelphia: W. B.
Saunders Company.

O'Donnell, J. M. (1999). Involvement of African American fathers in kinship foster
care services. *Social Work, 44,* 428-441.

Ogden, T. H. (1982). *Projective identification and psychotherapeutic technique.* New York: Jason Aronson Inc.

O'Hare, T. (1995). Mental health problems and alcohol abuse: Co-occurrence and gender differences. *Health and Social Work, 20,* 207-214.

Olkin, R. (1999). *What psychotherapists should know about disability.* New York: The Guilford Press.

Omin, R. (1989). To die in treatment: An opportunity for growth, consolidation and healing. *Clinical Social Work Journal, 17,* 325-336.

O'Neill, J. V. (1999). Substance abuse: The common thread. *NASW News, 44* (7), p. 3.

O'Neill, J. V. (2000a). Drugs-pregnancy brief filed. *NASW News, 45* (3), p. 7.

O'Neill, J. V. (2000b). Surgeon general publishes a must-read. *NASW News, 45* (5), p. 5.

Orlin, M. (1995). The Americans with Disabilities Act: Implications for social services. *Social Work, 40,* 233-239.

Osofsky, J. D. (1997). Children and youth violence: An overview of the issues. In J. D. Osofsky (Ed.), *Children in a violent society* (pp. 3-8). New York: The Guilford Press.

Oster, G. and Caro, J. (1990). *Understanding and treating depressed adolescents and their families.* New York: John Wiley and Sons.

Panic disorder: Part I (1990). *The Harvard Mental Health Letter, 7* (3), pp. 1-4.

Panic disorder: Part II (1990). *The Harvard Mental Health Letter, 7* (4), pp. 1-3.

Pannor, R. and Baran, A. (1984). Open adoption as standard practice. *Child Welfare, 43,* 245-250.

Paret, I. H. and Shapiro, V. B. (1998). The splintered holding environment and the vulnerable ego: A case study. In A. J. Solnit, P. B. Neubauer, S. Abrams, and A. S. Dowling (Eds.), *The psychoanalytic study of the child, Vol. 53* (pp. 300-324). New Haven: Yale University Press.

Parks, C. A. (1998). Lesbian parenthood: A review of the literature. *American Journal of Orthopsychiatry, 68,* 376-389.

Parson, E. R. (1995). Post-traumatic stress and coping in an inner-city child: Traumatogenic witnessing of interparental violence and murder. In A. J. Solnit, P. B. Neubauer, S. Abrams, and A. S. Dowling (Eds.), *The psychoanalytic study of the child, Vol. 50* (pp. 272-307). New Haven: Yale University Press.

Partida, J. (1996). The effects of immigration on children in the Mexican-American community. *Child and Adolescent Social Work Journal, 13,* 241-254.

Patterson, S. L., Germain, C. B., Brennan, E. M., and Memmott, J. (1988). Effectiveness of rural natural helpers. *Social Casework, 5,* 272-279.

Pavenstedt, E. (Ed.) (1967). *The drifters: Children of disorganized lower-class families.* Boston: Little, Brown and Company.

Pear, R. (1999a). Few seek to treat mental disorders, a U.S. study says. *The New York Times,* December 13, pp. A1, A26.

Pear, R. (1999b). More Americans were uninsured in 1998, U.S. says. *The New York Times,* October 4, pp. A1, A24.

Pear, R. (2000). Medicare spending for care at home plunges by 45 percent. *The New York Times,* April 21, pp. A1, A18.

Pérez Foster, R. (1999). An intersubjective approach to cross-cultural clinical work. *Smith College Studies in Social Work, 69,* 269-291.

Pérez Foster, R., Moskowitz, M., and Javier, R. A. (1996). Introduction. In R. Pérez Foster, M. Moskowitz, and R. A. Javier (Eds.), *Reaching across boundaries of culture and class: Widening the scope of psychotherapy* (pp. xiii-xvii). Northvale: Jason Aronson Inc.

Perloff, J. D. and Jaffee, K. D. (1999). Late entry into prenatal care: The neighborhood context. *Social Work, 44,* 116-128.

Perry, B. (1997). Incubated in terror: Neurodevelopmental factors in the "cycle of violence." In J. D. Osofsky (Ed.), *Children in a violent society* (pp. 124-149). New York: The Guilford Press.

Pfeffer, C. (1988). Modalities of treatment for suicidal children. In S. Lesse (Ed.), *What we know about suicidal behavior and how to treat it* (pp. 359-370). Northvale: Jason Aronson Inc.

Phillips, R. S. C. (1999). Intervention with siblings of children with developmental disabilities from economically disadvantaged families. *Families in Society: The Journal of Contemporary Human Services, 80,* 569-577.

Piaget, J. (1952). *The origins of intelligence in children.* New York: International Universities Press.

Piaget, J. (1995a). The first year of life of the child. In H. E. Gruber and J. J. Vonèche (Eds.), *The essential Piaget: An interpretive reference and guide* (pp. 198-214). New York: Basic Books.

Piaget, J. (1995b). Judgment and reasoning in the child. In E. H. Gruber and J. J. Vonèche (Eds.), *The essential Piaget: An interpretive reference and guide* (pp. 89-117). New York: Basic Books.

Piaget, J. and Inhelder, B. (1995). The growth of logical thinking from childhood to adolescence. In H. E. Gruber and J. J. Vonèche (Eds.), *The essential Piaget: An interpretive reference and guide* (pp. 405-444). New York: Basic Books.

Pies, R. and Keast, E. K. (1995). Cultural factors in psychiatric syndromes. *Psychiatric Times, 12* (January), 14-17.

Pill, C. J. and Zabin, J. L. (1997). Lifelong legacy of early maternal loss: A women's group. *Clinical Social Work Journal, 25,* 179-196.

Pinderhughes, E. B. (1983). Empowerment for our clients and for ourselves. *Social Casework, 64,* 331-338.

Postpartum disorders (1989). *The Harvard Medical School Mental Health Letter, 5* (11), pp. 1-3.

Post-traumatic stress: Part I (1991). *The Harvard Mental Health Letter, 7* (8), pp. 1-4.

Post-traumatic stress: Part II (1991). *The Harvard Mental Health Letter, 7* (9), pp. 1-4.

Poynter-Berg, D. (1986). Getting connected: Institutionalized schizophrenic women. In A. Gitterman and L. Shulman (Eds.), *Mutual aid groups and the life cycle* (pp. 263-281). Itasca, IL: F. E. Peacock Publishers, Inc.

Pray, J. E. (1991). Respecting the uniqueness of the individual: Social work practice with a reflective model. *Social Work, 36,* 80-85.

Prizant, B. M., Wetherby, A. M., and Roberts, J. E. (2000). Communication problems. In C. H. Zeanah Jr. (Ed.), *Handbook of infant mental health,* Second edition (pp. 282-297). New York: The Guilford Press.

Proctor, C. D. and Groze, V. K. (1994). Risk factors for suicide among gay, lesbian, and bisexual youths. *Social Work, 39*, 504-513.

Proctor, E. K. (1983). New directions for work with parents of retarded children. In F. J. Turner (Ed.), *Differential diagnosis and treatment in social work,* Third edition (pp. 511-519). New York: The Free Press.

Purdum, T. S. (1997). Tapes left by 39 in cult suicide suggest comet was sign to die. *The New York Times,* March 28, pp. A1, A11.

Puryear, D. A. (1984). Crisis intervention. In F. G. Guggenheim and M. F. Weiner (Eds.), *Manual of psychiatric consultation and emergency care* (pp. 33-41). New York: Jason Aronson Inc.

Putnam, F. W. (1997). *Dissociation in children and adolescents: A developmental perspective.* New York: The Guilford Press.

Queralt, M. (1996). *The social environment and human behavior: A diversity perspective.* Boston: Allyn & Bacon.

Racial and ethnic classifications used in Census 2000 and beyond (2000). Washington, DC: United States Census Bureau, Population Division, Special Population Staff. Available online at <http://www.census.gov/population/www/socdemo/race/racefactcb.html>.

Ramirez III, M. (1998). *Multicultural/multiracial psychology: Mestizo perspectives in personality and mental health.* Northvale: Jason Aronson Inc.

Rapoport, L. (1970). Crisis intervention as a mode of treatment. In R. W. Roberts and R. H. Nee (Eds.), *Theories of social casework* (pp. 265-311). Chicago: The University of Chicago Press.

Rathbone-McCuan, E. and Stokke, D. L. (1997). Lesbian women and substance abuse. In S. L. A. Straussner and E. Zelvin (Eds.), *Gender and addictions: Men and women in treatment* (pp. 167-196). Northvale: Jason Aronson Inc.

Ratnesar, R. (1998a). Lost in the middle. *Time, 152,* September 14, pp. 60-64.

Ratnesar, R. (1998b). A place at the table. *Time, 152,* October 12, p. 38.

Rauch, J. B. and Black, R. B. (1995). Genetics. In R. L. Edwards and J. G. Hopps (Eds.), *Social work encyclopedia*, Nineteenth edition, Vol. 2 (pp. 1108-1117). Washington, DC: NASW Press.

Rayfield, D. (1997). *Anton Chekhov: A life.* New York: Henry Holt and Company.

Rees, W. D. (1975). The bereaved and their hallucinations. In B. Schoenberg, I. Gerber, A. Wiener, A. H. Kutscher, D. Peretz, and A. C. Carr (Eds.), *Bereavement: Its psychosocial aspects* (pp. 66-71). New York: Columbia University Press.

Regehr, C., Marziali, E., and Jansen, K. (1999). A qualitative analysis of strengths and vulnerabilities in sexually assaulted women. *Clinical Social Work Journal, 27,* 171-184.

Regulus, T. A. (1995). Gang Violence. In R. L. Edwards and J. G. Hopps (Eds.), *Social work encyclopedia*, Nineteenth edition, Vol. 2 (pp. 1045-1054). Washington, DC: NASW Press.

Reiner, B. S. and Kaufman, I. (1959). *Character disorders in parents of delinquents.* New York: Family Service Association of America.

Remnick, D. (1998). Bad Seeds. *The New Yorker,* July 20, pp. 28-33.

Richardson, L. (1998). Wave of laws aimed at people with HIV. *The New York Times,* September 25, pp. A1, A25.

Richman, J. M. and Bowen, G. L. (1997). School failure: An ecological-interactional-developmental perspective. In M. W. Fraser (Ed.), *Risk and resilience in childhood: An ecological perspective* (pp. 95-116). Washington, DC: NASW Press.

Richman, J. M., Rosenfeld, L. B., and Bowen, G. L. (1998). Social support for adolescents at risk of school failure. *Social Work, 43,* 309-323.

Riebschleger, J. L. (1991). Families of chronically mentally ill people: Siblings speak to social workers. *Health and Social Work, 16* (2), 94-103.

Rimer, S. (1998a). Families bear a bigger share of caring for the frail elderly. *The New York Times,* June 8, pp. A1, A18.

Rimer, S. (1998b). For aged, dating game is numbers game. *The New York Times,* December 28, pp. A1, A18.

Rimer, S. (1998c). Paradoxes are a recurring theme at an annual conference on gerontology. *The New York Times,* November 27, p. A20.

Rimer, S. (1999). Caring for elderly kin is costly, study finds. *The New York Times,* November 27, p. A8.

Rimer, S. and Bonner, R. (2000). Whether to kill those who killed as youths. *The New York Times,* August 22, pp. A1, A16.

Robbins, S. P. (1995). Cults. In R. L. Edwards and J. G. Hopps (Eds.), *Social work encyclopedia,* Nineteenth edition, Vol. 1 (pp. 667-677). Washington, DC: NASW Press.

Robin, R. W., Rasmussen, J. K., and Gonzalez-Santin, E. (1999). Impact of childhood out-of-home placement on a southwestern American Indian tribe. *Journal of Human Behavior in the Social Environment, 2* (1/2), 69-89.

Robinson, R. L. (1997). Men and gambling. In S. L. A. Straussner and E. Zelvin (Eds.), *Gender and addictions: Men and women in treatment* (pp. 469-492). Northvale: Jason Aronson Inc.

Roche, T. (2000). A refuge for throwaways. *Time, 155,* February 21, pp. 50-51.

Rohde, D. (1998). An addict who is a father, too. *The New York Times,* June 14, pp. 35, 37.

Rose, E. (1996). Introduction from the founding chair of the National Study Group on Social Work and Psychoanalysis. In J. Edward and J. Sanville (Eds.), *Fostering healing and growth: A psychoanalytic social work approach* (pp. xvix-xx). Northvale: Jason Aronson Inc.

Rosenbaum, D. E. (1999). Health benefits bill shows power of the disabled. *The New York Times,* June 7, pp. A1, A18.

Rosenbaum, M. and Muroff, M. (1984). *Anna O.: Fourteen contemporary reinterpretations.* New York: The Free Press.

Rosenbloom, M. (1983). Implications of the Holocaust for social work. *Social Casework: The Journal of Contemporary Social Work, 64,* 205-213.

Rosenthal, E. (1998). In North Korean hunger, legacy is stunted children. *The New York Times,* December 10, pp. A1, A12.

Rosenthal, E. (1999). Women's suicides reveal rural China's bitter roots. *The New York Times,* January 24, pp. 1, 12.

Ross, J. M. (1984). Fathers in development: An overview of recent contributions. In R. Cohen, B. Cohler, and S. Weissman (Eds.), *Parenthood: A psychodynamic perspective* (pp. 373-390). New York: The Guilford Press.

Rossman, P. (1982). Psychotherapeutic approaches with depressed, acting out adolescents: Interpretive tactics and their rationale. In S. Feinstein, J. Looney, A. Schwartzberg, and A. Sorosky (Eds.), *Adolescent psychiatry: Developmental and clinical studies: Vol. X* (pp. 455-468). Chicago: The University of Chicago Press.

Rotheram-Borus, M. and Bradley, J. (1991). Triage model for suicidal runaways. *American Journal of Orthopsychiatry, 61,* 122-127.

Rutter, M. (1975). *Helping troubled children.* London: Penguin Books.

Saari, C. (1999). Intersubjectivity, language, and culture: Bridging the person/environment gap? *Smith College Studies in Social Work, 69,* 221-237.

Sachs, S. (1999a). Conference confronts the difficulties of being Muslim and gay. *The New York Times,* May 30, p. 22.

Sachs, S. (1999b). Drug and alcohol projects rooted in the old country. *The New York Times,* June 16, p. A25.

Sack, K. (1998). Hate groups in U.S. are growing, report says. *The New York Times,* March 3, p. A1.

Sack, K. (1999). HIV peril and rising drug use. *The New York Times,* January 29, p. A8.

Sackheim, G. (1974). Dream analysis and casework technique. *Clinical Social Work Journal, 2,* 29-35.

Sacks, O. (1989). *Seeing voices: A journey into the world of the deaf.* Berkeley: University of California Press.

Sacks, O. (1990). Neurology and the soul. *The New York Review of Books, 37,* November 22, pp. 44-50.

Saleebey, D. (Ed.) (1992). *The strengths perspective in social work practice.* New York: Longman.

Sameroff, A. J. and Fiese, B. H. (2000). Models of development and developmental risk. In C. H. Zeanah Jr. (Ed.), *Handbook of infant mental health,* Second edition (pp. 3-19). New York: The Guilford Press.

Sanville, J. (1994). Editorial. *Clinical Social Work Journal, 22,* 131-136.

Satel, S. L. (1999). Real help for the mentally ill. *The New York Times,* January 7, p. A31.

Satir, V. (1967). *Conjoint family therapy.* Palo Alto: Science and Behavior Books.

Schaefer, D. S. and Pozzaglia, D. (1986). Coping with a nightmare: Hispanic parents of children with cancer. In A. Gitterman and L. Shulman (Eds.), *Mutual aid groups and the life cycle* (pp. 297-311). Itasca, IL: F. E. Peacock Publishers, Inc.

Schaffer, H. R. (1994). Early experience and the parent-child relationship: Genetic and environmental interactions as developmental determinants. In B. Tizard and V. Varma (Eds.), *Vulnerability and resilience in human development: A festschrift for Ann and Alan Clarke* (pp. 39-53). London: Jessica Kingsley Publishers.

Schamess, G. (1996). Ego psychology. In J. Berzoff, L. M. Flanagan, and P. Hertz (Eds.), *Inside out and outside in: Psychodynamic clinical theory and practice in contemporary multicultural contexts* (pp. 67-101). Northvale: Jason Aronson Inc.

Schamess, G. (1999). Reflections on intersubjectivity. *Smith College Studies in Social Work, 69,* 188-200.

Scharff, D. and Scharff, J. (1987). *Object relations family therapy*. Northvale: Jason Aronson Inc.

Scharff, D. and Scharff, J. (1991). *Object relations couple therapy*. Northvale: Jason Aronson Inc.

Schlossberg, N. K. (1981). A model for analyzing human adaptation to transition. *The Counseling Psychologist, 9*, 2-18.

Schwaber, E. A. (1997). Reflections on the concept "the patient's psychic reality." In A. J. Solnit, P. B. Neubauer, S. Abrams, and A. S. Dowling (Eds.), *The psychoanalytic study of the child, Vol. 52* (pp. 42-53). New Haven: Yale University Press.

Schwartz, J. M., Jacobson, A. M., Hauser, S. T., and Dornbush, B. B. (1989). Explorations of vulnerability and resilience: Case studies of diabetic adolescents and their families. In T. F. Dugan and R. Coles (Eds.), *The child in our times: Studies in the development of resiliency* (pp. 134-156). New York: Bruner/Mazel.

Scott, J. (1998). Star professors, as a team, fail chemistry. *The New York Times,* November 21, pp. A1, A17.

Seasonal affective disorder (1993). *The Harvard Mental Health Letter, 9* (8), 1-4.

Seelye, K. Q. (1999). Citing "primitive" hatreds, Clinton asks Congress to expand hate-crime law. *The New York Times,* April 7, p. A18.

Segal, U. A. (1991). Cultural variables in Asian Indian families. *Family in Society: The Journal of Contemporary Human Services, 72*, 233-241.

Seifer, R. and Dickstein, S. (2000). Parental mental illness and infant development. In C. H. Zeanah Jr. (Ed.), *Handbook of infant mental health,* Second edition (pp. 145-160). New York: The Guilford Press.

Seiffge-Krenke, I. (1997). "One body for two": The problem of boundaries between chronically ill adolescents and their mothers. In A. J. Solnit, P. B. Neubauer, S. Abrams, and A. S. Dowling (Eds.), *The psychoanalytic study of the child, Vol. 52* (pp. 340-355). New Haven: Yale University Press.

Self-Help groups—Part I (1993). *The Harvard Mental Health Letter, 9* (9), pp. 1-3.

Self-Help groups—Part II (1993). *The Harvard Mental Health Letter, 9* (10), pp. 1-4.

Seligman, S. (1994). Applying psychoanalysis in an unconventional context: Adapting infant-parent psychotherapy to a changing population. In A. J. Solnit, P. B. Neubauer, S. Abrams, and A. S. Dowling (Eds.), *The psychoanalytic study of the child, Vol. 49* (pp. 481-500). New Haven: Yale University Press.

Sengupta, S. (2000a). Youth court of true peers judges firmly. *The New York Times,* June 4, pp. 1, 32.

Sengupta, S. (2000b). Youths leaving foster care with few skills or resources. *The New York Times,* March 28, pp. A1, A25.

Shannon, K. (2001). Perry signs hate-crimes bill into law. *Amarillo Globe-News,* May 12. Available online at <http://www.amarillonet.com/stores/051201/tex_perry.shtml>.

Shapiro, E. (1978). The psychodynamics and developmental psychology of the borderline patient: A review of the literature. *The American Journal of Psychiatry, 135*, 1305-1315.

Shapiro, J. R. and Applegate, J. S. (2000). Cognitive neuroscience, neurobiology and affect regulation: Implications for clinical social work. *Clinical Social Work Journal, 28*, 9-21.

Shapiro, V. and Gisynski, M. (1989). Ghosts in the nursery revisited. *Child and Adolescent Social Work, 6,* 18-37.

Shonkoff, J. P., Lippitt, J. A., and Cavanaugh, D. A. (2000). Early childhood policy: Implications for infant mental health. In C. H. Zeanah Jr. (Ed.), *Handbook of infant mental health,* Second edition (pp. 503-518). New York: The Guilford Press.

Shulman, L. and Gitterman, A. (1986). The life model, mutual aid, and the mediating function. In A. Gitterman and L. Shulman (Eds.), *Mutual aid groups and the life cycle* (pp. 3-22). Itasca, IL: F. E. Peacock Publishers, Inc.

Siebold, C. (1991). Termination: When the therapist leaves. *Clinical Social Work Journal, 19,* 191-204.

Silverman, K. (1991). *Edgar A. Poe: Mournful and never-ending remembrance.* New York: Harper Collins Publishers.

Silverman, P. R., Campbell, L., and Patti, P. (1994). Reunions between adoptees and birth parents: The adoptive parents' view. *Social Work, 39,* 542-549.

Singer, M. I., Bussey, J., Song, L.-Y., and Lunghofer, L. (1995). The psychosocial issues of women serving time in jail. *Social Work, 40,* 103-113.

Slaby, A. and McGuire, P. (1989). Residential management of suicidal adolescents. In B. Garfinkel and G. Northrup (Eds.), *Adolescent suicide: Recognition, treatment and prevention* (pp. 23-43). Binghamton, New York: The Haworth Press.

Sleep disorders—Part I (1994). *The Harvard Mental Health Letter, 11* (2), pp. 1-4.

Sleep-depriving jobs linked to accidents (1999). *The New York Times,* June 4, p. A22.

Smith, L. L. (1976). A general model of crisis intervention. *Clinical Social Work Journal, 4,* 162-171.

Smith, S. L. and Howard, J. A. (1994). The impact of previous sexual abuse on children's adjustment in adoptive placement. *Social Work, 39,* 491-501.

Smolowe, J. (1990). Last call for motherhood. *Time, Special Issue, Fall, 136,* p. 76.

Smolowe, J. (1997). A battle against biology; a victory in adoption. *Time, 143,* December 1, p. 46.

Smyth, N. and Miller, B. (1997). Parenting issues for substance-abusing women. In S. L. A. Straussner and E. Zelvin (Eds.), *Gender and addictions: Men and women in treatment* (pp. 123-150). Northvale: Jason Aronson Inc.

Sollors, W. (1986). *Beyond ethnicity: Consent and descent in American culture.* New York: Oxford University Press.

Solnit, A. J., Neubauer, P. B., Abrams, S., and Sowling, A. S. (Eds.), *The psychoanalytic study of the child, 50* (pp. 122-149). New Haven: Yale University Press.

Solomon, A. (1992). Clinical diagnosis among diverse populations: A multicultural perspective. *Families in Society: The Journal of Contemporary Human Services, 73,* 371-377.

Solomon, P. and Draine, J. (1995). Issues in serving the forensic client. *Social Work, 40,* 25-33.

Sontag, D. (1999). For a world apart, a lesson in social work. *The New York Times,* July 3, pp. A1, A5.

Sotomayor, M. (1997). Aging: Racial and ethnic groups. In R. L. Edwards, I. C. Colby, A. Garcia, R. G. McRoy, and L. Videka-Sherman (Eds.), *Social work en-

cyclopedia, Nineteenth edition, 1997 supplement (pp. 26-36). Washington, DC: NASW Press.

Spickard, P. R., Fong, R., and Ewalt, P. L. (1995). Undermining the very basis of racism—its categories. *Social Work, 40,* 581-584.

Spiegel, D. (1990). Breast cancer study shows psychotherapy improved survival. *The Psychiatric Times,* January, pp. 1, 17.

Spira, M. and Kenemore, E. (2000). Adolescent daughters of mothers with breast cancer: Impact and implications. *Clinical Social Work Journal, 28,* 183-195.

Statements that Heaven's Gate released over the years (1997). *The New York Times,* March 28, p. A12.

St. Clair, M. (1986). *Object relations and self psychology: An introduction.* Monterey: Brooks/Cole Publishing Company.

Steinberg, J. (2000). An unrelenting drive, and a Harvard degree. *The New York Times,* May 17, pp. A1, A20.

Steiner, S. J. (1995). Understanding HIV and AIDS: Preparing students for practice. *Journal of Social Work Education, 31,* 322-336.

Steinhauer, J. (1999a).When babies come in twos. *The New York Times,* November 29, p. A25.

Steinhauer, J. (1999b). Young, nonwhite, female and complacent about AIDS. *The New York Times,* September 1, p. A14.

Stern, D. N. (1985). *The interpersonal world of the infant: A view from psychoanalysis and developmental psychology.* New York: Basic Books, Inc.

Steroid use among teenage girls on the rise, studies find (1999). *The Providence Sunday Journal,* June 6, p. A12.

Stevens, W. K. (1998). Harmful heat is more frequent, especially at night, study finds. *The New York Times,* December 10, pp. A1, A18.

Stevens-Long, J. (1990). Adult development: Theories past and future. In R. Nemiroff and C. Colarusso (Eds.), *New Dimensions in Adult Development* (pp. 125-169). New York: Basic Books.

Stolberg, S. G. (1998). Eyes shut, black America is being ravaged by AIDS. *The New York Times,* June 29, pp. A1, A12.

Stolberg, S. G. (1999). Agreement allows new system for organ sharing. *The New York Times,* November 12, pp. A1, A25.

Stolberg, S. G. (2000). As the tiniest babies grow, so can their problems. *The New York Times,* May 8, pp. A1, A20.

Stolorow, R. D. and Atwood, G. E. (1987). *Psychoanalytic treatment: An intersubjective approach.* Hillsdale: Analytic Press.

Stolorow, R. D., Atwood, G. E., and Brandchaft, B. (1994). *The intersubjective perspective.* Northvale: Jason Aronson Inc.

Storr, A. (1988). *Solitude: A return to the self.* New York: The Free Press.

Strand, V. C. (1995). Single parents. In R. L. Edwards and J. G. Hopps (Eds.), *Social work encyclopedia*, Nineteenth edition, Vol. 3 (pp. 2157-2163). Washington, DC: NASW Press.

Straussner, S. L. A. and Zelvin, E. (Eds.) (1997). *Gender and addictions: Men and women in treatment.* Northvale: Jason Aronson Inc.

Strom, S. (1999). In Japan, mired in recession, suicides soar. *The New York Times,* July 15, pp. A1, A8.

Strom-Gottfried, K. (1997). The implications of managed care for social work education. *Journal of Social Work Education, 33,* 7-18.

Study sheds light on best treatments for ADHD (2000). *Psychiatric News,* January 21, p. 20.

Styron, W. (1990). *Darkness visible: A memoir of madness.* New York: Random House.

Styron, W. (1993). *The confessions of Nat Turner.* New York: Vintage Books.

Suit seeks to place retarded adults (1999). *The New York Times,* March 20, p. 23.

Sullivan, H. S. (1954). Preadolescence. In S. Perry and M. L. Gawel (Eds.), *The psychiatric interview: Vol. 1. The collected works of Harry Stack Sullivan* (pp. 245-262). New York: W. W. Norton.

Sun, A.-P. (2000). Helping substance-abusing mothers in the child-welfare system: Turning crisis into opportunity. *Families in Society: The Journal of Contemporary Human Services, 81,* 142-151.

Surgeon general opens campaign to counter rise in suicide (1999). *The New York Times,* July 29, p. A15.

Sutherland, S. (1989). *The international dictionary of psychology.* New York: Continuum.

Swarns, R. L. (1998). Hispanic mothers lagging as others escape welfare. *The New York Times,* September 15, pp. A1, A29.

Swarns, R. L. (1999). State overseer of troubled city child welfare agency has its own problems. *The New York Times,* January 8, p. A19.

Swenson, C. J. (1994). Freud's "Anna O.": Social work's Bertha Pappenheim. *Clinical Social Work Journal, 22,* 149-163.

Szalita, A. B. (1974). Grief and bereavement. In S. Arieti (Ed.), *American handbook of psychiatry: Vol. 1,* Fourth edition (pp. 673-684). New York: Basic Books, Inc.

Takahashi, K. (1990). Are the key assumptions of the "Strange Situation" universal? *Human Development, 33,* 23-30.

Talbot, M. (1998). Attachment theory: The ultimate experiment. *The New York Times Magazine,* May 24, pp. 24-30, 38, 46, 50, 54.

Talbot, M. (2000). A mighty fortress. *New York Times Magazine,* February 27, pp. 34-41, 68-69, 84-85.

Tamura, T. and Lau, A. (1992). Connectedness versus separateness: Applicability of family therapy to Japanese families. *Family Process, 31,* 319-340.

Tang, N. M. (1997). Psychoanalytic psychotherapy with Chinese Americans. In E. Lee (Ed.), *Working with Asian Americans: A guide for clinicians* (pp. 323-341). New York: The Guilford Press.

Tang, N. M. and Smith, B. L. (1996). The eternal triangle across cultures: Oedipus, Hsueh, and Gansea. In A. J. Solnit, P. B. Neubauer, S. Abrams, and A. S. Dowling (Eds.), *The psychoanalytic study of the child, Vol. 51* (pp. 562-579). New Haven: Yale University Press.

Tashjian, L. D. (1979). Failure in treatment of a borderline patient. *Psychiatric Opinion, 16* (7), 43-47.

Teen-agers learn AIDS Counseling (1999). *The New York Times,* May 9, p. 29.

Thomas, A. (1981). Current trends in developmental theory. *American Journal of Orthopsychiatry, 51,* 580-609.

Thomlison, B. (1997). Risk and protective factors in child maltreatment. In M. W. Fraser (Ed.), *Risk and resilience in childhood: An ecological perspective* (pp. 50-72). Washington, DC: NASW Press.

Thompson, C. L. (1996). The African-American patient in psychodynamic treatment. In R. Pérez Foster, M. Moskowitz, and R. A. Javier (Eds.), *Reaching across boundaries of culture and class: Widening the scope of psychotherapy* (pp. 115-142). Northvale: Jason Aronson Inc.

Thompson, G. (1999a). In Mexico, children, and promises, unkept. *The New York Times,* June 2, pp. A1, C30.

Thompson, G. (1999b). New clinics seek patients among lesbians, who often shun health care. *The New York Times,* March 30, p. A25.

Thyer, B. A. (1988). Radical behaviorism and clinical social work. In R. A. Dorfman (Ed.), *Paradigms of clinical social work* (pp. 123-148). New York: Brunner/Mazel Publishers.

Tizard, B. (1991). Intercountry adoption: A review of the evidence. *Journal of Child Psychology, Psychiatry, and Allied Disciplines, 32,* 743-756.

Toner, R. (1999). Long-term care merges political with personal. *The New York Times,* July 26, pp. A1, A11.

Toward nursing home reform (editorial) (1999). *The New York Times,* May 29, p. A26.

Trillin, C. (1999). Wanted: One egg (Ph.D. pref.). *Time, 153,* January 25, p. 20.

Trimble, D. (1986). Confronting responsibility: Men who batter their wives. In A. Gitterman and L. Shulman (Eds.), *Mutual aid groups and the life cycle* (pp. 229-243). Itasca, IL: F. E. Peacock Publishers, Inc.

Tully, C. T. (1995). Lesbians overview. In R. L. Edwards and J. G. Hopps (Eds.), *Social work encyclopedia,* Nineteenth edition, Vol. 2 (pp. 1591-1596). Washington, DC: NASW Press.

Turrini, P. (1996). Glossary. In J. Edward and J. Sanville (Eds.), *Fostering healing and growth: A psychoanalytic social work approach* (pp. 443- 467). Northvale: Jason Aronson Inc.

Twin babies spared death as tribe forgoes ritual (1999). *Providence Sunday Journal,* October 10, p. A14.

Upham, F. (1973). *Ego analysis in the helping professions.* New York: Family Service Association of America.

Urdang, E. (1964). An educational project for first-year students in a field placement. *Social Casework, 45,* 10-15.

Urdang, E. (1974). *Becoming a social worker: The first year.* Unpublished manuscript. Boston College Graduate School of Social Work.

Urdang, E. (1979). In defense of process recording. *Smith College Studies in Social Work, 50,* 1-15.

Urdang, E. (1994). *Self-perceptions of the beginning field instructor: The experience of supervising a social work intern.* Unpublished doctoral dissertation. Simmons College School of Social Work, Boston, MA.

Urdang, E. (1999). The influence of managed care on the MSW social work student's development of the professional self. *Smith College Studies in Social Work, 70,* 3-25.

Vaillant, G. E. (1993). *The wisdom of the ego.* Cambridge: Harvard University Press.

Vastola, J., Nierenberg, A., and Graham, E. H. (1986). The lost and found group: Group work with bereaved children. In A. Gitterman and L. Shulman (Eds.), *Mutual aid groups and the life cycle* (pp. 75-90). Itasca, IL: F. E. Peacock Publishers, Inc.

Verhovek, S. H. (1998). 2 die, despite domestic-violence screen. *The New York Times,* December 14, p. A12.

Verhovek, S. H. (1999). Gun control laws gaining support in many states. *The New York Times,* May 31, pp. A1, A9.

Vonk, M. E., Simms, P. J., and Nackerud, L. (1999). Political and personal aspects of intercountry adoption of Chinese children in the United States. *Families in Society: The Journal of Contemporary Human Services, 80,* 496-505.

Vonnegut, M. (1975). *The Eden Express: A personal account of schizophrenia.* New York: Praeger Publishers.

Wachtel, P. L. (1977). *Psychoanalysis and behavior therapy: Toward an integration.* New York: Basic Books, Inc.

Wade, N. (2000). Genetic code of human life is cracked by scientists: A shared success. *The New York Times,* June 27, pp. A1, A21.

Wagner, G. (1991). When a parent is abusive. In H. Jackson (Ed.), *Using self psychology in psychotherapy* (pp. 243-259). Northvale: Jason Aronson Inc.

Wakschlag, L. S. and Hans, S .L. (2000). Early parenthood in context: Implications for development and intervention. In C. H. Zeanah Jr. (Ed.), *Handbook of infant mental health,* Second edition (pp. 129-144). New York: The Guilford Press.

Wallace, J. (1992). The value of alcoholism treatment. *The Harvard Mental Health Letter, 8* (11), pp. 4-5.

Walters, K. L. (1999). Urban American Indian identity attitudes and acculturation styles. *Journal of Human Behavior in the Social Environment, 2* (1/2), 163-178.

War on domestic abuse gains ground (1999). *The Providence Sunday Journal,* June 13, p. A9.

Warn, D. J. (1997). Recovery issues of substance-abusing gay men. In S. L. A. Straussner and E. Zelvin (Eds.), *Gender and addictions: Men and women in treatment* (pp. 385-410). Northvale: Jason Aronson Inc.

Watts-Jones, D. (1992). Cultural and integrative therapy issues in the treatment of a Jamaican woman with panic disorder. *Family Process, 31,* 105-113.

Watzlawick, P., Beavin, J. H., and Jackson, D. D. (1967). *Pragmatics of human communication: A study of interactional patterns, pathologies, and paradoxes.* New York: W. W. Norton and Company.

Weaver, H. N. (1999). Health concerns for Native American youth: A culturally grounded approach to health promotion. *Journal of Human Behavior in the Social Environment, 2,* 127-143.

Weinreb, L. and Rossi, P. H. (1995). The American homeless family shelter "system." *Social Service Review, 69,* 86-107.

Wells, S. J. (1995). Child abuse and neglect overview. In R. L. Edwards and J. G. Hopps (Eds.), *Social work encyclopedia,* Nineteenth edition, Vol. 1 (pp. 346-353). Washington, DC: NASW Press.

Welu, T. C. (1975). Pathological bereavement: A plan for its prevention. In B. Schoenberg, I. Gerber, A. Wiener, A. H. Kutscher, D. Peretz, and A. C. Carr (Eds.), *Bereavement: Its psychosocial aspects* (pp. 139-149). New York: Columbia University Press.

Westerfelt, A. and Yellow Bird, M. (1999). Homeless and indigenous in Minneapolis. *Journal of Human Behavior in the Social Environment, 2* (1/2), 145-162.

Westermeyer, J. (1985). Psychiatric diagnosis across cultural boundaries. *American Journal of Psychiatry, 142,* 798-805.

Whitaker, B. (2000). Deaths of unwanted babies bring plea to help parents. *The New York Times,* March 6, pp. A1, A19.

White, J. (1997). "I'm just who I am." *Time, 151,* May 5, pp. 32-36.

White House will offer plan to cut illegal drug use in half (1999). *The New York Times,* Feb. 8, p. A19.

Whitley, D. M., White, K. R., Kelley, S. J., and Yorke, B. (1999). Strengths-based case management: The application to grandparents raising grandchildren. *Families in Society: The Journal of Contemporary Human Services, 80,* 110-119.

Whittaker, J. K., Kinney, J., and Tracy, E. M. (1990). Family preservation services and education for social work practice: Stimulus and response. In Whittaker, J. K., Kiney, J., Tracy, E. M., and Booth, C. (Eds), *Reaching high-risk families: Intensive preservation in human services* (pp. 1-9). New York: Aldine de Gruyter.

Wijnberg, M. H. and Reding, K. M. (1999). Reclaiming a stress focus: The hassles of rural, poor single mothers. *Families in Society: The Journal of Contemporary Human Services, 80,* 506-515.

Wilentz, A. (1987). Teen suicide: Two death pacts shake the country. *Time, 129,* March 23, pp. 12-13.

Wilgoren, J. (1999). Abstinence is focus of U.S. sex education. *The New York Times,* December 15, p. A16.

Wilgoren, J. (2000). Effort to curb binge drinking in college falls short. *The New York Times,* March 15, p. A 16.

Williams, A. L. (1997). Skin color in psychotherapy. In R. Pérez Foster, M. Moskowitz, and R. A. Javier (Eds.), *Reaching across boundaries of culture and class: Widening the scope of psychotherapy* (pp. 115-142). Northvale: Jason Aronson Inc.

Williams, J. H., Ayers, C. D., and Arthur, M. W. (1997). Risk and protective factors in the development of delinquency and conduct disorder. In M. W. Fraser (Ed.), *Risk and resilience in childhood: An ecological perspective* (pp. 140-170). Washington, DC: NASW.

Williams, M. (1999). Flak in the great hair war. *The New York Times,* October 13, p. A20.

Winchester, S. (1998). *The professor and the madman: A tale of murder, insanity, and the making of the Oxford English Dictionary.* New York: Harper Collins Publishers.

Winerip, M. (1999a). After years adrift, sanity in a jail cell. *The New York Times,* June 3, p. A21.

Winerip, M. (1999b). Bedlam on the streets: Increasingly, the mentally ill have nowhere to go. That's their problem—and ours. *New York Times Magazine,* pp. 42-49, 56, 65-66, 70.

Winnicott, D. (1965). *The maturational processes and the facilitating environment: Studies in the theory of emotional development.* Madison: International Universities Press.

Winters, W. and Maluccio, A. (1988). School, family, and community: Working together to promote social competence. *Social Work in Education, 10,* 207-217.

Witkin, S. (1998). Chronicity and invisibility. *Social Work, 43,* 293-295.

Witkin, S. (1999). Taking humor seriously. *Social Work, 44,* 101-104.

Wolf, E. S. (1988). *Treating the self: Elements of clinical self psychology.* New York: The Guilford Press.

Wolf, E. S. (1994). Selfobject experiences: Development, psychopathology, treatment, therapeutic process, and technique. In S. Kramer and S. Akhtar (Eds.), *Mahler and Kohut: Perspectives on development, psychopathology, and technique* (pp. 67-96). Northvale: Jason Aronson Inc.

Wolfe, T. (1999). *A man in full.* New York: Bantam Books.

Wolman, B. B. (Ed.) (1973). *Dictionary of behavioral science.* New York: Van Nostrand Reinhold Company.

Wong, L. and Mock, M. R. (1997). Asian American young adults. In E. Lee (Ed.), *Working with Asian Americans: A guide for clinicians* (pp. 196-207). New York: The Guilford Press.

Wood, B., Watkins, J. B., Boyle, J. T., Nogueira, J., Zimands, E., and Carroll, L. (1989). The "psychosomatic family" model: An empirical and theoretical analysis. *Family Process, 28,* 399-417.

Woods, F. and Hollis, F. (1990). *Casework: A psychosocial therapy,* Fourth edition. New York: McGraw-Hill Publishing Company.

Wren, C. S. (1998). Alcohol and drug use by teen-agers declines, reports says. *The New York Times,* December 20, p. 45.

Wren, C. S. (1999). Arizona finds cost savings in treating drug offenders. *The New York Times,* April 21, p. A16.

WuDunn, S. (1999). Child abuse has Japan rethinking family autonomy. *The New York Times,* August 15, pp. 1, 8.

Wyche, K. and Rotheram-Borus, M. (1990). Suicidal behavior among minority youth in the United States. In A. Stiffman and L. Davis (Eds.), *Ethnic issues in adolescent mental health* (pp. 323-338). Newbury Park: Sage Publications.

Yardley, J. (1999). A flurry of baby abandonment leaves Houston wondering why. *The New York Times,* December 26, p. 14.

Zambelli, G. and Clark, E. (1994). Parentally bereaved children: Problems in school adjustment and implications for the school social worker. *School Social Work Journal, 19* (Fall), 1-15.

Zastrow, C. and Kirst-Ashman, K. K. (1997). *Understanding human behavior and the social environment,* Fourth edition. Chicago: Nelson-Hall Publishers.

Zayas, L. H. (1987). Psychodynamic and developmental aspects of expectant and new fatherhood: Clinical derivatives from the literature. *Clinical Social Work Journal, 15,* 8-21.

Zayas, L. H., Kaplan, C., Turner, S., Romano, K., and Gonzalez-Ramos, G. (2000). Understanding suicide attempts by adolescent Hispanic females. *Social Work, 45,* 53-63.

Zeanah, C. H. (1991). Guidelines suggested for assisting parents following perinatal loss. *The Psychiatric Times Medicine and Behavior,* July, pp. 1, 12.

Zeanah, C. H. and Scheeringa, M. S. (1997). The experience and effects of violence in infancy. In J. Osofsky (Ed.), *Children in a violent society* (pp. 97-123). New York: The Guilford Press.

Zeanah Jr., C. H. (Ed.) (2000). *Handbook of infant mental health,* Second edition. New York: The Guilford Press.

Zipper, I. N. and Simeonsson, R. J. (1997). Promoting the development of young children with disabilities. In M. W. Fraser (Ed.), *Risk and resilience in childhood: An ecological perspective* (pp. 244-264). Washington, DC: NASW Press.

Index

HAWORTH Social Work Practice in Action
Carlton E. Munson, PhD, Senior Editor

DIAGNOSIS IN SOCIAL WORK: NEW IMPERATIVES by Francis J. Turner. (2002). "This book is a useful resource for scholars and clinicians involved in clinical social work. It is thoughtfully written and well researched, and a timely additional to the professional literature." *Kathleen J. Farkas, PhD, Associate Professor, Mandel School of Applied Social Sciences, Case Western Reserve University, Cleveland, OH*

HUMAN BEHAVIOR IN THE SOCIAL ENVIRONMENT: INTERWEAVING THE INNER AND OUTER WORLDS by Esther Urdang. (2002). "This book will serve as a superb introduction to human behavior, normal and pathologic, not only for graduate social work students, but also for anyone who is curious about the vicissitudes of the human condition....The students who use this book will be lucky, indeed." *Calvin A. Colarusso, MD, Clinical Professor of Psychiatry, University of California at San Diego*

THE USE OF PERSONAL NARRATIVES IN THE HELPING PROFESSIONS: A TEACHING CASEBOOK by Jessica Heriot and Eileen J. Polinger. (2002). "More than anything else, social work students need examples to connect theories with everyday practice. Here's a book that provides those examples. This book is not only valuable for teaching, it's also an absorbing and instructional pleasure to read." *Leon Ginsberg, PhD, Carolina Distinguished Professor, University of Maryland School of Social Work, Baltimore*

CHILDREN'S RIGHTS: POLICY AND PRACTICE by John T. Pardeck. (2001) "Courageous and timely . . . a must-read for everyone concerned not only about the rights of America's children but also about their fate." *Howard Jacob Kerger, PhD, Professor and PhD Director, University of Houston Graduate School of Social Work, Texas*

BUILDING ON WOMEN'S STRENGTHS: A SOCIAL WORK AGENDA FOR THE TWENTY-FIRST CENTURY, SECOND EDITION by K. Jean Peterson and Alice A. Lieberman. (2001). "An indispensable resource for courses in women's issues, social work practice with women, and practice from a strengths perspective." *Theresa J. Early, PhD, MSW, Assistant Professor, College of Social Work, Ohio State University, Columbus*

ELEMENTS OF THE HELPING PROCESS: A GUIDE FOR CLINICIANS, SECOND EDITION by Raymond Fox. (2001). "Engages the reader with a professional yet easily accessible style. A remarkably fresh, eminently usable set of practical strategies." *Elayne B. Haynes, PhD, ACSW, Assistant Professor, Department of Social Work, Southern Connecticut State University, New Haven*

SOCIAL WORK THEORY AND PRACTICE WITH THE TERMINALLY ILL, SECOND EDITION by Joan K. Parry. (2000). "Timely . . . a sensitive and practical approach to working with people with terminal illness and their family members." *Jeanne A.Gill, PhD, LCSW, Adjunct Faculty, San Diego State University, California, and Vice President Southern California Chapter, AASWG*

WOMEN SURVIVORS, PSYCHOLOGICAL TRAUMA, AND THE POLITICS OF RESISTANCE by Norma Jean Profitt. (2000). "A compelling argument on the importance of political and collective action as a means of resisting oppression. Should be read by survivors, service providers, and activists in the violence-against-women movement." *Gloria Geller, PhD, Faculty of Social Work, University of Regina, Saskatchewan, Canada*

THE MENTAL HEALTH DIAGNOSTIC DESK REFERENCE: VISUAL GUIDES AND MORE FOR LEARNING TO USE THE DIAGNOSTIC AND STATISTICAL MANUAL (DSM-IV) by Carlton E. Munson. (2000). "A carefully organized and user-friendly book for the beginning student and less-experienced practitioner of social work, clinical psychology, of psychiatric nursing . . . It will be a valuable addition to the literature on clinical assessment of mental disorders." *Jerold R. Brandell, PhD, BCD, Professor, School of Social Work, Wayne State University, Detroit, Michigan and Founding Editor, Psychoanalytic Social Work*

HUMAN SERVICES AND THE AFROCENTRIC PARADIGM by Jerome H. Schiele. (2000). "Represents a milestone in applying the Afrocentric paradigm to human services generally, and social work specifically. . . . A highly valuable resource." *Bogart R. Leashore, PhD, Dean and Professor, Hunter College School of Social Work, New York, New York*

SOCIAL WORK: SEEKING RELEVANCY IN THE TWENTY-FIRST CENTURY by Roland Meinert, John T. Pardeck and Larry Kreuger. (2000). "Highly recommended. A thought-provoking work that asks the difficult questions and challenges the status quo. A great book for graduate students as well as experienced social workers and educators." Francis K. O. Yuen, DSW, ACSE, Associate Professor, Division of Social Work, California State University, Sacramento

SOCIAL WORK PRACTICE IN HOME HEALTH CARE by Ruth Ann Goode. (2000). "Dr. Goode presents both a lucid scenario and a formulated protocol to bring health care services into the home setting. . . . this is a must have volume that will be a reference to be consulted many times." *Marcia B. Steinhauer, PhD, Coordinator and Associate Professor, Human Services Administration Program, Rider University, Lawrenceville, New Jersey*

FORSENIC SOCIAL WORK: LEGAL ASPECTS OF PROFESSIONAL PRACTICE, SECOND EDITION by Robert L. Barker and Douglas M. Branson. (2000). "The authors combine their expertise to create this informative guide to address legal practice issues facing social workers." *Newsletter of the National Organization of Forensic Social Work*

SOCIAL WORK IN THE HEALTH FIELD: A CARE PERSPECTIVE by Lois A. Fort Cowles. (1999). "Makes an important contrition to the field by locating the practice of social work in health care within an organizational and social context." *Goldie Kadushin, PhD, Associate Professor, School of Social Welfare, University of Wisconsin, Milwaukee*

SMART BUT STUCK: WHAT EVERY THERAPY NEEDS TO KNOW ABOUT LEARNING DISABILITIES AND IMPRISONED INTELLIGENCE by Myrna Orenstein. (1999). "A trailblazing effort that creates an entirely novel way of talking and thinking about learning disabilities. There is simply nothing like it in the field." *Fred M. Levin, MD, Training Supervising Analyst, Chicago Institute for Psychoanalysis; Assistant Professor of Clinical Psychiatry, Northwestern University, School of Medicine, Chicago, IL*

CLINICAL WORK AND SOCIAL ACTION: AN INTEGRATIVE APPROACH by Jerome Sachs and Fred Newdom. (1999). "Just in time for the new millennium come Sachs and Newdom with a wholly fresh look at social work. . . . A much-needed uniting of social work values, theories, and practice for action." *Josephine Nieves, MSW, PhD, Executive Director, National Association of Social Workers*

SOCIAL WORK PRACTICE IN THE MILITARY by James G. Daley. (1999). "A significant and worthwhile book with provocative and stimulating ideas. It deserves to be read by a wide audience in social work education and practice as well as by decision makers in the military." *H. Wayne Johnson, MSW, Professor, University of Iowa, School of Social Work, Iowa City, Iowa*

GROUP WORK: SKILLS AND STRATEGIES FOR EFFECTIVE INTERVENTIONS, SECOND EDITION by Sondra Brandler and Camille P. Roman. (1999). "A clear, basic description of what group work requires, including what skills and techniques group workers need to be effective." *Hospital and Community Psychiatry (from the first edition)*

TEENAGE RUNAWAYS: BROKEN HEARTS AND "BAD ATTITUDES" by Laurie Schaffner. (1999). "Skillfully combines the authentic voice of the juvenile runaway with the principles of social science research." *Barbara Owen, PhD, Professor, Department of Criminology, California State University, Fresno*

CELEBRATING DIVERSITY: COEXISTING IN A MULTICULTURAL SOCIETY by Benyamin Chetkow-Yanoov. (1999). "Makes a valuable contribution to peace theory and practice." *Ian Harris, EdD, Executive Secretary, Peace Education Committee, International Peace Research Association*

SOCIAL WELFARE POLICY ANALYSIS AND CHOICES by Hobart A. Burch. (1999). "Will become the landmark text in its field for many decades to come." *Sheldon Rahan, DSW, Founding Dean and Emeritus Professor of Social Policy and Social Administration. Faculty of Social Work, Wilfrid Laurier University, Canada*

SOCIAL WORK PRACTICE: A SYSTEMS APPROACH, SECOND EDITION by Benyamin Chetkow-Yannov. (1999). "Highly recommended as a primary text for any and all introductory social work courses." *Ram A. Cnaan, PhD, Associate Professor, School of Social Work, University of Pennsylvania*

CRITICAL SOCIAL WELFARE ISSUES: TOOLS FOR SOCIAL WORK AND HEALTH CARE PROFESSIONALS edited by Arthur J. Katz, Abraham Lurie, and Carlos M. Vida. (1997). "Offers hopeful agendas for change, while navigating the societal challenges facing those in the human services today." *Book News Inc.*

SOCIAL WORK IN HEALTH SETTINGS: PRACTICE IN CONTEXT, SECOND EDITION edited by Tobra Schwaber Kerson. (1997). "A first-class document . . . It will be found among the steadier and lasting works on the social work aspects of American health care." *Hans S. Falck, PhD, Professor Emeritus and Former Chair, Health Specialization in Social Work, Virginia Commonwealth University*

PRINCIPLES OF SOCIAL WORK PRACTICE: A GENERIC PRACTICE APPROACH by Molly R. Hancock. (1997). "Hancock's discussions advocate reflection and self-awareness to create a climate for client change." *Journal of Social Work Education*

NOBODY'S CHILDREN: ORPHANS OF THE HIV EPIDEMIC by Steven F. Dansky. (1997). "Professional sound, moving, and useful for both professionals and interested readers alike." *Ellen G. Friedman, ACSW, Associate Director of Support Services, Beth Israel Medical Center, Methadone Maintenance Treatment Program*

SOCIAL WORK APPROACHES TO CONFLICT RESOLUTION: MAKING FIGHTING OBSOLETE by Benyamin Chetkow-yanoov. (1996). "Presents an examination of the nature and cause of conflict and suggests techniques for coping with conflict." *Journal of Criminal Justice*

FEMINIST THEORIES AND SOCIAL WORK: APPROACHES AND APPLICATIONS by Christine Flynn Salunier. (1996). "An essential reference to be read repeatedly by all educators and practitioners who are eager to learn more about feminist theory and practice" *Nancy R. Hooyman, PhD, Dean and Professor, School of Social Work, University of Washington, Seattle*

THE RELATIONAL SYSTEMS MODEL FOR FAMILY THERAPY: LIVING IN THE FOUR REALITIES by Donald R. Bardill. (1996). "Engages the reader in quiet, thoughtful conversation on the timeless issue of helping families and individuals." *Christian Counseling Resource Review*

SOCIAL WORK INTERVENTION IN AN ECONOMIC CRISIS: THE RIVER COMMUNITIES PROJECT by Martha Baum and Pamela Twiss. (1996). "Sets a standard for universities in terms of the types of meaningful roles they can play in supporting and sustaining communities." *Kenneth J. Jaros, PhD, Director, Public Health Social Work Training Program, University of Pittsburgh*

FUNDAMENTALS OF COGNITIVE-BEHAVIOR THERAPY: FROM BOTH SIDES OF THE DESK by Bill Borcherdt. (1996). "Both beginning and experienced practitioners . . . will find a considerable number of valuable suggestions in Borcherdt's book." *Albert Ellis, PhD, President, Institute for Rational-Emotive Therapy, New York City*

BASIC SOCIAL POLICY AND PLANNING: STRATEGIES AND PRACTICE METHODS by Hobart A. Burch. (1996). "Burch's familiarity with his topic is evident and his book is an easy introduction to the field." *Readings*

THE CROSS-CULTURAL PRACTICE OF CLINICAL CASE MANAGEMENT IN MENTAL HEALTH edited by Peter Manoleas. (1996). "Makes a contribution by bringing together the cross-cultural and clinical case management perspectives in working with those who have serious mental illness." *Disabilities Studies Quarterly*

FAMILY BEYOND FAMILY: THE SURROGATE PARENT IN SCHOOLS AND OTHER COMMUNITY AGENCIES by Sanford Weinstein. (1995). "Highly recomended to anyone concerned about the welfare of our children and the breakdown of the American family." *Jerold S. Greenberg, EdD, director of Community Service, College of Health & Human Performance, University of Maryland*

PEOPLE WITH HIV AND THOSE WHO HELP THEM: CHALLENGES, INTEGRATION, INTERVENTION by R. Dennis Shelby. (1995). "A useful and compassionate contribution to the HIV psychotherapy literature." *Public Health*

THE BLACK ELDERLY: SATISFACTION AND QUALITY OF LATER LIFE by Marguerite Coke and James A. Twaite. (1995). "Presents a model for predicting life satisfaction in this population." *Abstracts in Social Gerontology*

NOW DARE EVERYTHING: TALES OF HIV-RELATED PSYCHOTHERAPY by Steven F. Dansky. (1994). "A highly recommended book for anyone working with persons who are HIV positive. . . . Every library should have a copy of this book." *AIDS Book Review Journal*

INTERVENTION RESEARCH: DESIGN AND DEVELOPMENT FOR HUMAN SERVICE edited by Jack Rothman and Edwin J. Thomas. (1994). "Provides a useful framework for the further examination of methodology for each separate step of such research." *Academic Library Book Review*

CLINICAL SOCIAL WORK SUPERVISION, SECOND EDITION by Carlton E. Munson. (1993). "A useful, thorough, and articulate reference for supervisors and for 'supervisees' who are wanting to understand their supervisor or are looking for effective supervision...." *Transactional Analysis Journal*

IF A PARTNER HAS AIDS: GUIDE TO CLINICAL INTERVENTION FOR RELATIONSHIPS IN CRISIS by R. Dennis Shelby. (1993). "A welcome addition to existing publications about couples coping with AIDS, it offers intervention ideas and strategies to clinicians." *Contemporary Psychology*

GERONTOLOGICAL SOCIAL WORK SUPERVISION by Ann Burack-Weiss and Frances Coyle Brennan. (1991). "The creative ideas in this book will aid supervisiors working with students and experienced social workers." *Senior News*

THE CREATIVE PRACTITIONER: THEORY AND METHODS FOR THE HELPING SERVICES by Bernard Gelfand. (1988). "[Should] be widely adopted by those in the helping services. It could lead to significant positive advances by countless individuals." *Sidney J. Parnes, Trustee Chairperson for Strategic Program Development, Creative Education Foundation, Buffalo, NY*

MANAGEMENT AND INFORMATION SYSTEMS IN HUMAN SERVICES: IMPLICATIONS FOR THE DISTRIBUTION OF AUTHORITY AND DECISION MAKING by Richard K. Caputo. (1987). "A contribution to social work scholarship in that it provides conceptual frameworks that can be used in the design of management information systems." *Social Work*

Order a copy of this book with this form or online at:
http://www.haworthpressinc.com/store/product.asp?sku=4533

HUMAN BEHAVIOR IN THE SOCIAL ENVIRONMENT
Interweaving the Inner and Outer Worlds

_____in hardbound at $129.95 (ISBN: 0-7890-0716-9)

_____in softbound at $59.95 (ISBN: 0-7890-1522-6)

COST OF BOOKS_____

OUTSIDE USA/CANADA/
MEXICO: ADD 20%____

POSTAGE & HANDLING_____
(US: $4.00 for first book & $1.50
for each additional book)
Outside US: $5.00 for first book
& $2.00 for each additional book)

SUBTOTAL_____

in Canada: add 7% GST____

STATE TAX____
(NY, OH & MIN residents, please
add appropriate local sales tax)

FINAL TOTAL____
(If paying in Canadian funds,
convert using the current
exchange rate, UNESCO
coupons welcome.)

❑   **BILL ME LATER:** ($5 service charge will be added)
(Bill-me option is good on US/Canada/Mexico orders only;
not good to jobbers, wholesalers, or subscription agencies.)

❑ Check here if billing address is different from
shipping address and attach purchase order and
billing address information.

Signature_____

❑ **PAYMENT ENCLOSED: $**_____

❑ **PLEASE CHARGE TO MY CREDIT CARD.**

❑ Visa   ❑ MasterCard   ❑ AmEx   ❑ Discover
❑ Diner's Club   ❑ Eurocard   ❑ JCB

Account # _____

Exp. Date_____

Signature_____

Prices in US dollars and subject to change without notice.

NAME_____
INSTITUTION_____
ADDRESS_____
CITY_____
STATE/ZIP_____
COUNTRY_____ COUNTY (NY residents only)_____
TEL_____ FAX_____
E-MAIL_____

May we use your e-mail address for confirmations and other types of information? ❑ Yes ❑ No
We appreciate receiving your e-mail address and fax number. Haworth would like to e-mail or fax special
discount offers to you, as a preferred customer. **We will never share, rent, or exchange your e-mail address
or fax number.** We regard such actions as an invasion of your privacy.

Order From Your Local Bookstore or Directly From
The Haworth Press, Inc.
10 Alice Street, Binghamton, New York 13904-1580 • USA
TELEPHONE: 1-800-HAWORTH (1-800-429-6784) / Outside US/Canada: (607) 722-5857
FAX: 1-800-895-0582 / Outside US/Canada: (607) 722-6362
E-mail: getinfo@haworthpressinc.com
PLEASE PHOTOCOPY THIS FORM FOR YOUR PERSONAL USE.
www.HaworthPress.com

BOF02